Progress in Infertility and Transvaginal Sonography

Progress in Infertility and Transvaginal Sonography

Edited by

Sadhana Desai
Gautam Allahbadia

CBS

CBS PUBLISHERS & DISTRIBUTORS

New Delhi - 110 002 (INDIA)

ISBN : 81-239-0423-1

First Edition : 1996

Production Director : Vinod Jain

Published by:

Satish Kumar Jain for CBS Publishers and Distributors
4596/1A, 11 Darya Ganj, New Delhi - 110 002 (India)

Laser Typeset at:

Rafah Typesetters
Delhi-110092

Printed at:

Tara Art Printers
Noida (U.P.)

To the Bombay Hospital Trust.
This work could not have been completed
without its active support and encouragement.

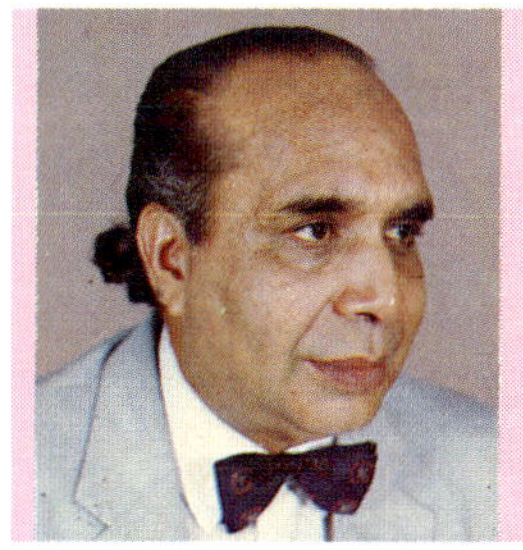

Foreword

Whatever the demographic policy of the Government and regardless of the aims proclaimed and/or pursued by the society, the individual family perceives its freedom to procreate as the most basic human right. Nothing more vividly demonstrates the importance of fertility to the individual than the reaction by and to those who do not have children. The grief of a woman who has failed to bear a live-born child is no less in modern society than it was for our forefathers. During the last few years formidable progress has been made in the fields of infertility management and reproductive biology. Sophisticated combination of genetic engineering with molecular biology techniques enabled identification of genes controlling the production and function of numerous hormones, growth factors and their specific receptors. Developments in organic chemistry facilitated manufacture of new artificial hormones more potent and active than their natural models. The assisted reproduction techniques have been refined and numerous new modifications were introduced. Reproductive medicine has entered a new era carrying promise of great advancement and opening of new horizons. All of the above relevant to clinical practice in our subcontinent has been covered in this textbook.

Transvaginal sonography in the form available to us today combines the advantages of endoscopy and sonography. The next light-reflecting surface, once the limit of endoscopy, represents no barrier to ultrasound. A whole range of both diagnostic and therapeutic procedures can be sonographically guided. Blood flow in vessels lying deep in the lesser pelvis can now be measured by means of vaginal duplex sonography. So much material has now been published that it has become almost impossible for any one individual to sift out what is directly relevant to his own work, and it is with this in mind that this book was planned. The book is intended not only to describe the progress in the field at the Bombay Hospital Institute of Medical Sciences, but also to take stock of developments so far. Today, it is clear that vaginosonography has become established as an integrative gynaecological/obstetrical investigation, and for this reason thc authors have laid special emphasis on the practical utility of vaginal ultrasound in the field.

I sincerely hope that this volume will assist obstetricians, gynaecologists and ultrasonologists to familiarise themselves with the subject and to apply the information gleaned to the benefit of their patients.

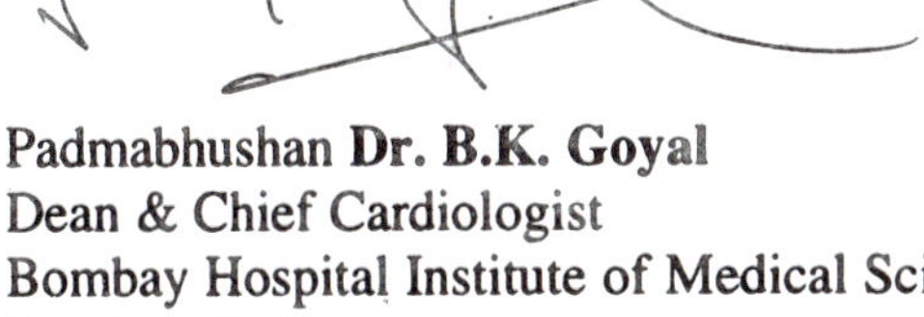

Padmabhushan **Dr. B.K. Goyal**
Dean & Chief Cardiologist
Bombay Hospital Institute of Medical Sciences
Bombay, India

Preface

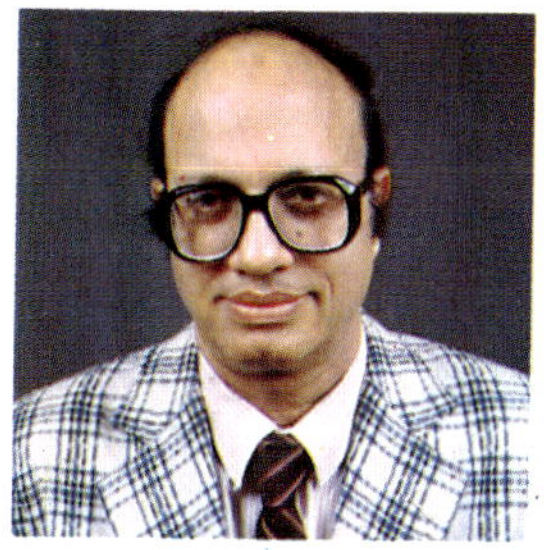

More than 25 years ago, when ultrasound diagnostic methods were first introduced into gynaecology and obstetrics, few of the pioneers of these techniques suspected what importance sonographic diagnosis was destined to assume. Most cultures regard children as an extension of self, as bearers and perpetuators of the family name and tradition as well as an expansion of one's hopes, aims and strivings. The inability to procreate is thus always perceived as a denial of basic rights, an injustice and a disappointment, sometimes bordering on grief. It is obvious that the primary task of the physician caring for infertile women is to diagnose the main cause (or causes) of infertility in each individual couple in order to be able to institute appropriate therapy within a reasonable time.

The core of this book is comprised of the compilation of various papers presented at the **Update on Infertility & Transvaginal Sonography** hosted by the Bombay Hospital Institute of Medical Sciences. Our aim was to bring to the practitioners of women's health care, advances that will place them in the vanguard of infertility management and transvaginal sonography. Some of the material contained in the following pages has never before appeared in print, and I am certain that the reader will find the data as exciting as I did reading it. We believe that the material contained in this book represents the state of the art as we now know it, and we feel duty bound to share this information with our colleagues.

The co-existence and vital importance of transvaginal sonography in follicular sizing, in vitro fertilisation, and ectopic pregnancy identification (and possible treatment) is obvious to all. The transvaginal route provides a new diagnostic pathway for early as well as later fetal development and fetal blood flow. The potential of colour Doppler flow becomes even more exciting. In charting new areas, one needs to consider the potential use of this modality for women in their post-reproductive years. Can the colour flow probe document the earlier presence of ovarian neoplasms? This area needs exploration. Will the value of this device remain limited to the hands of the specialist in sonography, or will it become part of the clinician's diagnostic and therapeutic armament at patient office visits? To reach this latter plateau (if it should be reached), we must educate more clinicians to use transvaginal sonography well, and to actively study whether the clinician's hands and judgement can be improved by the vaginal probe. The reader of this textbook will benefit from the writings of excellent clinicians who present a compendium of good data and good illustrations.

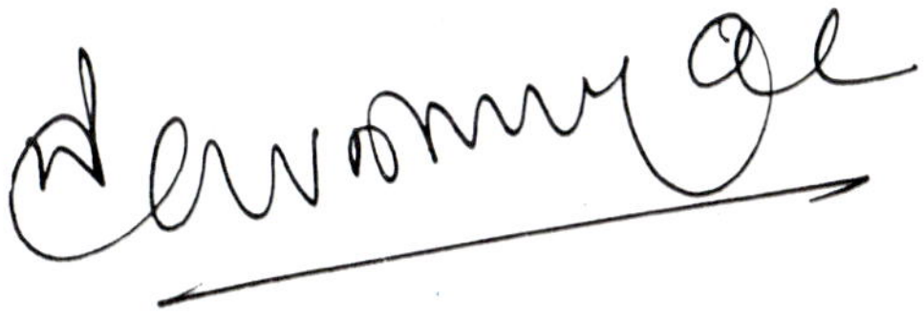

Dr. P.B. Pai Dhungat
Consultant Obstetrician & Gynaecologist
Bombay Hospital Institute of Medical Sciences

Acknowledgements

We wish to express our appreciation to all of the contributing authors. The timely publication of this text was made possible only as a result of their cooperation and good nature in the face of endless calls and questions. We would like to thank Shri S.V. Mazumdar, General S.N. Samarth and Dr. D.P. Vyas for their support and encouragement for this project. A special thanks to Commodore R.P. Rai for his help in getting the administrative problems sorted out. We would also like to thank Mr. N. Kishore, our telecommunications officer, whose help in getting the manuscripts delivered in time went beyond the call of duty.

In addition, Dr. Gautam Allahbadia is grateful to Kody Elcot Ltd., Madras for the technical support required for the Fukuda Denshi Ultrasound Unit used by him. Appreciation is also expressed to Masters Medical Equipment, New Delhi & Bombay for monitoring the image quality of the ultrasound plates from their Sony Thermal Paper Printers used for completion of the manuscripts.

List of Contributors

Gautam Allahbadia

Hon. Asstt. Consultant, Department of Obstetrics & Gynaecology, Bombay Hospital Institute of Medical Sciences
Consultant, Rotunda Nursing Home, Bombay, India

John Anderson

Technical Director, Sydney IVF Pte. Ltd., Sydney, Australia

Sudeep Banerjee

IVF & Assisted Reproduction Unit
Department of Obstetrics & Gynaecology
King George's Medical College, Lucknow, India

Benny Bartoov

Bar Ilan University, Ramat Gan, Israel

Shyam Baruah

Consultant Ultrasonologist, Downtown Hospital, Guwahati, Assam, India

M.R. Bharucha

Deputy Scientific Director
Serum Institute of India Research Foundation, Bombay, India

R.K. Bhathena

Consultant Obstetrician & Gynaecology
Parsee General & Masina Hospitals, Bombay, India

Tom Bourne

Lecturer, Department of Obstetrics & Gynaecology
King's College School of Medicine & Dentistry, London, UK

B.N. Chakravarty

Director, Institute of Reproductive Medicine, Calcutta, India

Ambrish Dalal

Chief, Department of Ultrasonography
Bombay Hospital & Medical Research Centre, Bombay, India

Adi Dastur

Hon. Associate Professor of Obstetrics & Gynaecology
Nowrosjee Wadia Maternity Hospital, Parel, Bombay, India

Sadhana Desai

Professor & Head, Department of Obstetrics & Gynaecology
Bombay Hospital Institute of Medical Sciences
Director, Fertility Clinic, Bombay, India

S. Ghosh Dastidar

Hon. Research Director, Assisted Reproductive Technology Program
Infertility Clinic & IVF Centre, Calcutta, India

Shashi Goyal

Hon. Associate Consultant, Bombay Hospital & Medical Research Centre, Bombay, India

Sulochana Gunasheela

Director, Gunasheela Surgical & Maternity Hospital, Bangalore, India

Mehroo Hansotia

Hon. Professor, Department of Obstetrics & Gynaecology
Nowrosjee Wadia Maternity Hospital, Parel
Director, Fertility Clinic, Bombay, India

Rajeev Jain

Department of Radiodiagnosis, All India Institute of Medical Sciences, New Delhi, India

Rajam Jaishankar

Director, Chemech Laboratories, Madras, India

Mukund Joshi

Hon. Prof., Department of Radiology, LTMMC & LTMGH, Sion, Bombay, India Consultant Ultrasonologist, Jaslok Hospital & Research Centre, Bombay, India

Prema Kania

Clinical Assistant, Department of Obstetrics & Gynaecology
Bombay Hospital & Medical Research Centre, Bombay, India

Alka Kriplani
Department of Radiodiagnosis, All India Institute of Medical Sciences, New Delhi, India

Pratap Kumar
Head, Manipal Assisted Reproduction Center
Kasturba Medical College & Hospital, Manipal, India

Chander Lulla
Consultant Ultrasonologist & Doppler Angiologist
Jaslok Hospital & Research Centre, Bombay, India

Bruno Lunenfeld
Professor Emeritus, Department of Life Sciences
Bar Ilan University, Ramat Gan, Israel

Jaideep Malhotra
Director, Malhotra Nursing Home, Agra, India

Narendra Malhotra
Director, Malhotra Nursing Home, Agra, India

Vijay Mangoli
Chief Embryologist, Fertility Clinic, Bombay, India

Champa Nariani
Professor, Department of Obstetrics & Gynaecology
Bombay Hospital Institute of Medical Sciences, Bombay, India

P.B. Pai Dhungat
Hon. Consultant Obstetrician & Gynaecologist
Bombay Hospital & Medical Research Centre, Bombay, India

Shailesh Raina
Consultant Urologist, Jaslok Hospital & Research Centre
Bombay, India

R. Rajan
Professor & Head, Department of Obstetrics & Gynaecology
Kottayam Medical College, Kottayam, Kerala, India

Kamini Rao
Medical Director, Bangalore Assisted Conception Centre, Bangalore, India

Sukhpal Sawhney
Department of Radiodiagnosis, All India Institute of Medical Sciences, New Delhi, India

Brij Saxena
Cornell University Medical College
The New York Hospital, New York, USA

Duru Shah
Hon. Associate Professor of Obstetrics & Gynaecology
Nowrosjee Wadia Maternity Hospital, Parel, Bombay, India

Geeta Shah
Consultant, N.M. Medical Centre, Bombay, India

Nilesh Shah
Director, N.M. Medical Centre, Bombay, India

R.K. Sharma
Army Medical Corps, India

Lakshmi Singh
Associate Professor & Incharge, IVF & Assisted Reproduction Unit
Department of Obstetrics & Gynaecology
King George's Medical College, Lucknow, India

Mukul Singh
Cornell University Medical College
The New York Hospital, New York, USA

Asha Singhal
Professor, Department of Obstetrics & Gynaecology
Bombay Hospital Institute of Medical Sciences, Bombay, India

Rakesh Sinha
Consultant Endoscopic Surgeon, H.N. Hospital, Bombay, India

Karuna Taneja
Department of Radiodiagnosis, All India Institute of Medical Sciences, New Delhi, India

S. Thatte
Associate Professor
Department of Urology, Bombay Hospital Institute of Medical Sciences, Bombay, India

Satish Tibrewala
Consultant Infertologist
Assistant Professor, Bombay Hospital Institute of Medical Sciences, Bombay, India

Prakash Trivedi
Consultant Endoscopic Surgeon, Jaslok Hospital & Research Centre, Bombay, India

Rajeshwar Upadhyay
IVF & Assisted Reproduction Unit
Department of Obstetrics & Gynaecology
King George's Medical College, Lucknow, India

Simon Wood
Senior Lecturer, Department of Obstetrics & Gynaecology
University of Exeter, Exeter, UK

Kusum Zaveri
Associate Hon. Prof., Department of Obstetrics & Gynaecology
Grant Medical College & Sir JJ Hospital, Bombay, India

Contents

Section F : General

Section G : Medically Assisted Conception

Section H : Male Factor

Section I : Surgery

PLATE 1

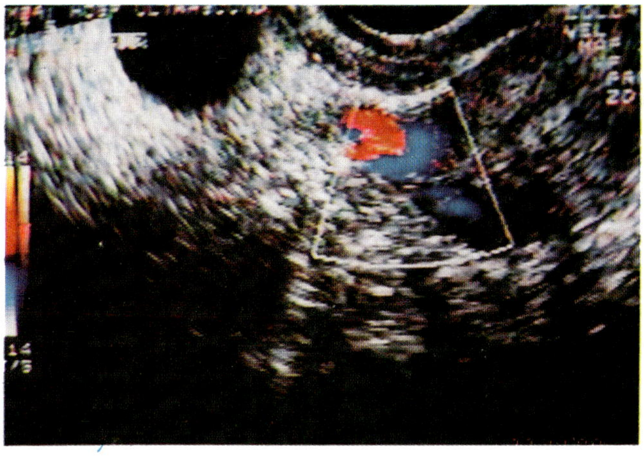

Fig. 1.2. The uterine vasculature seen at the level of the junction between the cervix and the body of the uterus.

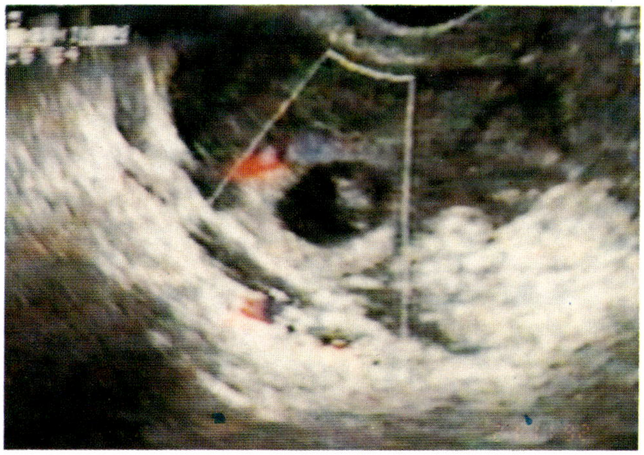

Fig. 4.8. Transvaginal colour Doppler sonogram. Another live ampullary ectopic pregnancy with peritrophoblastic blood flow seen clearly.

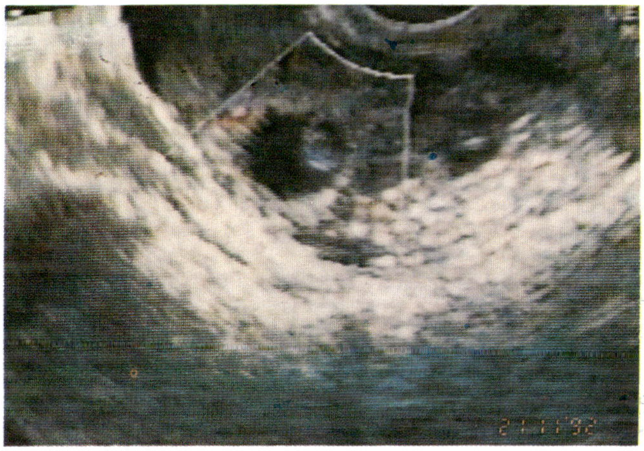

Fig. 4.6. Transvaginal colour Doppler sonogram. Live ampullary ectopic pregnancy.

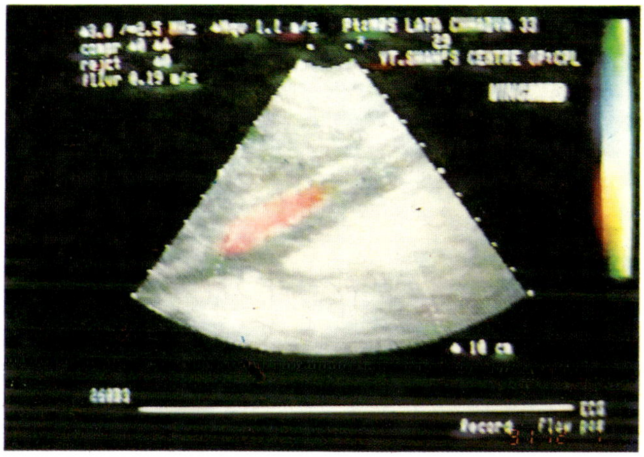

Fig. 5.13. The left internal iliac vessel outlined with colour Doppler.

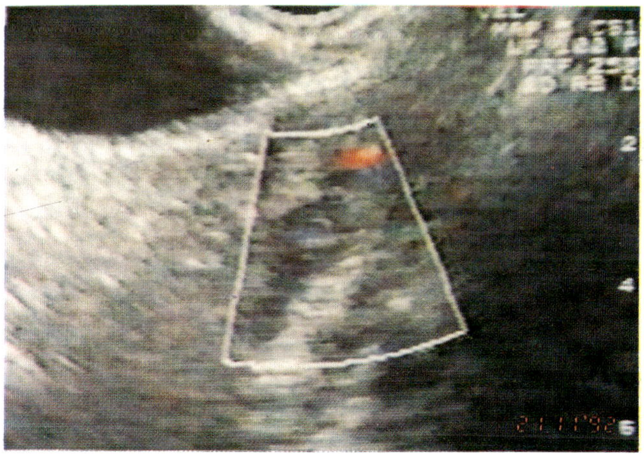

Fig. 4.7. Transvaginal colour Doppler sonogram. Live isthmo-ampullary ectopic pregnancy.

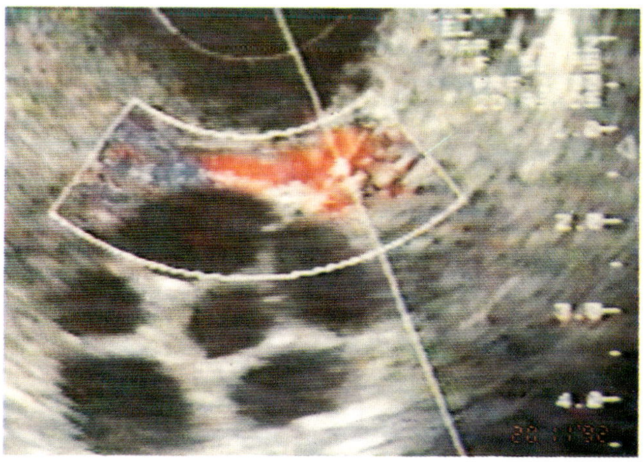

Fig. 5.14. The 2 mm volume cursor insonating the ovarian artery.

PLATE 2

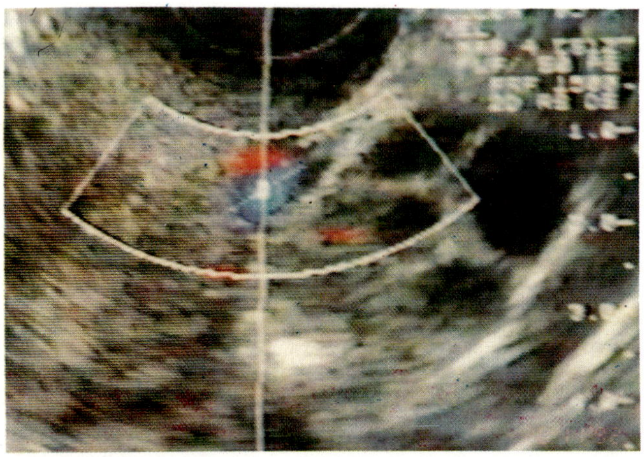

Fig. 5.15. The 2 mm volume cursor insonating the medial branch of the ovarian blood supply.

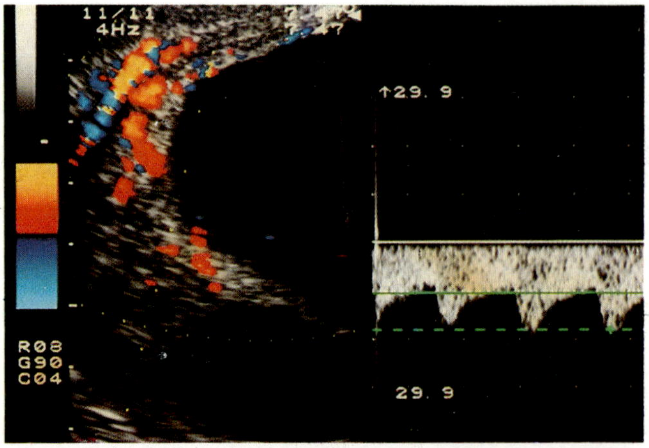

Fig. 5.18. Ovarian bilocular cystic structure with septal blood flow.

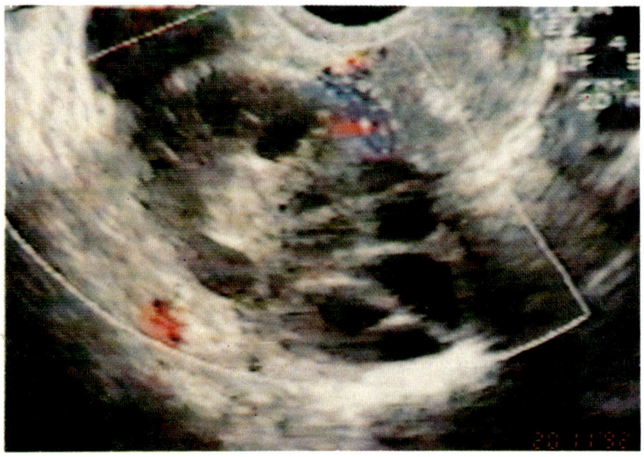

Fig. 5.16. The Doppler anatomic window narrowed down to outline the ovarian blood flow.

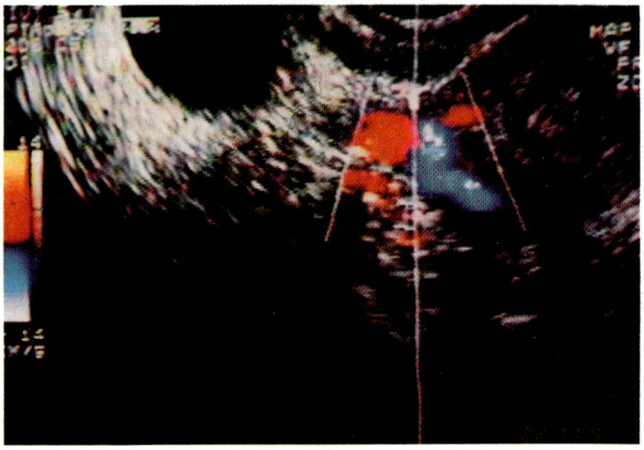

Fig. 5.19. The uterine artery at the level of isthmus being insonated.

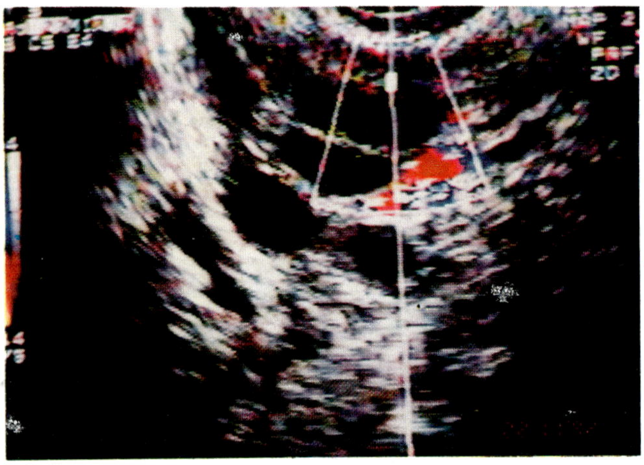

Fig. 5.17. The intraovarian blood flow seen clearly on this plate.

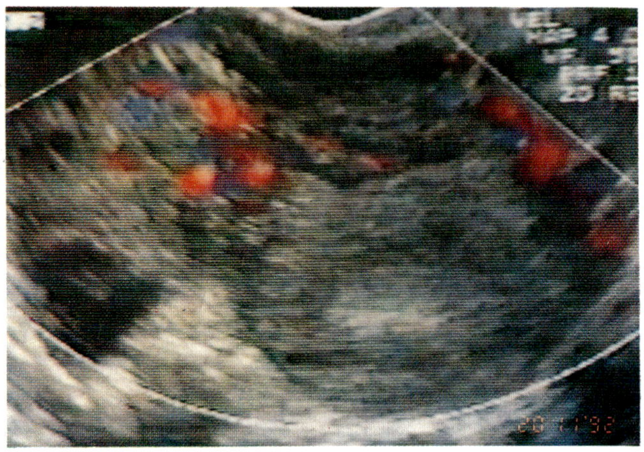

Fig. 5.20. The arcuate vasculature seen clearly within the Doppler anatomic window.

PLATE 3

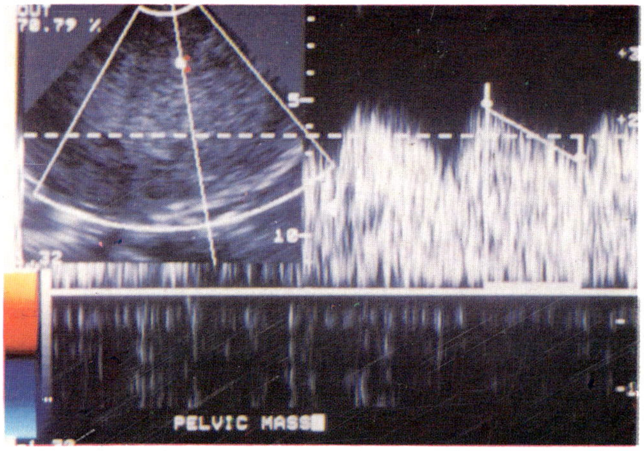

Fig. 5.21. Colour Doppler ultrasound of the pelvis showing an ovary with a PI and RI of 0.3.

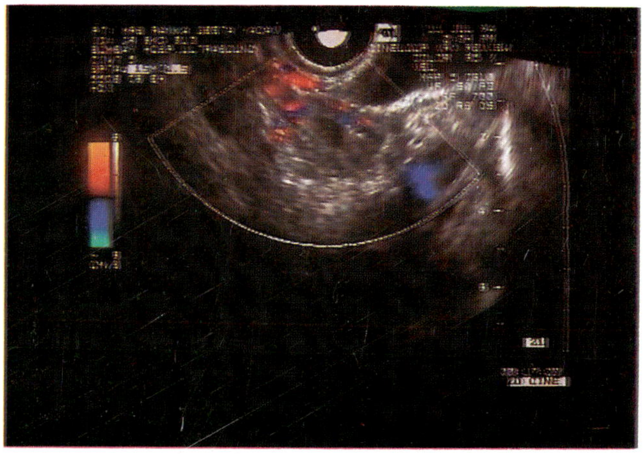

Fig. 11.1. Transvaginal colour Doppler sonogram. Plate shows a tubal ectopic pregnancy with peritrophoblastic flow seen clearly.

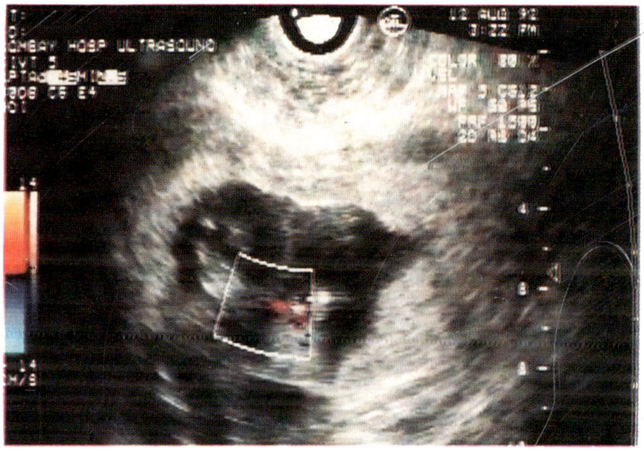

Fig. 7.2. Needle piercing the cardiac region of the fetus under guidance of colour Doppler ultrasonography.

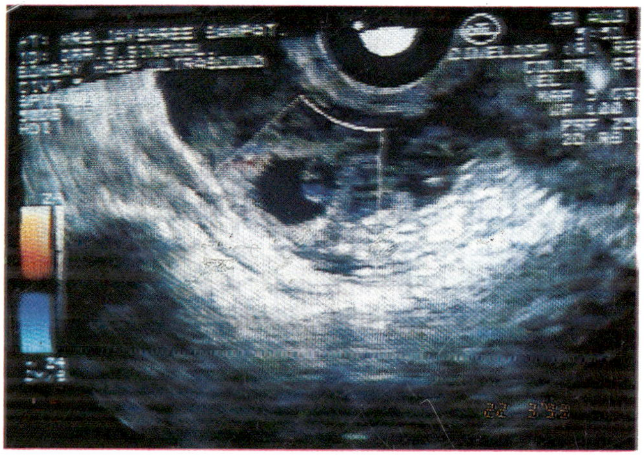

Fig. 11.2. Transvaginal colour Doppler sonogram. Plate shows a live ampullary ectopic pregnancy.

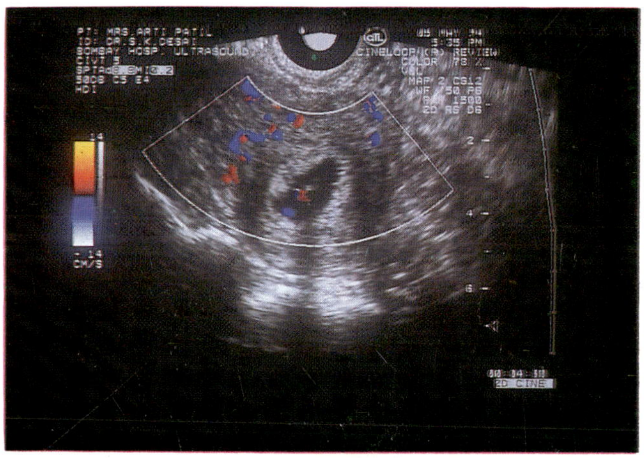

Fig. 9.14. Transvaginal colour Doppler aided saline infusion sonography of the uterine cavity. Plate shows a small endometrial polyp with its blood supply in its stalk well visualised. The arcuate vasculature is also seen in the sonogram.

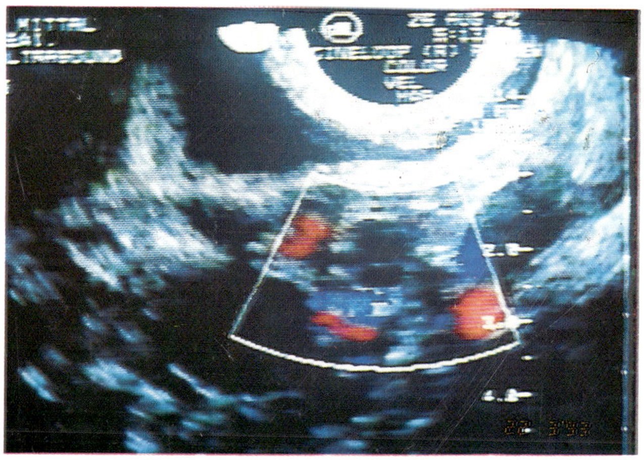

Fig. 11.3. Transvaginal colour Doppler sonogram. Peritrophoblastic flow seen around an early unruptured tubal ectopic pregnancy.

PLATE 4

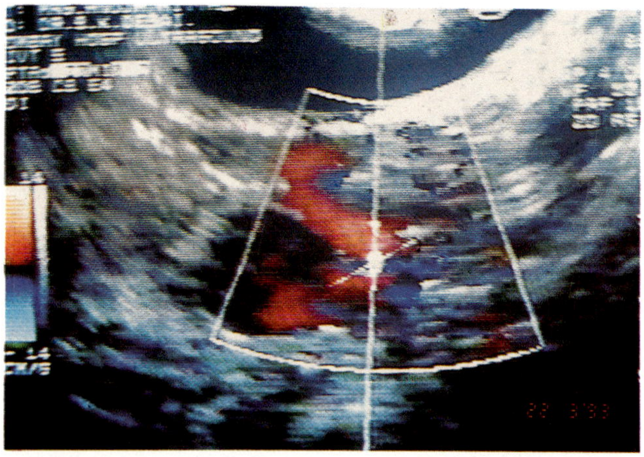

Fig. 11.4. Transvaginal colour Doppler sonogram. The 2 mm volume cursor insonating the peritrophoblastic blood flow in the same case as in Fig. 11.3.

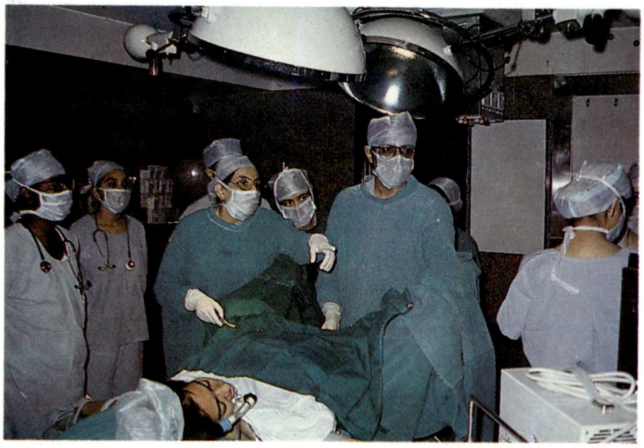

Fig. 11.7. The operating room setup for the procedure with the patient under GA.

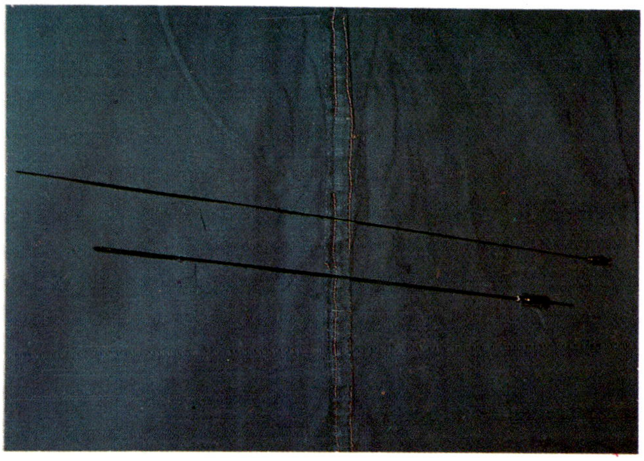

Fig. 11.5. The twin needle used for the procedure with the attached suction/injection syringe.

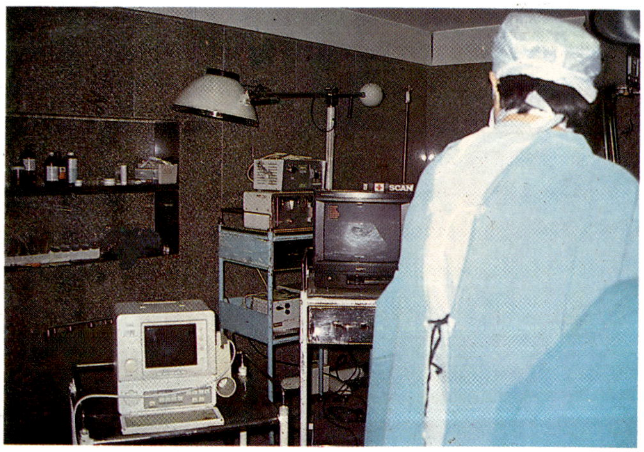

Fig. 11.8. The portable ultrasound unit along with the additional TV monitor seen with the procedure in progress.

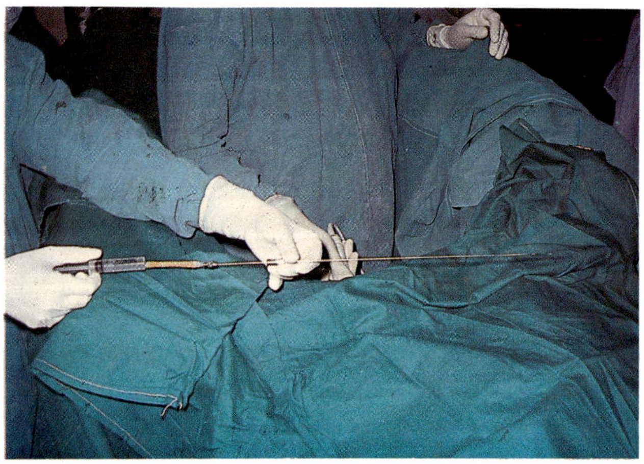

Fig. 11.6. The dismantled customised double needles; 17 gauge and 21 gauge.

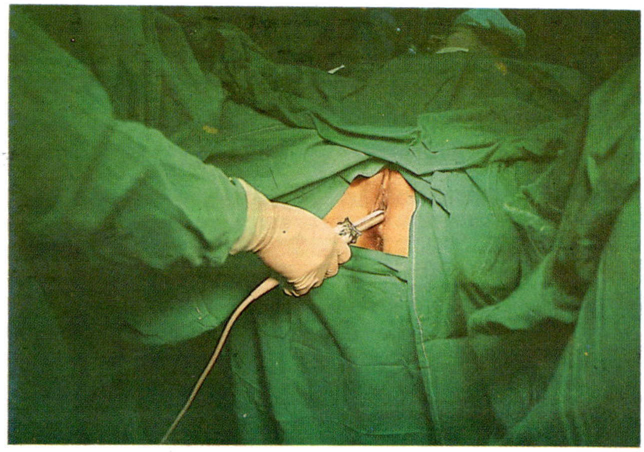

Fig. 11.9. The transvaginal probe with attached biopsy guide. A check scan in progress.

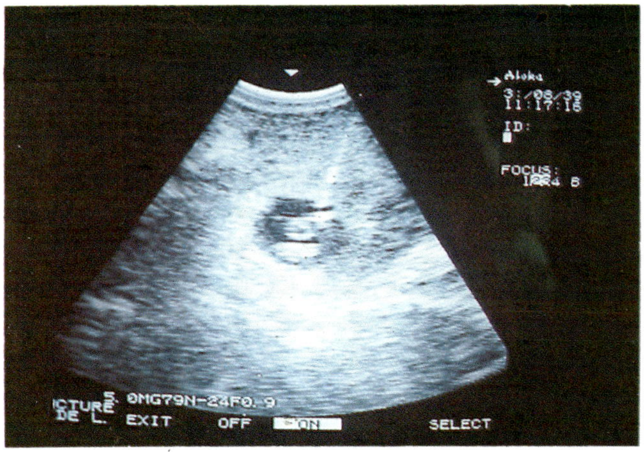

Fig. 11.10. An ectopic sac with the needle directed into the fetal pole.

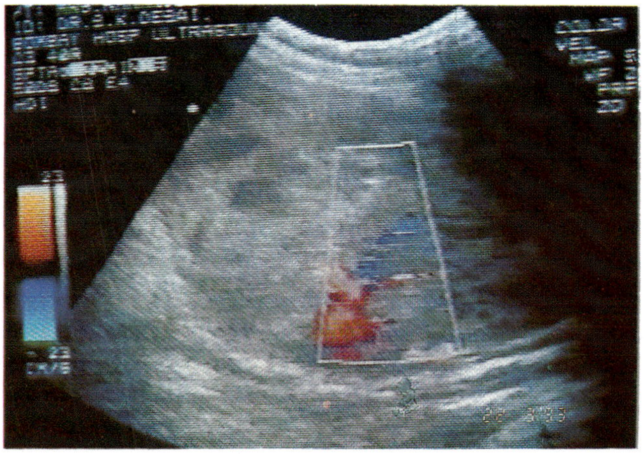

Fig. 18.4. Vascular signals seen clearly in the right ovary.

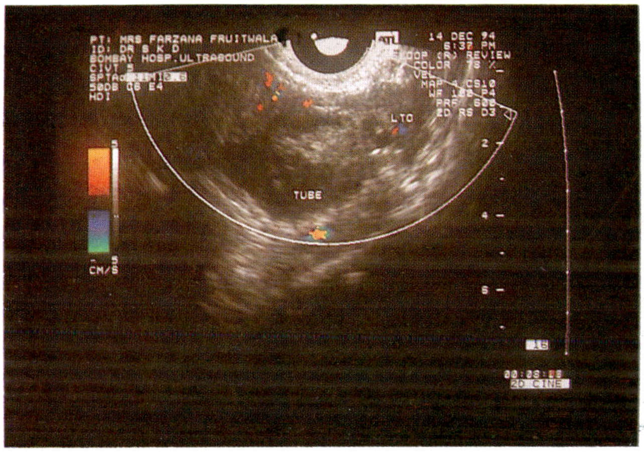

Fig. 11.11. Transvaginal colour Doppler sonogram. Plate shows a left sided hematosalpinx with left ovary seen separately.

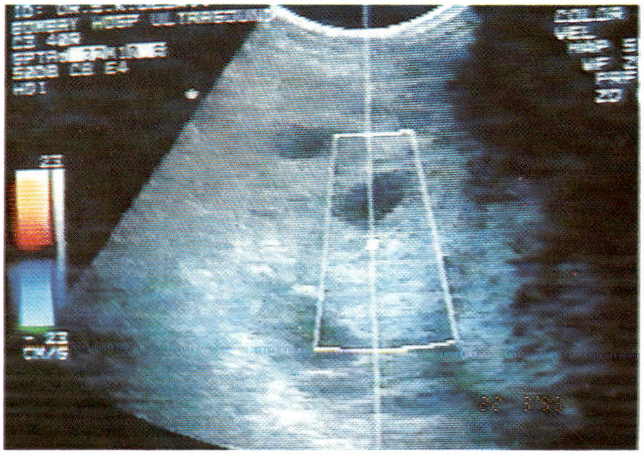

Fig. 18.5. Absence of blood flow to the torsed ovary detected by colour Doppler ultrasonography.

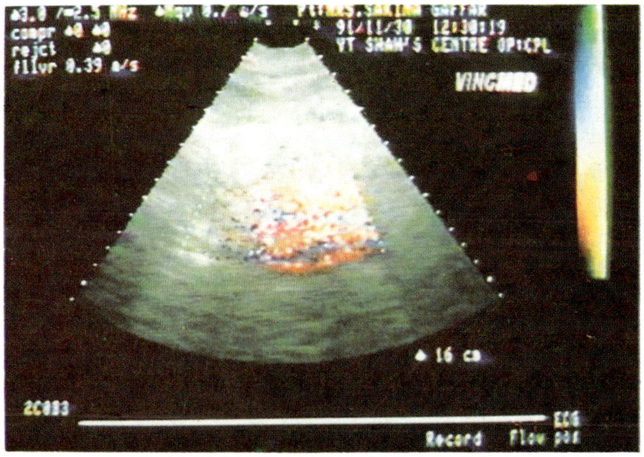

Fig. 18.3. Abdominal color Doppler sonosalpingography. Free peritoneal spill depicted as colour 'bruit'.

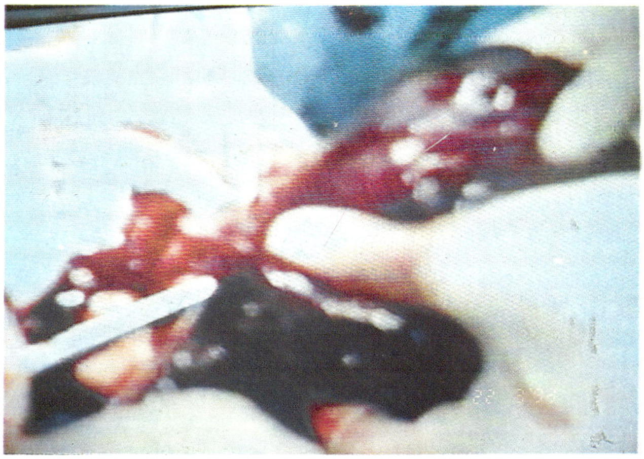

Fig. 18.6. The torsed necrotic ovary being removed at surgery.

PLATE 6

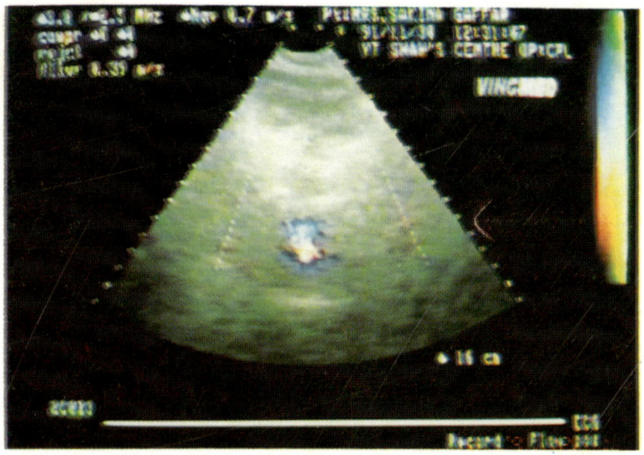

Fig. 20.1. Abdominal colour Doppler. The beginning of the peritoneal spill.

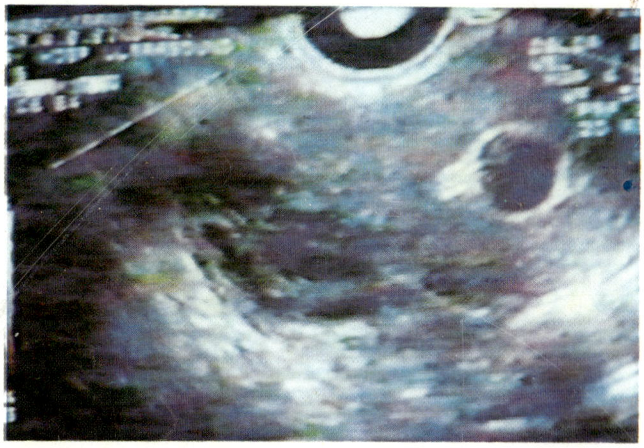

Fig. 20.4. TVCD. Transverse view of the uterus with Foley bulb before injection of saline. Also seen is part of the right ovary.

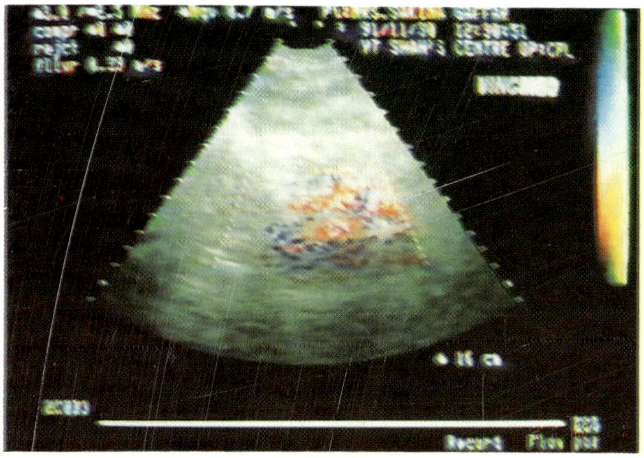

Fig. 20.2. Abdominal colour Doppler. Free spill from the left tube.

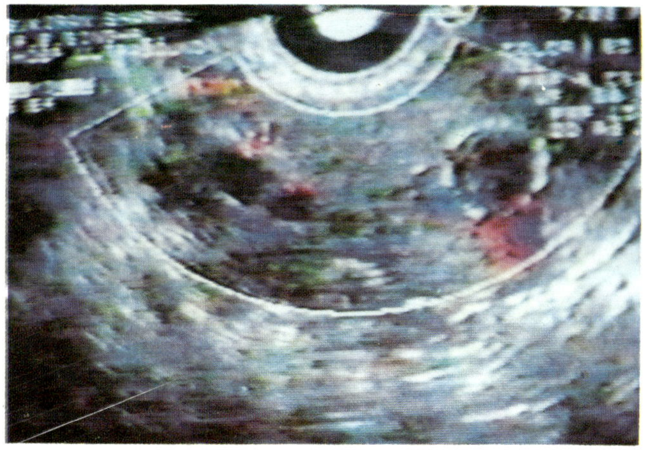

Fig. 20.5. TVCD. Beginning of free peritoneal spill from right tube.

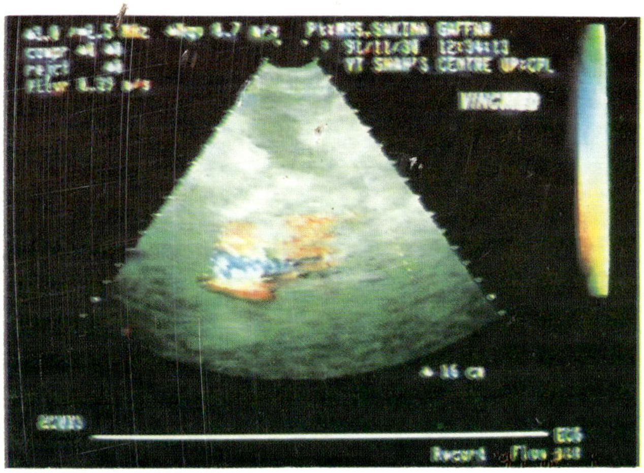

Fig. 20.3. Abdominal colour Doppler. Free spill from the right tube.

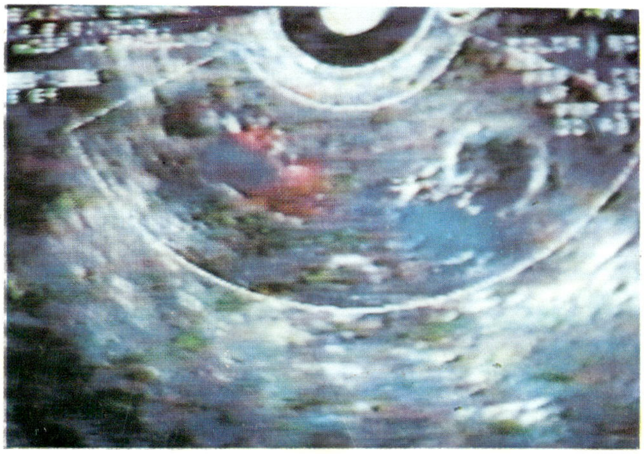

Fig. 20.6. TVCD. Free spill from right tube. Plate taken 45 seconds after Fig. 20.5.

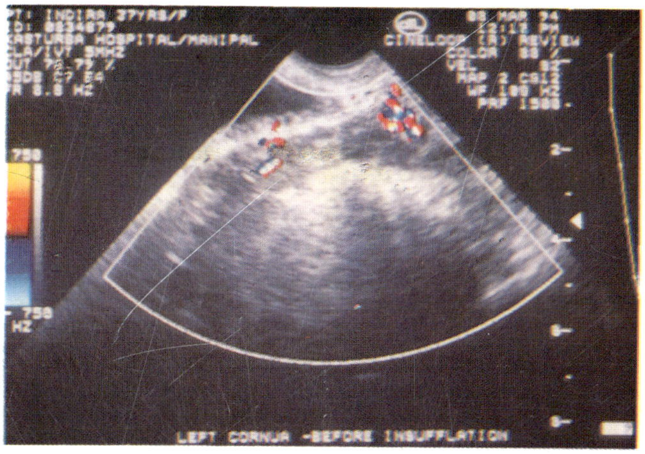

Fig. 20.7. TVCD. Beginning of free peritoneal spill in another patient.

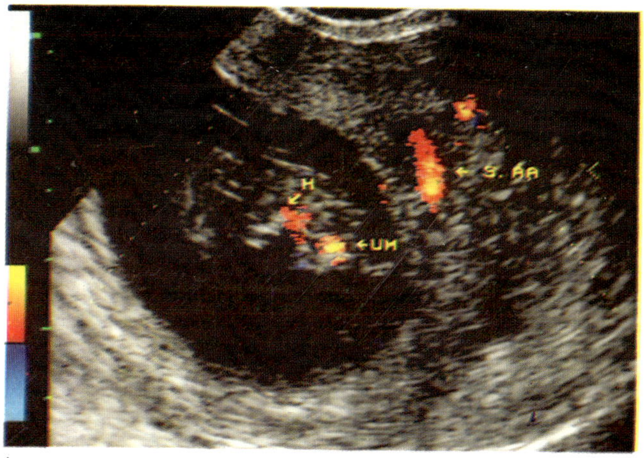

Fig. 21.2. The fetal heart, umbilical cord flow and spiral arterial blood flow depicted clearly here.

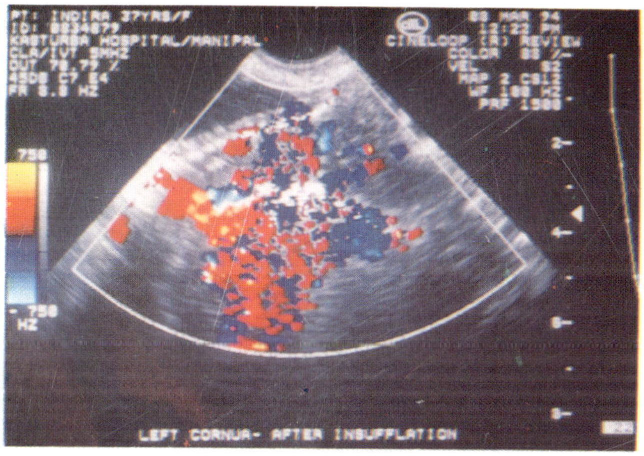

Fig. 20.8. TVCD. Free spill in the same patient as in Fig 20.7.

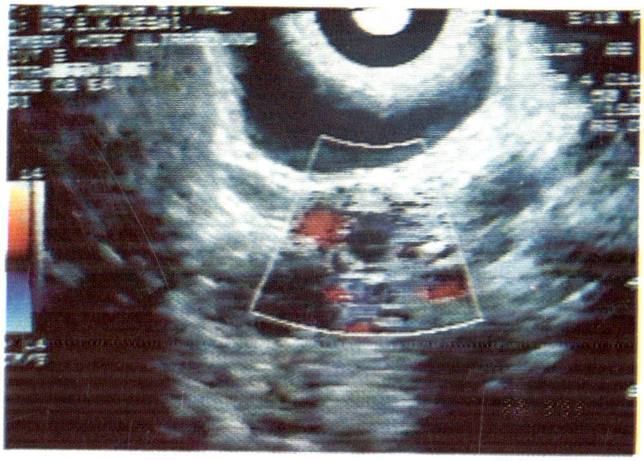

Fig. 21.3. Peritrophoblastic blood flow seen clearly in this ampullary ectopic pregnancy.

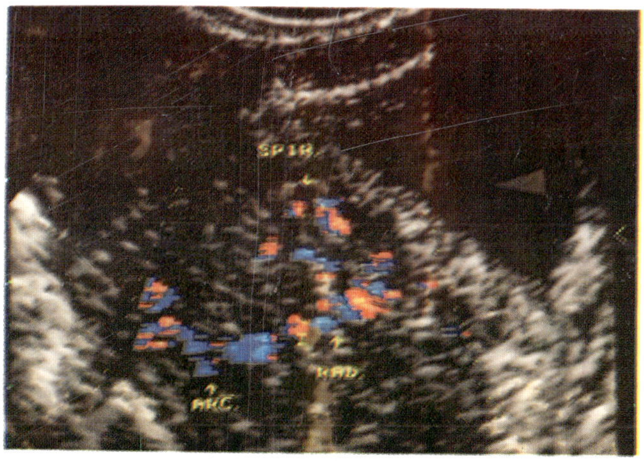

Fig. 21.1. Colour Doppler sonogram depicting the spiral, radial and arcuate vasculature clearly.

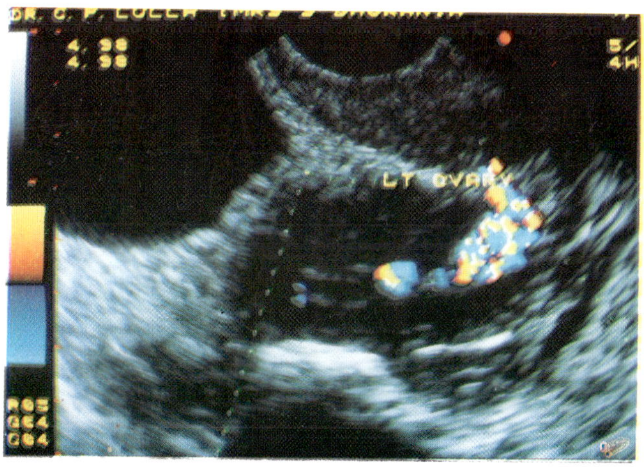

Fig. 22.1. Colour Doppler sonogram outlining the main ovarian artery.

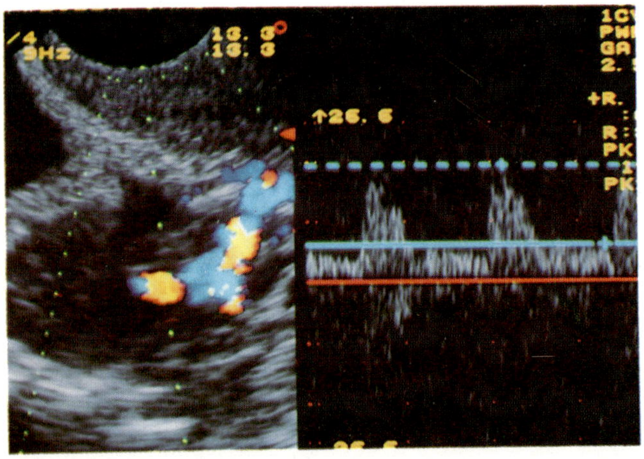

Fig. 22.2. Colour Doppler sonogram highlighting the low diastolic ovarian flow in the beginning of the cycle.

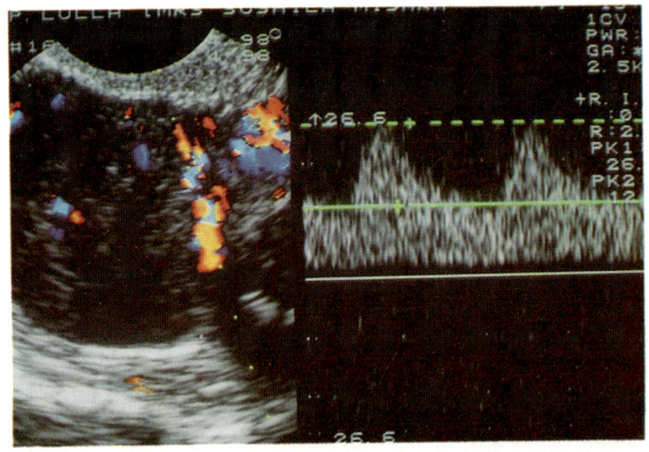

Fig. 22.5. Low impedance blood flow seen immediately post-ovulation.

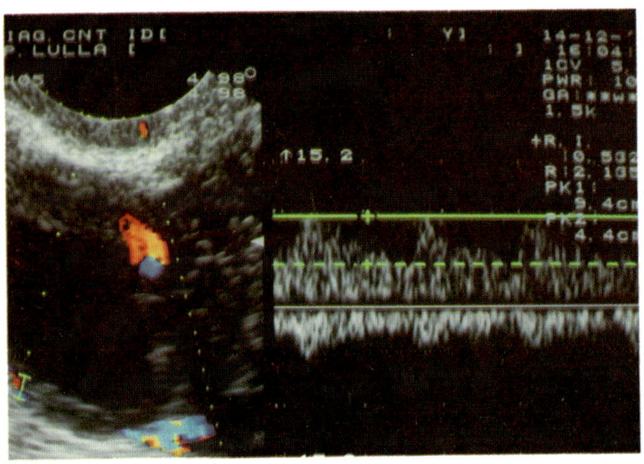

Fig. 22.3. Colour Doppler sonogram showing the low impedance ovarian blood flow around a dominant follicle.

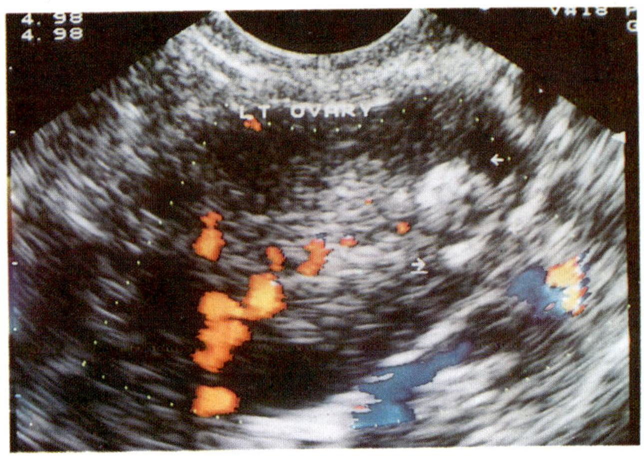

Fig. 22.6. Corpus luteum vascularity seen in this plate.

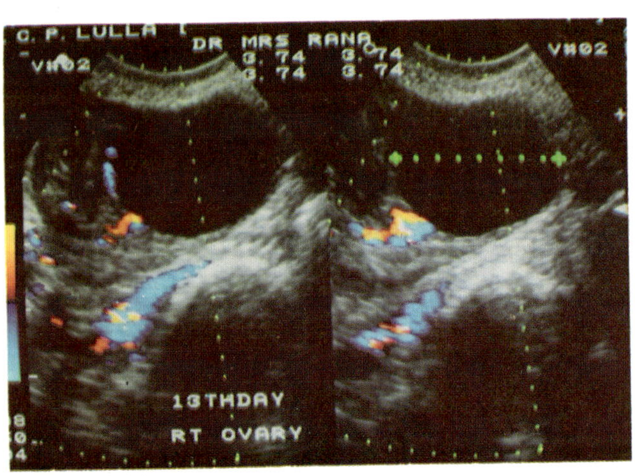

Fig. 22.4. Colour Doppler sonogram showing perifollicular blood flow on day 13. Also seen is the right hypogastric vessel.

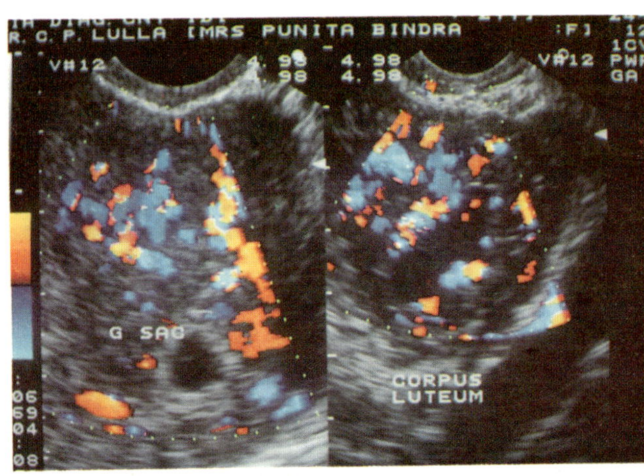

Fig. 22.7. Colour Doppler sonogram showing peritrophoblastic flow around an early gestational sac. Corpus luteal flow seen on the right.

PLATE 9

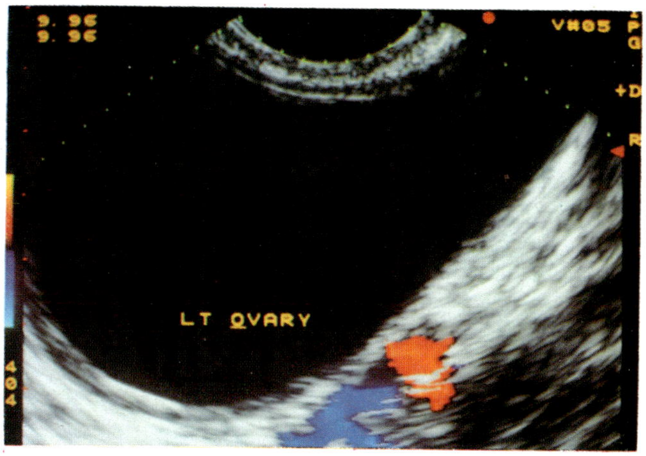

Fig. 22.8. Colour Doppler sonogram showing perifollicular blood flow around an unruptured luteinized follicle.

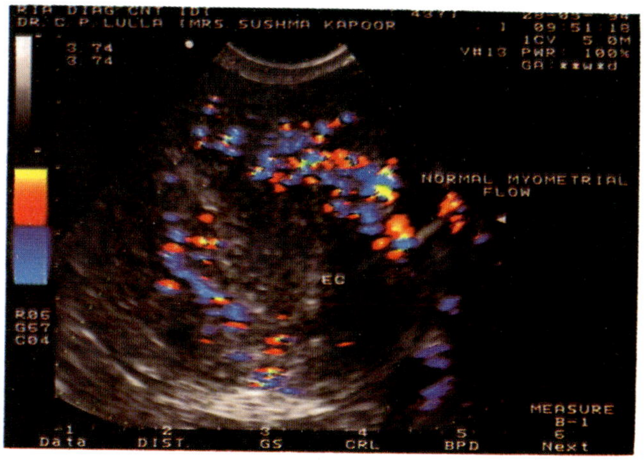

Fig. 22.11. Arcuate blood flow.

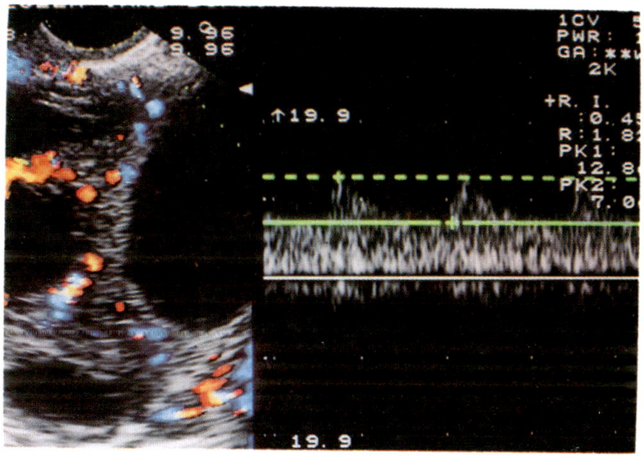

Fig. 22.9. Colour Doppler sonogram showing low impedance intra-ovarian blood flow in a stimulated cycle.

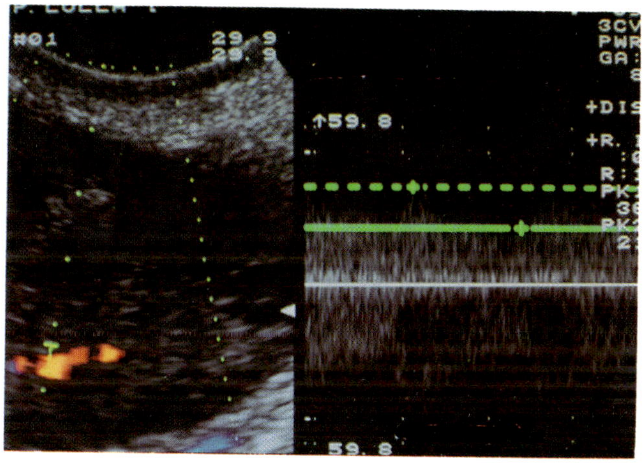

Fig. 22.12. Colour Doppler sonogram showing low impedance uterine blood flow.

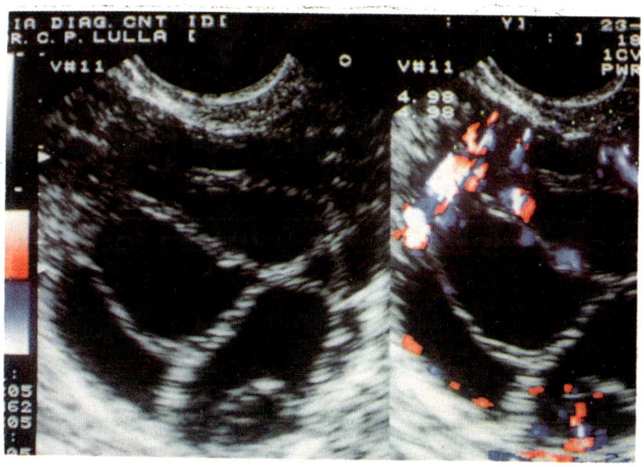

Fig. 22.10. Colour Doppler sonogram showing intra-follicular blood flow in a gonadotropin cycle.

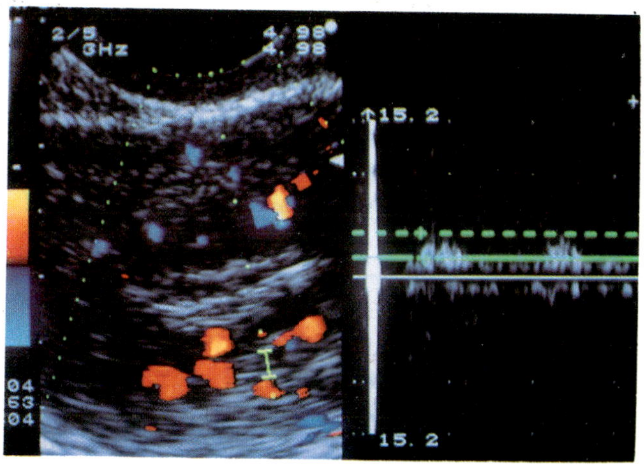

Fig. 22.13. Colour Doppler sonogram showing low impedance arcuate blood flow.

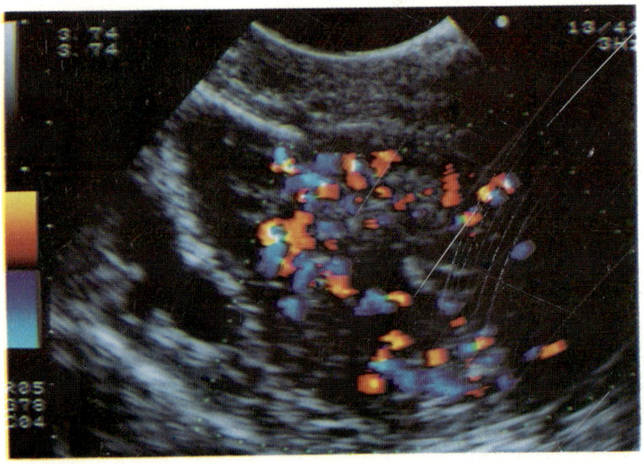

Fig. 22.14. Increased uterine perfusion in the follicular phase.

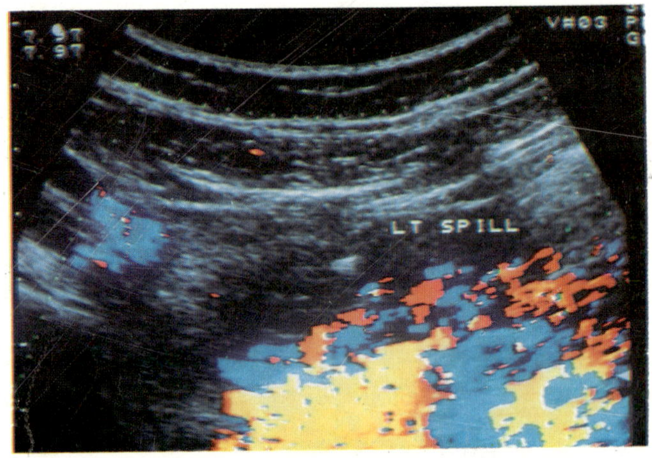

Fig. 22.17. Colour Doppler sonosalpingography showing free peritoneal spill.

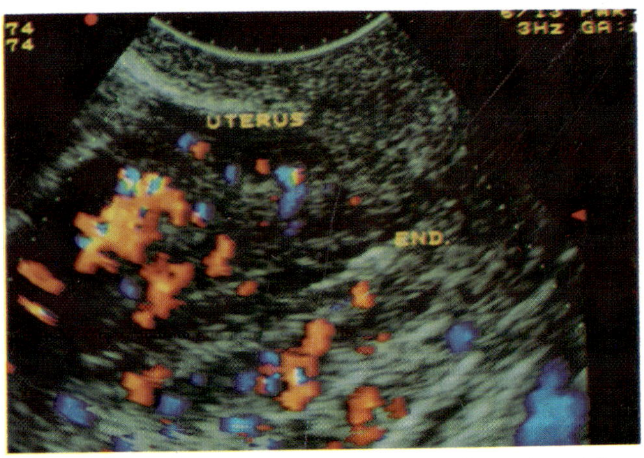

Fig. 22.15. Decreased uterine perfusion in the peri-ovulatory period.

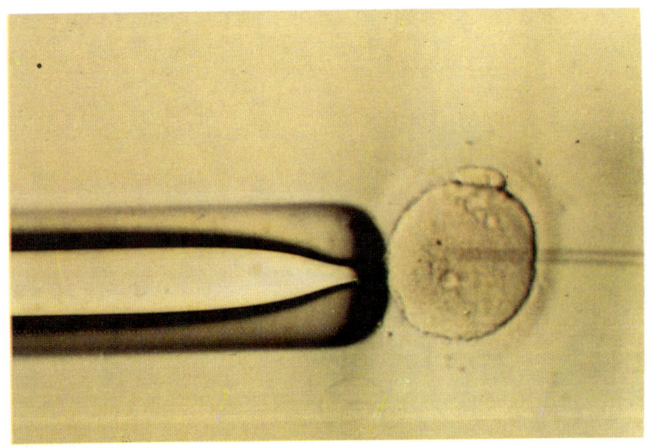

Fig. 37.3. Intracytoplasmic microinjection of single spermatozoon using microinjection pipette (right) while the left microholding pipette immobilises the oocyte (polar body at 12 o'clock position) — microphotograph taken at author's lab.

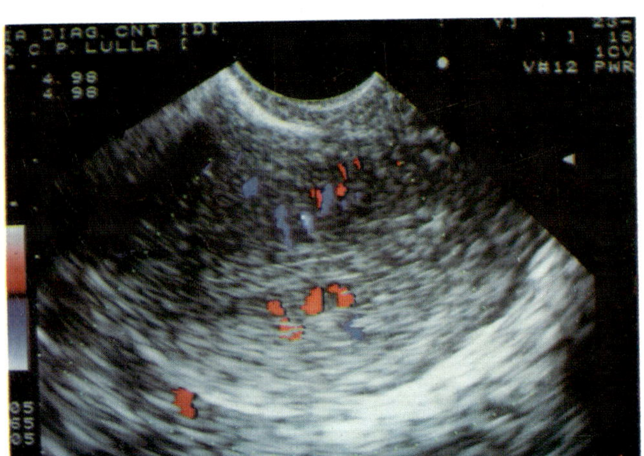

Fig. 22.16. Poor uterine perfusion in a stimulated cancelled IVF cycle.

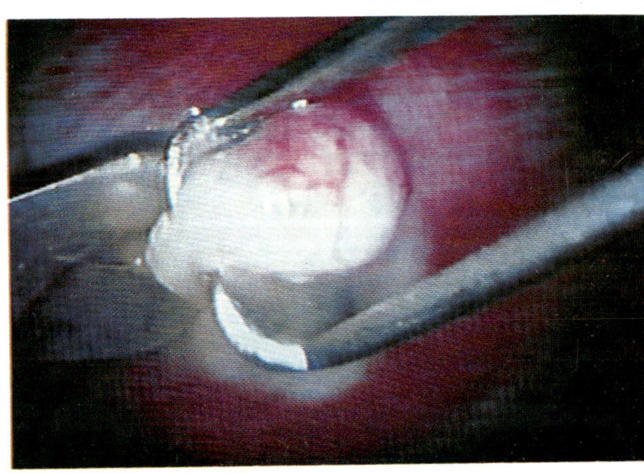

Fig. 44.1. The myoma is being held steady with the grasping forceps while bipolar cauterisation is being done at the base.

PLATE 11

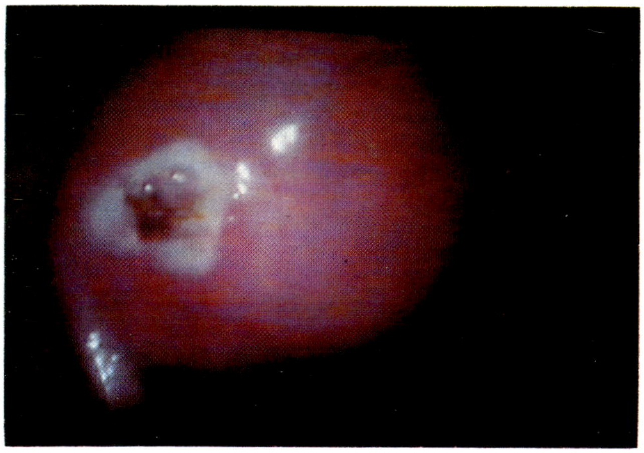

Fig. 44.2. Bed of the excised myoma now coagulated

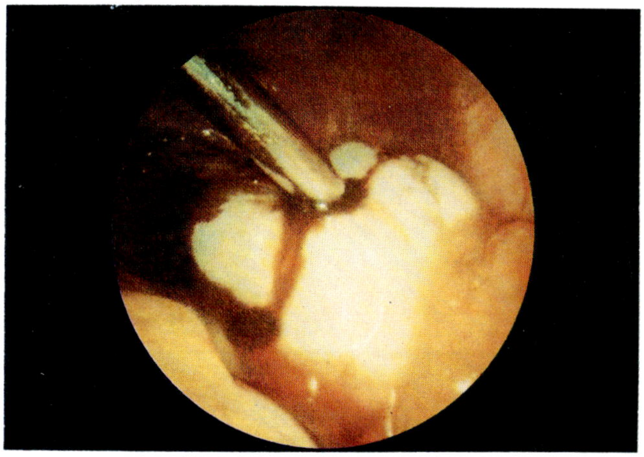

Fig. 45.2. Ovarian cyst is washed out with saline solution.

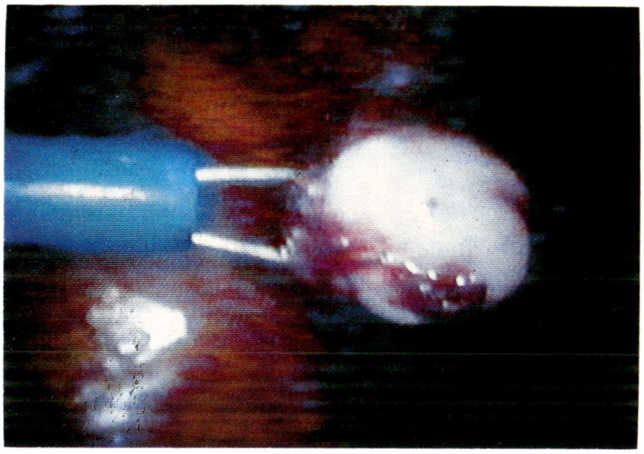

Fig. 44.3. Excised myoma being removed through the 10 mm portal.

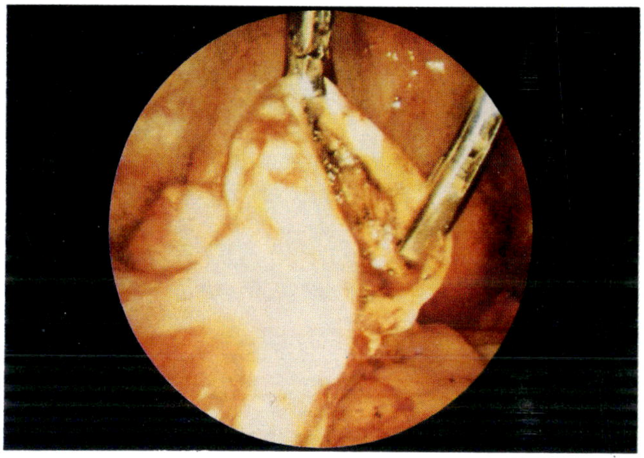

Fig. 45.3. Ovarian closure with fibrin glue.

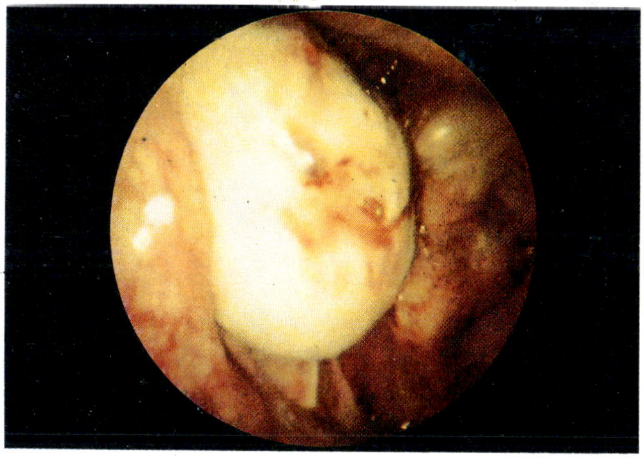

Fig. 45.1. Ovarian endometrioma less than 3 cm in diameter.

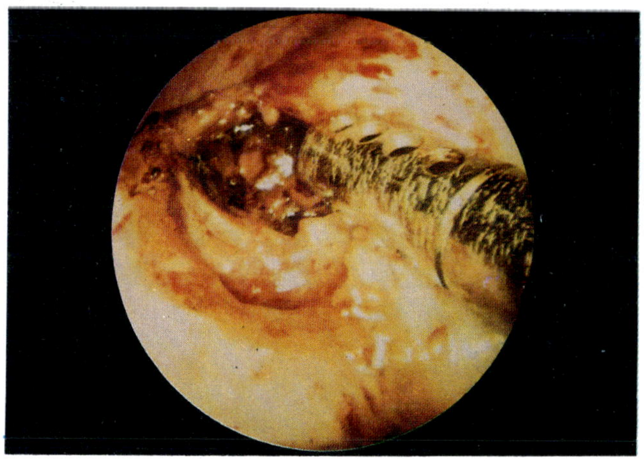

Fig. 45.4. The mucosal lining being vaporised.

PLATE 12

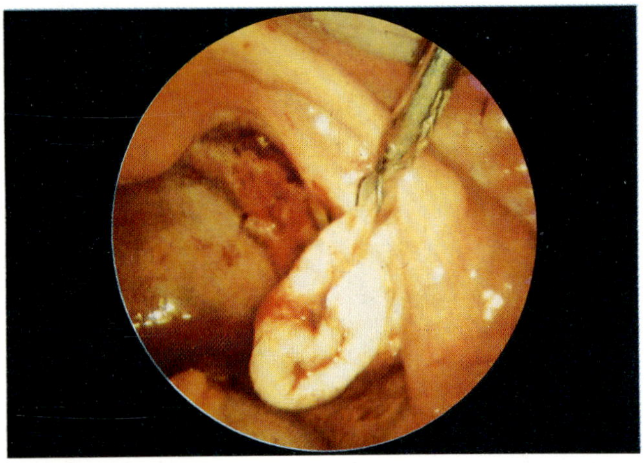

Fig. 45.5. Edges of ovarian cyst wall approximated with atraumatic forceps.

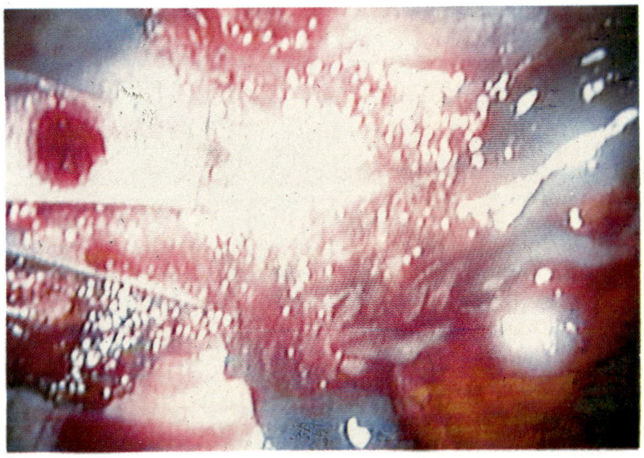

Fig. 46.3. The coagulated segment of the tube being cut with the help of the unipolar scissors.

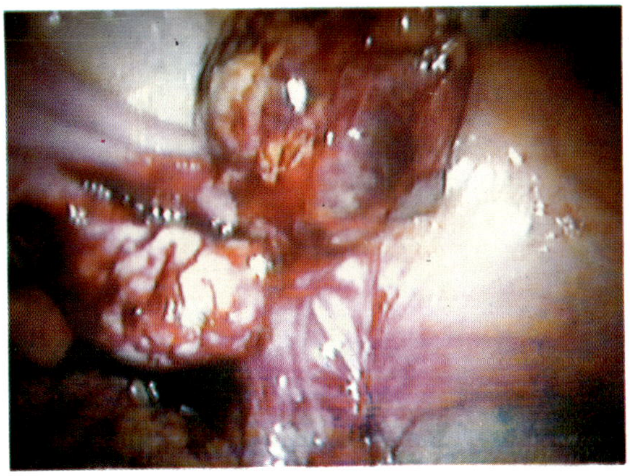

Fig. 46.1. A chronic ectopic pregnancy seen on the right. The ovary is seen to the left.

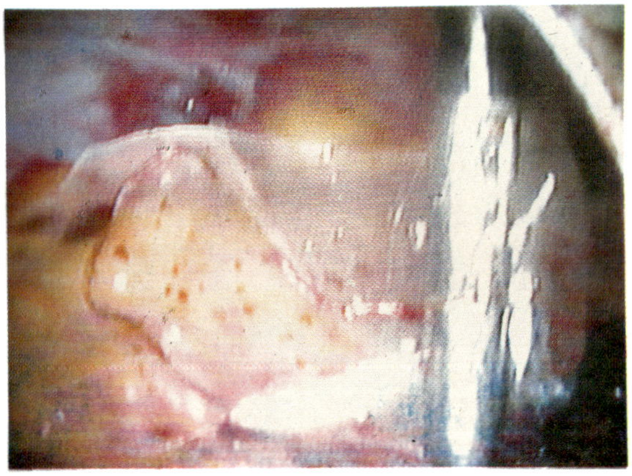

Fig. 46.4. An endo-bag being used to remove the chronic ectopic mass out of the peritoneal cavity.

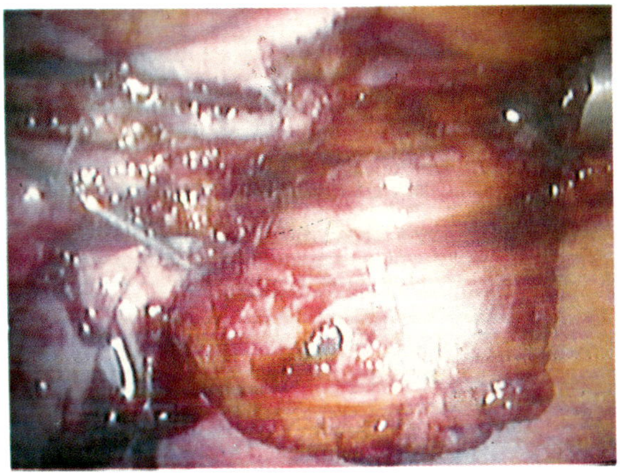

Fig. 46.2. Bipolar coagulation forceps being applied to the proximal tube. Ectopic pregnancy is being held with a grasping forceps.

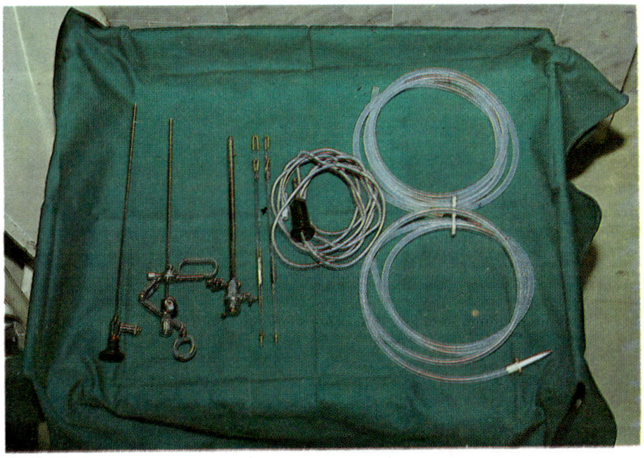

Fig. 47.1. Resectoscope instruments.

PART I

Transvaginal Sonography

CHAPTER

1

Introduction to Transvaginal Sonography

Adi Dastur

Physics of transvaginal sonography

The physics of transvaginal sonography is centered around small high frequency transducers or transducer arrays which can be placed in close proximity to the female pelvic organs but provide a relatively small field of view.

There is a wide variety of transducer designs ranging from long and thin to short and thick, from round to rectangular and from straight to angled.

Probes vary in length from the short ones of Brüel and Kjaer to the longer ones of Elscint, Siemens, Acuson and Diasonics just to name a few. The longer ones measure about 8″ in the length of the intracavity portion but seldom is more than 2-3″ actually inserted. A problem with the very long and angled probes is that they may be difficult to position to see the fundus of the acutely anteverted uterus because the handle hits the top of the bed or stretcher. This can be overcome by placing a foam wedge under the pelvis.

The shape of the probe head varies from small and round to large and rectangular. The former is most easily introduced into the introitus and easily moved within the vagina. The latter is more difficult to introduce and more cumbersome to manoeuvre inside the vagina. Most of the probes have straight handles but in some the handles are angled 30 degrees. The angled ones have an advantage in positioning to see the fundus and the lateral pelvic sidewall.

The transducer may be either *mechanical* with one or more elements which oscillates or rotates or *phased array* with the linear or curved crystal array. The variation of the mechanical type is to use two or even three crystals, a low frequency one for better penetration and a higher frequency for better resolution.

The sound beam may be directed either out of the probe, from the side or from the angle between. End-fire transducers may be either mechanical type or a curved linear array at the end of the probe. The area of interest remains in view as the transducer is rotated 90°. Off-axis probes are usually angled 20° to 30°, in theory to have the beam perpendicular to the long axis of the uterus, however this does not keep the area of interest in the field of view when the transducer is rotated 90°.

The frequencies used vary from 3.5 to 7.5 MHz with some manufacturers incorporating two and even three frequencies in one probe. The higher frequency obviously gives somewhat better resolution but at the expense of penetration. The lower frequencies of 3.5 or even 5.0 MHz are too low to give the degree of resolution that is needed in examining an early gestational sac or embryo. The dual frequency probes may add greater flexibility than the single crystal ones. The best axial resolution of a 3.5 MHz crystal is 0.67 mm and that of a 5.0 MHz crystal is 0.32 mm.

The field of view varies widely between transducers from 75° to 360°. A 90° sector provides an adequate field of view in most cases. The transducers with a 360° field of view have the disadvantage of having too much information without the ability to magnify the area of interest such as the small early gestational sac. It is important to remember that with this high resolution tool one must magnify the image and the area of interest to maximize the diagnostic return. The ideal field of view in our hand is usually 6 cm with 4 and even 2 cm frequently being used. Some of the phased array heads or single crystal ones are steerable either mechanically or electrically giving an even wider field of view and therefore a more versatile probe.

The focal zone of a single crystal is fixed and depends upon its frequency and diameter. For phased linear and curvilinear arrays the focal zone is dynamically variable. It is usually 1.5 cm to 2.5 cm from the transducer face. The absorption of sound at high frequencies does not allow for visualization of deeper structures. At 2 cm depth with 6.5 MHz there is 12.5% of the original sound energy that returns to the transducer; this compares with 20% at 5.0 MHz and 37% at 3.5 MHz. Large uterine and ovarian masses may not be adequately viewed endovaginally and a concomitant transvesical study is needed.

The technique of transvaginal examination

The flat ultrasound examination table is appropriate for most *in-line* transducer probes with an end-firing scanhead. Angled probes, however require a gynaecological examination table. A 15 to 20 cm thick foam cushion placed under the pelvis allows free movement to the examiner's hand to achieve maximum angling.

An important prerequisite for transvaginal sonography examination is a thorough and complete emptying of the urinary bladder, for three reasons.

1. A full bladder may *occupy* most of the screen and displace important *target organs* to be scanned.
2. Sound waves passing through the bladder filled with low impedance fluid create the well-known effect of enhancement (this high-echo area interferes with a proper gain setting).
3. A full bladder distorts pelvic anatomy by compressing pelvic organs and displacing possible ovarian and tubal pathology beyond the reach of the transducer.

After insertion of the transducer probe, the required gain curve and magnification are selected to obtain the best possible image on the screen.

To obtain image in various directions, planes, and depths, three main manipulations of the probe are possible :

1. *Titling* or *angling* the shaft by its handle so as to point the tip of the probe in any direction in the pelvis.
2. *Pushing-pulling* the whole probe to bring a deeper or a closer organ into the focal origin or actually into the focal length.
3. *Rotating* the handle slowly along the longitudinal axis of the probe to change the scanning plane along a 360° range.

In addition to these manual manipulations of the probe, the symmetrically end-firing *fan* of the beam can be titled in an off-axis scanning direction by the appropriate electronic controls. Thus, scanning of the whole pelvis is possible.

The first structure on the path of the vaginal probe to its final place of scanning the pelvis is the cervix. If the cervix has to be scanned it may be done as the probe penetrates 2.5-3 cm into the vagina, 2-3 cm before the tip of the probe reaches the cervix itself. This prevents the picture from being obscured by air that may be trapped in the fornices at the end of a prolonged or a repeated examination. The cervix may also be examined after locating the uterus and then pulling the probe slowly outward. Cystic structures adjacent to the cervical canal and external os are frequently seen. They represent endocervical cysts and Nabothian cysts. Cervical pregnancy should always be kept in mind and looked for if ectopic pregnancy is suspected.

The most prominent landmark in the pelvis is usually the uterus (Fig. 1.1). If the uterus is anteverted and anteflexed, the first cross-section to be seen is the cervix. A slow upward scan will reveal the body and finally the fundus of the uterus. With the same sequence (scanning from the back to the front) in a retroverted

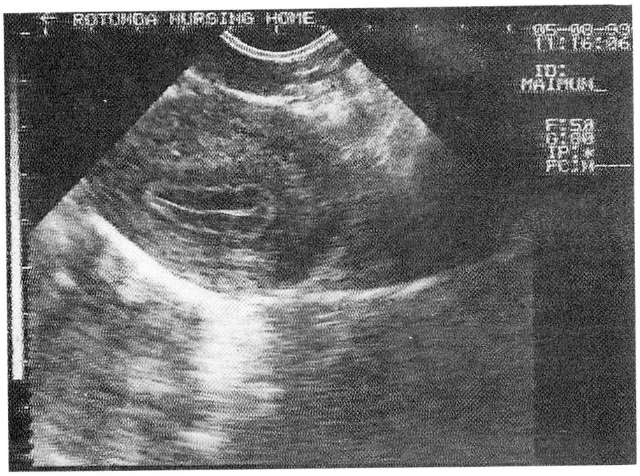

Fig. 1.1. Uterus in a transverse section. The triple layer pattern appreciated here.

uterus, the fundus is visualised first and the cervix last. The transverse or horizontal scan should be followed by the vertical scanning plane, which will reveal the entire uterus with its endometrial lining. Scanning of the lateral uterine margin on either side reveals the ingoing, outgoing and pulsating vascular pockets at the level of the junction between the cervix and the body of the uterus (Fig. 1.2 – Plate 1). Blood flow measurements of the uterine artery and vein may be done using this site.

After the uterus and its contents are examined, the pouch of Douglas should be sought. In many cases there is some free fluid present in the cul-de-sac. This minimal amount of fluid may be detected. Free fluid outlines the posterior wall of the uterus and sometimes even the ovaries.

The tip of the transducer should now be pointed towards the side of the uterus to visualize the adnexa. The ovaries are the most prominent landmark of the adnexa. They are distinct because of their relatively lower echogenic texture as well as different-sized Graafian follicles. The follicles appear as echo-free, translucent, round structures from several millimeters to 2 cm in diameter (Fig. 1.3). During the reproductive years these follicles serve as the sonographic *markers* of the ovaries; after menopause it is hard to find the ovaries because the above-described *markers* (*i.e.*, the follicles) are not present and the ovaries themselves undergo atrophy. If the ovaries are visualized in the postmenopausal patient, this should be clearly mentioned in the sonographic report and the workup of the case is advisable.

If the uterus and the ovaries are localised, the tubes may be scanned. They should be sought under the

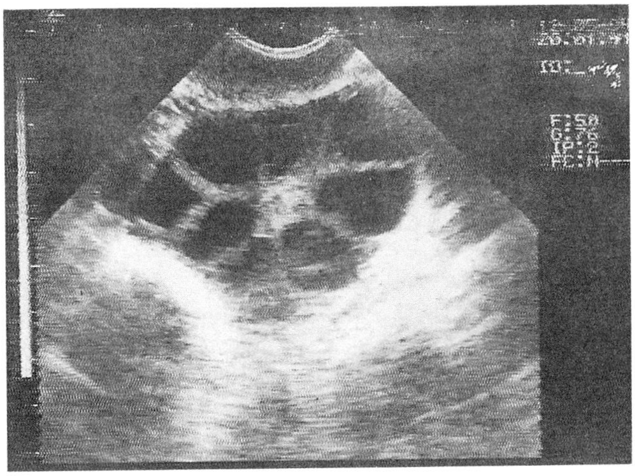

Fig. 1.3. Multiple follicular development in a stimulated cycle.

imaginary horizontal plane drawn at the level of the endometrial line at the side of the uterus. If found, they are usually behind the ovaries or in the cul-de-sac. If they are normal and healthy or no fluid surrounds them, they cannot be visualized. If pathological (*e.g.*, dilated, thick, fluid-filled, or housing gestational sac), they are usually outstanding and easily recognised (Figs. 1.4, 1.5 and 1.6).

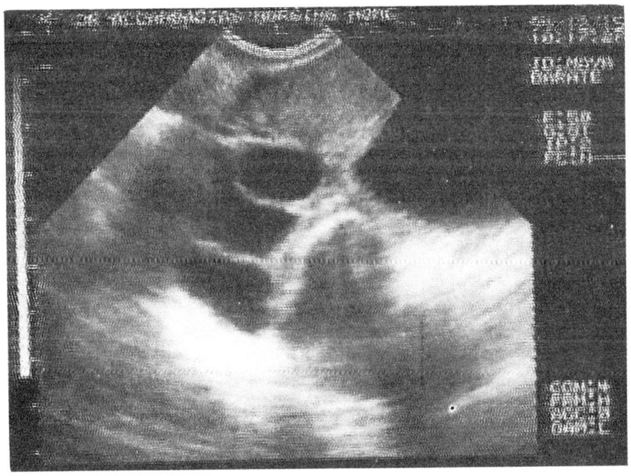

Fig. 1.4. Bilateral hydrosalpinges along with the uterus in a transverse plane. The left sactosalpinx shows the typical sacculations seen in a distended tube.

The next step is to look for space-occupying lesions in the pelvis. Since there is no specific place to direct our attention, the entire pelvis must be systematically *covered* by imaginary horizontal and vertical coordinates, and a thorough search should be made along these planes.

On the horizon exists the question whether this new technology may be used to understand and to identify

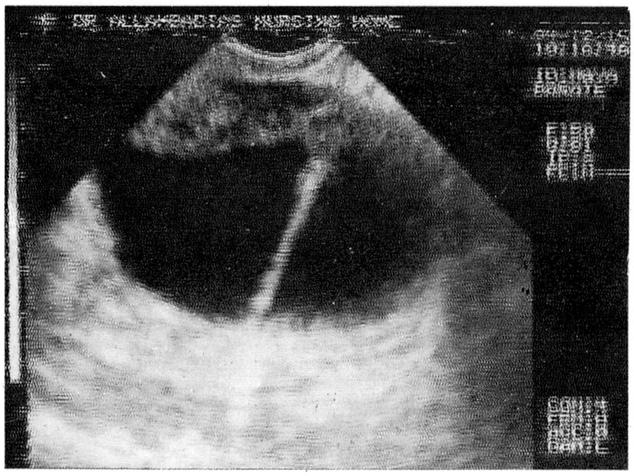

Fig. 1.5. A left-sided large hydrosalpinx.

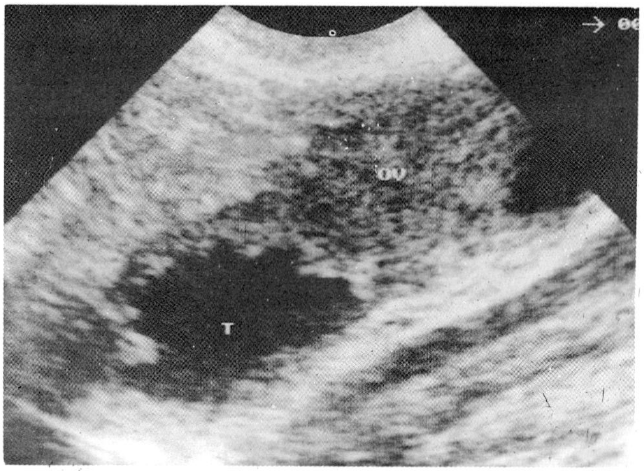

Fig. 1.6. Cross-section of a dilated tube. The wall is just slightly thickened, but the slightly prominent folds of the endosalpinx give the cog wheel sign, suggestive of a chronic sactosalpinx.

earlier the growth of ovarian neoplasms, a class of malignancies that throughout this clinician's lifetime have shown little therapeutic improvement, perhaps because of delays in recognition.

Hence the transvaginal approach has become a standard of care for all gynaecologists. A new doorway into understanding and improved patient care has been opened. Endovaginal colour Doppler imaging has opened further vistas in gynaecological diagnosis. Indeed the vaginal probe should and will be used, without much ado as routinely as the classical vaginal speculum of James Marion Sims.

CHAPTER

2

Sonoembryology : Transvaginal Sonography in Early Pregnancy

Pratap Kumar

The recent past has shown dramatic changes in our concepts concerning evaluation of early pregnancy due to transvaginal sonography.

Fertilization occurs in the fallopian tube when an oocyte released from an ovarian follicle comes in contact with sperm. Cleavage occurs in the first day; after 3 days, a 16-cell morula enters the uterus. The morula then further differentiates into a fluid-filled sphere, the outer layer of which is made of trophoblasts, cells that will ultimately develop into the chorionic membrane and fetal portion of the placenta. This blastocyst remains free within the uterus for another 2 days, and then implants into and invades the endometrium. As early chorionic villi develop, β-hCG is produced in detectable levels, with a positive pregnancy test occuring after 3 weeks menstrual age. The blastocyst is still less than 1 mm in size, and is not detectable by ultrasound. Growth is rapid at this phase, with the gestational sac reaching 1 mm at 4 weeks, 3 mm at 32 days, and 5 mm at 35 days.

Within the blastocyst, the inner cell layer gives rise to the amnion, embryonic yolk sac, embryo, and umbilical cord. During the fourth menstrual week, a bilaminar embryonic disk has formed along one edge of the blastocyst, with fluid-filled cavities on either side of this disk. At this stage, the smaller amniotic cavity lies near the trophoblastic layer (developing placenta), while the yolk sac is projected into the chorionic space (Fig. 2.1). The yolk sac is larger than the amniotic sac and more evident, initially seen at 36 to 40 days (about 1 week after identification of a gestational sac). When the amniotic cavity can be identified, the *double bleb sign* is present, made up of yolk sac and amnion on either side of the developing embryo (Fig. 2.2). The

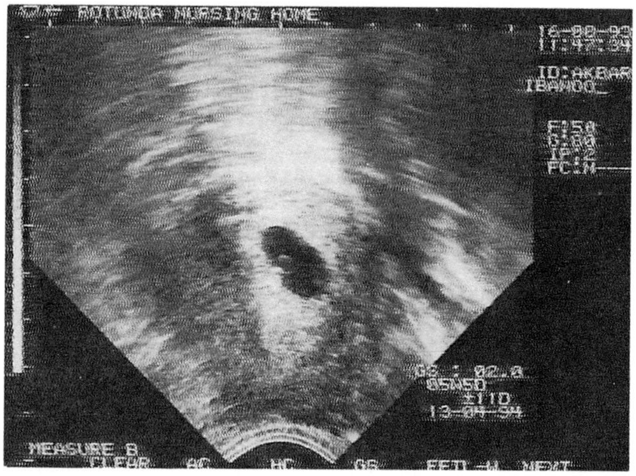

Fig. 2.1. A five week five day gestational sac. Yolk sac seen clearly.

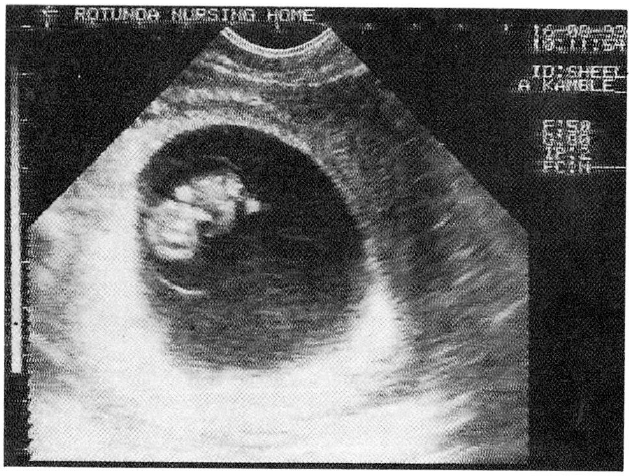

Fig. 2.2. The amnion seen clearly around the fetus.

sonographic significance of the yolk sac must be emphasized. When it is seen within an intrauterine fluid collection, the diagnosis of intrauterine gestation can be made with a high degree of certainty. The yolk sac reaches about 5 mm in diameter and disappears at about 9 weeks of gestation. An abnormally large yolk sac may indicate an abnormal pregnancy.

At about day 40, an embryo can be identified. Only rarely is an embryo seen without cardiac activity because the heart begins to contract at about day 37. More commonly, cardiac activity is observed with TVS prior to adequate embryonic definition because the embryo can be adjacent to the wall of the gestational sac and not be discernible clearly.

During the 2 weeks following the appearance of the yolk sac, there is infolding of the bilaminar embryo and growth of the amniotic cavity. The yolk sac is pinched off and becomes an extra amniotic structure tethered by the vitelline duct. A stalk can be identified attaching the embryo to the developing placenta. This is the early umbilical cord. The growing amniotic membrane begins to fuse with chorionic membrane in the mid-first trimester, and fusion of these membranes is not complete until at least the 12th week, and often as late as the 16th week. The expected TVS depiction of the amniotic membrane as a free structure should not be misinterpreted as subchorionic haemorrhage or residual amniotic cavity from demise of a twin.

Initial research has now been published suggesting the timing and early appearance of fetal structures by TVS. Early limb buds project laterally from the embryonic torso in a coronal plane in the eighth week (Fig. 2.3). In the ensuing 3 weeks, further development of joints allows rotation of limbs into the expected para-sagittal plane; extremity components — forearm, upper arm, thigh, and leg — can be resolved sonographically. Hands can be seen and fingers counted in the twelfth week.

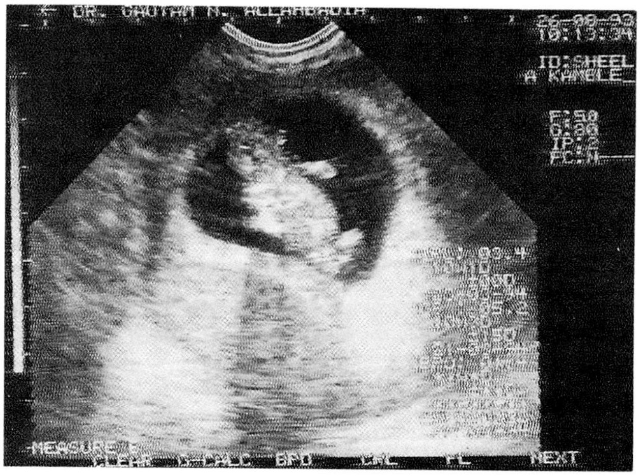

Fig. 2.3. Early limb buds seen clearly in this nine week fetus.

Although significant facial development occurs during the mid-first trimester, the characterization of facial features is difficult before the tenth week because of the curled configuration of the fetus. We have shown the developing orbit at 8 weeks. Using TVS other bony structures, such as mandible and maxilla, are recognizable at 10 weeks, with soft tissue elements (nose, lips) seen at 12 weeks. Because facial and limb abnormalities may be manifestations of genetic syndromes, appreciation of the expected appearance of these structures may be helpful in identifying patients at risk for transmitting genetic disorders.

Beginning in the seventh week, the developing spine can be imaged. The parallel lines of the developing neural tub are demonstrable on coronal sections. At 7 weeks, the fetal brain is seen as a single ventricle (telencephalon) that is subsequently partitioned by the falx. By the ninth week, the more familiar configuration of lateral ventricles filled predominantly with echogenic choroid plexus is apparent. Also identifiable during the eighth to tenth week is a small cystic space in the posterior cranium, representing the hindbrain (rhombencephalon) (Fig. 2.4).

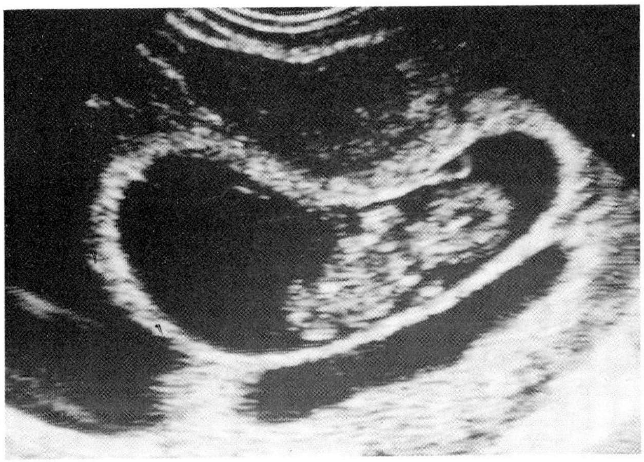

Fig. 2.4. Rhombencephalon seen clearly here.

Normal migration of midgut into the umbilical cord occurs during the 9th to 11th week. During this time, the midgut grows disproportionately with respect to the abdominal cavity. During the 11th week, the bowel returns to the abdominal cavity, completing a 270° counter-clockwise rotation that creates the normal orientation of bowel. By TVS, normal midgut herniation may be recognized as a broad-based structure filled with echogenic fetal bowel attached to the abdominal wall. Until 14 weeks when bowel loops can be expected to have re-entered the abdominal cavity, the diagnosis of omphalocele or gastroschisis should not be entertained.

In assessing patients during early pregnancy, we have found that sequential examinations with TVS every 3 days will allow progression through the milestones of gestational sac, yolk sac, embryo, and heartbeat. The interval for an individual patient will depend upon the clinical setting. In a patient who is at high risk for ectopic pregnancy, TVS may facilitate diagnosis of an ectopic pregnancy before clinical signs are present, permitting tubal salvage surgery or ablation with chemotherapeutic agents to be performed.

In a patient who presents with bleeding in the first trimester, TVS can be extremely useful in establishing that the gestation is normal with observation of the embryo and heartbeat. When the bleeding is attributable to subchorionic hemorrhage, the extrachorionic fluid collection can be easily identified in most patients, even when small. When bleeding is related to threatened abortion or embryonic demise, size discrepancy between the gestational sac, yolk sac, and embryo can suggest abnormal outcome of the pregnancy, even when an embryo with a heartbeat is seen. In this latter instance, however, the finding of cardiac activity supersedes all other signs of abnormal pregnancy and follow-up studies rather than dilatation and curettage is indicated. It has been our experience, as well as that of others, that the shape of the sac may not correlate well with viability since uterine contractions and unusual sac positions can create unusual shapes in early pregnancy particularly by TVS. The empty-bladder transvaginal technique obviates contour abnormality of the sac due to compression by a full bladder and permits the true sac configuration to be evaluated.

Transvaginal sonography has the unique ability to evaluate the first trimester of pregnancy with greater accuracy than previous techniques. Early embryonic anatomy can easily be identified due to the high resolution and proximity of the probe to the uterus.

The yolk sac when normal is a very regular circular structure (4 mm diameter) within the sac (Fig. 2.5). It has a very bright echogenic rim around a sonolucent

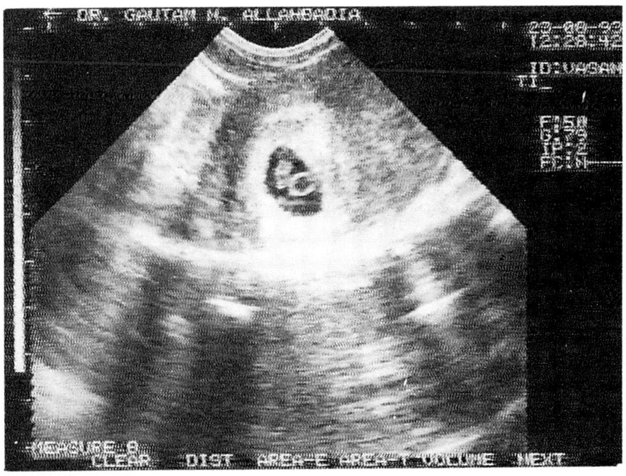

Fig. 2.5. A normal bright echogenic circular yolk sac seen clearly. The fetal pole can also be appreciated here.

centre. In abnormal pregnancies, the yolk sac may be enlarged, irregular or sometimes described as *floating*. Major sonographic criteria for predicting non-viability include sac size more than 2 cm without yolk sac or more than 2.5 cm without an embryo. However with TVS, gestational sac as small as 0.6 to 0.9 cm can be expected to demonstrate a yolk sac. Cardiac activity, which may be noticed before an embryo can be defined, should be seen when sacs are more than 0.9 cm.

CRL is more precisely measured with transvaginal sonography since the concern about errors like with transabdominal sonography (not identifying the longest diameter, including the limbs, yolk sac or part of uterine wall) are no longer a real consideration with transvaginal sonography (Fig. 2.6).

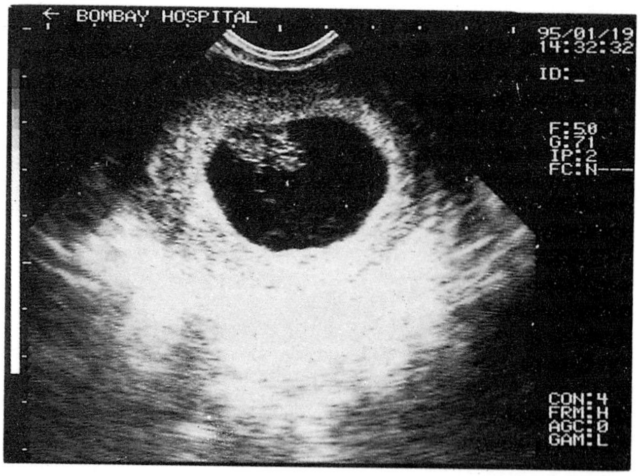

Fig. 2.6. A transvaginal sonogram of a seven week fetus.

CHAPTER

3

Transvaginal Ultrasound for Abortions and Anomalies in the First Trimester

Duru Shah

Introduction

Transvaginal sonography is gradually replacing transabdominal ultrasonography for most of the first trimester problems because of improved image and its ability to detect ectopic pregnancies as early as 1 week after a missed period. Besides, the convenience of being able to perform ultrasound examinations without the need for a full bladder, makes it a technique preferred by patients. This is especially because, in the first trimester bladder filling becomes difficult due to frequency of micturition, which is a well-established symptom of early pregnancy.

The normal intrauterine pregnancy

Kratochwil[1] was the first to describe the detection of pregnancy as early as the first week after missing menses (that is 3 weeks after ovulation or 5 weeks after the last period). Thus with the use of transvaginal ultrasound it is possible to image a gestation in the uterus within a day of a missed period. Thus by 4 weeks and 1 day the uterine cavity shows a thickened endometrium with the gestation sac seen as a 2 to 3 mm echo-free structure surrounded by a reflective trophoblastic ring (Fig. 3.1). This gives rise to the *double decidual sac* sign, *crescent* sign or *decidual chorionic sac* (DCS) sign, which are all terms used to describe the appearance of a normal gestation sac in which the decidua parietalis appears to diverge and surround a portion of the chorionic sac. Controversy exists over the cause of the DCS sign, but its reliability has been demonstrated in the differentiation of intrauterine pregnancy from ectopic pregnancy where the DCS sign does not occur. However, the DCS sign is only present in two-thirds of all normal pregnancies. Thus, when present it may be of value, when absent it is of less diagnostic significance. More often than not, the gestation sac is located in an eccentric position within the uterine cavity (Fig. 3.2); the presence of an echo-free space in a central position is more likely to be a pseudosac, which should make one suspect the presence of an ectopic gestation. Besides, in patients who have

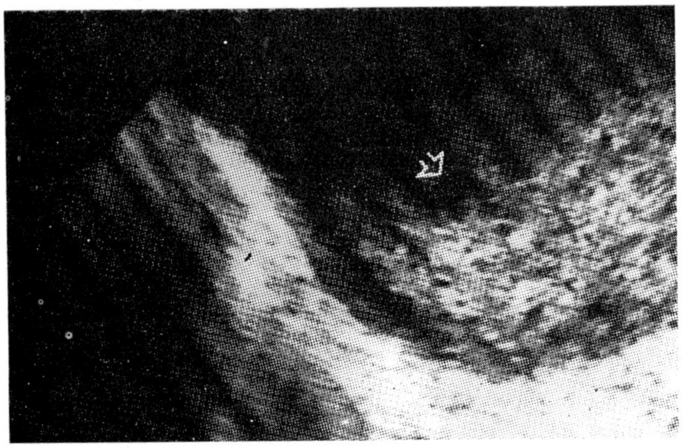

Fig. 3.1. Implanted gestation at 4 weeks 2 days (3 × 2 mm — open arrow). The serum β-hCG subunit level at this time was 600 mIU/ml (First Reference Standard).

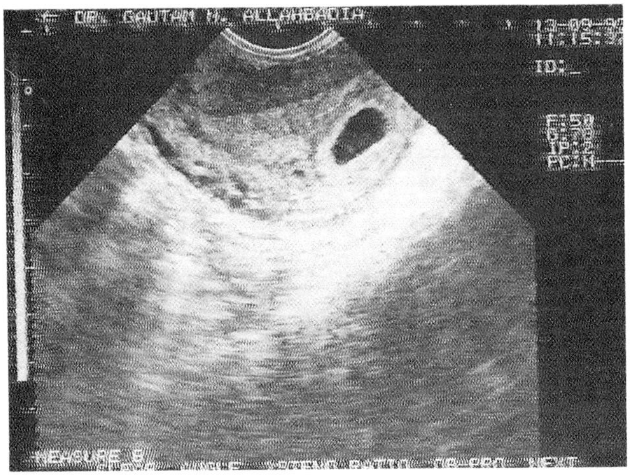

Fig. 3.2. An eccentrically implanted gestational sac.

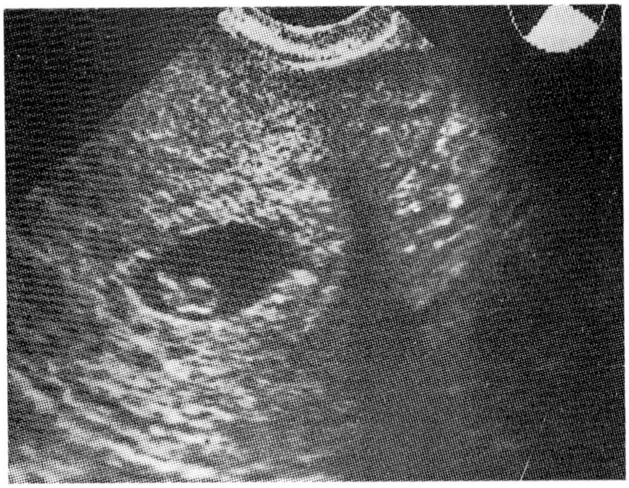

Fig. 3.3. 6 week intrauterine pregnancy. The embryo is approximately the same size as the yolk sac (5 mm). Cardiac pulsation is always seen in live embryos at this stage. Note the lacunar areas in the lateral wall of the gestational sac.

had a past history of ectopic gestation, a scan performed at the first sign of pregnancy helps to rule out an ectopic gestation in the present pregnancy.

By 5 weeks the yolk sac is demonstrated and it now measures between 3 and 4 mm. The gestation sac is double the size of the yolk sac. These two sacs become visible as two small bubbles or blebs, giving rise to the *double bleb sign*. By five and a half weeks, cardiac activity is seen at the edge of the yolk sac and the embryo appears as three thin lines located between the yolk sac and the chorionic plate. The gestation sac has a mean diameter of approximately 1 cm at this stage.

By 6 weeks the embryo is the same size as the yolk sac, which has a diameter of 4 to 5 mm (Fig. 3.3). At this stage, one can identify the region where the placenta will develop, in the form of lacunar structures on one side of the gestation sac. By this time, cardiac activity can almost be demonstrated in all patients by transvaginal sonography (TVS) as compared to transabdominal ultrasound in which cardiac activity can be detected in only 17% to 60% of patients at 6 weeks[2]. A gradual increase in foetal heart rate (FHR) during the first few weeks of pregnancy has been reported by several investigators[3]. DuBose *et al.*[4] reported that FHR can be used in the clinical setting to provide an estimate of embryonic age and that it correlates highly with CRL for embryos younger than 9 menstrual weeks. In the study by Rotsztejn and co-workers[5] the mean heart rate was 108 on days 26 to 30 after conception (5 weeks 4 days from LMP) in embryos of mean size 3 mm. The FHR gradually increased, reaching a maximum of 177 on days 51 to 55 (9 weeks from LMP) in embryos of 23 mm; it decreased to 156 on days 76 to 80 (12 weeks 5 days from LMP) in embryos of 62 mm. This interesting observation has been correlated with the β-hCG level pattern of the 1st trimester of pregnancy and was termed highly significant in single as well as multiple pregnancies.

At 7 weeks, the embryo measures 7 mm in length and the yolk sac 5 mm in diameter. It becomes possible to differentiate the head from the body, the former appearing larger than the latter. The heart rate at this stage is 120 beats per minute[6] and Doppler signals can be detected (Fig. 3.4).

At 8 weeks gestational age, the embryo measures 1 cm which is twice the diameter of the yolk sac which remains at 5 mm for the rest of the first trimester of pregnancy (Fig. 3.5). The head and yolk sac seem to be of equal size at this stage due to the presence of a single cerebral ventricle which almost simulates a second yolk sac. Embryonic movements, limb buds and development of the central nervous system are all landmarks

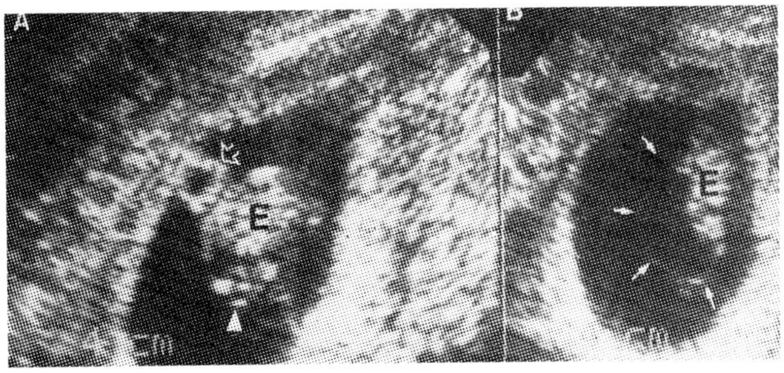

Fig. 3.4. Serial sections of the pregnant uterus 7 weeks 3 days. (**A**) Extra embryonic yolk sac (open arrow) and *curled up* embryo (E) are shown. The head is marked by an arrowhead. (**B**) Subsequent but parallel section of the same. The amnion is shown (arrows).

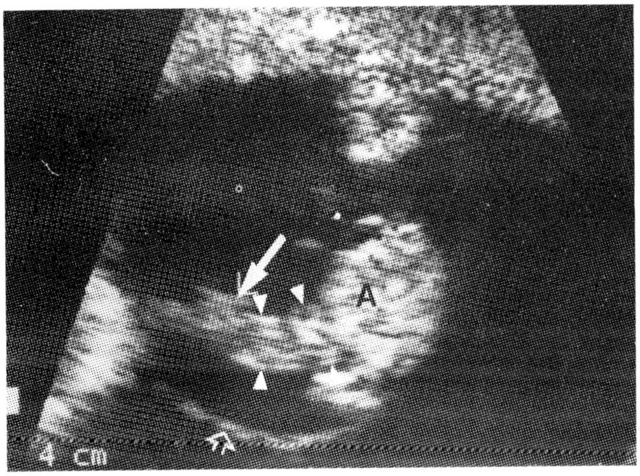

Fig. 3.5. Abdominal insertion of the cord (arrow) is shown at 8 weeks 4 days. Its approach is from the left. Before it reaches the Abdomen (A) it becomes somewhat more echogenic and thicker. This area (marked by arrowhead) is consistent with the physiologic midgut herniation into the cord at this gestation. The amnion is marked by an open arrow.

seen during this stage of development. Besides, the placental site becomes easily distinguishable and the umbilical cord insertion can be traced to both the placental and embryonic ends.

By the 9th week, the crown-rump length is greater than 2 cm, the limb buds are more prominent, the umbilical cord pulsations are marked and peristalsis may be seen in the physiological umbilical hernia. Intracranial anatomy gets more differentiated with the appearance of the falx cerebrum and the spine can be identified (Figs. 3.6 and 3.7).

By 10 weeks, organogenesis is complete and the fetal heart, stomach, urinary bladder and kidneys may be identified, if they have grown to be larger than 2 to 3 mm in size. Movements of the limbs and trunk help in the visualisation of most of these structures (Fig. 3.8).

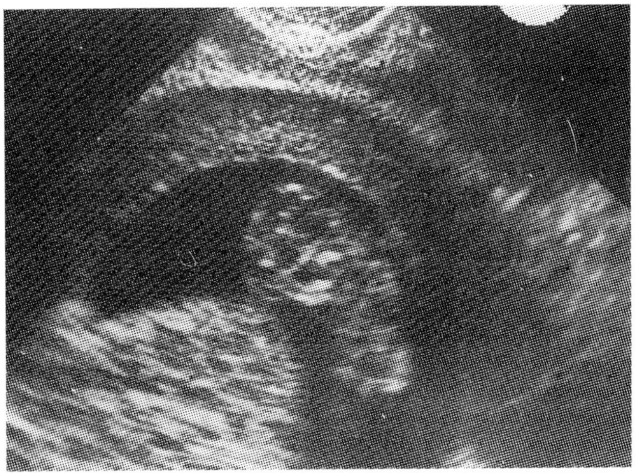

Fig. 3.6. A 9½ week intrauterine pregnancy. There is early differentiation of intracranial anatomy.

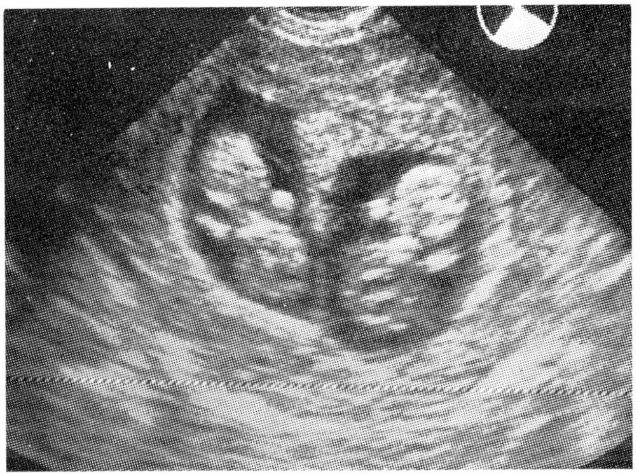

Fig. 3.7. Normal 9 week twin pregnancy. Both embryos and sacs are of equal size. Limb buds seen.

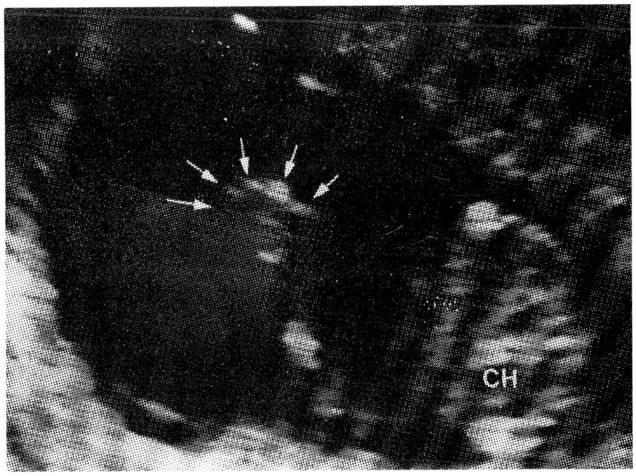

Fig. 3.8. Fetus of 10 weeks 2 days. Arm, forearm and hand are imaged (arrows), the fingers can be counted. CH = cross-section of the chest.

The movements of the limbs increase in the eleventh week and there are frequent *jumps* involving sudden, violent movements particularly of the trunk and lower limbs, the fetus propelling itself through the amniotic fluid and then subsequently sinking down again. The yolk-sac gradually disappears and the physiological umbilical hernia starts to reduce and finally disappears by 12 weeks.

After 10 weeks gestational age, the uterus enlarges out of the true pelvis and the transvaginal probe may not be able to identify structures beyond 8 cm of the transducer. The combination of abdominal and transvaginal scanning at this stage, using the same 5 MHz transducer by both routes, can help to image all the structures very satisfactorily, during the first trimester. A simple scheme of anatomic landmarks and their correlation with gestational age is shown in Table 3.1.

Table 3.1. Chronological assessment of structures in early pregnancy

Ultrasound findings	*Gestational age*
Gestation sac	4 weeks
Yolk sac	5 weeks
Cardiac pulsation	6 weeks
Embryonic movements	7 weeks
Head and limb buds	8 weeks
Yolk sac and head equal in size	8 weeks
Falx cerebri	9 weeks

The demonstration that the above sequence of developmental events is taking place at a normal rate, is a more reliable prognostic indicator of viability of the pregnancy, rather than a single ultrasound finding on one occasion.

Embryonic viability

The most reliable sign of viability is the demonstration of an embryonic heartbeat, which can be detected in most patients by 5½-6 weeks by transvaginal ultrasound. The demonstration of an embryonic heartbeat not only confirms a live intrauterine pregnancy but, irrespective of other ancillary signs, is of prognostic significance, with a low likelihood of spontaneous abortion (2% to 4%) after confirmation of a viable embryo. But if cardiac activity is not detected, then the following factors are taken into consideration.

Gestation sac size and growth

Charts correlating gestation sac size with gestational age are well established. A gestational sac too small for the menstrual age implies pregnancy failure. However, this interpretation is only possible if the approximate date of conception is known. Hence, it is very specific and sensitive in cases where ovulation is being monitored or following assisted reproductive technology. Robinson suggests that a gestation sac whose volume is greater than 2.5 ml and which does not contain a visible embryo is not viable[7]. This gestation sac volume/embryo relationship has been variously reported between 2.5 and 5 ml[8].

The assessment of gestation sac growth in normal pregnancies reveals a mean diameter growth rate of 1.2 mm per day. This compares with 0.25 mm per day in cases of blighted ovum. A sac that fails to double in volume each week between weeks five and eight is suggestive of gestational failure[9]. However, assessment of gestation sac growth is of limited diagnostic value, because in cases of embryonic demise (missed abortion) a gestation sac may continue to grow at a normal rate. Hence it is important to correlate the growth of the gestation sac and crown-rump length.

Gestation sac morphology

Various signs have been described as indicating a good progress for pregnancy outcome. Of these the intradecidual sign and the double decidual sac (DDS) sign or chorionic decidual reaction are best known. The absence of these signs indicates a poor prognosis for pregnancy outcome. However, these characteristics of early gestation sacs are not seen in all normal pregnancies, the DDS being observed in 75% of pregnancies. Moreover, these signs may also be present in pregnancies which subsequently fail.

The normal sac has a uniform round or oval shape. In missed abortion it is often distorted, angulated and irregular (Fig. 3.9). The presence of a normal-looking shape of the gestation sac is useful as a supportive diagnostic criterion of embryo viability. Occasionally, the sac even though normal, may appear flattened due to Braxton Hicks contractions, associate uterine fibroids, or uterine anomalies such as bicornuate uterus.

Hormone pregnancy tests and β-hCG

An intrauterine gestation sac is visible by vaginal ultrasound with serum levels of 700-800 mIU/ml or more[10]. Although this may be useful in the demonstration or diagnosis of ectopic pregnancy, its volume in the prognostication of embryo viability has not been confirmed. Low levels of β-hCG in the presence of a normal-appearing gestation sac could suggest an

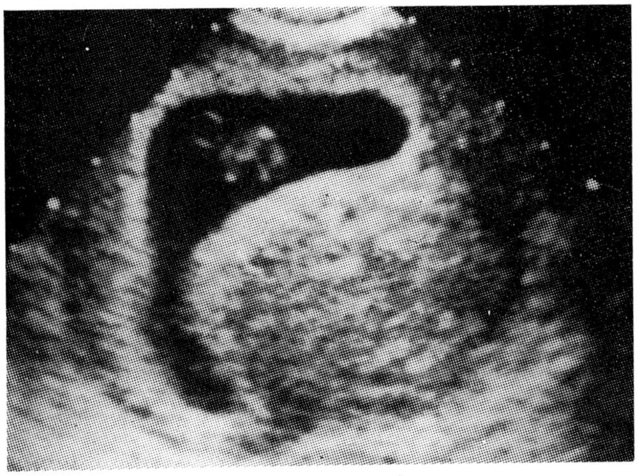

Fig. 3.9. An abnormally enlarged gestational sac. Note the embryo that is rather curled up in position and the sac measures more than six times the size of the embryo. Trisomy 18 was detected on chrosome examination of the embryo.

abnormal intrauterine gestation or a failing corpus luteum.

In an unpublished study by the author, serial measurements of CRL and β-hCG were carried out at weekly intervals in 30 consecutive conceptions, resulting from infertility treatment. The day of exogenous hCG and follicular rupture on sonography was known in each case. The earliest detection of an intrauterine gestational sac was on the 20th post-hCG day when the β-hCG level was 760 mIU/ml. All gestational sacs could be identified by the 24th post-hCG day when the mean β-hCG level was 2,685 ± 272 mIU/ml. The fetal pole could be first identified on the 24th post-hCG day (β-hCG level 2,518 mIU/ml). And it was detectable in all pregnancies by the 33rd post-hCG day (mean β-hCG level 23,810 ± 8,075 mIU/ml). The fetal cardiac activity was first detected on the 28th post-hCG day when the mean β-hCG level was 9,208 ± 5,145 mIU/ml and was recorded in all normal pregnancies by post-hCG day 35 (mean β-hCG level 26,987 ± 12,921 mIU/ml).

3 of the 30 pregnancies did not complete the first trimester. There was no cardiac activity noted at any time in them and β-hCG levels remained lower than normal.

Low implantation

The site of implantation of the gestation sac in the uterus is of doubtful importance in determining foetal outcome. A low implantation has been reported to have a poor prognosis[11], while others indicate it may only be a minor risk factor for placenta praevia rather than a predictor of early foetal loss.

Pregnancy failure

The incidence of spontaneous abortions varies between 20% and 30% in spontaneous or assisted conception pregnancies[12]. The rate seems to be higher in pregnancies achieved after ovulation induction or assisted reproductive technology, due to the earlier diagnosis of pregnancy made in all patients under treatment. On the other hand, in spontaneous conceptions such early pregnancy losses are misdiagnosed as delayed periods.

Transvaginal ultrasound has its greatest impact in the diagnosis of threatened abortion and missed abortion.

Threatened abortion

Due to the earlier detection of cardiac activity, transvaginal ultrasound has an edge over abdominal imaging. Besides, the presence of small retroplacental bleeds are also detected much earlier due to better imaging of the implantation site (Fig. 3.10).

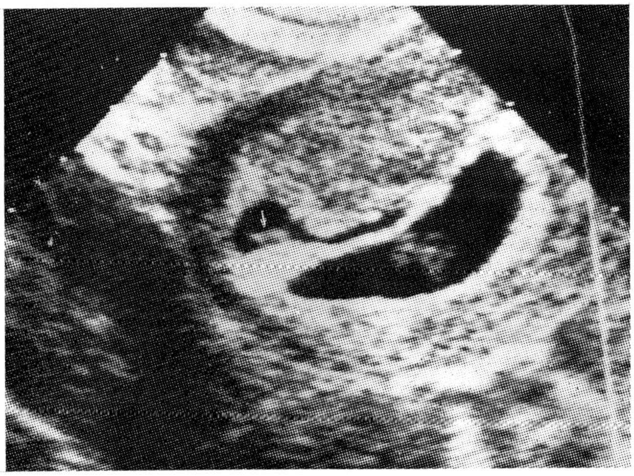

Fig. 3.10. Retroplacental bleed.

Retroplacental bleeds can be demonstrated in patients undergoing early pregnancy monitoring after ART treatment. These bleeds may be associated with low levels and low rates of rise in β-hCG levels. The retroplacental bleed or subchorionic hemorrhage corresponds with partial placental detachment in later pregnancy. The outcome of pregnancy is not related to the size of the bleed. About 50% of such pregnancies result in missed abortions or blighted ova.

Another prediction of poor outcome that is seen with transvaginal, but not with abdominal ultrasound, is the presence of large vascular spaces surrounding the whole gestation sac, with absence of embryo and retroplacental bleed. It may be a late consequence of retro-implantation bleeding.

The use of transvaginal colour Doppler in the prognosis of early pregnancy has been documented by studying the flow in the corpus luteum. A viable corpus luteum has a low resistance bed with relatively high diastolic flow, whereas diastolic flow is reduced or absent with failure of corpus luteum.

Inevitable abortion

Once a clinical diagnosis is made, it could be confirmed by ultrasound.

Features seen on ultrasound are :

(i) Gestation sac separate from the endometrium.
(ii) Embryo and intraluminal blood present low in the uterus with a dilated cervical canal.
(iii) Fetal cardiac activity may or may not be present.

Missed abortion and blighted ovum

Blighted ovum is a gestation sac without an embryo. Approximately half of all gestation sacs do not contain an embryo, or the embryo may be too small to resolve. An empty gestation sac may also be seen in very early pregnancy, but in order to differentiate between a blighted ovum and early pregnancy, one should take the other ancillary factors such as gestation sac morphology, etc., into consideration. Though gestation sac size does seem to have some prognostic value in the diagnosis of abnormal early gestation, it is particularly important in multiple pregnancies[13]. A small sac (mean diameter 50% of the co-existing sacs) is more likely to undergo spontaneous resorption. This condition described as the *vanishing twin* occurs in approximately 10% of twin pregnancies and 25% of triplet or quadruplet pregnancies, improving pregnancy outcome in the final analysis. There exists a possibility that overdiagnosis of vanishing twin is made due to a misdiagnosis. A distorted second gestation sac can resemble subchorionic hemorrhage, implantation bleeds, or a pseudo second sac. The vanishing twin does not seem to affect the outcome of the surviving twin, which usually proceeds to term.

Incomplete abortion

The appearances on ultrasound of an incomplete abortion are relatively non-specific. Blood, clots and products of conception in the uterine cavity are responsible for the variable appearances seen which range from echo-free to highly reflective on sonography. Hence diagnosis based only on ultrasound is difficult and one has to combine the clinical setting with the ultrasound picture.

In summary, the principal uses of transvaginal ultrasound in the abnormal first trimester are in providing a rapid assessment of fetal heart activity, accurate localisation of the implantation site, the detection of implantation defects and prognostic indicators such as intramural blood flow, which can avoid prenatal tests being blamed for spontaneous abortion. The superior imaging of blood clot and debris in and around the gestation sac improves the confidence in making a diagnosis of embryonic death. The limited use of Doppler should be stressed.

Congenital anomalies

The potential for ultrasound diagnosis of abnormalities earlier than the second trimester is extremely attractive. Organogenesis is completed by 12 weeks of gestation. Theoretically, therefore, some of the structural abnormalities which we now diagnose at 18 weeks scan might be demonstrable earlier.

Quashie *et al.*[14] observed that it is possible to demonstrate most of the major fetal structures by 13 weeks gestation and detection of fetal anomalies can be accomplished much earlier than with the trans-abdominal screening alone.

Skull ossification begins before 12 weeks and therefore the diagnosis of anencephaly is possible at this stage, though the diagnosis has been missed on an ultrasound scan performed at 10 weeks. The remainder of neural tube abnormalities have not yet been reliably diagnosed on ultrasound in the first trimester. Visualisation of the cerebellum in the first trimester might allow the earlier detection of the Chiari II malformation associated with spina bifida. However, as yet the chronology of migration of the foetal cerebellum in this condition is not known.

Abdominal abnormalities have been reported with use of TVS in the first trimester. The demonstration of omphalocele has been made in a 12 week gestation, with a soft tissue mass noted anterior to the abdomen. The association of this with an abdominal diameter significantly smaller than the biparietal diameter, allowed the diagnosis to be made[14]. Such a diagnosis should be made with caution, because of the normal extra-abdominal position of the embryonic gut which may remain outside the anterior abdominal wall till as late as 12 weeks gestation in 20% of cases[15].

The appearance of embryonic kidneys as early as 9 weeks of gestation offers the potential for diagnosis of severe abnormalities of the renal tract by the demonstration of abnormally dilated collecting systems, or distended bladders[16].

As the limbs can be measured by the end of the 12th

week, dwarfism, if detected at this stage, could prevent the emotional trauma if diagnosis is made during the latter part of pregnancy. However, many forms of short-limbed dwarfism are associated with normal limb bone lengths in the first trimester, the reduced growth of the limbs being manifest later.

Cystic hygromas can be detected in the first trimester. If present, they are an indication for chromosome testing even when transient, since most of these are associated with trisomy 21 or 18[17].

Other structural abnormalities seem unlikely to be diagnosed in the first trimester, at least for the present. The lateral ventricles, for example occupy most of the intracranial hemidiameter making the early diagnosis of hydrocephalus difficult, though not, impossible. Choroid plexus cysts have been demonstrated at 12 weeks, and although none have been shown to be associated with chromosomal abnormalities, this remains a potential source of information.

Evaluation of the heart in the first trimester, except for the demonstration of variation in heart rate, awaits documentation of embryological development. So also is the case with other structural abnormalities. Though detection of other deformities and anomalies has been reported[16] these are difficult situations where it is impossible to confirm the diagnosis after pregnancy termination by curettage in the first trimester. This raises difficult ethical issues with the risk of normal pregnancies being terminated because of misdiagnosis.

There is no doubt that the introduction of transvaginal probes operating at high frequencies can yield clear images for diagnostic use in the first and early second trimester fetus. At present there are too few studies large enough to prove the statistical significance of a first trimester malformation workup by transvaginal sonography.

Acknowledgment

The author would like to thank Dr. Anita Santamaria for her help during the preparation of this chapter.

REFERENCES

1. Kratochwil A, Eisenhut L. Der frutieste nachweis der fetalen herzaktion during ultraschall. Geburtshilfe Frauen Heilkd 1967; 27 : 176-8.
2. Schillinger H. Detection of heart action and active movements of the human embryo by ultrasonic time motion techniques. Eur J Obstet Gynecol Reprod 1976; 6 : 333-9.
3. Schenker L, Astle C, Reed K. Embryonic heart rate before the seventh week of pregnancy. J Reprod Med 1986; 31 : 333-5.
4. DuBose TJ, Cunyus JA, Johnson LF. Embryonic heart rate and age. J Diagn Med Sonography 1990; 6 : 151-7.
5. Rotsztejn D, Ran N, Dmowski W. Correlation between fetal heart rate, crown-rump length and beta chorionic gonadotropin levels during the first trimester of well-timed conceptions resulting from infertility treatment. Fertil Steril 1993; 59 : 1169-73.
6. Rempen A. Diagnosis of viability in early pregnancy with vaginosonography. J Ultrasound Med 1990; 9 : 711-3.
7. Robinson HP. Gestation sac volumes as determined by sonar in the first trimester of pregnancy. Hum Reprod 1975; 2 : 739-40.
8. Nyberg DA, Leing FC, Filly RA. Threatened abortion : Sonographic distinction of normal and abnormal gestation sacs. Radiology 1986; 158 : 397-8.
9. Nyberg DA, Mack LA, Leing FC. Distinguishing normal from abnormal gestation sac growth in early pregnancy. J Ultrasound Med 1987; 6 : 23-5.
10. Dickey RP, Gasser RF. Ultrasound evidence for variability in the size and development of normal human embryos before the tenth post-insemination week after assisted reproductive technologies. Human Reprod 1993; 8 : 331-7.
11. Mantoni M. Ultrasound studies of patients with bleeding in early pregnancy. Dan Med Bulletin 1987; 34 : 250-5.
12. Hertz JB. Diagnostic procedure in threatened abortion. Obstet Gynecol 1984; 66 : 223-6.
13. Schatts R, Brandsma G, Cleveringa LM. Evidence of asynchronous implantation in IVF multiple pregnancies. Hum Reprod 1988; 3 : 7-9.
14. Quashie C, Weiner S, Bolobnese R. Efficacy of first trimester transvaginal sonography in detecting normal fetal development. Am J Perinat 1992; 9 : 209-13.
15. Curtis JA, Watson L. Sonographic diagnosis of omphalocele in the first trimester of fetal gestation. J Ultrasound Med 1988; 7 : 97-9.
16. Butic M, Podobnik M, Korenic B. First trimester diagnosis of low obstruction uropathy : An indicator of initial renal function in the fetus. JCU 1987; 15 : 537-8.
17. Rottem S, Bronstein M. Transvaginal sonographic diagnosis of congenital anomalies between 9 weeks and 16 weeks menstrual age. JCU 1990, 18 : 307-8.

CHAPTER

4

Ectopic Pregnancy and Transvaginal Sonography

Narendra Malhotra and Jaideep Malhotra

Introduction

The incidence of ectopic pregnancy has markedly increased in the last two decades and even in the USA, 6-11% of all maternal deaths are due to ectopic pregnancy (leading cause of death in the first trimester of pregnancy). The increasing incidence of ectopic pregnancy has been attributed to an increase in pelvic inflammatory disease, use of I.U.C.D.'s, fallopian tube surgery and also our improved ability to diagnose an ectopic pregnancy.

Because of the variability of symptoms and morphologic presentations, ectopic pregnancy is still difficult to diagnose at times. In our country usually the presentation is of classical ruptured ectopic (60%); another 25% cases present with chronic ectopic and only 15% cases present to us before rupture. It is these 15% cases in which diagnosis is of paramount importance because here conservative surgical management and non-surgical management may have a role.

Transabdominal sonography (TAS) has proved disappointing in the diagnosis of ectopic pregnancy. Transvaginal sonography (TVS) cannot eliminate all problems but offers great advantage in positively diagnosing extrauterine gestation. The place of ultrasound in the overall approach to the patient with suspected ectopic pregnancy (EP) has undergone significant evolution since diagnosis of ectopic pregnancy was first described sonographically about 25 years ago. Initially, ultrasound was used to directly visualise ectopic masses[1]. Later, recognition of the non-specificity of sonographic adnexal findings prompted the use of ultrasound to primarily exclude patients with intrauterine pregnancy[2-4]. Today with transvaginal ultrasound we can not only identify the ectopic mass but also characterize it for therapeutic planning[5-6].

Materials and methods

We have been using transabdominal sonography (TAS) for the last 9 years for obstetrics and gynaecology and using transvaginal scanning (TVS) for the past 4 years.

In the last 9 years we have scanned over 8000 cases and have picked up 5 cases of unruptured ectopic pregnancies (4 by TVS and 1 by TAS) and 20 cases of ruptured ectopic pregnancies and 5 cases of chronic ectopic pregnancies as adnexal masses. We have missed the diagnosis of ectopic pregnancy in two cases by TAS in the early period of our scanning (1985-86). The ultrasound machines being used at our hospital are the Pie Medical Scanner 1120 and the Network Nebula 202.

Sonographic findings of ectopic pregnancy by transvaginal sonography[7] (Figs. 4.1, 4.2 and 4.3)

A. Intrauterine findings
   1. Empty uterus or thickened endometrium.
   2. Central hypoechoic area.
   3. A sac-like structure (pseudogestational sac).
   4. Very rarely a concurrent intrauterine pregnancy (Figs. 4.4 and 4.5).

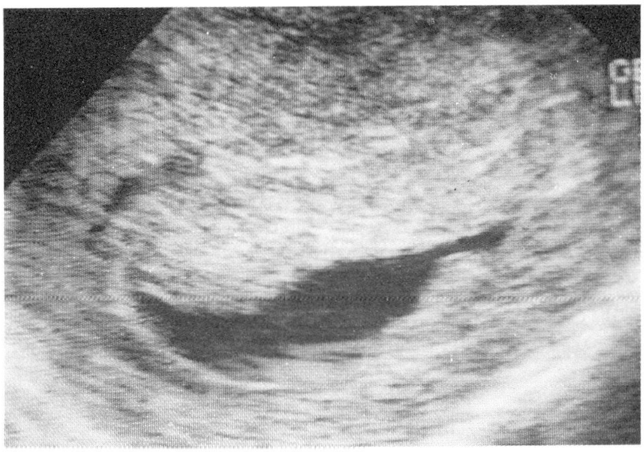

Fig. 4.1. Pseudogestational sac of an ectopic pregnancy.

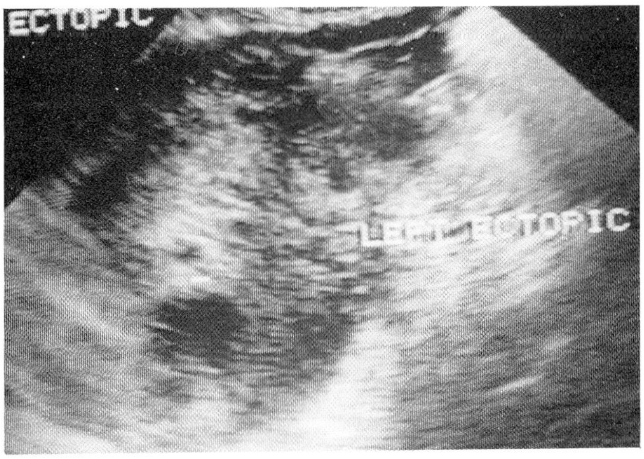

Fig. 4.2. A left sided ectopic pregnancy before local methotrexate injection.

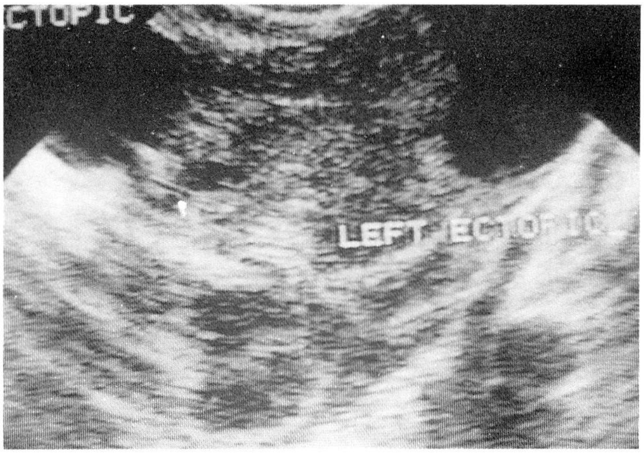

Fig. 4.3. Same patient as in Fig. 4.2. Plate taken 10 days post-injection.

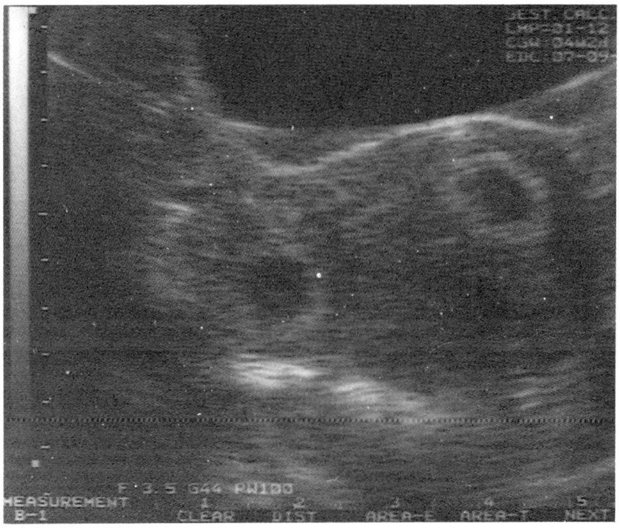

Fig. 4.4. An abdominal sonogram showing an heterotopic pregnancy.

Axioms

a. Best evidence against an ectopic is the presence of intrauterine pregnancy.

b. Absence of a detectable intrauterine pregnancy in pregnant women without symptoms significantly increases the likelihood of an ectopic.

c. Consider ectopic whenever intrauterine contents do not resemble a normal intrauterine pregnancy.

B. Extrauterine findings
   1. Adnexal masses.
   2. Living extrauterine embryo in an unruptured sac.
   3. Extra uterine gestational sac.
   4. Cul-de-sac findings.

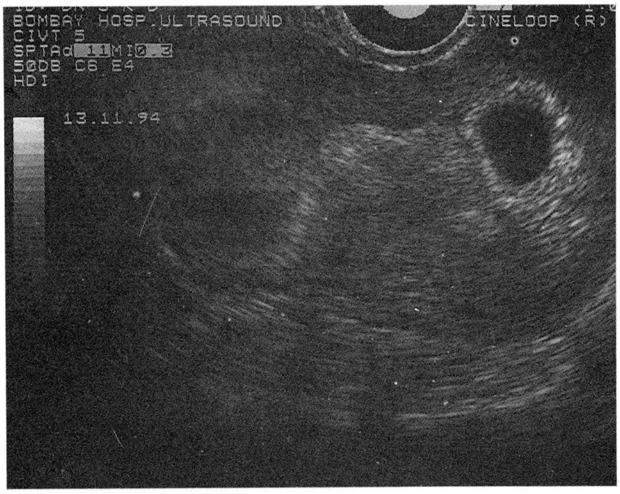

Fig. 4.5. Vaginal sonogram of the same case as in Fig. 4.4. An intrauterine gestational sac seen concurrently visualised with a cornual pregnancy.

C. Other ectopic pregnancies
   1. Heterotopic pregnancy (coexisting intra- and extra-uterine) (Figs. 4.4 and 4.5).
   2. Interstitial pregnancy.
   3. Rudimentary horn pregnancy.
   4. Ovarian pregnancy.
   5. Cervical pregnancy.
   6. Abdominal (peritoneal pregnancy).

Overview of sonographic signs[8]

The sonographic workup of possible ectopic pregnancy includes both negative and positive signs.

1. Negative signs
   a. Intrauterine pregnancy.
      1. Living intrauterine embryo.
      2. Gestational sac with yolk sac.
      3. Double decidual sac signs.
2. False negative signs
   a. Intrauterine pseudogestational sac.
3. Indirect positive signs
   a. Empty uterus sign.
   b. Free pelvic and abdominal fluid.
4. Direct positive signs
   a. Adnexal pregnancy.
      1. Living embryo.
      2. Tubal or adnexal ring.
      3. Complex or solid mass.
   b. Abdominal pregnancy.

Negative sonographic signs

Intrauterine pregnancy

When considering an ectopic pregnancy, the first branch in the sonographic decision tree is whether or not there is evidence of an intrauterine pregnancy essentially ruling out the possibility of an ectopic pregnancy. This was originally based on a calculated incidence for heterotopic pregnancy of 1 in 30,000 pregnancies[9]. However, based on the currently increased incidence of ectopic pregnancy in general, heterotopic pregnancy is now estimated to occur as frequently as 1 : 10,000 pregnancies[10].

One strategy to deal with this problem is not to confirm intrauterine pregnancy until a embryo with cardiac activity is demonstrated, although this can delay diagnosis for 1 to 2 weeks. Actually, embryonic development can be recognized even earlier, before demonstration of the embryo itself, through demonstration of a yolk sac. The yolk sac is consistently demonstrable in normal intrauterine pregnancy by transabdominal sonography in a gestational sac of 2 cm in diameter[11] and by transvaginal sonography in a gestational sac of 0.6-0.8 cm[12].

False negative sonographic signs

Pseudogestational sacs (Fig. 4.1)

Pseudogestational sacs[13] are intrauterine fluid sacs surrounded by decidual reaction that simulate the sonographic appearance of true gestational sacs and are found in 8-29% of patients with ectopic pregnancies[14]. Identification of the double decidual sac sign or of embryonic development often is helpful in differentiating pseudogestational sacs from normal intrauterine gestational sacs, but may prove problematic in distinguishing pseudo-gestational sacs from the sacs of failed or failing intrauterine pregnancy. Colour Doppler sonography has provided us with new diagnostic information to differentiate pseudogestational sacs from gestational sacs of intrauterine pregnancy, both normal and failing[15].

Indirect positive signs

Empty uterus sign and the discriminatory zone

Demonstration of an empty uterus in a patient known to be pregnant, is one of the oldest signs of ectopic pregnancy. After introduction of the highly sensitive radioimmunoassay hCG test, hormonal pregnancy testing became positive two weeks prior to sonographic demonstration of the intrauterine gestational sac. Application of the empty uterus sign in conjunction with a positive radioimmunoassay pregnancy test therefore risked misdiagnosing normal intrauterine pregnancy as ectopic pregnancy in the two weeks prior to visualization of the normal sac.

Nonvisualisation of an intrauterine sac, together with a serum hCG above the discriminatory zone, indicated an abnormal pregnancy, either a spontaneous abortion or an ectopic pregnancy. As sonographic resolution has improved the discriminatory zone has continued to fall, now at 1,000 mIU/ml (IRP) with transvaginal sonography[12].

Free pelvic and abdominal fluid

Pelvic fluid may fulfill two functions in sonographic diagnosis : as a primary, though indirect, sonographic sign of ectopic pregnancy, and as a supporting sign, increasing the specificity of the other adnexal findings. Pelvic fluid functions as a relatively specific sign of ectopic pregnancy only when it is found in large volume or when it is echogenic. As a primary sign, echogenic fluid (representing hemoperitoneum indicates ectopic pregnancy with a specificity of 25 to 59 percent[9].

Direct positive signs

Adnexal pregnancy

Live extrauterine embryo. Demonstration of a live adnexal embryo is the most specific sonographic sign, though not a particularly sensitive sign of ectopic pregnancy. The sensitivity of this sign, however, has increased over the years, probably due to earlier presentation and diagnosis and due to the superior resolution of transvaginal sonography.

Tubal or adnexal ring. A live adnexal embryo is always found within a gestational sac. The sac, termed as adnexal or tubal ring because of its location, has a characteristic appearance with no live embryo within. As in the case of the intrauterine gestational sac, the tubal ring consists of an anechoic central fluid sac and an echogenic thick rim. Tubal rings without live embryos (with or without yolk sacs) are seen in 28-44% of ectopic pregnancies via transvaginal scanning[5]. The potential exists, however, for similar sonographic appearances to cause tubal rings and corpus luteum cysts to be confused with one another.

Complex or solid masses. Complex or solid adnexal masses are found with transvaginal sonography in 22-45% of cases of ectopic pregnancies[5,15]. It is imperative to pay close attention to the ovaries during the evaluation of all adnexal masses for possible ectopic pregnancy. Failure to demonstrate a distinct ipsilateral ovary in addition to the visualized mass may indicate that the mass is ovarian in origin.

Abdominal pregnancy

Sonographic diagnosis of abdominal pregnancy presents a challenge. The diagnosis may be missed 25% of the time or more, and often is delayed until late in pregnancy.

Colour and pulsed Doppler sonography for ectopic pregnancy (Figs. 4.6, 4.7 and 4.8 – all on Plate 1)

Colour and pulsed Doppler ultrasound adds physiologic information to the sonographic workup of possible ectopic pregnancy thereby increasing the sonographic diagnostic sensitivity for ectopic pregnancy, normal early intrauterine pregnancy, and failed early intrauterine pregnancy. Diagnostic sensitivity increased from 71 to 87% for ectopic pregnancy, from 24 to 59% for failed intrauterine pregnancy, from 90 to 99% for normal intrauterine pregnancy, and from 62 to 82% for all diagnoses when transvaginal sonography was augmented with colour Doppler sonography in our series. The combined use of colour and pulsed Doppler and two-dimensional imaging solves the following sonographic problems in the ectopic pregnancy workup.

1. Differentiation of pseudogestational and gestational sac.
2. Differentiation of the empty uterus sign into either intrauterine pregnancy (normal and abnormal) or no intrauterine pregnancy (with a greatly increased chance of ectopic pregnancy).
3. Identification of the site of the corpus luteum.
4. Assistance in detection and confirmation of the nature of adnexal ectopic pregnancies.

Conclusion

Transvaginal sonography dramatically improved our ability to detect and manage abnormal pregnancy and ectopic gestations.

REFERENCES

1. Kobayashi M, Hellman LM, Fillisti LP. Ultrasound : An aid in the diagnosis of ectopic pregnancy. Am J Obstet Gynecol 1969; 103 : 1131-40.
2. Lawson TL. Ectopic pregnancy criteria and accuracy of ultrasound diagnosis. AJR 1978; 131 : 153-6.

3. Pelosi MA. The value of pelvic ultrasound in the diagnosis of ectopic pregnancy. Diag Gynecol Obstet 1981; 3 : 337-46.
4. Bradley WG, Fiske CE, Filly RA. The double sac sign of early intrauterine pregnancy : Use in exclusion of ectopic pregnancy. Radiology 1982; 143 : 223-6.
5. Cacciatore B. Can the status of tubal pregnancy be predicted with transvaginal sonography? A prospective comparison of sonographic, surgical and serum hCG findings. Radiology 1990; 177 : 481-4.
6. Stovall TG, Ling FW, Buster JE. Outpatient chemotherapy of unruptured ectopic pregnancy. Fertil Steril 1989; 51 : 435-8.
7. Timor-Tritsch IE, Yeh MN, Peisner DB. The use of transvaginal ultrasonography in the diagnosis of ectopic pregnancy. Am J Obstet Gynecol 1989; 161 : 157-61.
8. Dasnefsky S, Lyons E, Levi C. Suspected ectopic pregnancy : Endovaginal and transvesical ultrasonography. Radiology 1988; 169 : 181-6.
9. DeVoe RW, Pratt JH. Simultaneous intrauterine and extrauterine pregnancy. Am J Obstet Gynecol 1948; 56 : 1119-26.
10. Bright DA, Gaupp FB. Heterotopic pregnancy : A re-evaluation. J Am Board Fam Pract 1990; 164 : 161-4.
11. Nyberg DA, Mack LA, Laing FC. Distinguishing normal from abnormal gestational sac growth in early pregnancy. J Ultrasound Med 1987; 7 : 23-7.
12. Bree RL, Edwards M, Bohm VM. Transvaginal sonography in the evaluation of normal early pregnancy : Correlation with hCG level. AJR 1989; 153 : 75-9.
13. Mueller CE. Intrauterine pseudogestational sac in ectopic pregnancy. J Clin Ultrasound 1979; 7 : 133-6.
14. Marks WM, Filly RA, Callen PW. The decidual cast of ectopic pregnancy : A confusing ultrasonographic appearance. Radiology 1979; 133 : 451-4.
15. Emerson DS, Cartier MS, Altieri LA, Felker RE, Smith WC, Stovall TG, Gray LA. Diagnostic efficacy of endovaginal color flow Doppler in an ectopic pregnancy screening program. Radiology 1991; 183 : 413-20.

CHAPTER

5

Role of Transvaginal Sonography in Gynaecologic Infertility

Ambrish Dalal

Sonography has a vital role to play in diagnosis and management of infertility related to gynaecological disorders. Its major applications are :

1. Follicular monitoring (cycle evaluation).
2. Follicular aspiration (oocyte retrieval).
3. Embryo transfer.

The main causes of gynaecological infertility are occlusive tubal disease, endometriosis, ovulation disorders, luteal phase abnormalities, cervical factors, pelvic varicosities and unexplained infertility[1-3]. Structural abnormalities of the uterus like myomas, septate uterus, undeveloped or hypoplastic uterus, etc., may also contribute towards causing infertility. Sonography has decisively helped in diagnosing most of these factors and therefore becomes an integral part of the workup and management of gynaecologic infertility.

In addition to this, sonographic guidance has also been sought in oocyte retrieval, embryo transfers in difficult cases and in transcervical cannulation of fallopian tubes for SIFT, GIFT and ZIFT procedures.

With the advent of high resolution transvaginal transducers and colour Doppler evaluation of cyclical changes in the endometrium and evaluation of corpus luteal blood flow have helped in diagnosis of luteal phase inadequacy[4].

Instrumentation

Conventional real time sector scanners have been used for abdominal sonography using 3.5 MHz or 5.0 MHz transducers. However in recent years transvaginal transducers have outdated the use of abdominal scanning, especially in gynaecological disorders. Endovaginal transducers allow a more detailed depiction of the uterus and ovaries for several reasons. As these structures are closer to the transducers during transvaginal examination, it is possible to use a higher frequency beam (between 5.0 and 7.5 MHz) which gives far superior resolution. Secondly, as the beam does not have to traverse through the abdominal wall, there is less beam scattering. Thirdly transvaginal examination avoids the interference from interposed bowel loops as in case of abdominal scanning. Last but not the least, full bladder is not required for transvaginal scanning relieving the patient's inconvenience.

Thus the superior resolution offered by transvaginal transducers allows us to visualise the morphological changes occurring in the maturing follicles and endometrium which was not possible with abdominal scanning[5].

Follicular monitoring

Serial sonographic monitoring of a cycle helps depict the changes in the maturity of a Graafian follicle (Figs. 5.1 to 5.5). Although the maturity of the oocyte can only be indirectly inferred by the size of the follicle and associated endometrial development, associated knowledge of estradiol values provide a fairly accurate assessment of the presence or absence and number of

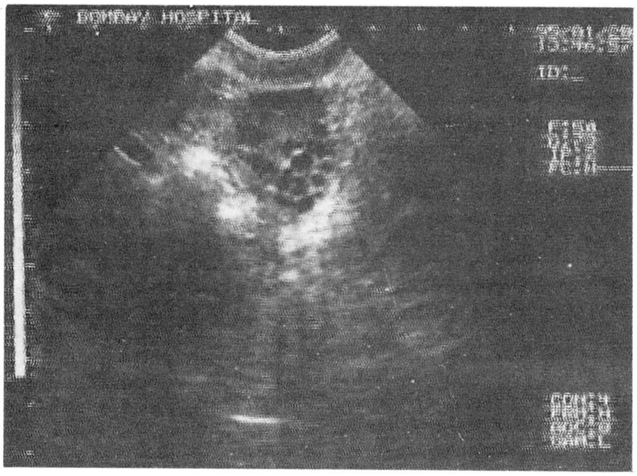

Fig. 5.1. A polycystic ovary with multiple small follicles on day 8.

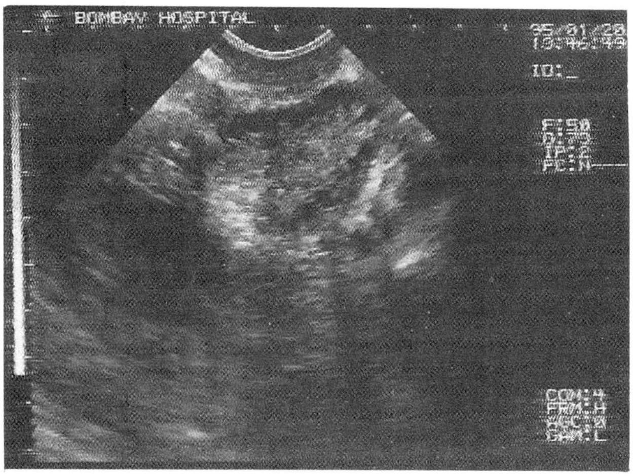

Fig. 5.2. A polycystic ovary with peripherally distributed small follicles.

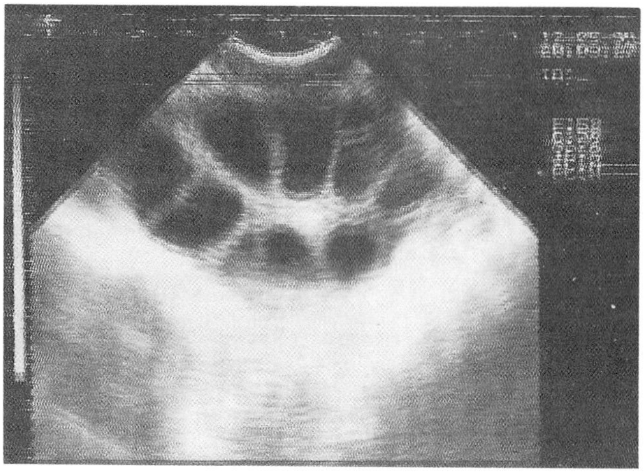

Fig. 5.3. Ovary on day 11 of a gonadotropin stimulated cycle.

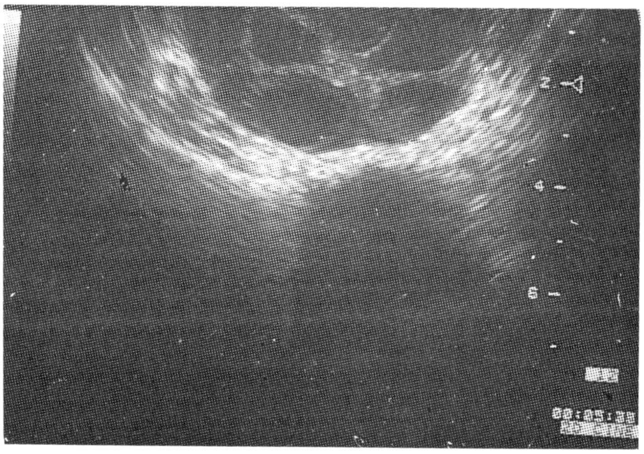

Fig. 5.4. Multiple follicles.

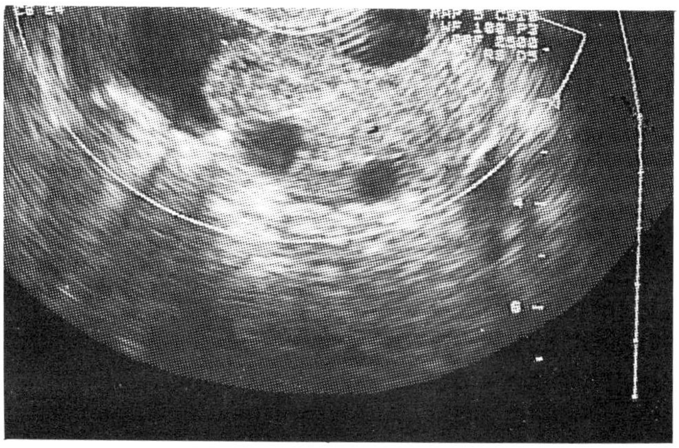

Fig. 5.5. Follicular rupture with fluid in the cul-de-sac.

mature oocytes. Anatomic information gained by serial sonography allows us to depict the side of ovulation, time of ovulation, number of growing follicles in stimulated cycles and the rate of growth of follicles[6]. This helps us in better management of induced cycles. Luteinized unruptured follicle (L.U.F.) syndrome can be a cause of unexplained infertility. In this disorder there is failure of rupture of follicle and the oocyte remains trapped within the follicle. This condition can be observed as a failure of a mature follicle to deflate on serial sonographic examinations[7-11].

Spontaneous cycle evaluation

It is not uncommon to observe more than one follicle to grow up to the size of about 10 mm in the early phase of the menstrual cycle beyond which one of these dominates and grows at the rate of 1.5 to 2 mm per day, while the others regress[12]. As the follicle matures more fluid is elaborated in its centre and number of granulosa cells lining the inner wall of the follicle increases. An oocyte which measures less than 0.1 mm cannot be visualised on sonography, but it gets surrounded by a cluster of granulosa cells which forms a complex termed cumulus oophorus which may be occasionally visible in the periovulatory phase[13-16]. Around this time of the cycle low level intra-follicular echoes may be visible. These are probably from the cluster of granulosa cells that shear off the wall and are floating in the follicular fluid in the preovulatory period[17]. As the follicle reaches maturity, its dimension reaches between 18 to 24 mm. Since this is a rather large range, it is not possible to predict an impending ovulation judging by the size alone. However it is observed that the preovulatory size is fairly constant in the same individual from cycle to cycle in spontaneous non-stimulated cycles[18]. After ovulation the follicular wall becomes irregular as the follicle collapses (deflates) and if sonographic examination is done within 4 to 6 hours of rupture a small amount of peritoneal fluid in the cul-de-sac may be visualised. It is not uncommon to see a very small amount of fluid (1-3 cc) around the ovary just prior to ovulation and this should not be mistaken for a sign of ovulation[19].

Induced cycles

Ovulation induction is indicated in patients whose infertility is attributed to ovulation abnormalities and in IVF/ET. These patients are examined and followed more closely and on a daily basis in order to carefully monitor follicular development and to adjust the dose of medication to achieve optimal stimulation. As hMG contains both FSH and LH, a spontaneous LH surge is less frequent with hMG stimulation and therefore hCG at a proper time is required to induce final maturation. Sonographic delineation of follicular size is crucial because hCG is best administered between the size of 17-19 mm[20].

Sonography has an important role to play in decreasing the likelihood of hyperstimulation. This can occur in various degrees of severity in cases of ovulation induction. Ovarian hyperstimulation is uncommon in women whose ovaries show several (up to 5-6) large follicles (over 15 mm) but tends to occur when there are more than 11 to 12 medium-sized or intermediate-sized follicles (Fig. 5.6). Associated assessment of E_2 levels is a must in these cases and

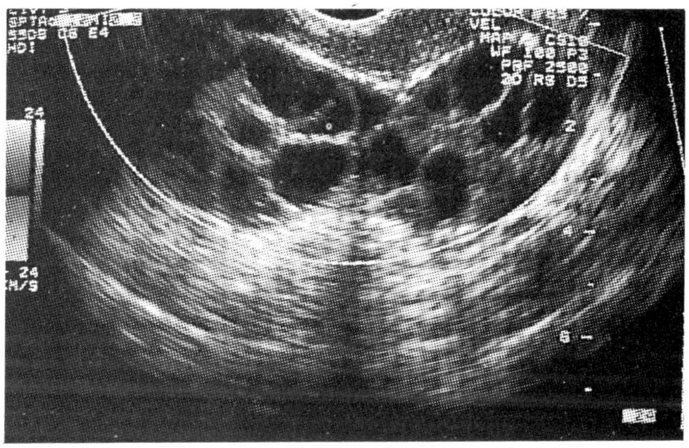

Fig. 5.6. Bilaterally hyperstimulated ovaries.

withdrawal of hCG in patients with more number of follicles per ovary may help avoid hyperstimulation[21,22]. Most of the severe cases of hyperstimulation have been described to have occurred between 4-7 days of hCG administration in patients with more than 11-12 intermediate-sized follicles. Some patients who have been stimulated and get pregnant also stand a risk of hyperstimulation, though such cases are rarely encountered. This is probably a reflection of the closer monitoring that these patients receive. Aspiration and drainage of these follicles may also account for diminished incidence of hyperstimulation in IVF cases[23].

Patients undergoing stimulation should be examined early before the commencement of stimulation to identify the presence of functional cysts. These cysts may represent previously unruptured follicles which have not totally regressed. It is postulated that a larger cyst may cause compression to the ovarian blood supply rendering the remaining ovarian tissue to be less responsive to hormonal therapy[24]. Some authors have recommended aspiration of cysts over the size of 2 cm prior to stimulation for IVF if one does not wish to skip that particular cycle[25-27] (Figs. 5.7 and 5.8).

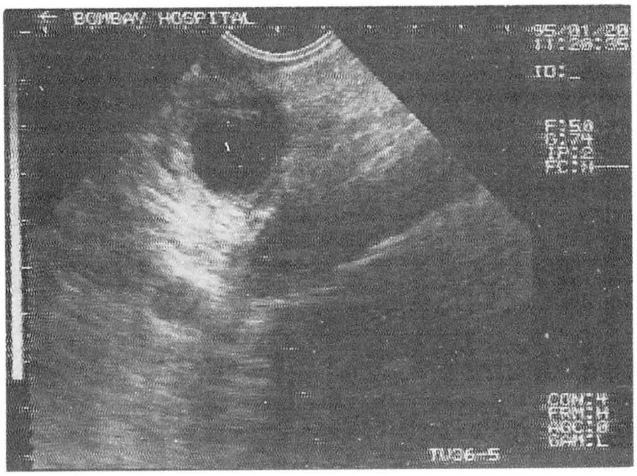

Fig. 5.7. A 3 cm residual cyst seen just prior to aspiration.

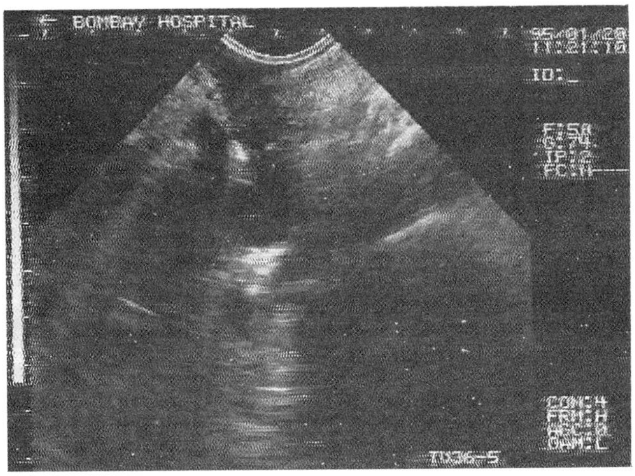

Fig. 5.8. A needle seen inside the partially aspirated cyst.

Sonography can be helpful in avoiding or decreasing the incidence of multiple gestation. However in my opinion it is difficult to predict multiple gestation in stimulated cycles. Clearly, when there are more than four mature follicles the chance of multiple gestation beyond twins does exist.

Ultrasound guided follicle aspiration

This has now become the preferred route of choice for oocyte retrieval and all other methods have only historic importance except in some selected cases. As far as GIFT or ZIFT is concerned some centers have started doing ultrasound-guided fallopian tube transfers to avoid laparoscopy completely. Major advantages of this technique are :

1. Avoids or decreases exposure to general anaesthesia.
2. Avoids exposure of oocytes to gas used for anaesthesia.
3. Feasibility to perform an outpatient procedure.
4. Less chances of operative complications.
5. Better acceptability.

Endometrial assessment (Figs. 5.9 to 5.12)

Assessment of endometrial changes occuring during the cycle has been possible and more accurately done after the invention of endovaginal transducers. A new term of endometrial dynamics has evolved since then as one can observe the change in endometrial thickness and morphology in menstrual, proliferative, late proliferative (periovulatory) and secretory phase. Some attempts at grading the texture of endometrium and correlating it in prediction of achieving pregnancy in that particular cycle have been made[28-34].

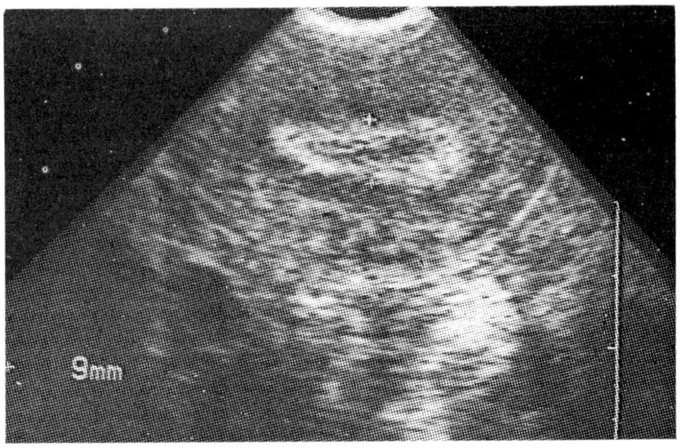

Fig. 5.9. Early postovulatory endometrium (induced cycle).

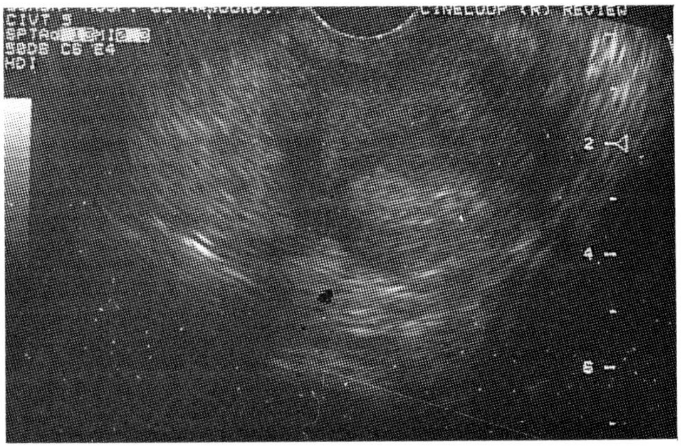

Fig. 5.10. Secretory phase endometrium (induced cycle).

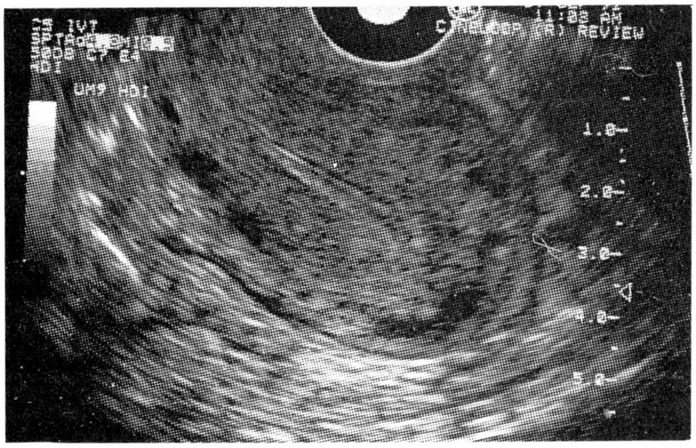

Fig. 5.11. Preovulatory endometrium (spontaneous cycle).

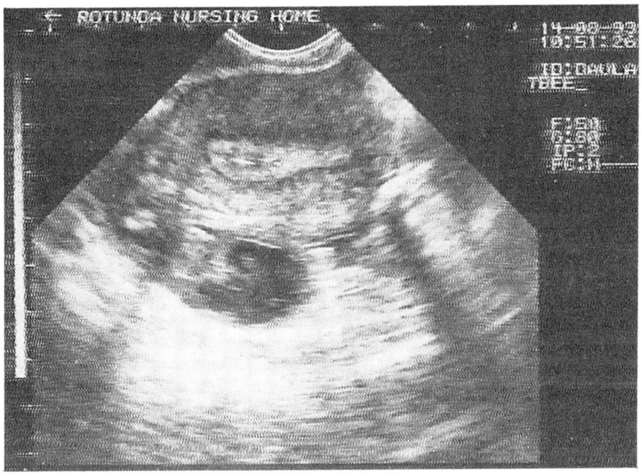

Fig. 5.12. Late secretory phase endometrium. Also seen is the corpus luteum in the right ovary.

In spontaneous and induced cycles, sonographic appearance of endometrium varies according to the phase of development[35]. In the menstrual phase it is thin and slit-like with broken echogenic interfaces and its thickness measures 1-5 mm. In the proliferative phase it thickens and becomes isoechoic or slightly hyperechoic measuring between 5-9 mm. In late proliferative or periovulatory phase it has a multilayer appearance. The inner hypoechoic area probably represents oedema in the compact layer of endometrium while the outer hyperechoic ring represents an area of increased vascularity near the outer myometrium[29,31]. Periovulatory endometrial thickness is generally around 12 ± 2 mm with thickness being about 2 mm more in properly induced cycles[36]. In the secretory phase it thickens further and achieves a width between 9-16 mm with increased echogenicity attributed to increased mucus and glycogen content in the glands as well as an increased number of interfaces created by tortuous glands[28,33]. Some workers have tried to measure total endometrial volume but the interpretation of the studies have not yet shown encouraging results[37]. Some workers have also tried to grade the endometrium according to its echogenicity and have felt that the most echogenic type of periovulatory endometrium stands a better chance of achieving pregnancy[32].

The inner third of the myometrium demonstrates a subtle contractile pattern best appreciated when a magnified midsagittal view of the endometrial canal is recorded on videotape and played back at five times the regular speed[38,39]. Subendometrial contractions propagate from the internal cervical os to the uterine fundus during the periovulatory period, but reverses direction during menses. The frequency of subendometrial contractions also peaks during the preovulatory phase. Some workers have speculated that the symmetric pattern of subendometrial contractions assists sperm transport, and the asymmetric waves serve to maintain the blastocyst within the uterine fundus[38,39].

Sonography may have a role in further evaluation of patients with luteal phase inadequacy. It is conceivable that these patients have an underdeveloped endometrium which could be characterised sonographically as thinner and less echogenic than expected.

Colour Doppler with spectral analysis (Figs. 5.13 and 5.14 – both on Plate 1, 5.15 to 5.20 – all on Plate 2, 5.21 – Plate 3, and 5.22 to 5.24)

Until now we had availability of gray scale USG which gave only anatomic information. With the advent of transvaginal colour Doppler it may be possible to understand the physiologic dimension of blood flow to the organs concerned. We already know that structural changes that occur in the uterus and ovary during the

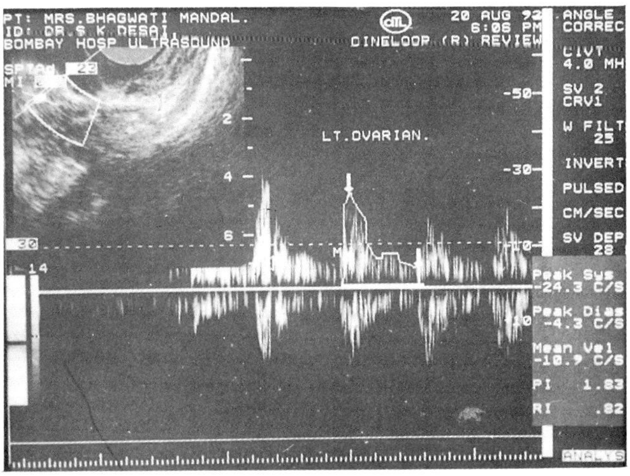

Fig. 5.22. The left ovarian artery showing a PI of 1.83 and an RI of 0.82.

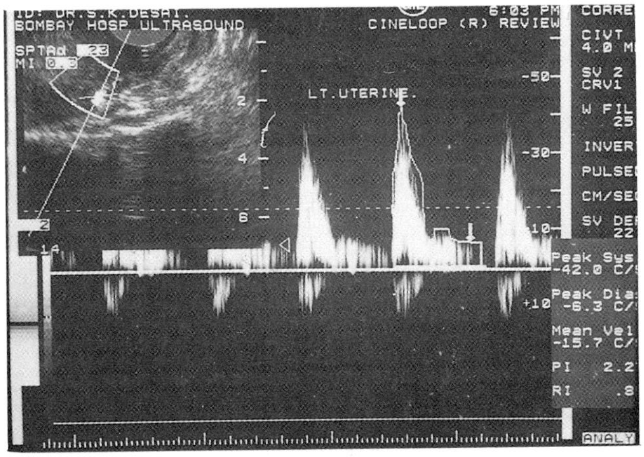

Fig. 5.23. The left uterine artery showing a PI of 2.2 and an RI of 0.8.

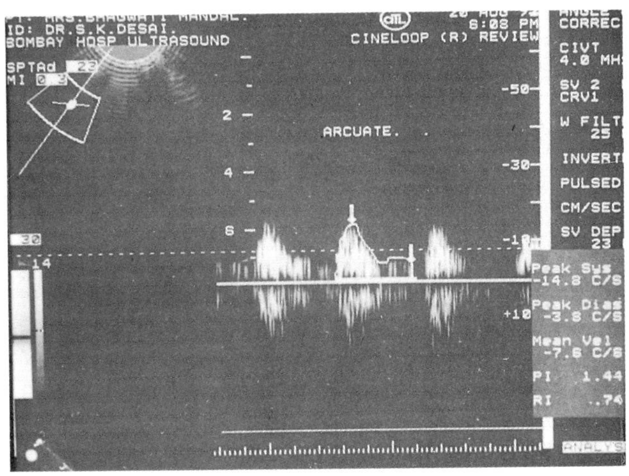

Fig. 5.24. The arcuate vessels showing a PI of 1.44 and an RI of 0.74.

menstrual cycle are associated with increased vascularity[40-44]. This increased angiogenesis is considered to be a prerequisite for these structural changes to occur. With increasing estrogen concentration during the follicular phase there is an associated increased blood flow to the uterus which can be serially observed on transvaginal colour Doppler examination. It is now possible to measure the change in blood flow that occurs during the follicular phase on serial examination in ovarian, main uterine and arcuate vessels. In the initial phase of the cycle there is a high impedance waveform with low amplitude and absent or minimal diastolic flow[45]. As the follicles start growing, the ovary with the dominant follicle begins to show diastolic flow and increased amplitude. We have been measuring the Resistance Index (RI) and Pulsatility Index (PI) to standardise the procedure. Pulsatility Index (PI) is represented by peak systolic velocity — peak diastolic velocity divided by mean velocity and represents the blood flow. While Resistance Index (RI) is obtained by peak systolic velocity — peak diastolic velocity divided by peak systolic velocity and represents the resistance to the flow. Around the periovulatory period of the cycle the diastolic flow through the ovarian and uterine artery is increased thereby representing diminished resistance to the flow and therefore the resistive index through the ovarian vessels falls by about 0.04 to 0.08 representing that the ovulation is imminent[46]. Around this time the flow Pulsatility Index of the uterine artery increases and the diastolic flow through the arcuate vessels also increases and continues to do so until the twenty-first day along with the formation of corpus luteum.

One day after ovulation an ideal PI through the uterine artery may be between 2 and 2.5 and there should be a continuous diastolic flow through the arcuate arteries suggesting a low resistance continuous blood supply to the uterus and endometrium. A good corpus luteum waveform is represented by good diastolic flow with low RI values. Thus it is now possible to identify patients with corpus luteum deficiency by measuring corpus luteal flow[47].

Serial colour Doppler evaluation therefore can help us in a stimulated cycle evaluation in the better timing of hCG administration and therefore may help improve the results of IVF and GIFT procedures. It also gives us valuable information about uterine and endometrial blood flow thereby improving our understanding in cases of unexplained infertility[48,49]. It is also possible to time the embryo transfer as uterine receptivity can be better judged by assessment of uterine flow[50,51]. In patients with corpus luteal deficiency a colour Doppler examination may help define the patients requiring luteal support.

Thus with this much of understanding it may be logically possible to predict early increased perfusion associated with high E_2 levels in early prediction of hyperstimulation. It may also help us in deciding the timing of administration of hCG in cases of E_2/USG mismatch or utero-ovarian mismatch.

Thus transvaginal Doppler flow measurement being a non-invasive method that can be repeated as often as required may help throw an additional light in an otherwise complex dynamic daily changing physiology of the human menstrual cycle.

Summary

Sonography has become an integral part of infertility management and any attempt to treat patients of infertility without an indepth understanding of the subject may not be justified in times to come.

REFERENCES

1. Office of Technology Assessment : Report brief — Infertility : medical and social choices. Washington, OTA, US Congress, 1988.
2. Speroff L, Glass RH, Kase NG. Clinical gynecologic endocrinology and infertility, 4th edition, Baltimore, Williams & Wilkins, 1989.
3. Nyberg DA. Ultrasonography in reproductive endocrinology and infertility. In Soules MR (ed.) : Controversies in reproductive endocrinology and infertility, Elsevier, pp. 229-70, 1989.
4. Kurjak A. Ultrasound and infertility, Boca Raton, Fla, CRC Press, 1989.
5. Drugan A, Itskovitz J, Brandes JM. The use of transvaginal sonography in the diagnosis and treatment of infertility. In Timor-Tritsch IE, Rottem S (eds.) : Transvaginal sonography, 2nd edition, New York, Elsevier, 1991.
6. Gougeon A. Dynamics of follicular growth in the human : a model from preliminary results. Hum Reprod 1986; 1 : 81-7.
7. Cabau A, Bessis R. Monitoring of ovulation induction with human menopausal gonadotropin and human chorionic gonadotropin by ultrasound. Fertil Steril 1981; 36 : 178-82.
8. Mendelson EB, Friedman H, Neiman HL. The role of imaging in infertility management. AJR 1985; 144 : 415-20.
9. Check JH, Dietrich C, Houck MA. Ipsilateral versus contralateral ovary selection of dominant follicle in succeeding cycle. Obstet Gynecol 1991; 77 : 247-9.
10. Ritchie WGM. Ultrasound in the evaluation of normal and induced ovulation. Fertil Steril 1985; 43 : 167-81.
11. DeCherney AH, Laufer N. The monitoring of ovulation induction using ultrasound and estrone in women throughout the menstrual cycle. J Clin Endocrinol 1974; 38 : 1009-15.
12. Hamilton CJCM, Evers JLH, Tan FES, Hoogland HJ. The reliability of ovulation prediction by a single ultrasonographic follicle measurement. Hum Reprod 1987; 2 : 103-7.
13. Smith DH, Picker RH, Sinosich M, Saunders DM. Assessment of ovulation by ultrasound and estradiol levels during spontaneous and induced cycles. Fertil Steril 1980; 33 : 387-90.
14. McNatty KP, Smith DM, Makris A, Osathanondh R, Ryan KJ. The microenvironment of the human antral follicle : Interrelationships among the steroid levels in antral fluid, the population of granulosa cells, and the status of the oocyte in vivo and in vitro. J Clin Endocrinol Metab 1979; 49 : 851-60.
15. O'Herlihy C, De Crespigny L, Lopata A. Preovulatory follicular size : a comparison of ultrasound and laparoscopic measurements. Fertil Steril 1980; 34 : 24-6.
16. Mantzavinos T, Garcia JE, Jones HW. Ultrasound measurement of ovarian follicles stimulated by human gonadotropins for oocyte recovery and in vitro fertilization. Fertil Steril 1983; 40 : 461-5.
17. Eissa MK, Hudson K, Docker MF, Sawers RS, Newton JR. Ultrasound follicle diameter measurement : an assessment of interobserver and intraobserver variation. Fertil Steril 1985; 44 : 751-4.
18. Gonzalez DJ, Curson R, Parsons J. Transabdominal versus transvaginal ultrasound scanning of ovarian follicles : Are they comparable? Fertil Steril 1988; 50 : 657-9.
19. Davis JA, Gosink BB. Fluid in the female pelvis : cyclic patterns. J Ultrasound Med 1986; 5 : 75-9.
20. Ylostalo P, Lindgren PG, Nillius SJ. Ultrasonic measurement of ovarian follicles, ovarian and uterine size during induction of ovulation with human gonadotropins. Acta Endocrinol 1981; 98 : 592-8.
21. Eissa MK, Obhrai MS, Docker MF. Follicular growth and endocrine profile in spontaneous and induced conception cycles. Fertil Steril 1986; 45 : 191-6.
22. Blankstein J, Shalev J, Saadon T. Ovarian hyperstimulation syndrome : prediction by number and size of preovulatory ovarian follicles. Fertil Steril 1987; 47 : 597-602.
23. Navot D, Relou A, Birkenfeld A. Risk factors and prognostic variables in the ovarian hyperstimulation syndrome. Am J Obstet Gynecol 1988; 159 : 210-5.
24. Tummon IS, Henig I, Radwanska E. Persistent ovarian cysts following administration of human menopausal and chorionic gonadotropins : an attenuated form of ovarian hyperstimulation syndrome. Fertil Steril 1988; 49 : 244-8.
25. Hornstein MD, Barbieri RL, Ravnikar VA, McShane PM. The effects of baseline ovarian cysts on the clinical response to controlled ovarian hyperstimulation in an in vitro fertilization program. Fertil Steril 1989; 52 : 437-40.
26. Thatcher SS, Jones E, DeCherney AH. Ovarian cysts decrease the success of controlled ovarian stimulation and in vitro fertilization. Fertil Steril 1989; 52 : 812-6.
27. Tal J, Paz B, Samberg I, Lazarov N, Sharf M. Ultrasonographic and clinical correlates of menotropin versus sequential clomiphene citrate : Menotropin therapy for induction of ovulation. Fertil Steril 1985; 44 : 342-9.
28. Forrest TS, Elyaderani MK, Muilenburg MI. Cyclic endometrial changes : US assessment with histologic correlation. Radiology 1988; 167 : 223-7.

29. Brandt TD, Levy EB, Grant TH, Marut E, Leland J. Endometrial echo and its significance in female infertility. Radiology 1985; 157 : 225-9.
30. Fleischer AC, Kalemeris GC, Entman SS. Sonographic depiction of the endometrium during normal cycles. Ultrasound Med Biol 1986; 12 : 271-7.
31. Wiczyk HP, Janus CL, Richards CJ. Comparison of magnetic resonance imaging and ultrasound in evaluating follicular and endometrial development throughout the normal cycle. Fertil Steril 1988; 49 : 969-72.
32. Gonen Y, Casper RF, Jacobson W, Blankier J. Endometrial thickness and growth during ovulation stimulation : a possible predictor of implantation in in vitro fertilization. Fertil Steril 1989; 52 : 446-50.
33. Gonen Y, Casper RF. Prediction of implantation by the sonographic appearance of the endometrium during ovarian stimulation for IVF. J In Vitro Fert Embryo Transf 1990; 7 : 146-52.
34. Fleischer AC, Herbert CM, Hill GA, Kepple DM, Worrell JA. Transvaginal sonography of the endometrium during induced cycles. J Ultrasound Med 1991; 10 : 93-5.
35. Gonen Y, Calderon I, Dirnfeld M, Abramowicz H. The impact of sonographic assessment of the endometrium and meticulous hormonal monitoring during natural cycles. Ultrasound Obstet Gynecol 1991; 1 : 122-6.
36. Schulman A, Schulman N, Weinglass L, Bahary C. Ultrasonic assessment of the endometrium as a predictor of estrogen status in amenorrheic patients. Hum Reprod 1989; 4 : 616-9.
37. Deichert U, Hackeloer BJ, Daume E. The sonographic and endocrinologic evaluation of the endometrium in the luteal phase. Hum Reprod 1986; 4 : 219-22.
38. DeVries K, Lyons EA, Ballard G, Levi CS, Lindsay DJ. Contractions of the inner third of the myometrium. Am J Obstet Gynecol 1990; 162 : 679-82.
39. Abramowicz JS, Archer DF. Uterine endometrial peristalsis — a transvaginal ultrasound study. Fertil Steril 1990; 54 : 451-4.
40. Taylor KJW, Burns PW, Wells PNT, Conway DI, Hull MGR. Ultrasound Doppler flow studies of the ovarian and uterine arteries, Br J Obstet Gynaecol 1985; 92 : 240-6.
41. Bourne TH, Jurkovic D, Waterstone J. Intrafollicular blood flow during human ovulation. Ultrasound Obstet Gynecol 1991; 1 : 53-9.
42. Collins W, Jurkovic D, Bourne TH, Kurjak A, Campbell S. Ovarian morphology, endocrine function, and intrafollicular blood flow during the periovulatory period. Hum Reprod 1991; 6 : 319-26.
43. Scholtes MCW, Wladimiroff JW, Van Rijen HJM, Hop WCJ. Uterine and ovarian flow velocity waveforms in the normal menstrual cycle : a transvaginal Doppler study. Fertil Steril 1989; 52 : 981-5.
44. Deutinger J, Reinthaller A, Berneschek G. Transvaginal pulsed Doppler measurement of blood flow velocity in the ovarian arteries during cycle stimulation and after follicle puncture. Fertil Steril 1989; 51 : 466-70.
45. Hata K, Hata Senoh D. Change in ovarian arterial compliance during the human menstrual cycle assessed by Doppler ultrasound. Br J Obstet Gynaecol 1990; 97 : 163-6.
46. Picker RH, Smith DH, Tucker MH, Saunders DM. Ultrasonic signs of imminent ovulation. J Clin Ultrasound 1983; 11 : 1-2.
47. Baber RJ, McSweeney MB, Gill RW, Transvaginal pulsed Doppler ultrasound assessment of blood flow to the corpus luteum in IVF patients following embryo transfer. Br J Obstet Gynaecol 1988; 95 : 1226-30.
48. Goswamy RK, Steptoe PC. Doppler ultrasound studies of the uterine artery in spontaneous ovarian cycles. Hum Reprod 1988; 3 : 721-6.
49. Goswamy RK, Williams G, Steptoe PC. Decreased uterine perfusion — a cause of infertility. Hum Reprod 1988; 3 : 955-9.
50. Sterzik K, Crab D, Sasse V. Doppler sonographic findings and their correlation with implantation in an in vitro fertilization program. Fertil Steril 1989; 52 : 825-8.
51. Steer CV, Mills S, Campbell S, Mason BL, Tan SL, Collins WP, Crayford T. The use of transvaginal color flow imaging after in vitro fertilisation to identify optimum uterine conditions before embryo transfer. Fertil Steril 1992; 57 : 372-6.

CHAPTER

6

Positive Contrast Sonography of the Fallopian Tubes

Gautam Allahbadia, Sadhana Desai, Prema Kania and Simon Wood

Introduction

Burns[1] in the first edition of his *Principles of Midwifery*, published in 1809, recognised "impervious" fallopian tubes as a cause of subfertility. The demonstration of tubal patency, utilizing many different approaches (Table 6.1), has been the major method of assessing tubal function. The main tools in the diagnosis of tubal disorders so far have been hysterosalpingography (HSG) and chromolaparoscopy. Chromolaparoscopy, although it permits a direct evaluation of the oocyte-reception process, involves drawbacks such as the need for anaesthesia and surgical intervention. All the same, normal fallopian tube function is currently determined by the majority of physicians by demonstrating patency and a normal visual appearance at endoscopy[2].

Radiographic HSG, which is frequently utilized for primary tubal diagnostics and applications such as the pre-operative localisation of tubal occlusions, involves radiation exposure risks and is not feasible in patients with idiosyncrasies to X-ray contrast agents[3], the use of anaesthesia being optional. Patient's fear of anaesthesia, surgery or radiation exposure, combined with the need for stationary treatment and the objective risks of intervention, have led to the recommendation that the examination of the tubal passage be given last priority in sterility diagnostics[4].

This approach may lead to long periods of expensive attempts at treatment with ovulation inducing drugs before the patient is finally referred to a hospital for tubal diagnosis. This situation calls for a low risk method for early detection of tubal passage disorders, one that would possibly even be suited for ambulatory application.

With the exception of pathologically altered fallopian tubes such as sactosalpinges, it has not been possible so far to visualise normal tubes with ultrasonic methods without the tubes being surrounded by fluid medium that is negative contrast sonography[5]. The author has proposed a tubal patency test that reports on

Table 6.1.

Transcervical
Gas (insufflation) (18)
Contrast media
Radio-opaque (19)
Echogenic (10)
Hydrotubation
Dye
Culdoscopy (20)
Culdocentesis (21)
Laparoscopy (22)
Radiolabelled gas (23)
Microsphere migration
Non-radiolabelled (24)
Radiolabelled albumin (25)
Phenosulphonpthalein (26)
Direct cannulation
Blind (27)
Guided
Hysteroscopic (28)
Ultrasonic
Fluoroscopic (29)

the exit of saline through the fimbrial end into the peritoneal cavity that can be visualised by transvaginal ultrasound[6] (Figs. 6.1 to 6.8). But even this technique cannot directly visualise the entire length of the tube. Experience has shown that intrauterine findings are easier to establish when the uterus is filled with a fluid, i.e., in haematometra or serometra[7] or by hydrohysterosonography[8]. Thus, a process of contrast-enhanced visualisation of uteri and fallopian tubes, combined

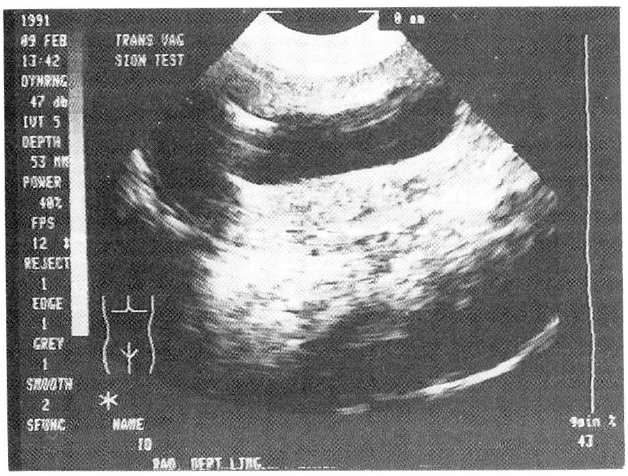

Fig. 6.1. The Sion test. Uterus with distended Foley bulb seen in sagittal plane.

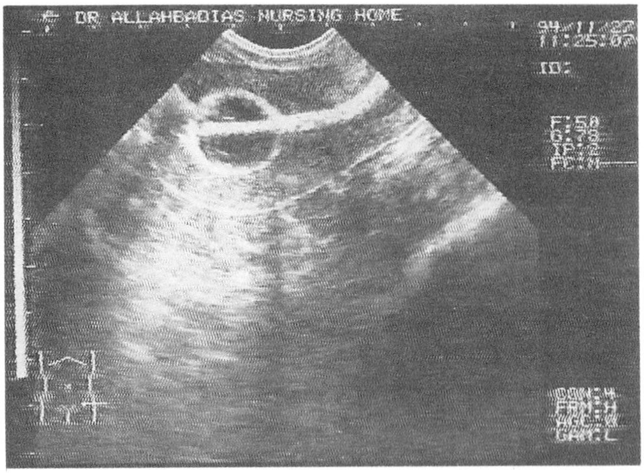

Fig. 6.2. The Sion test. Distended Foley bulb with stem of catheter seen clearly just before injection of saline.

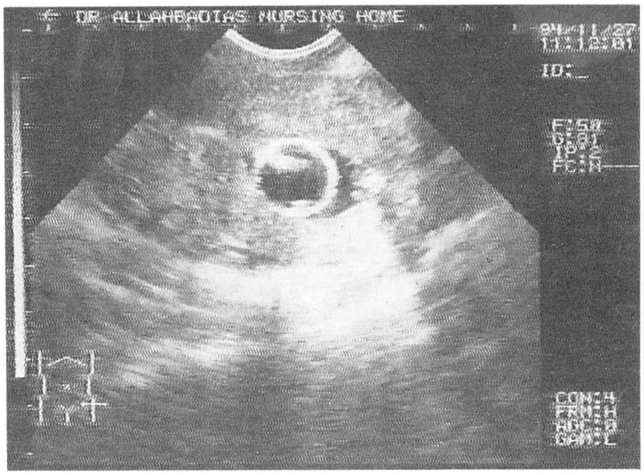

Fig. 6.3. The Sion test. Uterus seen in coronal plane. Plate taken at the beginning of injection of normal saline showing an endometrial polyp near the left tubal ostium.

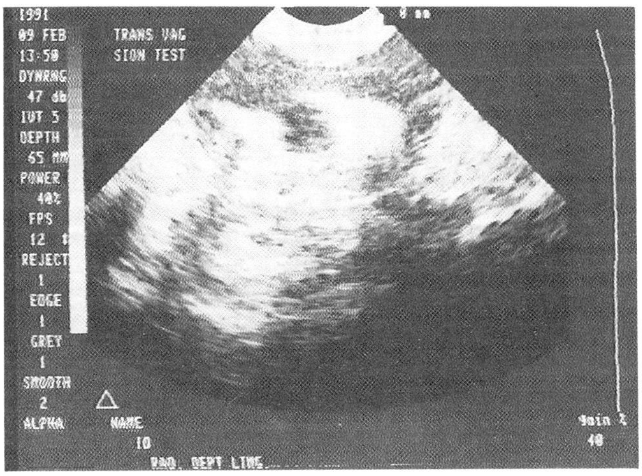

Fig. 6.4. The Sion test. Free peritoneal spill depicted on B-mode imaging : 'The waterfall sign'.

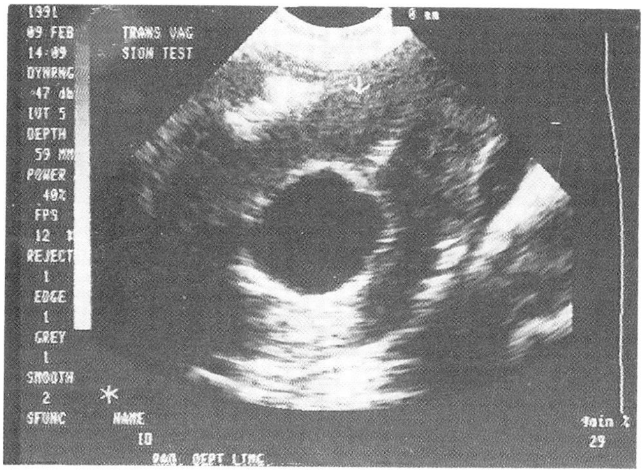

Fig. 6.5. The Sion test. Reflux seen clearly in the stem of the Foley catheter in a patient with bilaterally blocked tubes.

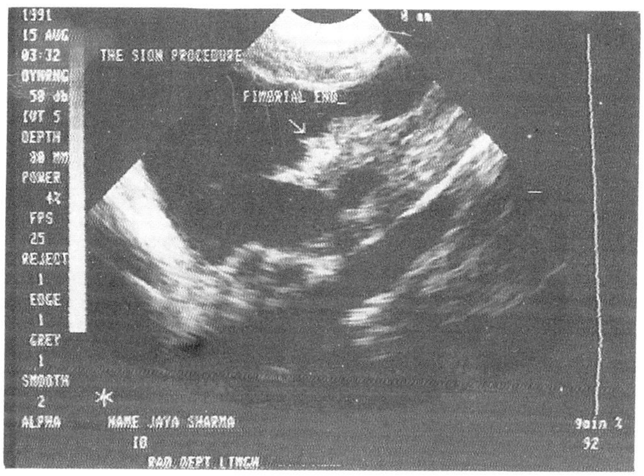

Fig. 6.6. The Sion procedure. Fimbrial end with fimbria ovarica seen clearly.

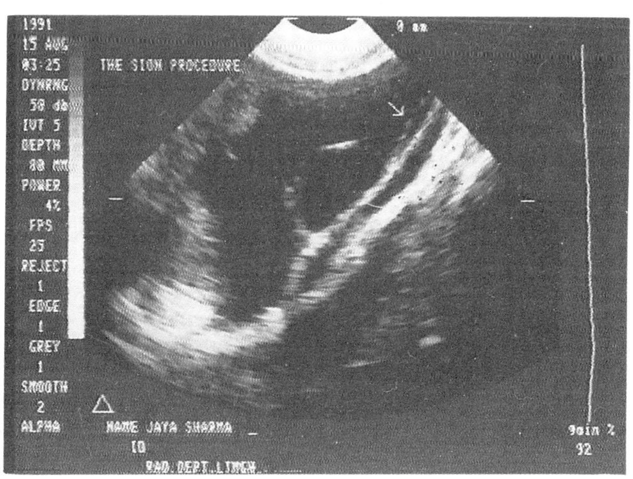

Fig. 6.7. The Sion procedure. Arrow points to filmy peri-adnexal adhesions.

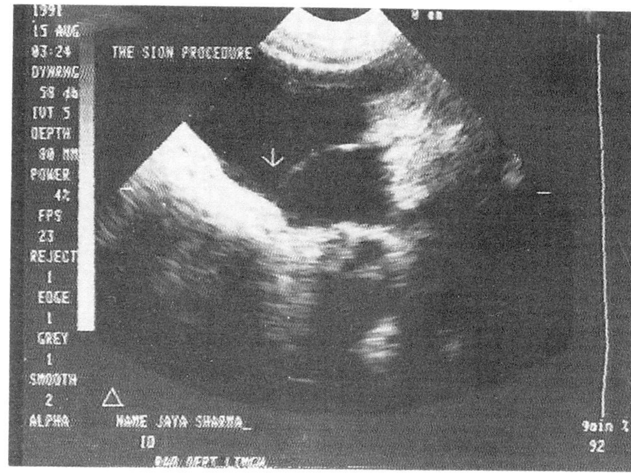

Fig. 6.8. The Sion procedure. Arrow points to a thin peritubal adhesion.

with vaginosonography, was very much required in our sterility diagnosis programme. Reports from the United Kingdom[9] and Germany[10] showed that apart from an improved demarcation of uterine wall structures, positive contrast sonography could visualise the entire length of fallopian tube as well as establish tubal patency. Transvaginal hysterosalpingo-contrast sonography (HyCoSy) was described by Deichert[10] as a new method for direct imaging of the tubal passage in tubal diagnostics. We, at the Bombay Hospital Institute of Medical Sciences have had limited experience with HyCoSy and all the images (Figs. 6.9 to 6.16) presented in this chapter are a part of the workshop during the ICIT '95 at Bombay.

Hysterosalpingo-contrast-sonography (HyCoSy)

For vaginal ultrasound images the 5/6.5 MHz panoramic

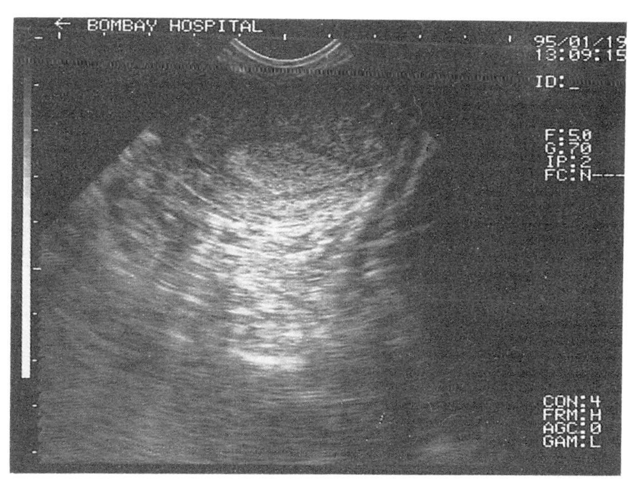

Fig. 6.9. HyCoSy. The left tubal ostium as seen when normal saline has been injected.

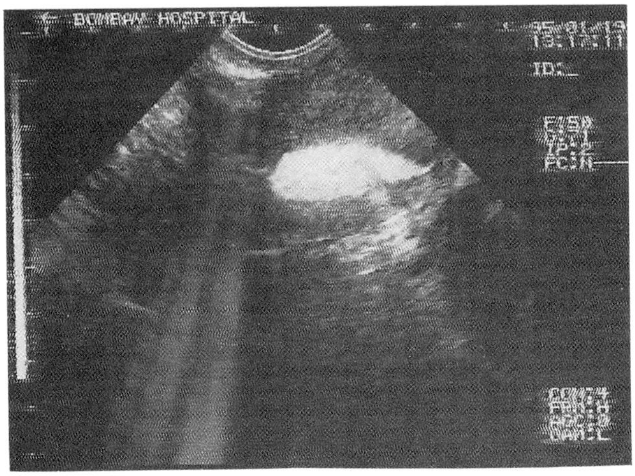

Fig. 6.10. HyCoSy. The left tubal ostium in the same patient when Echovist is injected.

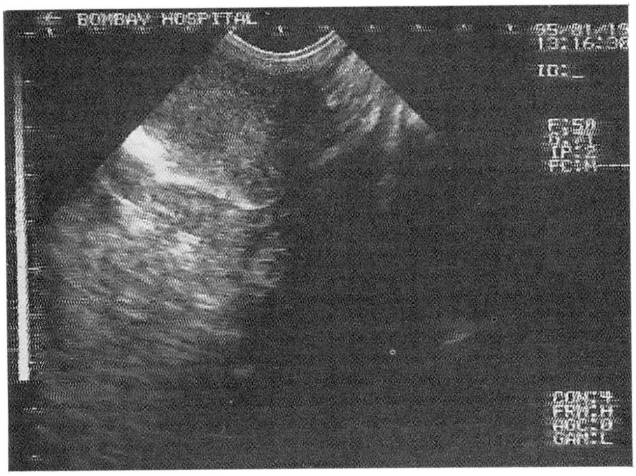

Fig. 6.11. HyCoSy. Part of the uterine cavity, the intramural portion, the isthmic portion and the ampullary portion of the left tube in the same patient as in Fig. 6.10 when more contrast is injected.

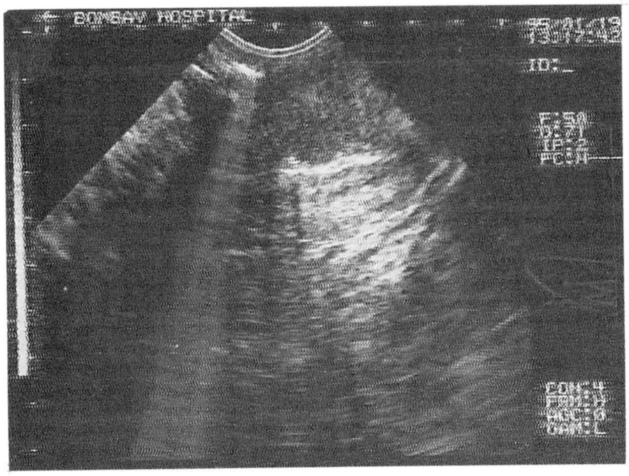

Fig. 6.12. HyCoSy. The endometrial cavity seen outlined with Echovist in between active injection.

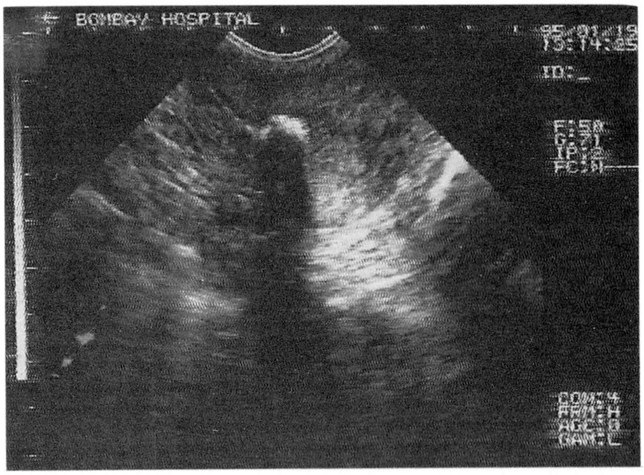

Fig. 6.13. HyCoSy. The right tubal spill now seen along with part of the uterine cavity.

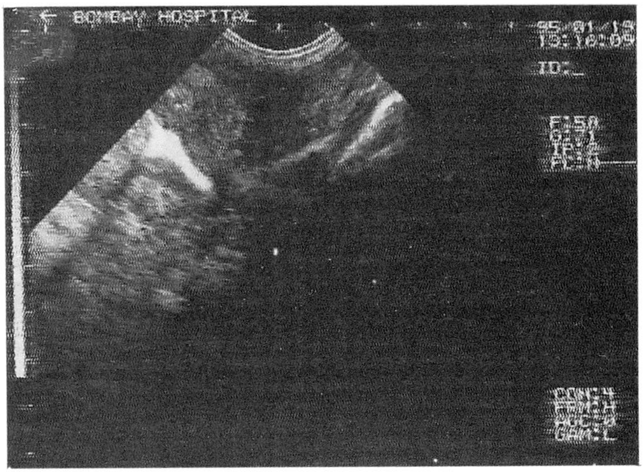

Fig. 6.14. HyCoSy. A left sided spill seen in another patient. Note that the proximal portion of the left tube is seen very clearly.

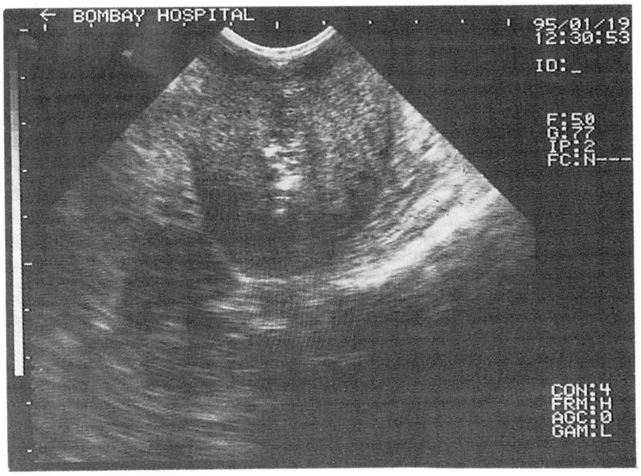

Fig. 6.15. HyCoSy. Post-injection picture with remains of the contrast along with some air seen in the uterine cavity.

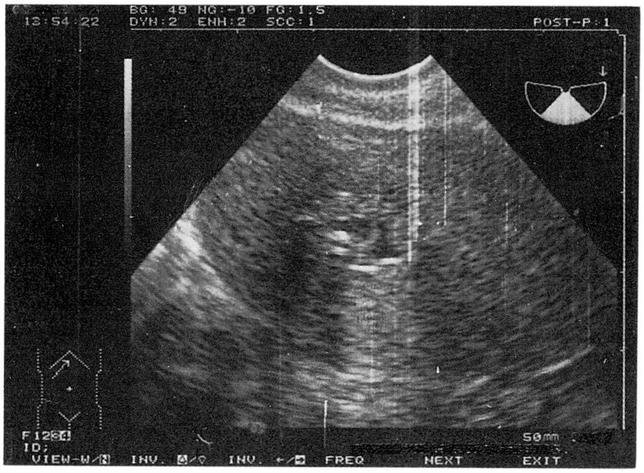

Fig. 6.16. HyCoSy. A localised area of intrauterine synechiae seen clearly in this plate.

scanner of Siemens Sonoline 500 and the 5 MHz scanner of Fukuda Denshi FF Sonic 4500 was used.

HyCoSy was employed in the following way : after vaginal disinfection with Betadine antiseptic solution (Win Medicare, New Delhi, India), an HSG catheter set was applied, or an 8F Foley catheter, introduced through the cervix and blocked with 1.5-2 ml saline, was used. Sterile saline was used as a low-echo negative contrast agent for the visualisation of the uterine cavity. With the HSG instruments or intracervical catheter in position, the vaginal sonographic examination was performed, including images of the uterus, the pouch of Douglas and both adnexal regions. Intermittent injection of the positive contrast agent Echovist (Schering, Germany) unfolded the uterine cavity. The uterine wall was evaluated with respect to smoothness or presence of irregularities. The unit was then set to image the adnexal junctions and more contrast agent was injected to observe its tubal passage.

The first part of the investigation used about 20-50 ml sterile normal saline while in the second part the tubal passage was imaged with a novel echocontrast (SH U 454, Echovist, Schering, Germany) applied in quantities up to 20 ml.

SH U 454 is a preparation presently undergoing clinical trials; it consists of a suspension of soluble galactose microparticles (50% < 2 millimicrons) in an aqueous 20% (w/v) solution of galactose, containing miniscule air bubbles of the order of several micrometres in size. Chemically, this product is pure galactose while, from the physical point of view, it constitutes an acoustically inhomogeneous suspension — microbubbles/microparticles — which exhibits dose-dependent, pronounced echogenic properties. Clinical trials of SH U 454 have so far been concentrated on echocardiography, where its good tolerance following i.v. injection has been demonstrated in > 700 patients[11].

Turbulent flow in the tubes, emergence of the contrast agent at the end of the fimbriae and an increased volume of retrouterine fluid were deemed to be indicators of an unobstructed tubal passage. The results were recorded on videotape as well as photographs, after which the conventional procedure was performed, i.e., HSG or chromolaparoscopy. Echovist is injected 1-2 ml at a time and the tubes are intermittently filled. The ultrasound probe is manipulated to detect signals from the intramural area, isthmus and ampulla of each tube (Fig. 6.11). A tube is considered to be patent if the flow of Echovist can be visualised using B-mode scanning for at least 5-10 seconds. Figs. 6.9 to 6.15 show examples of B-mode images observed during the HyCoSy procedure.

Patients were observed for about two hours after HyCoSy, and discharged home with instructions to report any side-effects that may occur over the next few days. The side-effects reported by patients included pain with cannulation and injection and one patient reported post-procedure abdominal cramps which were relieved by simple analgesics.

We agree with other investigators that training in ultrasound imaging is essential to use the echogenic contrast medium effectively. It also became clear that excessive distension of the self-retaining Foley balloon or volumes exceeding 50 ml caused side-effects such as cramps that were uncomfortable. All patients should be given pre-operative sedation and antispasmodics.

The sticky nature of the contrast medium outlined submucous fibroids well enough to assess the contours of the fibroids within the uterine cavity. This may obviate the need for hysteroscopy in patients where the extent of encroachment of individual fibroids could influence whether or not the patient would be suitable for hysteroscopic resection. It would also help in deciding whether pre-operative priming with drugs, such as GnRH analogs was indicated prior to hysteroscopic surgery.

Finally, the ability of vaginal ultrasound to image the ovaries, the uterine wall, cervix and adnexal structures in conjunction with contrast medium may relegate the laparoscopy and dye test to a secondary position. Just as most gynaecologists only perform HSG when laparoscopy and dye test findings indicate it, it may well follow that laparoscopy may be only performed in cases where vaginal ultrasound and HyCoSy are unable to provide all the information needed.

Discussion

Echocontrast in gynaecology was developed from two fortuitous and independent observations. In 1981, Nainini *et al.*[12] were the first to report that saline injected into the uterine cavity allowed intrauterine structures such as the endometrium to be observed with ultrasound. Occasionally this fluid could be observed in the pouch of Douglas, indicating that the fluid must have flowed through the fallopian tubes and hence that the tubes were patent. Some years later, Deichert *et al.*[7] noticed that in a naturally fluid-filled uterus, such as in the case of haematometra due to a uterus myomatosis, intrauterine structures are highlighted because of the surrounding fluid. Normal fallopian tubes are not visible by ultrasound, but in cases of tubal damage such as sactosalpinx, the tubes can be seen and a diagnosis made. The observations that fluid in the uterus and tubes could enhance the diagnostic power of ultrasound led to several investigators reporting that injecting fluid into the uterus could allow both intrauterine structures and tubal patency to be investigated using ultrasound[10,11,13,14,15]. Initially, saline or Ringer's solution was used as a contrast agent for this new technique. The results were, however, unpredictably reproducible with only the free peritoneal spill seen clearly. In 1986 a new ultrasound echoenhancing agent, Echovist, was undergoing trials in echocardiography as previously described and was picked up to assess tubal patency.

Results so far[10,11,13] indicate that HyCoSy shows significant promise in its ability to assess tubal patency, with the added benefits of being performed as an outpatient procedure that is well tolerated by patients. Our first patient at Bombay Hospital had a family history of allergy to iodine and was counselled for checking her tubal patency with Echovist. This particular patient had bilaterally patent tubes and in addition a localised area of intrauterine synechiae was also picked up clearly (Fig. 6.16). The combined experience of the investigators has revealed a number of points which contribute significantly to the understanding and appreciation of the procedure and what can be achieved with it. The potential exists for HyCoSy to be used as an initial screen of tubal patency so that the more extensive and more costly procedures of hysterosalpingography (HSG) and chromolaparoscopy can be reserved for those cases where they are irreplaceable.

Tubal patency is assessed to determine the course of treatment for infertility. If neither or only one tube is closed, ovarian stimulation is recommended; if both tubes are closed, the patient can be put forward to IVF or tubal surgery. A rapid well-tolerated outpatient procedure which can establish tubal patency — such as HyCoSy — might allow the patient to be assigned to the appropriate treatment at an earlier stage. This would have the dual benefits of saving time and cost, and would be particularly beneficial to the growing number of couples presenting at a later age.

REFERENCES

1. Burns J. Principles of Midwifery. Longman, Hurst, Rees & Orme, London, 1809, pp 131-32.
2. Blackwell RE. The infertility workup and diagnosis. J Reprod Med 1989; 34 : 81-6.
3. San Filipo JS, Yussman MA, Smith O. Hysterosalpingography in the evaluation of infertility : a six year review. Fertil Steril 1978; 30 : 636-43.
4. Runnebaum B, Rabe T. Gynakologische Endokrinologie. Springer Verlag, Berlin, 1987, pp 367-69.
5. Allahbadia G, Nalawade Y, Panjwani M, Vaidya P, Merchant S. The Sion Procedure. J Obstet Gynaecol India 1992; 42 : 814-8.
6. Allahbadia GN, Nalawade YV, Patkar VD, Niyogi GM, Shah PK. The Sion Test. Aust NZ J Obstet Gynaecol 1992; 32 : 67-70.
7. Deichert U, van de Sandt M, Daume E. Vaginale Hysterokontrastsonographie zur Differentialdiagnostichen Abklarung eines Pseudogestationsachs. Ultraschall Klin Prax 1987; 2 : 245-48.
8. Allahbadia G. Vaginosonography and the uterine tubes. Infertility and Transvaginal Sonography, Jaypee Brothers Medical Publishers, New Delhi, 1995 pp 250-52.
10. Deichert U, van de Sandt M, Daume E. Die vaginale hysterokontrastsonographie in ersatz oder erdazung zur differential diagnostichen hysterosalpingographie und chromolaparoscopie. Ultraschall Klin Prax 1989; 1 (Suppl) : 48-51.
11. Schlief R, Deichert U. Hysterosalpingo-contrast sonography of the uterus and fallopian tubes : results of a clinical trial of a new contrast medium in 120 patients. Radiology 1991; 178 : 213-215.
12. Nainini R, Chelo E, Branconi F. Dynamic echohysteroscopy : a new diagnostic technique in the study of female infertility. Acta Europ Fertil 1981; 12 : 165-71.
13. Deichert U, Schlief R, van de Sandt M. Transvaginal hysterosalpingo-contrast sonography (HyCoSy) compared with conventional tubal diagnostics. Hum Reprod 1989; 4 : 418-24.
14. Schurmann RJ, Neindorf HP, Schlief R. Efficacy and tolerance of hysterosalpingocontrast-sonography with a

saccharide based contrast agent in 425 patients. Radiology 1991; 181 : 89-91.

15. Venezia R, Zangara C. Echohysterosalpingography : new diagnostic possibilities with SH U 454. Acta Eur Fertil 1991; 22 : 279-82.
16. Deichert U, Schlief R, van de Sandt M. Transvaginal hysterosalpingo-contrast sonography of tubal patency with gray scale imaging and additional use of pulsed wave Doppler. Fertil Steril 1992; 57 : 62-67.
17. Stern J, Peters AJ, Coulam CB. Colour Doppler ultrasonography assessment of tubal patency : a comparison study with traditional techniques. Fertil Steril 1992; 58 : 897-900.
18. Rubin IC. The nonoperative determination of patency of fallopian tubes. J Am Med Assoc 1920; 75 : 661-7.
19. Cary WH. Note on determination of patency of fallopian tubes by the use of Collargol and X-ray shadow. Am J Obstet Dis Women Child 1914; 69 : 462-5.
20. Decker A. Culdoscopy. W.B. Saunders Co., Philadelphia, 1952.
21. Ansari AH. Tubal patency evaluation by the methylene blue test. Am J Obstet Gynecol 1969; 103 : 1170.
22. Gabos P. A comparison of HSG and endoscopy in evaluation of tubal function in infertile women. Fertil Steril 1976; 27 : 238-40.
23. Pertynski T, Jakubowski W, Stelmachow J. A scintographic method of examining the patency of oviducts using XE 133. Eur J Nuc Med 1977; 2 : 159-61.
24. Conil Serra V. A new method of exploration of tubal function. Proceedings of the First World Congress. Fertil Steril 1953; 2 : 116-18.
25. Iturralde M, Venter PF. Hysterosalpingo-radionuclide scintography (HERS). Semin Nucl Med 1981; 11 : 301-5.
26. Speck G. Phenolsulfonpthalein as a test for the determination of tubal patency. Am J Obstet Gynecol 1948; 55 : 1048-50.
27. Tyler Smith W. Further observations on the method of treating sterility by the removal of obstructions from the fallopian tubes. Lancet 1849; 2 : 116-9.
28. Novy MJ, Thurmond AS, Patton P. Diagnosis of cornual obstruction by transcervical fallopian tube cannulation. Fertil Steril 1988; 50 : 434-7.
29. Someshwar V. Fallopian tube recanalisation — A new hope for the infertile. Desai S, Allahbadia G (eds) Infertility and Transvaginal Sonography, Jaypee Brothers Medical Publishers, New Delhi, 1995 pp 127-31.

CHAPTER

7

Transvaginal Ultrasound in Selective Embryo Reduction for Multiple Pregnancy

Ambrish Dalal, Sadhana Desai and Gautam Allahbadia

Ovulation induction for the treatment of infertility is known to carry the risk of inducing multiple gestations. Various studies have shown an incidence of multiple gestation after induced ovulation ranging from 16-39%[1]. A large number of fetuses is associated with an increased frequency of maternal complications[2,3] and greater perinatal morbidity and mortality[2-9]. Mothers of triplets have a 20% rate of preeclampsia and a 35% risk of serious postpartum hemorrhage[10]. Complication rates for mothers of four or more fetuses are likely to be even higher. The ultimate outcome of multifetal gestations relates in part to the number of conceptuses and the quality of obstetric and neonatal care.

Multiple gestations can be controlled to some extent by reducing the number of embryos transferred to the uterus during in vitro fertilization (IVF), especially when facilities for embryo cryopreservation are available, or by withholding hCG during ovarian hyperstimulation therapy if the number of preovulatory follicles is too great[11]. Nevertheless, the possibility of multiple gestation still exists, and a means of controlling embryo development is of clinical importance. Some research workers[10] advocate that in young women undergoing IVF, under the age 35, with a high cleavage rate and morphologically good embryos; one should transfer only two embryos and cryopreserve the supernumeraries. Selective reduction of the number of fetuses represents one of the few options for increasing the likelihood of a successful outcome for patients with multifetal pregnancies (Fig. 7.1). The major potential benefit of embryo reduction is an increase in gestational age at birth and, thereby, a decrease in perinatal mortality and morbidity.

Selective reduction of the number of fetuses in a multiple gestation using transvaginal ultrasound[12,13] is a recent technological development and represents an important addition to the management of unplanned multiple pregnancy resulting from infertility treatment. First trimester fetal reduction may be performed using one of four techniques :

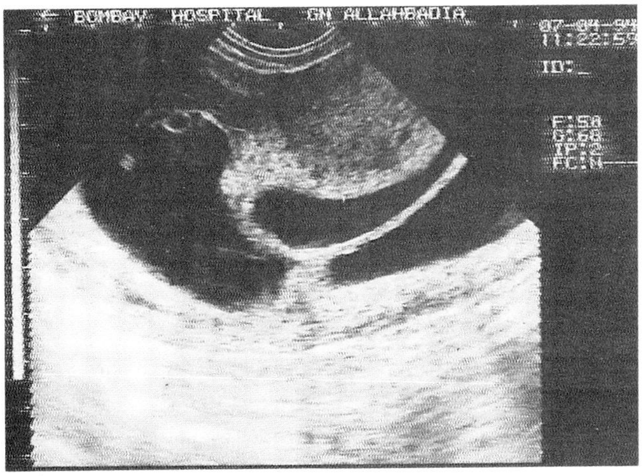

Fig. 7.1. Triplet pregnancy.

1. Cervical dilatation and transcervical aspiration of a gestational sac[14].
2. Transabdominal intrathoracic injection of potassium chloride[15-17] or other lethal substances[18], or direct needle trauma to the heart.
3. Transvaginal ultrasonographically guided aspiration of gestational sacs[19].
4. Transvaginal ultrasonographically directed intrathoracic injection of potassium chloride[20].

A report from Bombay recently described for the first time a completely new method of embryo reduction using colour Doppler ultrasonography[17] (Fig. 7.2 – Plate 3).

Transvaginal ultrasound guided fetal reduction may have several advantages over methods reported previously that involve the transabdominal[15] or transcervical approach[14]. The vaginal route is better for several reasons. The material used is the same as for oocyte recovery, localisation and guidance are easy, and the vaginal elasticity enables the optimal approach to the gestational sac and embryo. The proximity of the vaginal transducer to the pelvic organs makes the use of higher frequency probes (*e.g.*, 7.0 MHz) possible, thus enhancing resolution of the gestational sac and its contents. Even otherwise, the image definition is often better than when using an abdominal probe and obesity or commonly encountered abdominal scars are not an obstacle. The shorter puncture route and the more precise and accurate puncture procedure compared with the transabdominal approach reduce the risk of puncture to bowel or blood vessel or inadvertent damage to the other gestational sacs. This also allows the procedure to be performed at an earlier stage of pregnancy. Performing the procedure earlier in pregnancy may also make it easier for the couple to accept it. Itskowitz *et al.*[13] reported that it is feasible to do procedures as early as six weeks' gestation, although it is preferable to wait until eight weeks or longer to allow for occurrence of the natural phenomenon of the *vanishing twin* (Figs. 7.3 and 7.4).

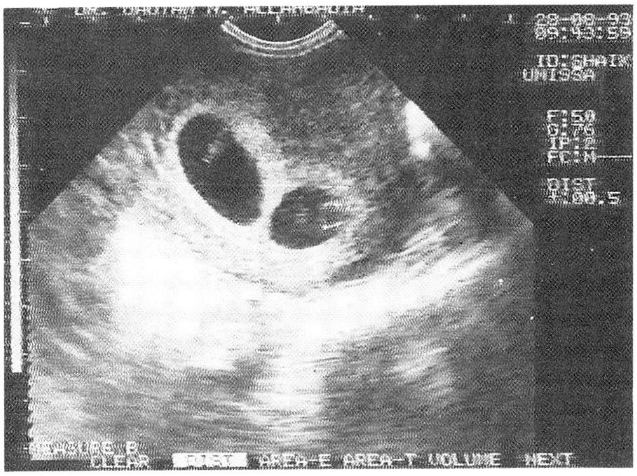

Fig. 7.3. A twin gestation with discrepancy in sac size. Cardiac flicker appreciable in both the fetuses at 7 weeks.

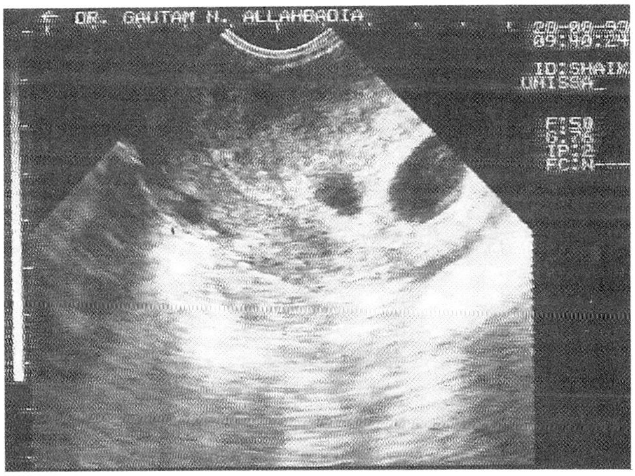

Fig. 7.4. Sonogram at 9 weeks shows a 'vanishing' sac.

Transvaginal selective reduction with the use of the *double needle* technique[20] is the method of choice for fetal reduction. Obviating the need for multiple uterine penetrations, the *double needle* method most probably reduces the risk of infection and uterine contractions. Although the risks associated with selective reduction, such as infection, septic abortion, bleeding, or damage to the gestational sacs, are known, the dearth of experience with the procedure to date makes it impossible to assess their frequency accurately. We believe that the major risk of this procedure is septic abortion resulting from the possible introduction of vaginal organisms into the injected fetal sac and the possibility that the entire pregnancy can be lost as a consequence.

Virtually all of the specialists now performing embryo reduction leave two viable embryos. While singleton pregnancies certainly have a greater chance of survival, the successful management of twin pregnancies is fairly routine. If a singleton pregnancy is left and a problem develops, the patient may have no surviving offspring. With twins, at least there is some hope that one fetus will survive even if a problem arises. Furthermore, the majority of these patients are previously infertile couples for whom a twin pregnancy may satisfy family planning desires.

In most of the series using gray scale ultrasonography, an ultrasound scan was performed the day after the procedure to confirm the death of the injected embryos. The procedure was repeated on the following day because of the persistence of embryonic life, despite initial signs of death. This was probably due to the poor quality of the ultrasound images after reduction, as previously reported[15,16,21]. With the new technique of colour flow mapping, fetal demise can be confirmed on table at the same sitting thus eliminating the doubt of persistence of cardiac activity in injected fetuses and the possibility of a second procedure on the same patient[17] (Fig. 7.2 – Plate 3).

The fetal heart is extraordinarily resilient to insults in utero. Attempts to achieve exsanguination in the second trimester, as well as direct needle trauma to the heart in the first, have failed to achieve permanent asystole[22]. We believe that a cardiotoxic drug should be injected right into the fetal heart in order to decrease the duration of the procedure and to increase its effectiveness. This can be best accomplished under transvaginal colour flow mapping. Potassium chloride is used in most of the series because the action is rapid and there is very little danger to the mother if small amounts of the potassium enter her bloodstream. The injection of air into the fetal heart should be discouraged with use of colour flow mapping because it greatly compromises the clarity of the colour flow image.

The major concern with using any cardiotoxic agent or air embolization is that in monochorionic twin pregnancies, a significant circulatory exchange might be present through placental anastomosis. In this situation, a lethal agent injected into the anomalous fetus could enter the circulation of the normal twin and result in death or permanent damage. Regardless of the method used, it is theoretically possible that unexplained death of the second twin could occur soon after the procedure, possibly because of vascular connections between the two fetal circulations, causing the living twin to *bleed out* into the circulation of its dead co-twin as a result of a marked decrease in peripheral resistance. Ischemic accidents are well documented in the surviving monozygotic twin after in utero death of the other fetus[23]. A rare complication that could also occur in the surviving twin are lesions related to disseminated intravascular coagulation from transchorionic transmission of thromboplastic material from the dead fetus. In monochorionic pregnancies, cerebral, renal, and cutaneous lesions have been described in the surviving twin after the spontaneous in utero death of its co-twin[24]. Use of transvaginal colour flow mapping at the time of reduction procedures could well avoid almost all the above mentioned complications. Transvaginal colour flow imaging should be able to delineate all the vascular connections between siblings in utero. Whenever colour flow imaging indicates the monozygotic vascular connections, one can leave both the twins unharmed and select other fetuses for reduction. Contrary to this view one can inject cardiotoxic agents into both the monoamniotic twins if quadruplets or more are present. We see no advantage in delaying the procedure beyond the 10th week of gestation, because if all the fetuses look healthy and are of appropriate size at the time, spontaneous losses in the next few weeks are unlikely. Furthermore, the later in pregnancy the termination is performed, the more probable it is that fetal resorption will be incomplete. This, in turn, may increase the chance that maternal disseminated intravascular coagulation will develop. Finally, the longer a patient waits to undergo a selective reduction, the greater may be the psychological difficulty of making the decision. Candidates for the procedure invariably undergo multiple ultrasound examinations that provide visual contact with their fetuses; this can evoke the type of emotional bonding that normally begins to develop after birth[25].

The use of embryo reduction technology should be guided by the couple's desires and ethical positions. Any form of abortion after infertility treatment is distressing. However, many women seek selective termination because they feel unable to cope with maternal and psychological problems associated with the simultaneous birth of four or more babies. The fact that an objective perinatal benefit can be expected from embryo reduction is of great moral relief to mothers who feel guilty about requesting selective termination. Preparing herself for the procedure is a severe mental strain on the anxious mother. Telling her on the following day that the procedure would have to be repeated puts her into unfathomable mental torture. The new technique using colour flow imaging would go a long way in achieving *complete* first time selective reduction procedures[17]. Because of the psychological and ethical drawbacks of embryo reduction, however, the main emphasis in limiting multiple gestations should be placed on improving the control of infertility therapies. Ending on an optimistic note, we have recent reports on the physical and mental development of co-sibs surviving selective reduction of multifetal pregnancies (Fig. 7.5) which emphasize that these babies are not handicapped and did not fall short of their matched controls in any way[26].

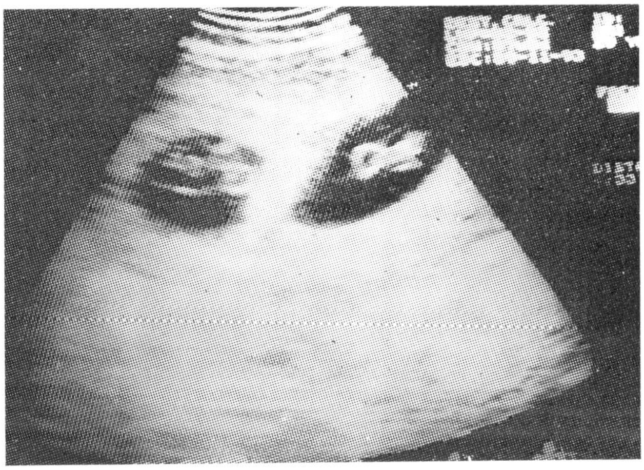

Fig. 7.5. Surviving twin co-sibs at 8 weeks gestation. Fetal poles and yolk sacs seen in both the gestational sacs.

The transvaginal selective embryo reduction technique under ultrasonic guidance, performed between 7 and 10 weeks of amenorrhoea and leaving two embryos in place is, in our opinion, a simple procedure, devoid of any risk to the mother, associated with a very low risk of infection and with no effect on the remaining fetuses. In our opinion, this procedure is necessary when there are four or more embryos, and it should also be proposed for triplet pregnancies. The incorporation of colour Doppler ultrasonography into the vaginal transducers will further enhance the ease and first time completion of vaginal multifetal reductions. Fetal reduction is still a palliative procedure for multifetal gestations, and all efforts should be made to prevent such pregnancies.

REFERENCES

1. Hobbins JC. Selective reduction — a perinatal necessity? N Engl J Med 1988; 316 : 1062-3.
2. Itzkowic D. A survey of 59 triplet pregnancies. Br J Obstet Gynaecol 1979; 86 : 23-8.
3. Syrop CH, Varner MW. Triplet gestation : Maternal and neonatal implications. Acta Genet Med Gemellol 1985; 34 : 81-8.
4. Daw E. Triplet pregnancy. Br J Obstet Gynaecol 1978; 85 : 505-9.
5. Michelewitz H, Kennedy J, Kawada C, Kennison R. Triplet pregnancies. J Reprod Med 1981; 26 : 243-6.
6. Ron-El R, Caspi E, Schreyer P, Weinrub Z, Areili S, Goldberg M. Triplet and quadruplet pregnancies and management. Obstet Gynecol 1981; 57 : 458-63.
7. Holeberg G, Biale Y, Lewenthal H, Insler V. Outcome of pregnancy in 31 triplet gestations. Obstet Gynecol 1982; 59 : 472-6.
8. Loucopoulos A, Jewelewicz R. Management of multifetal pregnancies : Sixteen years' experience at the Sloane Hospital for women. Am J Obstet Gynecol 1982; 143 : 902-5.
9. Botting BJ, Davies IM, Macfarlane AY. Recent trends in the incidence of multiple births and associated mortality. Arch Dis Child 1987; 62 : 941-50.
10. Vauthier-Brouzes D, Lefebvre G. Selective reduction in multifetal pregnancies : technical and psychological aspects. Fertil Steril 1992; 57 : 1012-6.
11. Schenker JG, Yarkoni S, Granat M. Multiple pregnancies following induction of ovulation. Fertil Steril 1981; 35 : 105-25.
12. Gonen Y, Blankier J, Casper RF. Transvaginal ultrasound in selective embryo reduction for multiple pregnancy. Obstet Gynecol 1990, 75 : 720-2.
13. Itskovitz J, Boldes R, Thaler I, Levron J, Rottem S, Brandes JM. First trimester selective reduction in multiple pregnancy guided by transvaginal sonography. J Clin Ultrasound 1990; 18 : 323-7.
14. Dumez Y, Oury JF. Method for first trimester selective abortion in multiple pregnancy. Contrib Gynecol Obstet 1986; 5 : 50-3.
15. Berkowitz RL, Lynch L, Chitkara U, Wilkins IA, Mehalek KE, Alvarez E. Selective reduction of multifetal pregnancies in the first trimester. N. Engl J Med 1988; 318 : 1043-7.
16. Evans MI, Fletcher JC, Zador IE, Newton BW, Quigg MH, Struyk CD. Selective first-trimester termination in octuplet and quadruplet pregnancies: clinical and ethical issues. Obstet Gynecol 1988; 71 : 289-96.
17. Desai SK, Allahbadia GN, Dalal AK. Selective reduction of multifetal pregnancies in the first trimester using colour Doppler ultrasonography. Hum Reprod 1993; 8 : 642-4.
18. Brandes JM, Itskovitz J, Timor-Tritsch IE, Drugan A, Frydman R. Reduction of the number of embryos in a multiple pregnancy : quintuplet to triplet. Fertil Steril 1987; 48 : 326-7.
19. Timor-Tritsch I, Rottem S, Thaler I. Review of

transvaginal ultrasonography : description with clinical application. Ultrasound Quart 1986; 6 : 1-7.

20. Shalev J, Frankel Y, Lipitz S, Serr DM, Goldman B, Mashiach S. Selective reduction of multifetal pregnancies. N. Eng J Med 1988; 319 : 949-50.
21. Macfarlane A, Price F, Daw EG, Botting B. Multiple pregnancy and assisted reproduction. Lancet 1987; ii, 1090.
22. Kanhai HHH, Van Rijssel EJC, Meerman RJ, Bennebrock Gravenhorst J. Selective termination in quintuplet pregnancy during first trimester. Lancet 1986; i, 1447-8.
23. Szymonowicz W, Preston H, Yu VYH. The surviving monozygotic twin. Arch Dis Child 1986; 61 : 454-6.
24. Enbom JA. Twin pregnancy with intrauterine death of one twin. Am J Obstet Gynecol 1987; 152 : 424-9.
25. Fletcher JC, Evans MI. Maternal bonding in early fetal ultrasound examination. N. Engl J Med 1983; 308 : 392-3.
26. Brandes JM, Itskovitz J, Scher A, Gershoni-Baruch R. The physical and mental development of co-sibs surviving selective reduction of multifetal pregnancies. Hum Reprod 1990; 5 : 1014-17.

CHAPTER

8

Transvaginal Sonography in Assisted Reproduction

Kamini Rao

The introduction of transvaginal sonography (TVS) has revolutionised our understanding of the reproductive organs. This is because the impedance that is caused by the fat and sub-cutaneous tissue is overcome. The transducer is closer to the pelvic organs and so higher frequencies can be used, reducing attenuation of the sound beam, resulting in improved overall image quality. Thus transvaginal sonography has been found to be more accurate than transabdominal sonography[1].

Ultrasound is used in almost all areas of IVF-ET programmes. It is used in follicular growth monitoring, egg retrieval, measurement of endometrial thickness, cyst aspiration and embryo transfer.

Ultrasound follicular monitoring is done using the transvaginal approach. Here the follicles are measured in three dimensions and a mean is taken to give us the diameter of the follicle. The endometrium is also a useful indicator during the monitoring of IVF cycles. The echo texture of the endometrium gives some idea about the secretory and proliferative phase of the endometrium.

Ultrasound directed follicle aspiration (UDFA) is now the preferred method of oocyte collection in many centres performing IVF-ET, in preference to laparoscopic retrieval[2]. Operators using UDFA techniques are convinced of its safety; no reports of serious sequelae have been published. Many patients undergoing the IVF-ET procedure have extensive pelvic disease or have had unsuccessful pelvic surgery. In view of this high incidence of pelvic adhesions, the risk of visceral perforation during laparoscopy may be increased[3]. Furthermore, laparoscopy is usually performed under general anaesthesia, which is also associated with morbidity and mortality. Although some centres use general anaesthesia for UDFA, they are now changing over to I.V. sedation with or without analgesia[4,5,6].

The first UDFA technique, using the transabdominal-transvesical route, was described in 1981[4]. Dellenbach *et al.*[7] introduced the transvaginal approach, scanning through the full bladder, which they thought was psychologically more acceptable to the patients. Parsons *et al.*[6] noted the improved visualisation of the needle that was at right angles to the ultrasound beam, but found access to the ovaries difficult with this transvaginal technique and hence described the perurethral technique. Feichtinger and Kemeter[8] described the use of the vaginal ultrasound probe to collect oocytes. This route is simpler to learn than the perurethral approach or abdominal approach and causes less discomfort but requires a vaginal probe that may not be available.

Vaginal ultrasonography has been used in the evaluation of polycystic ovaries and for the analysis of ovarian stroma and microcysts (Fig. 8.1). The vaginal

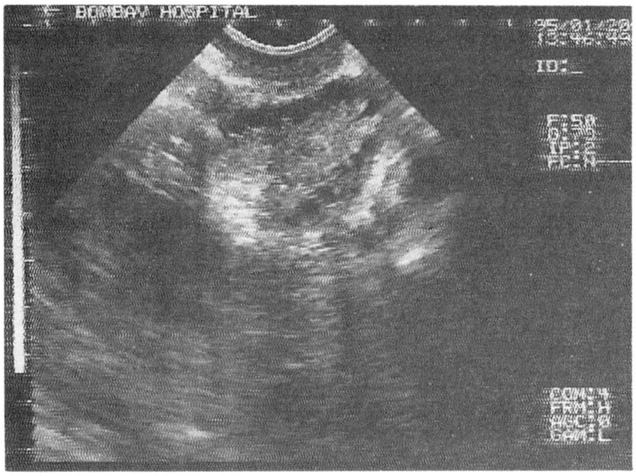

Fig. 8.1. A polycystic ovary seen here with microcysts distributed peripherally like a 'pearl necklace'.

route for the diagnosis of polycystic ovaries is particularly true when ovaries are deeply located within the pelvis/ in obese women in whom the progression of ultrasonography is impaired by the thickness of abdominal fat. Therefore, vaginal ultrasonography is particularly helpful in polycystic ovaries, which is more frequently associated with obesity than other anovulatory diseases.

The uterine corpus is an important structure in transvaginal sonography. It serves as a useful anatomical landmark for targeted organ imaging (Fig. 8.2). The endometrial appearance varies throughout the menstrual cycle. In the proliferative phase, the endometrial thickness increases and appears either iso- or hypoechoic. During the midcycle or periovulatory period, a characteristic trilaminar appearance occurs, while in the luteal phase, increasing tortuosity of the endometrial glands and glycogen accumulation result in a hyperechoic endometrium.

The thickness of the endometrium is measured from the echogenic interface of the junction of the endometrium and myometrium. This measurement represents two layers of endometrium. The hypoechogenic halo is

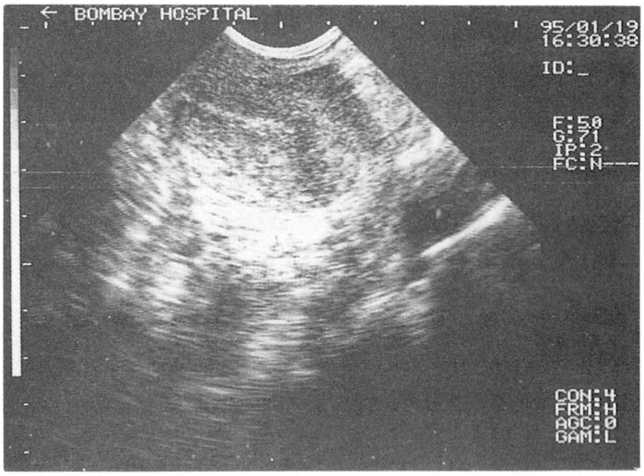

Fig. 8.2. A postmenstrual uterus seen in the sagittal plane.

not included in the measurement, as this represents the inner layers of compact and vascular myometrium. The average thickness of the endometrium is greater in the secretory phase (3.6 ± 4 mm) than in the proliferative phase (2.9 ± 1.0 mm)[9].

Transvaginal sonography may eliminate the subjectivity of the vaginal and rectal examination and provide a more objective assessment. The identification of ovaries through transvaginal sonography is made by using landmarks in association with the ovaries and identifying them; hence the need to have such landmarks (Figs. 8.3, 8.4 and 8.5). Many a time we find that patients come to us with corpus luteum cysts (Figs. 8.6 and 8.7) or retention cysts and transvaginal sonography helps us to tap these cysts and to effect ovulation.

In transvaginal egg pickup patients are more comfortable and the procedure is less painful. With transvaginal sonography the total number of follicles can be identi-

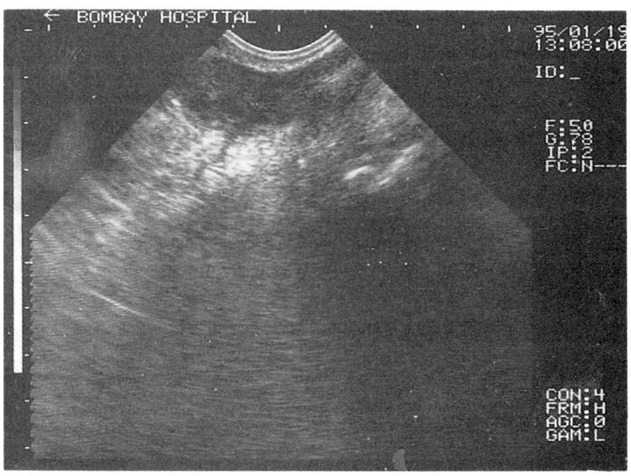

Fig. 8.3. An ovary with normal size, position and echotexture in the early proliferative phase.

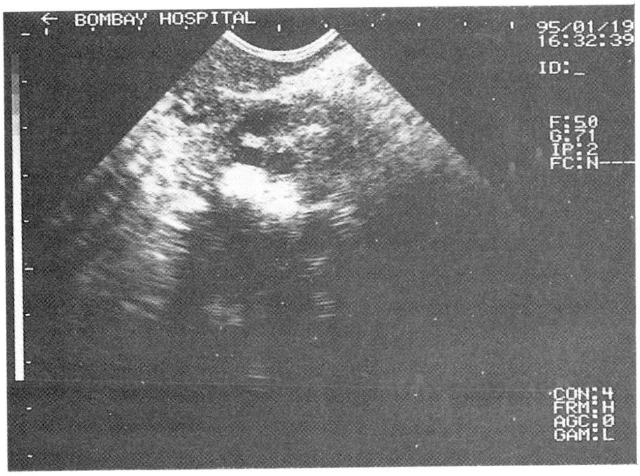

Fig. 8.4. An ovary with normal size, position and echotexture in the midproliferative phase.

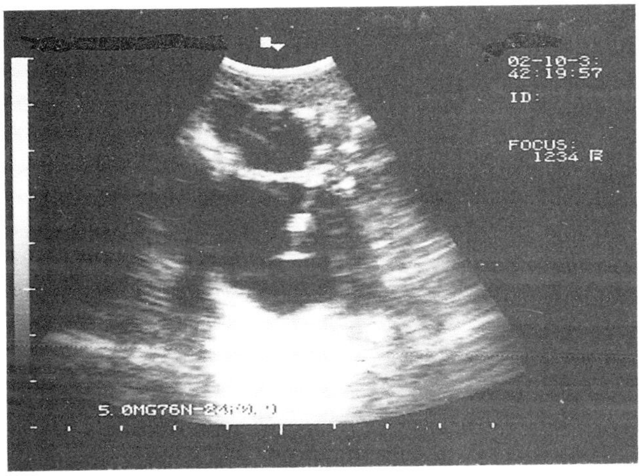

Fig. 8.5. A preovulatory follicle being aspirated in a spontaneous cycle.

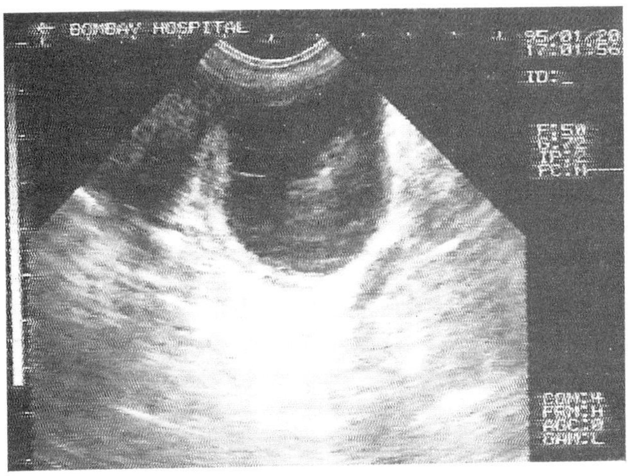

Fig. 8.6. Corpus luteum cyst.

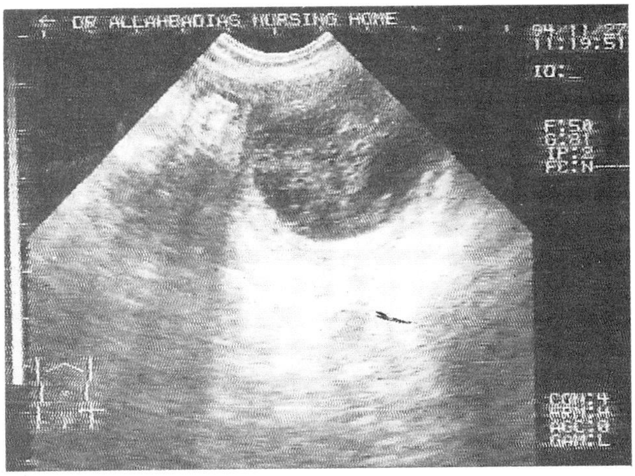

Fig. 8.7. Corpus luteum cyst.

fied and the eggs aspirated. Whereas in the laparoscopic technique, only surface follicles can be identified and therefore egg retrieval rate by the transvaginal approach is much better than through the abdominal approach.

Duplex Doppler sonography has assumed a useful role in vascular diagnosis. The vessel wall and lumen can be visualised with B-mode ultrasound while the Doppler mode permits flow to be demonstrated and measured. The Doppler effect describes the change in frequency of ultrasound scatter by red cells moving within a vessel.

If the ultrasound signal is transmitted along the axis of the vessel then the velocity of the red cells can be related to the shift in Doppler frequency. If the signal approaches the vessels at an angle, then the frequency of the reflected signal is reduced in proportion to the cosine of that angle. The signal reflected from a moving interface contains frequency as well as an amplitude information, therefore it is possible to process and display these data to show the relative motion of the target toward or away from the ultrasound transducer. Using transvaginal colour Doppler, Kurjak *et al.*[10] determined the normal flow pattern of pelvic vessels. Diastolic flow was absent or small and the value of the RI was > 0.5. In abnormal flow patterns, there was high diastolic flow and the RI was < 0.5. The same Doppler can be used to study the vascularity of the ovary and to avoid puncturing vessels at the time of egg retrieval, thus decreasing complications.

Conclusion

Transvaginal sonography has revolutionised our management of infertility particularly so in Assisted Reproductive

Techniques by way of increasing the efficacy of egg retrieval, bettering our understanding and in-depth knowledge of ovarian architecture and improving the pregnancy rate. In short transvaginal sonography is synonymous with Assisted Reproductive Techniques (ART).

REFERENCES

1. Tessler FN., Schiller VL, Perrella RR, Sutherland ML, Grant EG. Transabdominal versus endovaginal pelvic sonography : Prospective study. Radiology 1989; 170 : 553-6.
2. Edwards RG, Steptoe PC. Current status of in vitro fertilisation and implantation of human embryos. Lancet 1983; ii : 1265-6.
3. Royal College of Obs. & Gyn. : Gynaecological laparoscopy. In report on the confidential enquiry into Gynaecological Laparoscopy, (ed.) G Chamberlain, J Carron Brown. London, Royal College of Obs. & Gyn. 1978.
4. Lenz S, Lauritsen J, Kjellow M. Collection of human oocytes for in vitro fertilisation by ultrasonically-guided follicle puncture. Lancet 1981; i : 1163-4.
5. Lenz S, Lauritsen J. Ultrasonically-guided percutaneous aspiration of human follicles under local anesthesia : A new method of collecting oocytes for in vitro fertilisation. Fertil Steril 1982; 38 : 673-6.
6. Parsons J, Riddle A, Booker M, Sharma V, Goswamy R, Wilson L, Akkermans J, Whitehead M, Campbell S. Oocyte retrieval for in vitro fertilisation by ultrasonically-guided needle aspiration via the urethra. Lancet 1985; i : 1076-7.
7. Dellenbach P, Nisand I, Moreau L, Feger B, Plumere C, Gerlinger P, Brun B, Rumpler Y. Transvaginal sonographically controlled ovarian follicle puncture for egg retrieval. Lancet 1984; i : 1467-8.
8. Feichtinger W, Kemeter P. Transvaginal sector scan sonography for needle-guided transvaginal follicle aspiration and other applications in gynaecological routines and research. Fertil Steril 1986; 45 : 722-4.
9. Fleischer AC, Kalemeris GC, Entman SS. Sonographic depiction of the endometrium during normal cycles. Ultrasound Med Biol 1986; 12 : 271-7.
10. Kurjak A, Zalud I, Alfirevic Z, Jurkovic D. The assessment of abnormal pelvic blood flow by transvaginal color and pulsed Doppler. Ultrasound Med Bio 1990; 16 : 437-2.

CHAPTER

9

Saline Infusion Sonography of the Uterine Cavity

Gautam Allahbadia, Sadhana Desai and Ambrish Dalal

Introduction

Saline Infusion Sonography of the Uterine Cavity (SISCU) or sonographic uterine cavity visualisation by uterine cavity distension helps to distinguish true endometrial thickening from other intracavity pathological conditions, assuming the same sonographic appearance. This technique helps in tailoring the correct treatment in various conditions which manifest as abnormal uterine bleeding.

The importance of endovaginal sonography in diagnosing endometrial pathology, such as endometrial malignancy is well established and documented[1,2]. The indicators evaluated in sonography are endometrial thickness, tissue structure and invasion into myometrium and surrounding tissue. The presence of intrauterine fluid in such examinations is considered ominous and has been related to malignancy[3,4,5]. Endometrial cancer is the most prevalent malignancy in the genital tract[6]. It has been reported that the incidence of endometrial carcinoma in patients with postmenopausal bleeding ranged from 3.7% to 17.9%[7]. Ultrasonography allows the assessment of endometrial thickness and contour before endometrial sampling. Postmenopausal women should have virtually no endometrial tissue in vivo and inactive tissue on curettage. This should be represented by a thin echogenic line that results from the interface of two opposing sides of basal endometrium. Excessive thickness and irregular endometrial lining, as well as unusual patterns of endometrial structure demonstrated by sonography in postmenopausal women, are considered alerting signs, indicating further investigation[8]. The endometrial cavity is a potential space. Therefore, it is extremely difficult to distinguish between endometrial thickening and any intracavity growth by means of ultrasound.

Imaging of the uterine cavity has been traditionally accomplished either indirectly by HSG, or directly by hysteroscopy. These techniques are reportedly more accurate than ultrasound in the detection of intracavity abnormalities[9,10]. SISCU, was recently reported to improve uterine imaging and to assist in the diagnosis of various intrauterine abnormalities[11,12].

Technique

1 to 5 ml of sterile normal saline is injected through an infant feeding tube into the uterus to distend the endometrial cavity. As the sterile solution is injected, a continuous real time sonographic observation is done and images recorded on videotape as well as on a paper printer. The uterine wall is visualised with a 5.0 MHz transvaginal probe by zooming in on the endometrial lining. This technique allows detailed visualisation of the uterine cavity in both longitudinal and transverse planes. The endometrium is evaluated for the presence of polyps, submucous fibroids, intrauterine synechiae and foreign bodies. The concept for developing this technique at our Institute came when transvaginal ultrasound examination performed immediately after an HSG displayed a filling defect of the uterine cavity. On ultrasound, residual radiographic contrast material clearly outlined a hyperechoic endometrial polyp and localised its stalk, differentiating the filling defect from a submucous myoma. The principal author had also relevant experience in developing the "Sion Test" for transvaginal USG-aided tubal patency assessment (Fig. 9.1)[13] and the "Sion Procedure" which helps in demonstrating the peritubal environment (Fig. 9.2)[14]. Thereafter, we intentionally used fluid as intrauterine sonographic contrast material in subsequent suspected cases of uterine polyps (Fig. 9.3) or submucous myomas (Figs. 9.4 and 9.5). Transvaginal sonographic

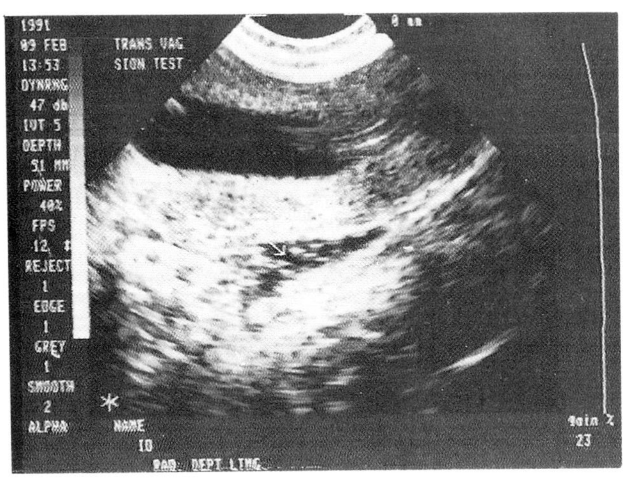

Fig. 9.1. The Sion Test. Plate shows the inflated Foley bulb within the uterine cavity pictured in a sagittal plane. Arrow points to the saline collection in the pouch of Douglas at the end of the test with obvious patency of at least one tube.

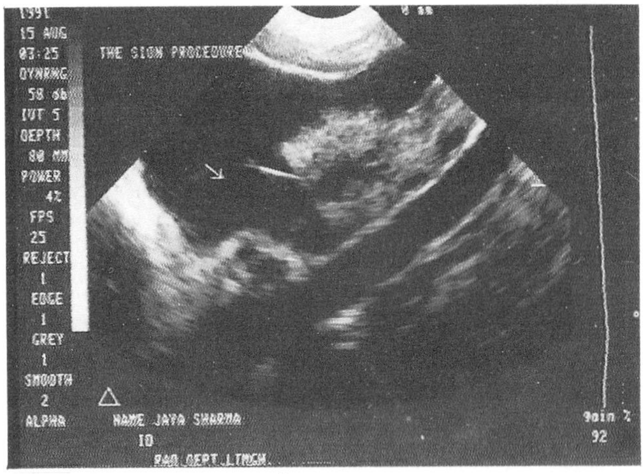

Fig. 9.2. The Sion Procedure. The fimbrial end of the tube seen clearly in this plate. Arrow points to a filmy perifimbrial adhesion.

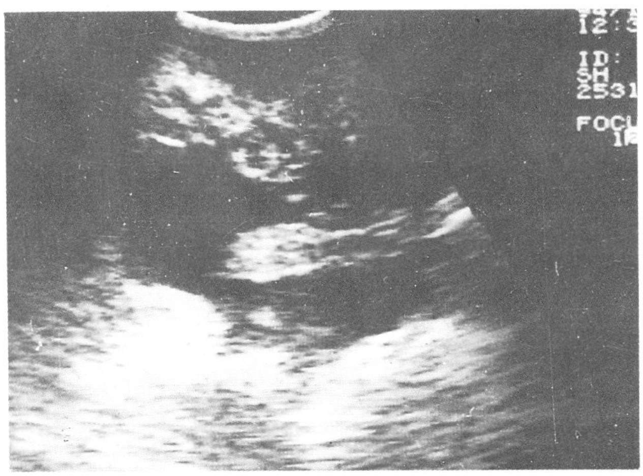

Fig. 9.3. SISCU. Plate shows an intrauterine endometrial polyp.

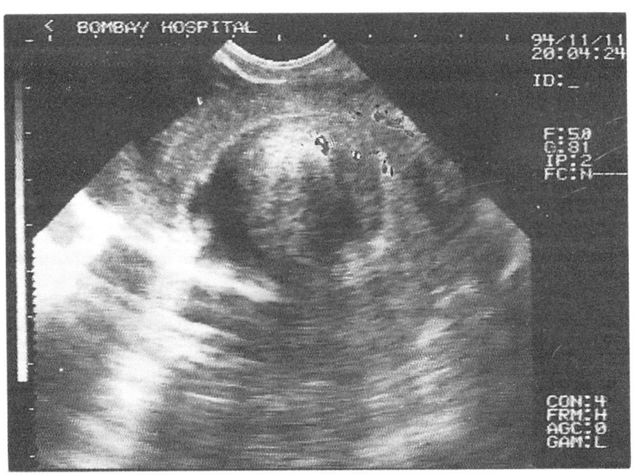

Fig. 9.4. SISCU. Plate shows a large submucous fibroid.

Fig. 9.5. Same fibroid specimen as in Fig. 9.4 after hysteroscopic removal.

screening, particularly in the late proliferative phase, should suggest the presence of most polyps as hyperechoic densities within the endometrial stripe (Fig. 9.6).

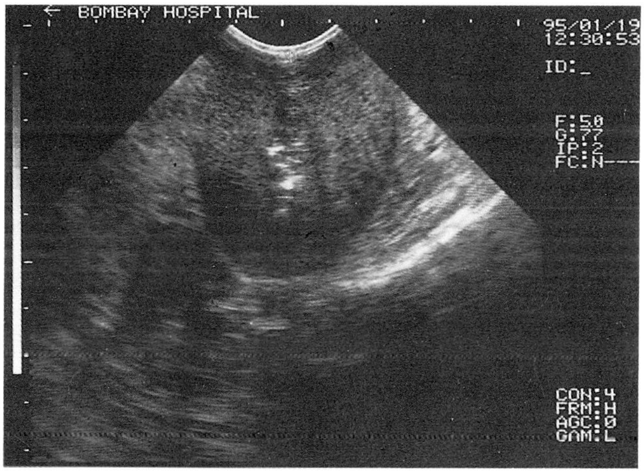

Fig. 9.6. TVS picture of an endometrial polyp in the proliferative phase without saline enhancement.

A densely hyperechoic, secretory lining tends to obscure visualisation. Although little has been accomplished in the incidental diagnosis of polyps during the last 20 years, SISCU can identify and localise suspected uterine polyps readily and inexpensively.

Discussion

In the beginning of 1994 we started performing SISCU in all patients posted for a diagnostic or therapeutic hysteroscopy. Our aim was to evaluate the benefits or pitfalls of SISCU as compared to TVS in the diagnosis of uterine cavity defects. The uterine cavity in each case was examined by TVS, SISCU and hysteroscopy in that order. Our impression was similar to other investigators[15,16] in that SISCU is superior to TVS in evaluating intrauterine pathology and should be considered a valuable advance in the evaluation of infertility and abnormal uterine bleeding. French investigators[17] evaluated the potential improvement of endovaginal ultrasound by injection of Echovist (Schering, Germany), a contrast product into the uterine cavity. They reported that the information obtained by SISCU was similar with those of HSG or hysteroscopy. The diagnosis of adenomyosis is especially evident with this new examination. The value of SISCU on middle-aged women with metorrhagia was evaluated by Mocsary *et al.*[18] along with a comparison of the histopathology. A strong positive correlation was found between positive histological findings and 3-D ultrasound technique was assessed in 1146 asymptomatic Austrian menopausal women in a prospective study[19]. The study proved that SISCU and/or 3-D ultrasound provides information on the exact location of any type of endometrial lesions.

There are limitations of current methods of evaluating the endometrial cavity, and a thickened endometrium visualised on routine TVS should always be investigated by the further instillation of normal saline into the uterine cavity (SISCU). The technique of saline instillation is simple, and impressive images are obtained (Figs. 9.7 to 9.13). We believe that this procedure should be a routine part of the ultrasound assessment of the uterus before any more invasive method is embarked upon as it will reveal both polyps and irregularities of the endometrial cavity. It can be particularly useful when the endometrial cavity is hard

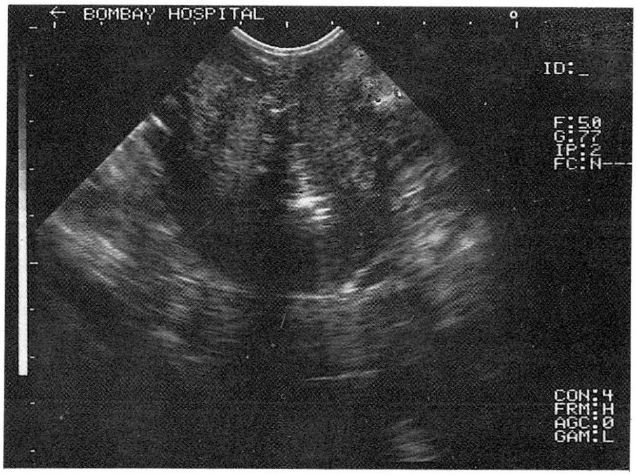

Fig. 9.7. SISCU. An embedded IUCD seen in the uterine cavity.

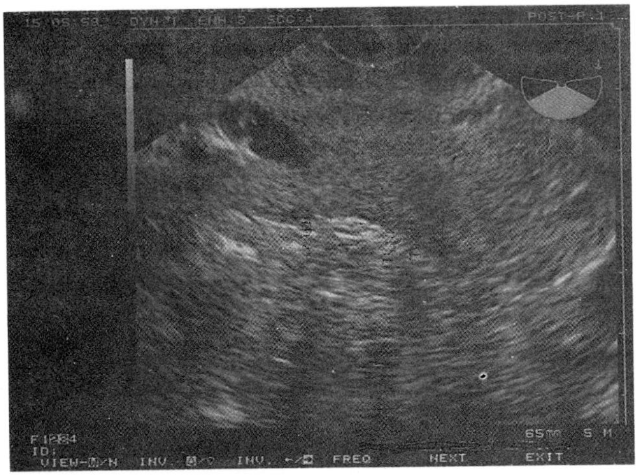

Fig. 9.8. SISCU. A bicornuate uterus with a normal uterine cavity visualised in the right horn.

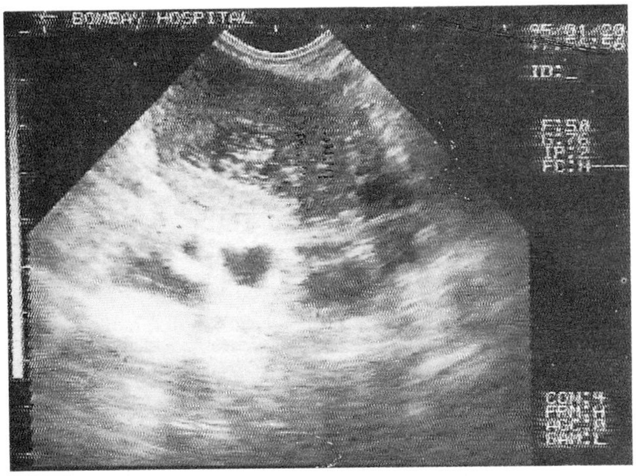

Fig. 9.9. SISCU. The turbulence of saline pictured as it enter the uterine cavity and separates the apposing endometrial lining.

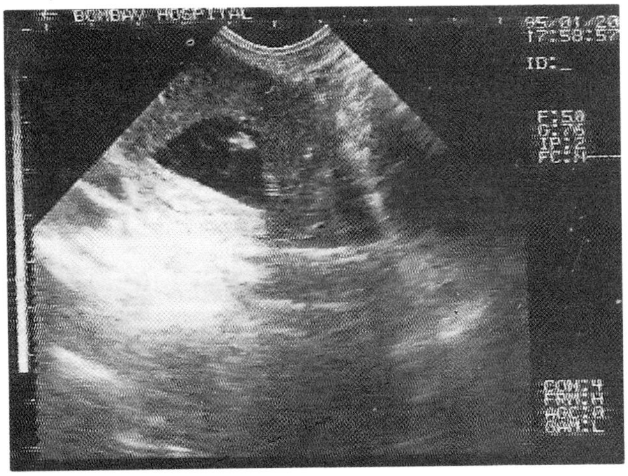

Fig. 9.10. SISCU. A small endometrial polyp seen clearly on the anterior margin.

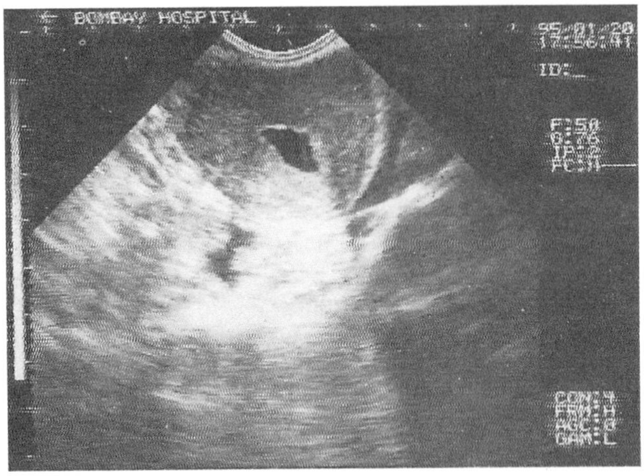

Fig. 9.11. SISCU. A normal postmenopausal cavity in a case with postmenopausal bleeding.

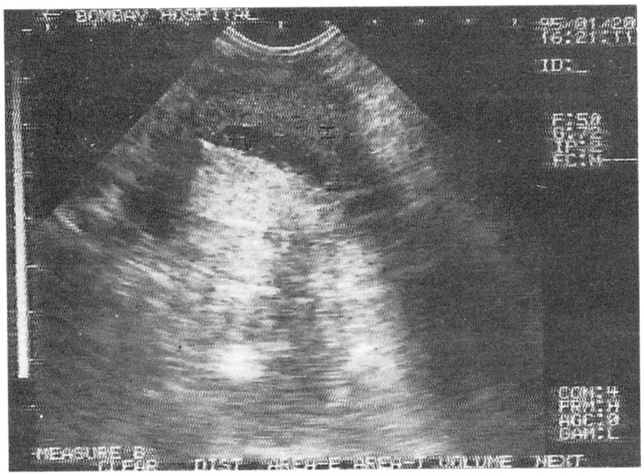

Fig. 9.12. SISCU. Normal uterine cavity in an infertile patient.

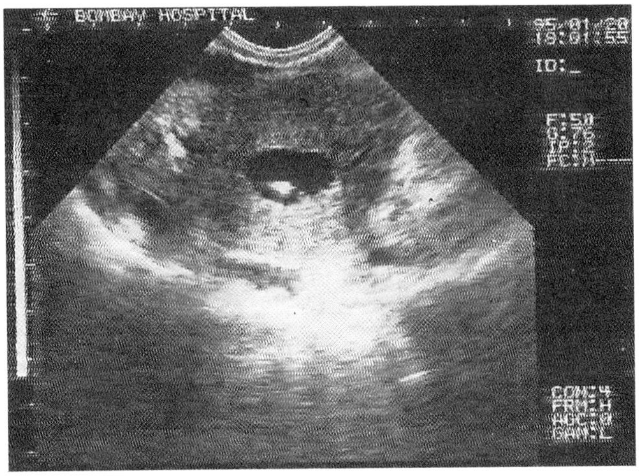

Fig. 9.13. SISCU. Small endometrial polyp seen clearly on the posterior surface of the cavity.

to visualise on initial B-mode ultrasonography. Addition of colour Doppler to SISCU further enhances the diagnostic capabilities of the vaginal probe and can help in planning out the therapeutic aspects of the pathology (Fig. 9.14 – Plate 3).

REFERENCES

1. Osmers R, Volksen M, Schauer A. Vaginosonography for early detection of endometrial carcinoma? Lancet 1990; 335 : 1569-71.
2. Goldstein SR, Natchigall M, Synder JR. Endometrial assessment by TVS before endometrial sampling in patients with postmenopausal bleeding. Am J Obstet Gynecol 1990; 163 : 119-23.
3. Brechenridge JW, Kurtz AB, Ritchie WGM, Macht EL. Postmenopausal uterine fluid collection indicator of carcinoma. Am J Radiol 1982; 139 : 529-34.
4. Laing FC, Filly RA, Marks WM, Brown TW. Ultrasonic demonstration of endometrial fluid collections unassociated with pregnancy. Radiology 1980; 137 : 471-4.
5. McCarthy KA, Hall DA, Kopans DB, Swann CA. Postmenopausal fluid collections : always an indicator of malignancy? J Ultrasound Med 1986; 5 : 647-9.
6. Silverberg E, Lubera J. Cancer Statistics. Cancer J Clin 1987; 39 : 3-10.
7. Merril JA. Management of postmenopausal bleeding. Clin Obstet Gynecol 1981; 24 : 285-8.
8. Granberg S, Wikland M, Karlsson B, Norstrom A, Friberg L. Endometrial thickness as measured by TVS for identifying endometrial abnormality. Am J Obstet Gynecol 1991; 164 : 47-52.
9. Siegler AM. Hysterosalpingography. Fertil Steril 1983; 40 : 139-42.
10. Wamstekar K. Hysteroscopy in the management of abnormal uterine bleeding in 199 patients. *In* Siegler AM and Lindemann HJ (eds) Hysteroscopy, Principles & Practice, Philadelphia, Lippincott, 1984.
11. Randolph JR, Ying MK, Maier DB, Schmidt ML. Comparison of real-time USG, HSG and laparoscopy/hysteroscopy in the evaluation of uterine abnormalities and tubal patency. Fertil Steril 1986; 46 : 828-32.
12. Parsons AK, Lense JJ. Sonohysterography for endometrial abnormalities : preliminary results. J Clin Ultrasound. 1993; 21 : 87-95.
13. Allahbadia GN, Nalawade YV, Patkar VD, Niyogi GM, Shah PK. The Sion Test. Aust NZ J Obstet Gynaecol 1992; 32 : 67-70.
14. Allahbadia GN, G, Nalawade Y, Panjwani M, Vaidya P, Merchant S. The Sion Procedure. J Obstet Gynaecol India 1992; 42 : 814-18.
15. Sadek A, Schitz HA, Istre O. The advantage of fluid scanning prior to hysteroscopy for menometorrhagia. Ultrasound Obstet Gynecol 1994; 4 : 84.
16. Rudigoz RC, Placenza JS, Gaucherand P. Study of uterine cavity by hysterosonography with saline solution safety and efficiency : 153 cases. Ultrasound Obstet Gynecol 1994; 4 : 100.
17. Favre R, Roy C. Potential use of echohysterography for uterine cavity abnormalities. Ultrasound Obstet Gynecol 1994; 4 : 89.
18. Mocsary P, Fabian A, Orosz L. The value of hysterosonography in middle-aged women with metorrhagia. Ultrasound Obstet Gynecol 1994; 4 : 79.
19. Chan L, Salameh WA, Mikola G, Potsch B. Ultrasound screening for endometrial pathology in the asymptomatic menopausal women : value of saline enhancement and 3-D ultrasound technique. Ultrasound Obstet Gynecol 1994; 4 : 150.

CHAPTER

10

Role of Transvaginal Sonography for Embryo Transfer

Lakshmi Singh, Sudeep Banerjee and Rajeshwar Upadhyay

Ultrasound-guided embryo transfer (ET) was performed in 17 patients and the technical and statistical advantages over the conventional technique of blind ET was compared to a control group of 36 patients. Though the study is too small to draw conclusions, yet it clearly indicates the advantages of the ultrasound-guided ET over the conventional procedure.

Introduction

Leeton (1984)[1] has attributed most of the human in vitro fertilization (IVF) failures to the ET procedure. Though, there are studies suggesting that the high failure rate may be due to the poor quality of the embryo[2] or uterine receptivity, yet there has hardly been many attempts made to modify the conventional technique.

Ultrasound (US), though a key component of all major IVF-ET programmes, has not yet found much recognition in the ET procedure. US-guided transfundal ET technique was first described by Lenz[3] and as per his reports, the technique was abandoned after 10 procedures failed to achieve any pregnancy. The idea of US-guided ET was promulgated by Strickler *et al.* in 1985[4] and Leong *et al.* in 1986[5]. After the advent of high frequency US with transvaginal US producing better resolution, transvaginal US-guided ET was done by Hurley *et al.*[6] in 1991 with very encouraging results.

A similar study was conducted by our unit to assess the efficacy of the procedure as described by Hurley *et al.*

The major aims of the study were :

1. To assess the precision of the positioning of the embryo transfer catheter in the uterus by blind clinical feel.
2. To observe if there was any significant variation between the pregnancy rates (PR) in the two procedures.
3. To evaluate the feasibility of the ultrasound-guided ET procedure.
4. To assess any other advantage or disadvantage in the ultrasound-guided ET procedure.

Materials and methods

53 ET procedures were done between March, 1993 and June 1994; of which 17 ET procedures were done under transvaginal US-guidance. The patients were randomly selected and no attempt was made to control the two groups for the variables, as it was found impractical.

Transfer technique

The pelvis was ultrasonographically assessed using the transvaginal US probe for its axis, and the degree of flexion of the uterus and the uterine length. The probe was then removed and a bivalve speculum was inserted, exposing the cervix. The cervix and the vagina was washed using Ham's F-10 culture medium. The outer cannula of the transfer catheter (Wallace) was inserted through the external cervical os. The inner cannula was then inserted through the internal cervical os by clinical feel, till it touched the fundus. The speculum was then removed and the transvaginal probe was inserted. The ET cannula was identified and moved approximately 1 cm away from the fundus. The embryos were now transferred, suspended in 30 μl of culture medium. Transfer was observed on the US monitor, and the embryos were identified by the agitation (bright echogenic spots) caused on the US monitor by the inter-embryonal air bubbles (Figs. 10.1 and 10.2).

ET in the control group was done by the conventional technique as described by Leeton[7]. No backflow of the embryos was observed in any of the cases as described by Leong *et al.*[5]

The catheter was checked microscopically to ensure that no embryos remained inside the catheter. The patient was then returned to the ward.

Results

Of the 17 patients in whom US-guided ET was attempted 6 patients (23.52%) conceived, of which 2 have aborted in the first trimester, as compared to 16 conceptions achieved out of the 36 ETs done by the conventional method. Of these 9 aborted in the first trimester and 2 have delivered and 5 are continuing with their pregnancy (19.44%).

The transfer catheter was not visualised in the first 2 cases on the US monitor. The failure could be attributed to the uterine axis lying parallel to the US beam. However, the catheter was clearly seen in all the subsequent transfers. We did not observe any discrepancy between the blind clinical positioning of the transfer cannula and then its confirmation by US, as described by Hurley *et al.*[6].

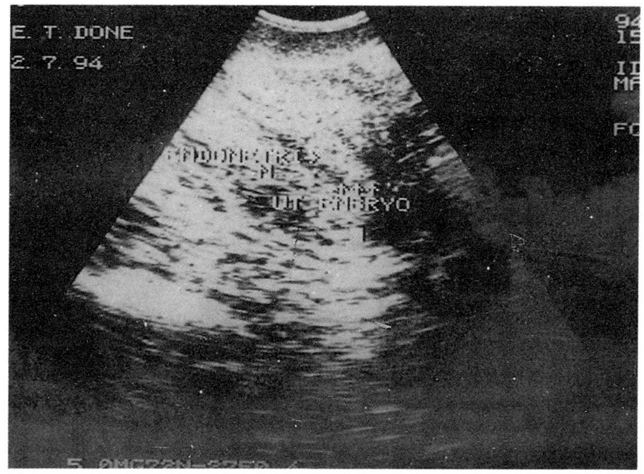

Fig. 10.1. US-guided ET catheter within the uterine cavity.

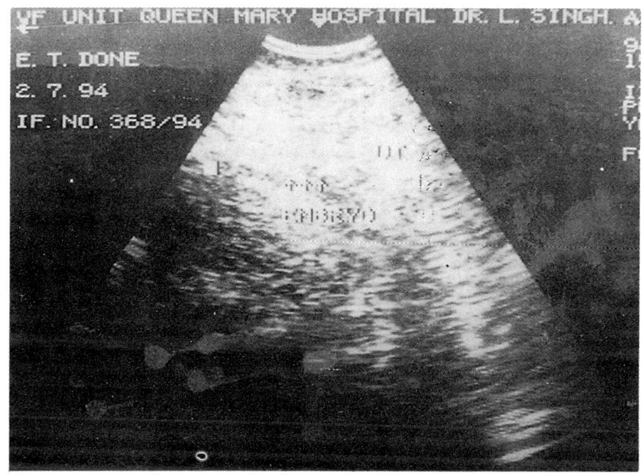

Fig. 10.2. Post-ET sonogram.

The pregnancy rate (PR) achieved in the control group during our study was 19.44% (7 out of 36) as compared to the US-guided transfer group who achieved a pregnancy rate of 22.52% (4 out of 17).

Discussion

The following conclusive observations were made by our study :

1. That the clinical assessment of the positioning of the transfer catheter has been fairly accurate.
2. That there was a significant increase in the PR by the US-guided embryo transfer (ET) group.
3. That the US-guided ET transfer is a feasible procedure and does not cause undue inconvenience to the clinician or the patient.
4. There may be a hypothetical disadvantage that by putting the transvaginal probe during ET, the

embryos might be dislodged from their original position in the uterine cavity.

5. Visualisation of the transfer process on the US monitor by the patients resulted in a reduced anxiety level in the patients from the US-guided ET group as compared to the control group.

However, this study is too small and further research is required to conclusively prove the advantage.

REFERENCES

1. Leeton J. Embryo transfer. In : In vitro fertilization and embryo transfer. Edited by A. Tronson. Edinburg, Churchill Livingstone, 1984, p. 197.
2. Speirs AJ. Changing the face of infertility. Am J Obs Gyn; 158 : 1390, 1988.
3. Lenz S, Leeton J, Rogers P, Trounson A. Transfundal transfer of embryos using ultrasound. J In Vitro Fert Embryo Transfer; 4 : 13, 1987.
4. Strickler R, Christianson C, Crane J, Curato A, Knight A, Yang V. Ultrasound guidance for embryo transfer. Fertil Steril; 38 : 156, 1982.
5. Leong M, Leung C, Tucker M, Wong C, Chan H. Ultrasound assisted embryo transfer. J In Vitro Fert Embryo Transfer; 3 : 383, 1986.
6. Hurley VA, Osborn JC, Leoni MA, Leeton J. Ultrasound-guided embryo transfer : a controlled trial. Fertil Steril; 55 : 559, 1991.
7. Leeton K, Trounson A, Jessup D, Wood C. The technique for human embryo transfer. Fertil Steril; 38 : 156, 1982.

CHAPTER

11

Vaginosonographic Salpingocentesis for Treatment of Ectopic Pregnancy

Gautam Allahbadia, Sadhana Desai and Ambrish Dalal

Introduction

Medical management of ectopic pregnancy (EP) was first proposed in 1982[1]. Several studies have been performed using parenteral methotrexate (MTX)[2-5], a cytostatic agent with a proven major antitrophoblastic activity. Recent advances in the diagnosis of pregnancy, using high resolution transvaginal sonography (TVS) and the beta subunit of hCG, provide a more accurate early diagnosis of ectopic pregnancy[6]. The addition of colour flow Doppler into the vaginal probes have further enhanced the process of diagnosis of this pathological condition (Figs. 11.1 to 11.3 – Plate 3, and 11.4 – Plate 4). MTX can be injected directly into the ectopic sac under vaginosonographic guidance, using the procedure originally described for oocyte collection in IVF programmes[7]. With TVS, the ectopic sac can now be seen in an estimated 70% of cases[8], allowing for local treatment. In an in vivo study of gravid rat oviducts injected with MTX versus normal saline solution, no toxicity of MTX was observed on the female reproductive tract[9]. The benefits of local versus parenteral MTX administration are a decrease in the systemic side-effects[10] and an increase in the local antitrophoblastic effect[11].

Procedure

After an informed consent, the patient is given general anaesthesia. With the patient in a lithotomy position, a customised 17 gauge needle is inserted into the needle guide, through the vaginal fornix, and up to the ectopic sac. Then a co-axial 21 gauge needle is passed through this first needle into the ectopic sac under TVS control (Figs. 11.5 and 11.6 – both on Plate 4). Serohematinic material is aspirated so that the sac collapses. If the cardiac flicker is present, 0.5 to 1.0 ml of KCl is injected in the region of the cardiac flicker or into the yolk sac if seen clearly and the disappearance of the heart beats is observed under TVS control. Then, a single 50 mg dose of MTX is injected into the sac. A check scan is performed to evaluate for any collection or persistence of the cardiac flicker (Figs. 11.7 to 11.9 – all on Plate 4, and 11.10 – Plate 5). Follow-up includes (1) serial β-hCG assays on day 1, 2, 5, 10 and 15 after treatment; and (2) clinical and TVS evaluation on days 5, 10 and 15. The patient is admitted and closely monitored until the dissolution of serum β-hCG to below 10 mIU/ml. The patient undergoes a transvaginal colour Doppler examination by one of the senior authors (AKD) about 48 hours after the procedure or, if required, earlier. This helps in charting the disappearance of peritrophoblastic flow and observing the well-being of the affected tube. Every case is followed up in an individualised fashion and not according to a fixed protocol. The follow-up guidelines mentioned above are gross guiding principles we follow to ensure that there is an uneventful decay of the serum β-hCG. An HSG is asked for at the end of 8-12 weeks after β-hCG levels are normal to evaluate the ipsilateral tubal function.

Discussion

The increasing frequency of diagnosing early undisturbed tubal pregnancy was a stimulus to adopt different lines of conservative treatment for this condition. Recent reviews have suggested that the therapeutic approach to ectopic pregnancy is changing as different clinical patterns of this disease are recognised. If a non-bleeding, unruptured tubal gestation with falling levels of β-hCG and no demonstrable fetal heart activity is diagnosed, it may need only careful observation or, at the most, systemic administration of MTX. Systemic administration of MTX was highly successful in the treatment of some cases of ectopic pregnancy; however, it has the drawback of toxic side effects[12]. Our results[12] indicate that local TVS-guided injection of MTX is effective in the majority of unruptured tubal gestations with rising β-hCG titres. It is a non-surgical alternative to classical and laparoscopic management that can be performed on stable patients with an early unruptured ectopic pregnancy. Comparison of various non-surgical procedures is indicative only, since no consensus yet exists for inclusion of patients. We believe that a definite diagnosis of tubal pregnancy can be reached in the majority of cases without resorting to laparoscopy. Furthermore, spontaneous resolution of ectopic pregnancy may have occurred in some cases without medical treatment[13].

Various protocols of non-surgical management of ectopic pregnancy have been reported[14]. Drugs with an indirect antitrophoblastic effect, including RU-486[15] and prostaglandins[16], administered systemically, have given disappointing results. The direct antitrophoblastic effect of MTX has been previously demonstrated in experimental studies[10]. A major disadvantage of parenteral MTX is the risk of side-effects[2]. Dermatitis, alopecia, stomatitis, pleuritis, vomiting, diarrhoea, and hepatic or bone marrow toxicity have been observed in up to 24% of cases[2]. In our experience with local MTX administration[12], we observed no systemic side-effects. Further trials are needed to determine the best indications for non-surgical management of ectopic pregnancy. A ruptured tube or significant hemoperitoneum are obvious contraindications. However, we have observed no relationship between gestational age, size of the adnexal mass, or initial β-hCG level and the outcome after MTX injection. The impact of local methotrexate on tubal patency and function is under evaluation. Avoiding a tuboperitoneal scar may be of benefit. However, potential disadvantages are (1) a delay in the termination of trophoblastic activity; (2) partial tubal obstruction by necrotic trophoblastic remnants; and (3) direct toxicity on the tube itself. Delayed HSG and laparoscopy may be considered in patients with infertility after successful conservative management. In a pregnant rat model, there was no observed toxicity on the genital tract mucosa with a local MTX injection[9]. However, MTX is known to produce inflammation when administered into serosae. Therefore, injection into the gestational sac must be carefully monitored to avoid leakage into the peritoneal cavity.

Tubal pregnancy itself can impair subsequent tubal patency and fertility. Tube blockage has been observed in 25-30% of patients after ectopic pregnancy, which did not require intervention[17,18], although Carp *et al.*[19] found preserved tubal patency in all of five patients who underwent hysterosalpingography after observation until tubal abortion or resorption occurred without other treatment. These observations are probably explained by tubal abortion or resorption of a "missed" ectopic gestation with recanalisation of the affected tube. After conservative surgery for tubal pregnancy, tubal patency is found in 46-60% of patients[20].

Conclusion

In the future the treatment of ectopic pregnancy may fit into one of the following categories :

1. The leaking (Fig. 11.11 – Plate 5) or ruptured or secondary abdominal pregnancy will still require laparotomy.
2. The unruptured, but missed, ectopic pregnancy with decreasing levels of β-hCG may be safely followed by TVS. Systemically or locally (by

TVS) injected MTX can be an alternative in these patients.

3. Selected early ectopic pregnancies with live conceptuses may be treated by the transvaginally performed puncture procedure as described above. Early TVS examinations of the high risk population to identify and classify ectopic gestation are advisable, so the best therapeutic approach can be selected. The transvaginally performed, sonographically directed puncture procedure represents an important addition to the treatment of this widespread complication.

REFERENCES

1. Tanaka T, Hayashi H, Kutsukawa T, Fujimoto S, Ichinoe K. Treatment of interstitial ectopic pregnancy with Methotrexate : report of a successful case. Fertil Steril 1982; 37 : 851-5.
2. Ory SJ, Villanueva AL, Sand PK, Tamura RK. Conservative management of ectopic pregnancy with methotrexate. Am J Obstet Gynecol 1986; 154 : 1299-1301.
3. Rodi IA, Sauer MV, Gorill MJ. The medical treatment of unruptured ectopic pregnancy with methotrexate and citrovorum factor preliminary experience. Fertil Steril 1986; 46 : 811-6.
4. Sauer MV, Gorill MJ, Rodi IA, Yeko TR, Greenberg LH. Nonsurgical management of ectopic pregnancy : an extended trial. Fertil Steril 1987; 48 : 752-6.
5. Stovall TG, Ling FW, Buster JE. Outpatient chemotherapy of unruptured ectopic pregnancy. Fertil Steril 1989; 51 : 435-6.
6. Fossum GT, Davajan V, Kletzky OA. Early detection of pregnancy with TVS. Fertil Steril 1988; 49 : 788-800.
7. Goldstein SR, Synder JR, Watson C, Danon M. Very early pregnancy detection with endovaginal ultrasound. Obstet Gynecol 1988; 72 : 200-204.
8. Feichtinger W, Kemeter P. Conservative treatment of ectopic pregnancy by transvaginal aspiration under sonographic control and methotrexate injection. Lancet 1987; 1 : 381-3.
9. Perrotez B, Menard A, Madelenat P. Effets tissulaires de l'injection in situ de methotrexate chez la rate gravide. Gynecologie. 1994; 56 : 752-9.
10. Hans LCF, van Kessel PH, Kock HCLV. Treatment of ectopic pregnancy with methotrexate. Eur J Obstet Gynaecol Reprod Biol 1987; 24 : 63-6.
11. Sand PK, Subblefield PA, Ory JS. Methotrexate inhibition of normal trophoblasts in vitro. Am J Obstet Gynecol 1986; 155 : 324-7.
12. Desai SK, Allahbadia GN, Dalal AK. Conservative management of tubal pregnancy. *In* Desai SK and Allahbadia GN (eds), Infertility & Transvaginal Sonography : Current Concepts. Jaypee Brothers Medical Publishers, New Delhi, 1994.
13. Dericks-Tan JSE, Scholz C, Taubert HD. Spontaneous recovery of ectopic pregnancy : a preliminary report. Eur J Obstet Gynaecol Reprod Biol 1987; 25 : 181-4.
14. Ory SJ. Nonsurgical treatment of ectopic pregnancy. Fertil Steril 1986; 46 : 767-9.
15. Kenigsberg D, Porte J, Hull M, Spitz IM. Medical treatment of residual ectopic pregnancy : Ru-486 and methotrexate. Fertil Steril 1987; 47 : 702-4.
16. Lindblom B, Kallfelt B, Hahlin M, Hamberger L. Local prostaglandin f2 alpha injection for termination of ectopic pregnancy. Lancet 1987; 1 : 776-8.
17. Ichinoe K, Wake N, Shinkai N. Nonsurgical therapy to preserve oviduct function in patients with tubal pregnancies. Am J Obstet Gynecol 1987; 156 : 484-7.
18. Garcia AJ, Aubert JM, Sama J. Expectant management of presumed ectopic pregnancies. Fertil Steril 1987; 48 : 395-400.
19. Carp HJA, Sen MD, Oeisner G. Fertility after non-surgical treatment of ectopic pregnancy. J Reprod Med 1985; 31 : 119-22.
20. Mitchell DE, McSwain HF, McCarthy JA, Peterson HB. Hysterosalpingographic evaluation of tubal patency after ectopic pregnancy. Am J Obstet Gynecol 1987; 157 : 618-21.

CHAPTER

12

Endoscopy and Endosonography

R. Rajan

By modern standards of gynaecological practice, clinical examination is too insufficient a method of pelvic diagnosis, which offers nothing more than basic information, and hence not preferred except in situations of huge pelvic masses such as big uterine myomas or huge ovarian tumors. On the contrary laparotomy is too invasive an approach which is not only obsolete as a diagnostic measure, but also is being fast replaced by endoscopic surgery as a therapeutic remedy. In between these two unacceptable extremes diagnostic endoscopies enjoy an enviable role, particularly when there are no big pelvic masses or when negative pelvic findings need to be confirmed such as in infertility practice. Laparoscopic and hysteroscopic diagnoses remain the most popular and ultimate in gynaecological diagnosis, so much so, it is not surprising that a gynaecological diagnosis is considered far from complete without a recourse to endoscopy.

With the current and promising developments in gynaecological sonography, particularly endopelvic sonography, a new dimension is added to pelvic diagnosis, and the compelling role of endoscopy is being quite often challenged. Apart from being a noninvasive and nonincisional diagnostic method endovaginal sonography provides for a panoramic cross-sectional study of the pelvic organs in which respect endoscopies are inferior. A close range inspection of the pelvic organs which provides for magnification with high resolution is the hallmark of endovaginal sonographic imaging. While this technology is certainly inferior to laparoscopy for diagnosis of peritoneal surface pathology; by various indirect strategies these problems are circumvented to a considerable extent. It is quite encouraging that pelvic diagnosis is being refined day by day without a recourse to endoscopic measures, and the latter is assigned a more meaningful role of being consigned to the therapeutic armamentarium. It is quite surprising that over a few minutes of medical time and that too in a most unassuming fashion a wealth of meaningful information

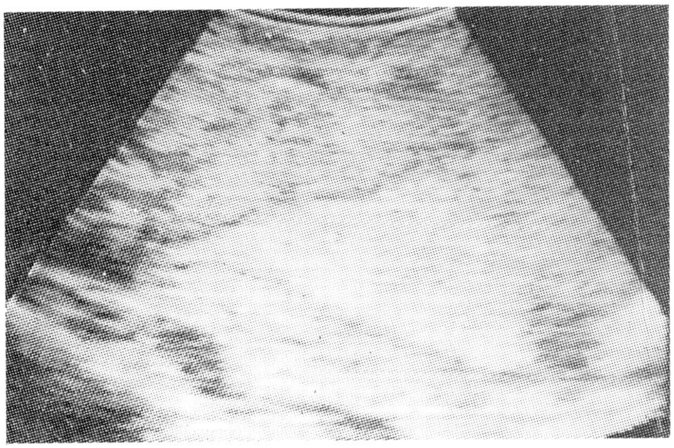

Fig. 12.1. Semicoronal section of uterus. The endometrium is imaged as a triangular structure, with both tubo-cornual regions identified. The proximal intramural tubal lumen is identified clearly on the left side.

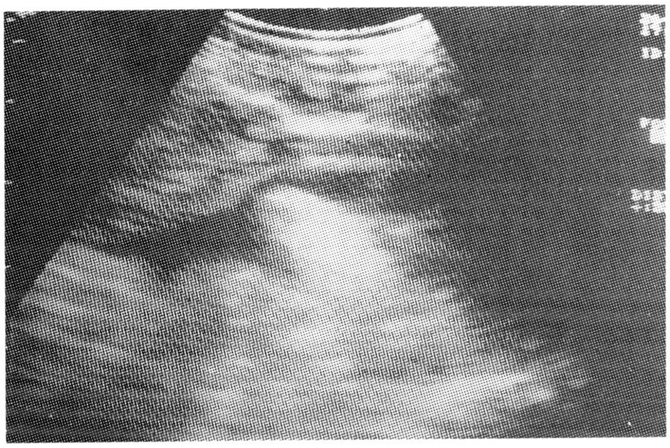

Fig. 12.2. The round ligament. The round ligament can be imaged as a cord-like structure seen extending from the uterus. The peritoneal fluid can be seen as an echo-free area surrounding the round ligament, and the intestines are imaged as echo-dense areas in the periphery.

is gathered by endopelvic sonography. At the first visit itself the patient is given a clear picture of the state of her pelvic organs, and thus the counselling becomes very effective.

Normal pelvic organs

Since the advent of endovaginal sonography, I feel that there is only very limited, if not negligible, diagnostic role for laparo/hysteroscopy in gynaecological practice, particularly the low risk subjects. The most popular indication for endoscopic diagnosis was to negate a pelvic pathology in an infertile subject. It is well recognised that the pelvic organs prove normal at endoscopy in 80 to 90% of infertile couples. I consider the pelvic organs normal at endovaginal sonography

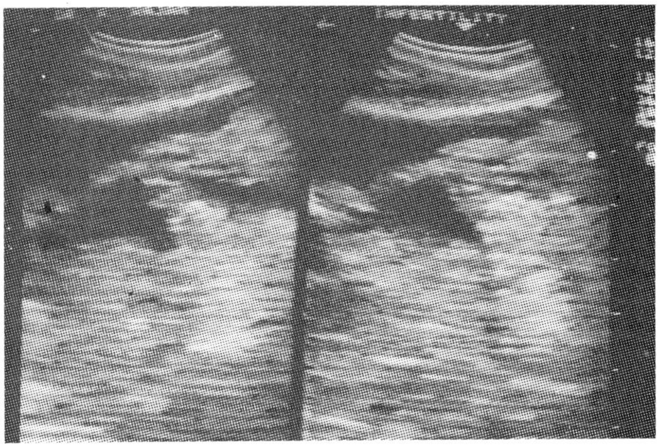

Fig. 12.3. Proximal fallopian tubal segment. The narrow echogenic strip seen surrounded by the echo-free fluid compartment is the proximal tubal segment which extends from the uterine cornua. Thee intestines are seen in the periphery as echogenic areas.

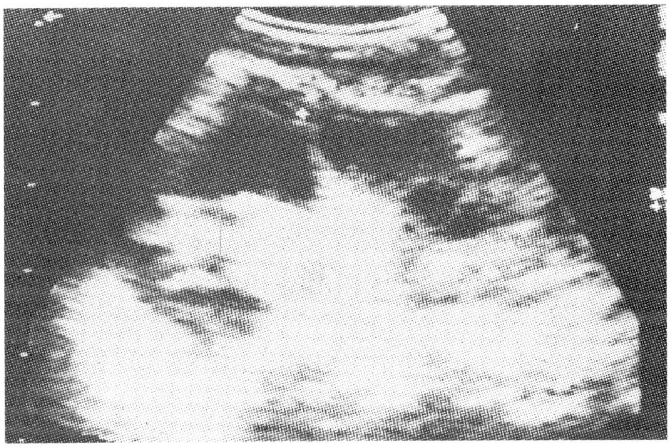

Fig. 12.4. Distal fallopian tubal segment. At sonosalpingography, following injection of around 250 ml of Ringer's lactate solution the tubal fimbria and ampulla remain clearly imaged. The fimbrial projections can be precisely seen and thus peritubal adhesions are excluded. The small cystic structure seen is the Morgagnian hydatid.

and negate a primary role for endoscopic diagnosis if the following criteria are satisfied :

1. The uterus and ovaries are imaged easily without any discomfort for the patient, and they appear normal in size and shape.
2. Free gliding of the pelvic organs by the endovaginal probe, and cradling of these organs, particularly the ovaries by the peristalsing intestines, whereby significant pelvic adhesions are excluded.
3. Cross-sectional studies of the cervix, cervical canal, endometrium, myometrium, and ovaries proving normal. The diagnostic accuracy of this

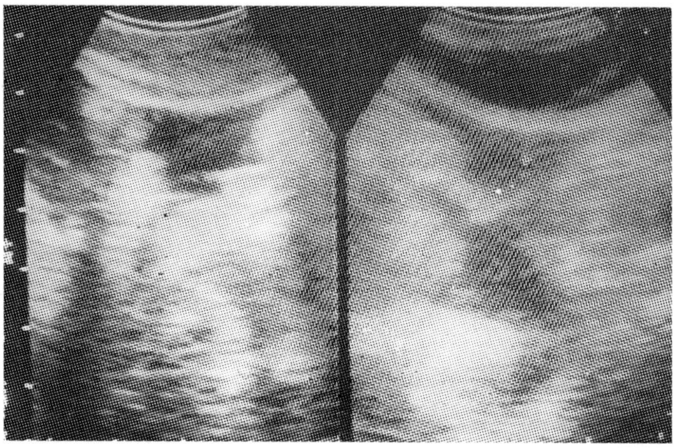

Fig. 12.5. Sonosalpingography. This is another picture clearly imaging the fallopian tube freely floating in the fluid medium (right picture). The intestines are nicely packed away by the fluid compartment, just as pneumoperitoneum keeps the intestine away at laparoscopy.

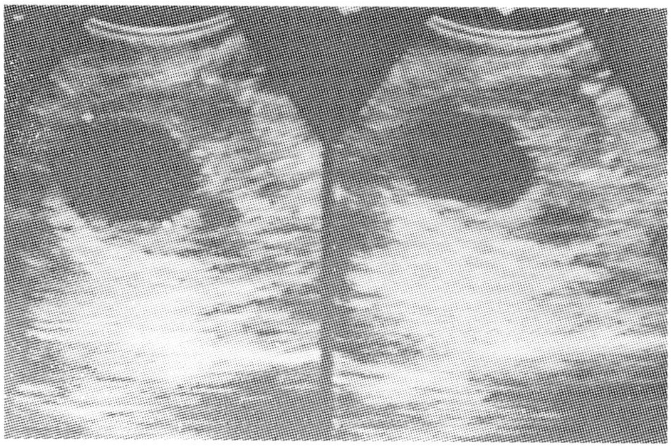

Fig. 12.6. Preovulatory follicle. Both pictures show the uniformly echo-free, well-defined preovulatory follicle, evidencing granulosa lining, and cumulus mass (in the lower part of the follicle). The follicular diameter is 20 mm.

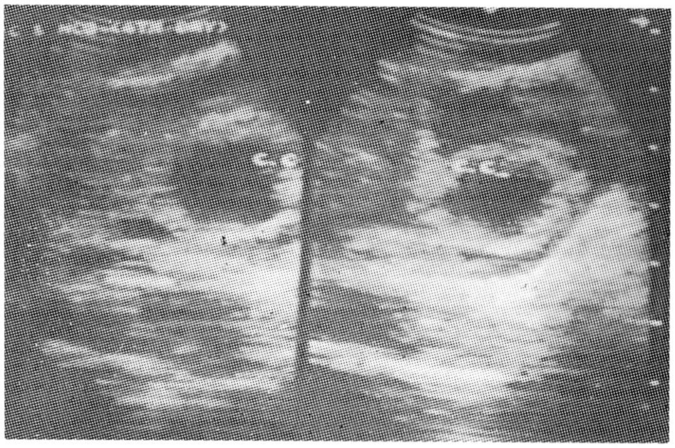

Fig. 12.7. Corpus luteum. Typical sonographic presentation of the corpus luteum. The irregular festooned echogenic structure could be seen with relatively echo-free cystic space in the middle. The adnexa is surrounded by an echo-free fluid, which is a common observation in the postovulatory period.

observation is 75.42%; and the false negative for normal pelvic findings of 24.58% can be significantly minimised by the following approach. Endosonosalpingography, particularly employing an injection of 200 to 250 ml volume of Ringer's lactate, provides for testing the tubal patency as well as excluding pelvic adhesions by locating the freely floating fimbrial and ampullary segments of the fallopian tubes and the ovaries. Tubal evaluation by sonography improves the accuracy to 81.33%. Presence of an adequate amount of fluid in the pelvic cavity nicely packs the intestines away from the pelvic organs, and provides for a clear imaging, in as much as what pneumoperitoneum does for laparoscopy.

If stage I endometriosis (few noncontributory endometrial peritoneal implants) diagnosed at laparoscopy is considered less relevant (particularly in a low risk group and parous subjects) accuracy of negative pelvic diagnosis is improved to 90%. Similarly, if many of the noncontributory minimal pelvic adhesions encountered at laparoscopy can also be ignored, the endopelvic diagnostic accuracy for normal pelvic organs becomes meaningful in 93.75%. When one compares this overwhelming predictive value of endosonography (93.75%) with the proven incidence of pelvic pathology (at laparoscopy) in only 10 to 20% for an infertile couple, the choice falls on endosonography as the first and the most decisive diagnostic measure.

Diagnosis of pelvic pathology

If the pelvic findings are inconclusive or if the patient belongs to the high risk category, endoscopic diagnosis should always be final and confirmatory. A pelvic pathology suspected at endopelvic scan was confirmed in 97.87% of occasions, and an adnexal pathology suspected was confirmed in 93.10%. Moreover, apart from suspecting pelvic disorders mandating endoscopy, endovaginal sonography could by itself be diagnostic. Among those subjects who had positive pelvic findings at sonography, such as uterine abnormalities, ovarian enlargements, tubal masses, and other pelvic findings, a clear and confirmed diagnosis of pelvic pathology could be arrived at sonography itself in 80% of situations. The conditions which are optimally diagnosed at endopelvic scan include :

Uterine. Myoma, adenomyosis, bicornuate or double uterus, septate or subseptate uterus, uterine or cervical polyps, trophoblastic disease and other early pregnancy complications and uterine adhesions.

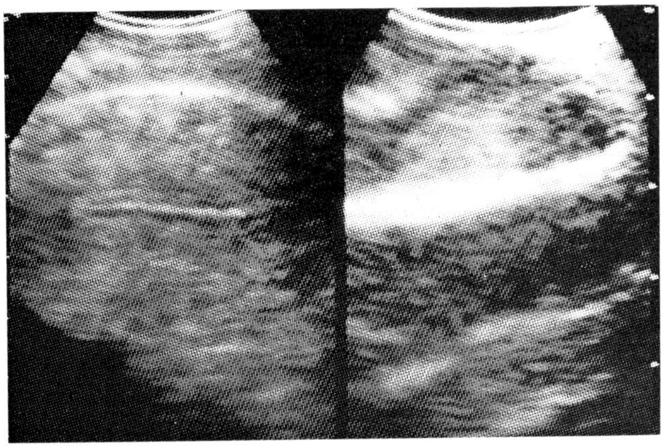

Fig. 12.8. Displaced copper device. The left picture shows the sagittal scan of the normal uterus, evidencing mid-proliferative endometrium. The right picture shows the cervical canal occupied by the copper device, seen as an echodense elongated structure.

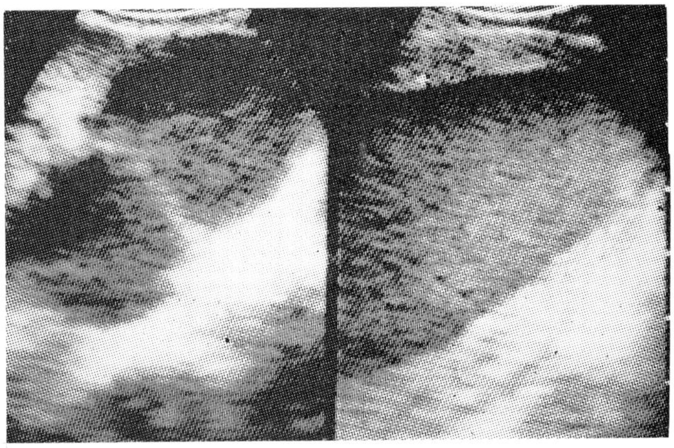

Fig. 12.10. Hematometra. The picture on the right side shows a uterine cavity hugely distended by a blood collection. The fine homogeneous echo-pattern of old blood collection is quite clearly appreciated. The picture on the left side is an hematosalpinx, showing old blood collection inside the dilated and distally blocked ampullary segment of the fallopian tube.

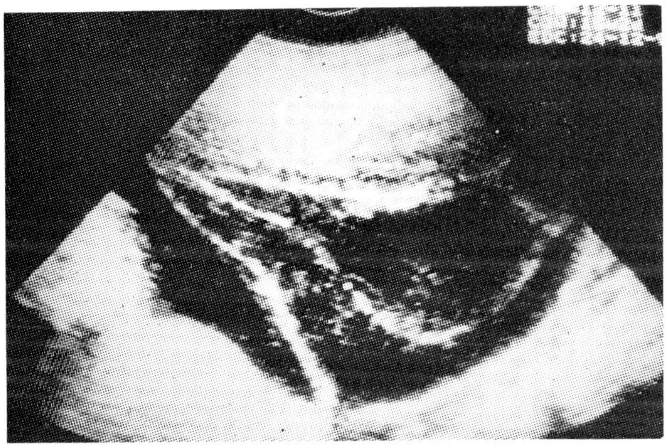

Fig. 12.9. Intrauterine synechiae. This is an early mid-gestation evidencing intrauterine adhesive bands in the lower uterine cavity. The placenta can be seen on the left side posteriorly. Intrauterine adhesions are not an uncommon observation in early pregnancy scans, nor are they harmful for the pregnancy.

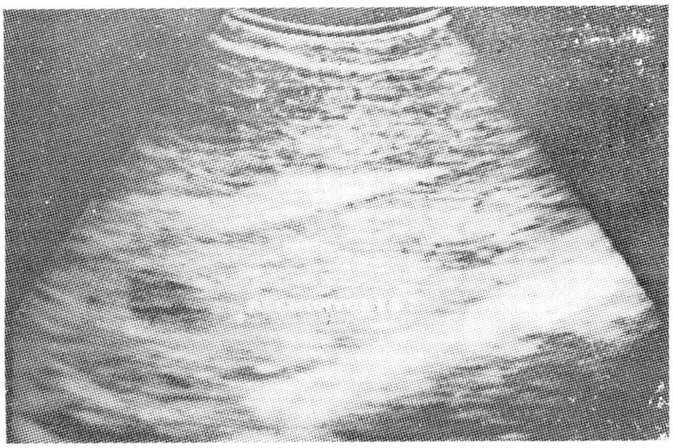

Fig. 12.11. Adenomyosis. Sagittal scan of the uterus showing the endometrial cavity line in the middle. The posterior myometrium evidences an echo-free cavity surrounded by relatively echogenic endometrial lining. This is one of the sonographic presentations of adenomyosis.

Ovarian. Functional cysts (which are managed expectantly, and hence must be differentiated from organic lesions), endometriomata, ovarian adhesions, different types of ovarian tumors (such as dermoid, mucinous cystadenoma, serous and papillary cystadenoma, solid tumors and frank malignancies), ovarian abscess, and paraovarian cysts.

Tubal. Ectopic gestation (intact and live, tubal mole, carneous mole, tubal abortion, pelvic hematocele), hydrosalpinx, hematosalpinx and tubal adhesions.

I feel if a definite diagnosis is made at endovaginal sonography there is no need for endoscopic confirmation, and the role of endoscopy now is only therapeutic. This is mostly applied to various tubal disorders and endometriosis managed at laparoscopy, and uterine anomalies and luminal fibroids operated hysteroscopically. Certain conditions such as pelvic adhesions and intrauterine synechiae suspected at sonography necessitate endoscopic confirmation and concurrent surgical correction.

Ectopic gestation

Since the popular application of endovaginal scanning early pregnancy surveillance, the incidence of ectopic gestation has been computed to be 5.48% among indicated scans. Tubal ectopic gestation is diagnosed with 80.43% accuracy at the first scan without a recourse to β-hCG study. Complementary β-hCG

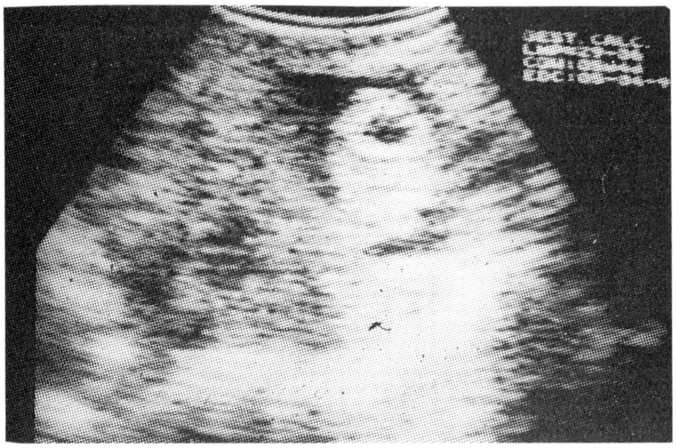

Fig. 12.12. Ectopic gestation. Ectopic gestation sac in a 5 weeks 4 days pregnancy is imaged in the form of a well-defined bright echogenic adnexal ring. The echo-free area surrounding the sac indicates minimal blood collection. Such smaller sacs of early ectopic gestations are ideally treated by parenteral administration of methotrexate.

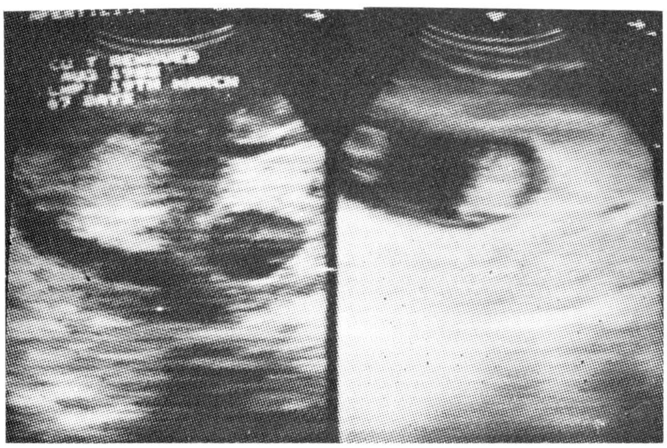

Fig. 12.13. Ectopic and intrauterine gestation. This is a 9 weeks + gestation occurring following use of copper device. The left picture evidences the adnexal ring of ectopic gestation, and the right picture shows the intrauterine gestation evidencing the fetal pole and the yolk sac. The ectopic gestation was surgically removed, and the intra-uterine gestation resulted in a normal term delivery.

monitoring and a review scan make 93.50% ectopic gestations diagnosable at endopelvic scan. A false negative diagnosis of 6.50% and a false positive diagnosis of 4.92% have been encountered among the 61 ectopic gestations studied over 2 years. Apart from the diagnostic role, endopelvic scanning can dictate the treatment strategy for ectopic gestation. More than 50% of ectopic gestations diagnosed do not deserve to be treated. Under these circumstances endopelvic scanning will identify those to be treated, and if so the optimal method as to whether surgical or medical (and whether intra-amniotic injection or parenteral therapy). We

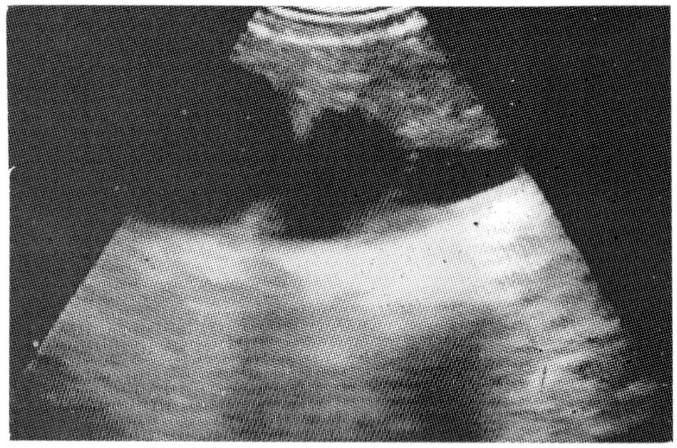

Fig. 12.14. Hydrosalpinx. The echo-free fluid-filed fallopian tube is clearly imaged at endosonography. 75% of the hydro-salpinges are diagnosed at endovaginal scanning.

prefer parenteral chemotherapy for very early ectopic gestations where the sac is too small to be approached for local instillation. Ectopic gestations present as organised carneous moles or blighted ovum in 61.11%, fresh blood moles in the process of spontaneous abortion in 11.11%, pelvic hematocele in 11.11%, in the process of fimbrial extrusion in 8.33% and with live fetal pole in 8.33%.

Another unique opportunity offered by endopelvic scanning is diagnosis of concurrent intrauterine and ectopic gestations. From a total of 1114 early pregnancy scans there have been 3 such cases (0.27%), and this constituted 4.92% of all the ectopic gestations. This study only proves that concurrent ectopic and intrauterine gestations are not that uncommon, and neither β-hCG monitoring nor laparoscopy could salvage and support such a diagnosis.

Hydrosalpinx and hematosalpinx

At least 68% of tubal swellings, usually hydrosalpinx, are diagnosed at endovaginal scan. Apart from their importance in infertile subjects, we see lot of subjects presenting with a pelvic mass following hysterectomies (no oophorectomy), and tubal sterilizations. In such subjects identifying the pelvic mass as tubal swelling and excluding an ovarian pathology (neoplasm) relieves the anxiety, and also avoids a major surgery. If tubal extirpation is considered mandatory I prefer endoscopic salpingectomy.

Pelvic endometriosis

In our infertility practice 77.50% of pelvic endo-metriosis have been diagnosed at endovaginal sono-graphy itself. The diagnostic clues employed are :

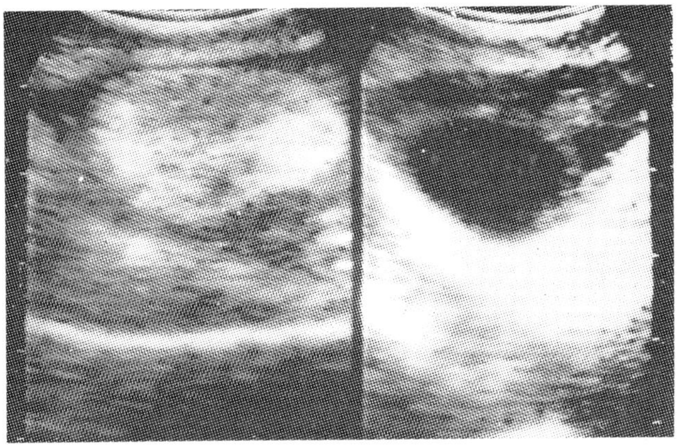

Fig. 12.15. **Dermoid cyst of ovary.** The picture on the right shows an uniform echogenic oval mass, clearly seen separate from the rest of the ovary. Calcification shows this echogenic pattern. This is one of the presentations of dermoid cyst. The left picture images the contralateral normal ovary, with a preovulatory follicle.

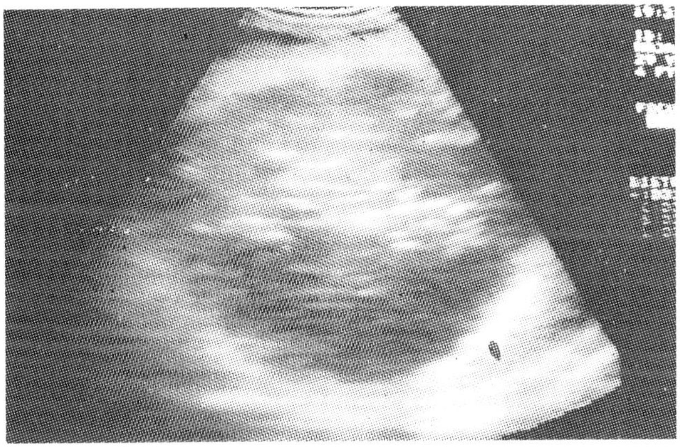

Fig. 12.16. **Dermoid cyst with sebum.** This big cyst could be seen to contain lot of prominent high level echogenic areas. This appearance is due to the presence of sebum in the dermoid tumor.

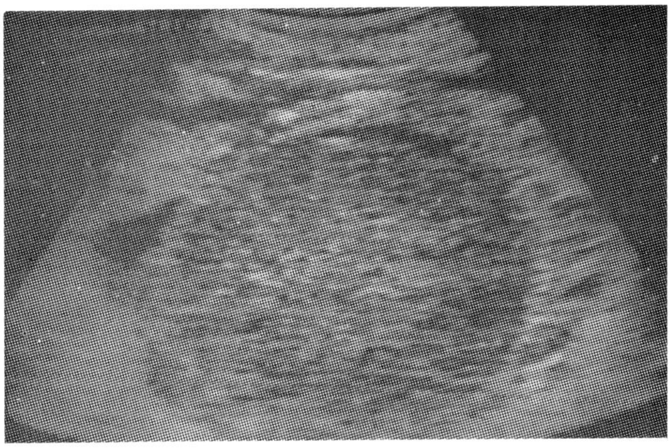

Fig. 12.17. **Endometrial cyst of the ovary.** The typical features are fine granular homogeneous echogenic content (old blood) uniformly distributed inside the cyst cavity. The clearly defined capsule can be seen in the periphery, indicating the enucleability of the cyst.

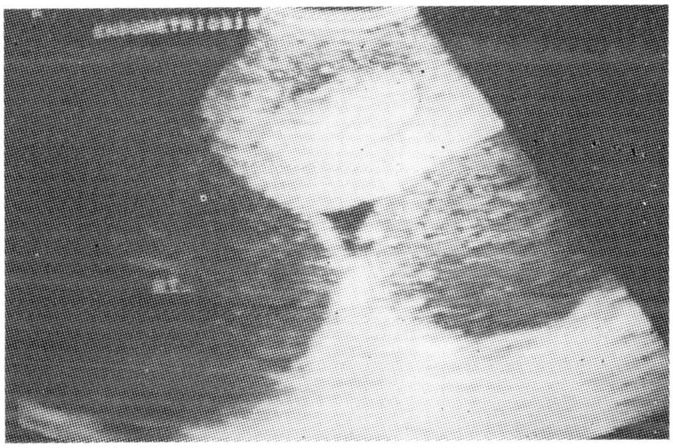

Fig. 12.18. **Bilateral ovarian endometriosis.** The uterus can be seen on top, with both ovaries evidencing the typical endometrial cysts remaining close to each other.

1. Typical sonographic features of endometrial cysts : well encapsulated oval or round cysts, with fine homogeneous, uniformly distributed, granular echo-pattern. The cysts could be multiple and bilateral. While this typical presentation is always confirmatory; endometrial cysts could occasionally present as clear cysts.
2. Evidence of pelvic adhesions, particularly ovarian adhesions to the posterior surface of the uterus.
3. Tubes remain free of adhesions, particularly the tubal fimbriae, as proved by freely floating fimbriae at endosonosalpingography.

Admittedly pelvic implants and noncontributory pelvic adhesions remain undetected by this approach, and hence the diagnostic accuracy of 77.50%. Nonetheless this false negative diagnosis is a lesser concern, since treatment of mild endometriosis (state I) does not significantly improve the fertility of the couple.

Since in our earlier study we have proved that 90% subjects with endometriosis have at least one tube normal, and 55% have both tubes normal, we prefer to initiate medical treatment (danazol), as a primary therapeutic measure, without a recourse to laparoscopic diagnosis. An average fertility rate of 30% has been achieved on exclusive medical therapy.

Ovarian enlargements

The majority of ovarian enlargements encountered are functional cysts, which are precisely diagnosed at endovaginal scan. Nonneoplastic conditions such as

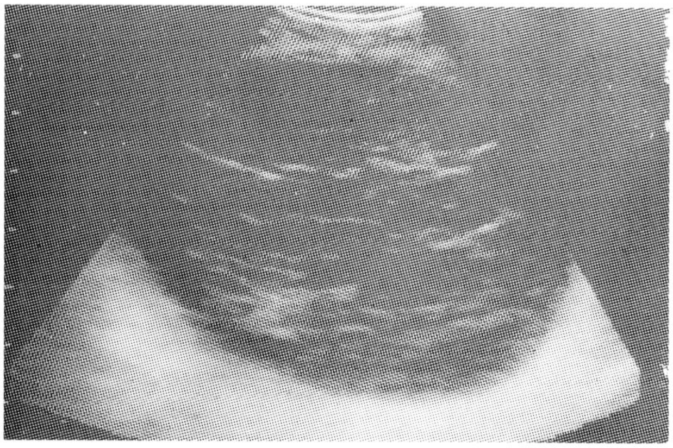

Fig. 12.19. Corpus luteal cyst. This is a functional cyst of the ovary, magnified to image the trabecular pattern which represents the organised blood collected inside the cyst. The cyst diameter is 4.5 cm.

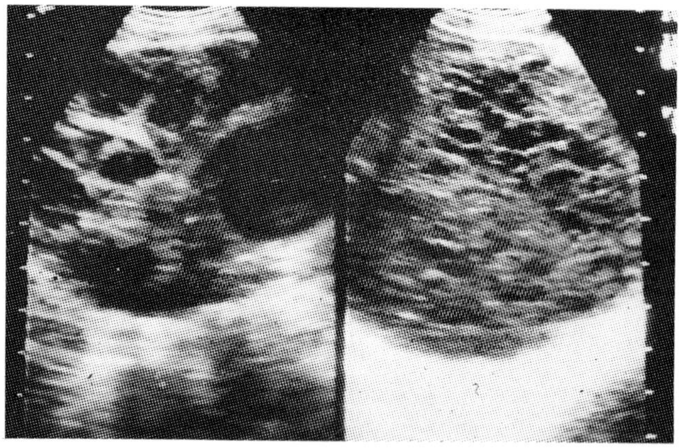

Fig. 12.21. Adenocarcinoma of the ovary. Adenocarcinoma of the ovary showing cystic areas, and areas of degeneration.

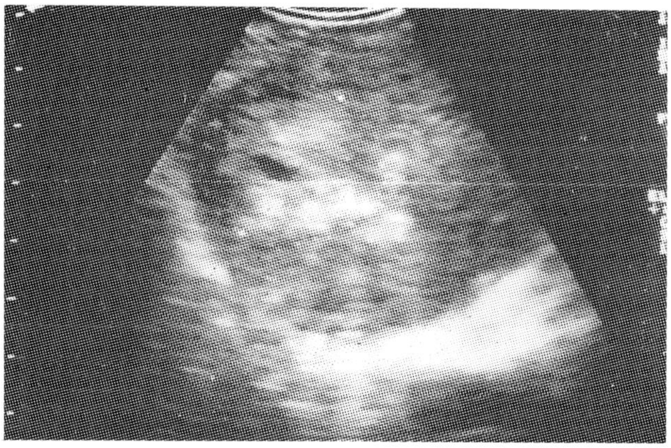

Fig. 12.20. Solid tumor of the ovary. This is a solid tumor of the ovary, evidencing one small cystic area. The malignant potential can be assessed by Doppler studies.

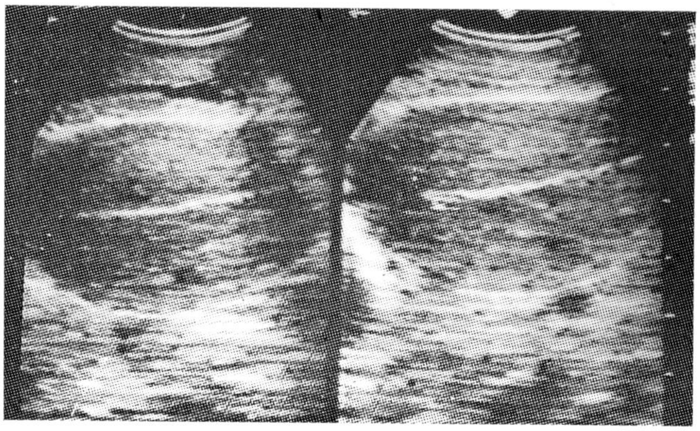

Fig. 12.22. Inactive endometrium. Both pictures show the normal uterus in the longitudinal scan, with the uniform myometrial texture. The endometrium is represented by the thin central echogenic line. There is no echo-free stroma surrounding the central cavity line evidencing poor estrogenic response.

endometrial cysts and ovarian abscesses are also optimally identified at scan. Benign tumors such as dermoids and mucinous cysts are again diagnosed accurately at scan, thus leaving only 30% of ovarian masses mandating further and detailed evaluation.

I prefer Doppler flow velocity studies at this stage. Cystic masses with absent flow velocity (particularly diastolic filling) could signify torsion. Among solid or cystic masses with high pulsatility indices, the potential for malignancy is high. Benign tumors usually present with a PI of 3 to 5. Moreover, the typical presentation of ascites, nodular masses and solid ovarian enlargement located at endovaginal scanning stand for a diagnosis of ovarian malignancy.

Cancer screening

We employ an endopelvic scan for ovarian and endometrial cancer screening in elderly, particularly postmenopausal subjects. Sonographic screening is quite simple, quick, noninvasive and convenient, and the predictive accuracy is comparable or superior to many invasive diagnostic measures. If both ovaries can be imaged and the volume measured is less than 4.6 ml then there is decreased suspicion of malignancy. However, if ovaries cannot be imaged on endopelvic scanning it is a good sign, provided abdominal scanning also confirms nonvisualisation of the ovaries. As regards the endometrium, an inactive endometrial pattern represented by a thin and poorly echogenic endometrial cavity line, measuring not more than 5 mm is encouraging. Presence of a thick endometrium, pyometra, polypoidal masses, or myometrial thickening and vascular areas will call for a detailed scrutiny. This approach eliminates the need for routine hysteroscopy

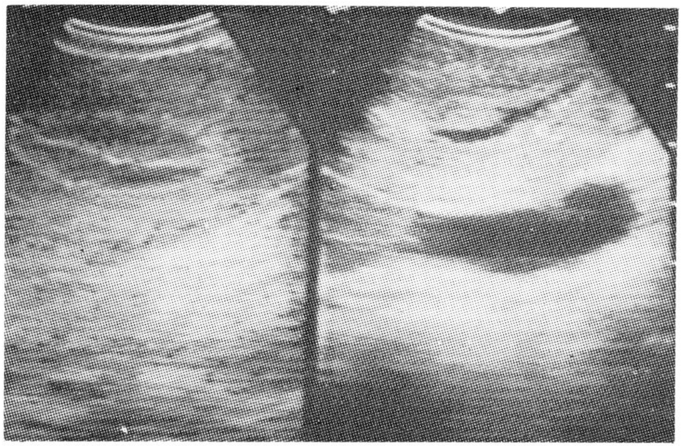

Fig. 12.23. Late proliferative endometrium. The picture on the left shows late proliferative endometrium measuring a thickness of 7 mm. The central cavity line is clearly imaged in the middle, which is surrounded by relatively echo-free stroma. The picture on the right shows the cervical canal, seen as an echo-free linear area with a diameter of 3 mm.

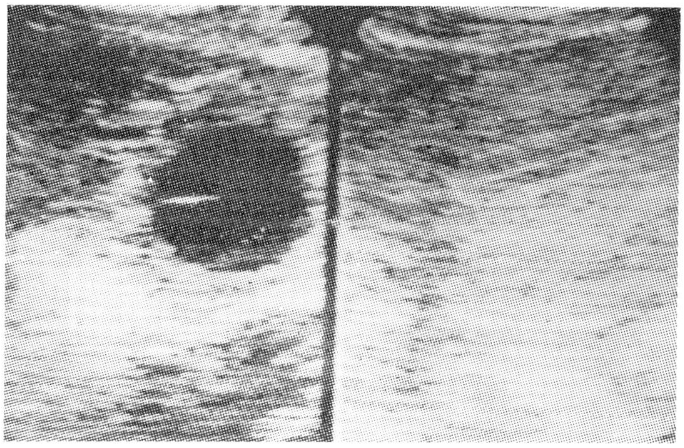

Fig. 12.24. Midproliferative endometrium. The picture on the left side is a dominant follicle showing granulosa lining surrounding the echo-free cystic space. On the right side the sagittal scan of the uterus shows the endometrium in midproliferative phase. The central cavity line is surrounded by more of echo-free stromal edema, indicting moderate estrogenic response.

and endometrial curettage or aspiration for diagnosis of postmenopausal bleeding.

The unique feature of this cancer screening program by endopelvic scanning which is not shared by any of the other screening techniques is that two organs, namely the ovaries and uterus can be concurrently studied by this simple method without any additional effort.

Uterus and endometrium

Endometrial dating by endosonography has practically

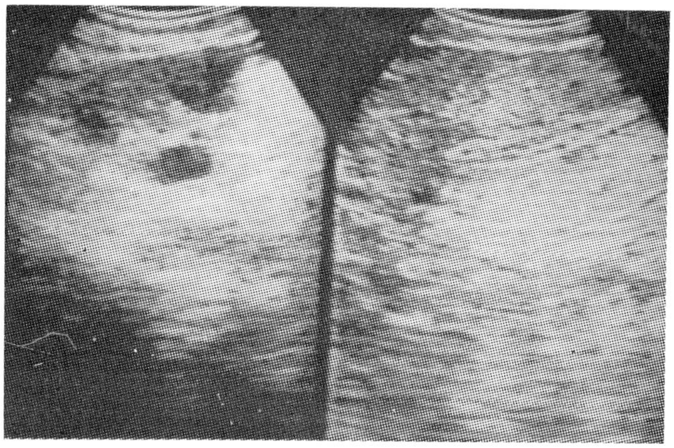

Fig. 12.25. Early proliferative endometrium. The picture on the right side shows longitudinal scan of the uterus. The central cavity line of the endometrium is surrounded by minimal echo-free stromal edema, indicating minimal estrogenic response. The endometrial thickness is hardly 2 mm.

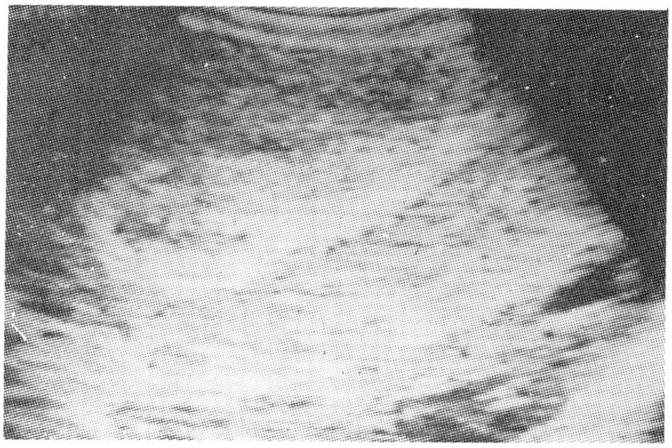

Fig. 12.26. Midsecretory endometrium. Sagittal scan of the uterus evidencing the thick echogenic endometrium which surrounds a central echo-free collection of endometrial secretion. The endometrial thickness measures 6 mm. This picture denotes midluteal phase of the cycle.

replaced endometrial biopsy and other methods of evaluating ovulation, follicular maturation and corpus luteal competency. Normal-looking endometrium, particularly the one that evidences the dynamic cyclic changes, is certified normal and healthy; and all endometrial diseases including Asherman's syndrome remain excluded on this score. Asherman's syndrome presents either with characteristic high density endometrial echoes, or a failure of endometrium to optimally respond to ovarian steroids.

Uterine anomalies, bicornuate versus subseptate, are discriminated easily, because endosonography is both a luminal and surface study for the uterus. Otherwise this much information is gathered only at a combined

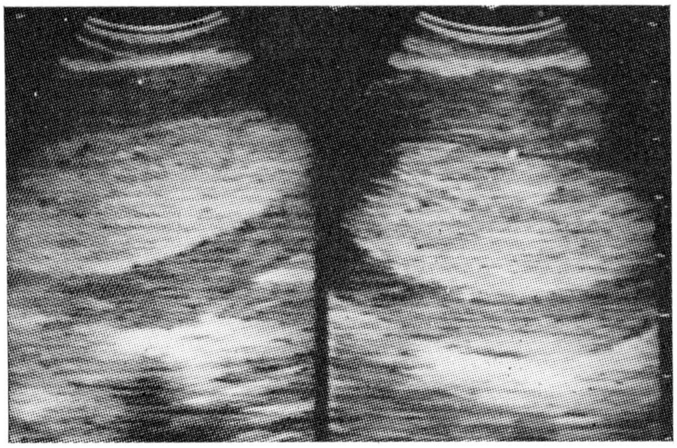

Fig. 12.27. Pseudodecidual endometrium. This is the transverse scan of the uterus imaging the endometrium as a bright echogenic thick structure measuring 8 mm in thickness. No endometrial cavity or secretions are discerned. This picture is consistent with the premenstrual pseudodecidual endometrial pattern, seen in the late luteal phase.

laparohysteroscopy. A word of caution is that even the mildest degree of uterine anomalies are located at endovaginal scanning and unnecessary and over-enthusiastic treatment for such conditions should be discouraged.

Uterine myomas, particularly the small-sized tumors, are clearly imaged at endovaginal scanning with the following benefits : (1) the number; (2) the size; (3) the exact location and the precise distance from the endometrial lining; and (4) scanning of kidneys for any pressure effect. This preoperative evaluation will optimise the surgical approach, whether it should be hysteroscopic or laparoscopic

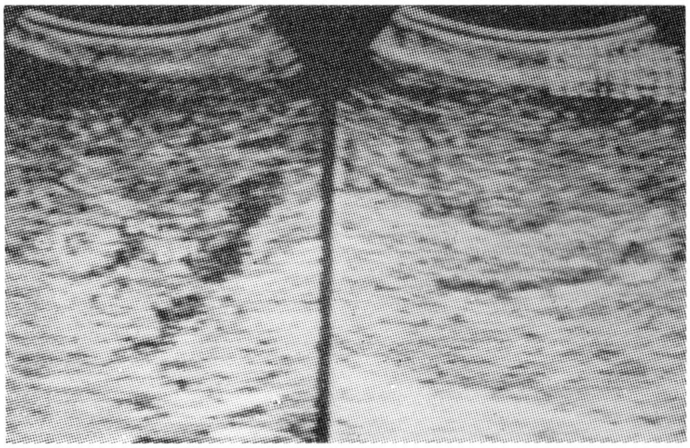

Fig. 12.28. Early pregnancy. The picture on the left shows the longitudinal scan of the uterus, evidencing very thick and bright decidua surrounding the early chorionic vesicle.

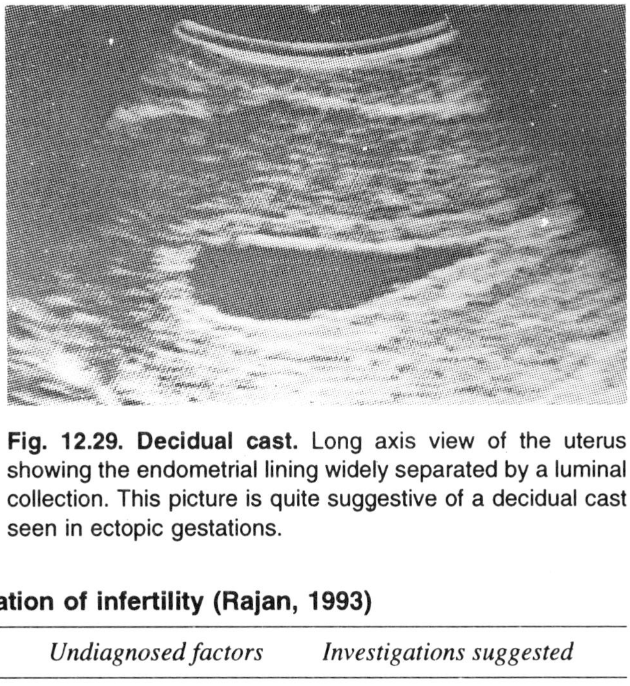

Fig. 12.29. Decidual cast. Long axis view of the uterus showing the endometrial lining widely separated by a luminal collection. This picture is quite suggestive of a decidual cast seen in ectopic gestations.

Table 12.1. Sonographic classification of infertility (Rajan, 1993)

Classification	*TVS diagnosis*	*Undiagnosed factors*	*Investigations suggested*
Normal pelvic organs	Uterus and ovaries normal and mobile; normal genitals	Tubal status; endocrine factor	HSG or sonosalpingography
Endocrine synchrony	Normal follicular and luteal phase	Tubal status	HSG or sonosalpingography
Pelvic pathology	Endometriosis, hydrosalpinx, ectopics, fibroids, uterine anomalies	Nil	No further investigations; operative laparoscopy, laparotomy, medical treatment
Endocrine infertility	P.C.O.D.; primary and secondary ovarian failure, ovulatory dysfunctions	Nil	Endocrine study : PRL, FSH, LH, T
Pelvic adhesions	Ovaries adherent and close to uterus	Inflammatory or endometriosis	Laparoscopy
Inconclusive	Indefinite findings and scan	Pelvic inflammatory disease, endometriosis, or normal	Laparoscopy and hysteroscopy

myomectomy, or by laparotomy. It also allows for counting the number of fibroids to be removed, and prevents unnecessary opening of the uterine cavity.

Endovaginal sonography has significantly influenced gynaecological diagnosis, and today endoscopy is only second in line in pelvic diagnosis. Many interventional endovaginal sonographic procedures, such as treatment of ectopics and aspiration of ovarian cysts are gradually emerging as an attractive and lesser invasive alternative to surgical endoscopies.

CHAPTER

13

Transvaginal Sonography and the Ovary

Ambrish Dalal

Pelvic sonography and development of transvaginal probes have changed the workup and management of gynaecological problems. Introduction of vaginal transducers have added a new dimension of sophistication to the diagnostic accuracy especially in visualising structural anatomy of the ovaries thus improving diagnostic accuracy or at least narrowing the differential diagnosis considerably. In addition, Doppler has allowed us an added understanding of the physiologic aspects of ovarian masses.

It is advisable to perform a transabdominal ultrasound examination at the first instance before doing a transvaginal examination as it provides a panoramic view of pelvic anatomy in a rapid manner so that one can focus the transvaginal study to a particular area of interest, thereby reducing the time of transvaginal examination. Sometimes large masses located beyond the reach of a transvaginal scanning field may be thus visualised. It may be advisable to ask the patient to empty her bladder before transvaginal examination. Visualisation of the ovarian anatomy with transvaginal sonography has almost completely replaced the per vaginum examination under anaesthesia which was commonly done in the past.

Normal ovary

Ovaries are typically located between the uterus and the pelvic sidewalls and antero-medial to the internal iliac vessels. However, the ovary is one of those mobile structures that one may find anywhere in the pelvis and sometimes can be located in the cul-de-sac, adjacent to the uterus or in the upper pelvis and may move with volume changes in the urinary bladder.

One may have difficulty in localising the ovary when it is situated in the extreme lateral or anterior position after an hysterectomy or in the postmenopausal patients. Use of colour Doppler may be helpful by tracing the ovarian artery to the ovary.

Normal ovarian size has been described by a number of authors and is approximately $2 \times 3 \times 4$ cm.

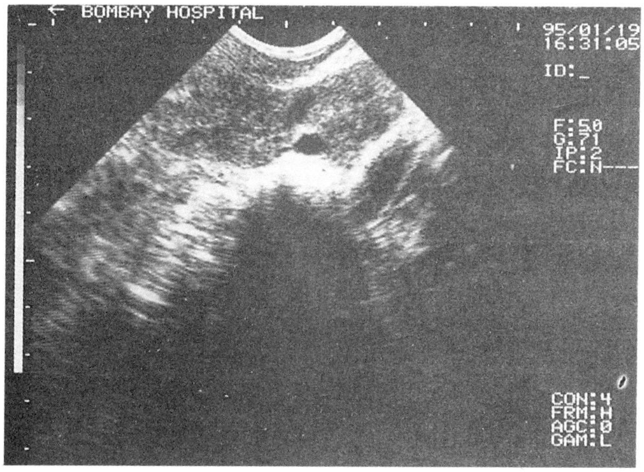

Fig. 13.1. The left ovary seen in the ovarian fossa between the uterus and pelvic sidewall.

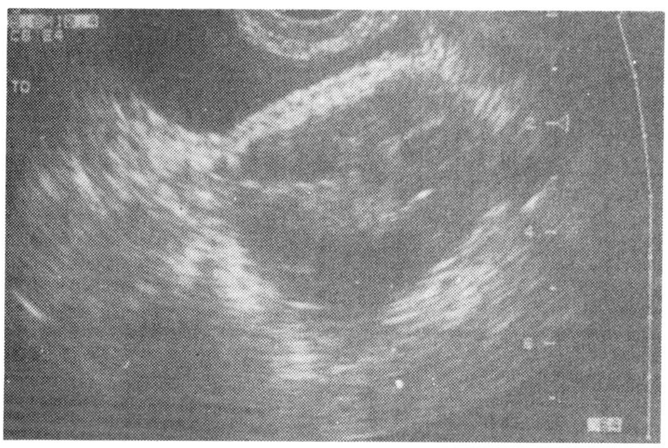

Fig. 13.2. Hyperstimulated ovary with multiple follicles.

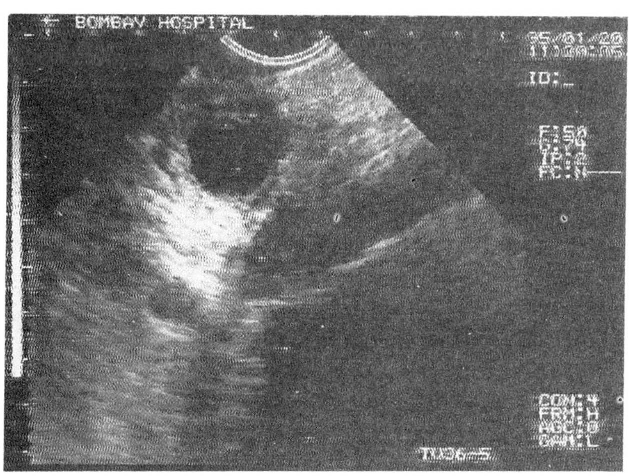

Fig. 13.3. The ovary seen with a small functional cyst with the puncture guide just before cyst aspiration on day 2 of the cycle.

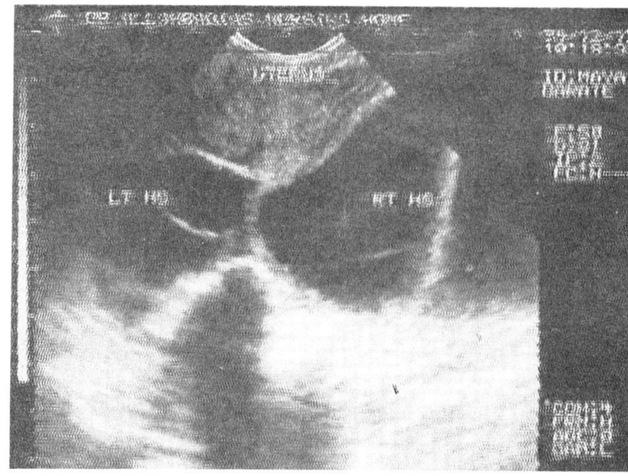

Fig. 13.4. Uterus and bilateral hydrosalpinges seen in a transverse plane.

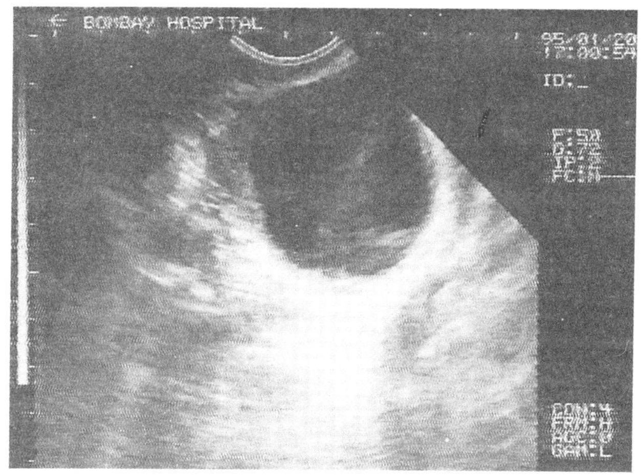

Fig. 13.5. Corpus luteum cyst.

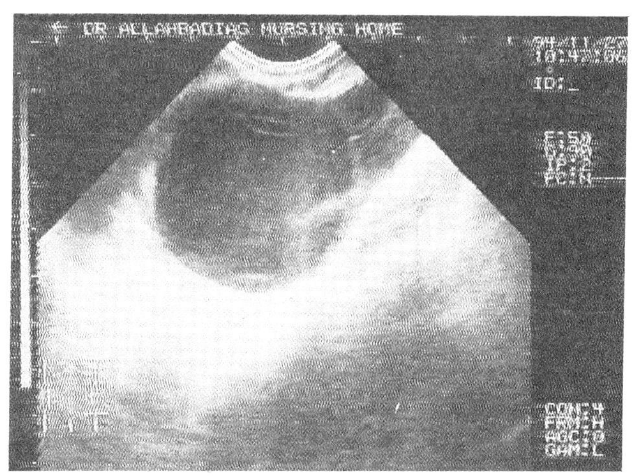

Fig. 13.6. Haemorrhagic cyst.

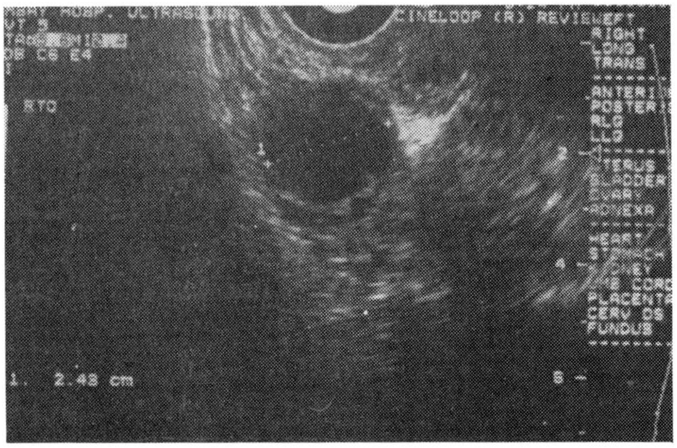

Fig. 13.7. Preovulatory mature follicle with cumulus and debris.

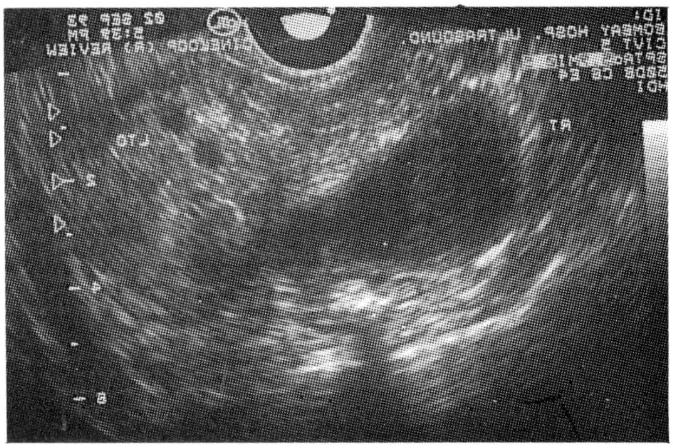

Fig. 13.8. Bilateral ovarian endometriomas. The right ovary is cystic with low level echoes while the left ovary has a more solid echogenic appearance and small secondary follicles.

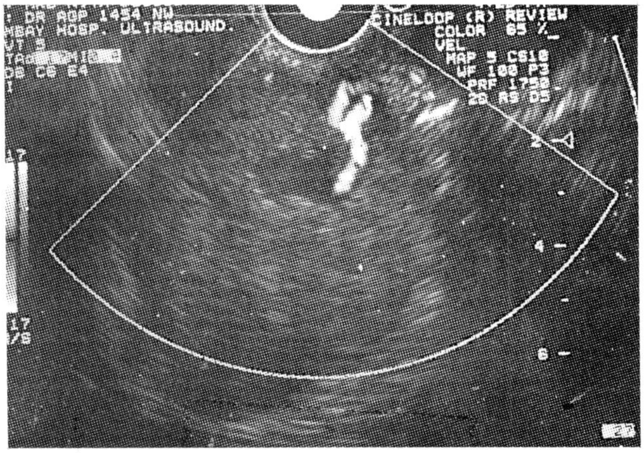

Fig. 13.9. Large solid ovarian mass with a large feeding vessel seen on colour Doppler ultrasonography.

Calculating ovarian volume has become an objective way of following the ovarian size, especially in postmenopausal patients. Normal ovarian size fluctuates with the phase of the menstrual cycle and is usually large in the ovary containing follicles. Pelvic veins and bowel loops are commonly seen adjacent to the ovaries and one must learn to identify them and not confuse them for ovarian cysts or hydrosalpinges.

Transvaginal sonography can accurately define the nature of ovarian masses which can be categorised into cystic, complex and solid massed depending on their sonographic appearance. A fourth category of 'ovarian enlargement' may also be considered for classification.

Ovarian masses

Functional cysts

Functional cysts are one of the most common abnormalities visualised in the ovaries which result from normal ovulatory processes. These include simple follicular cysts, corpus luteum cysts and haemorrhagic cysts. Most functional cysts measure less than 5 cm in diameter. These resolve within 1 to 2 menstrual cycles in the majority of cases.

Simple follicular cysts

An ovulatory follicle usually measures less than 2.5 cm in size. A follicle that fails to rupture may be larger in size but usually is less than 5 cm in diameter. These are usually asymtomatic but larger cysts may be associated with menstrual irregularities or occasionally be associated with pain. These may be complicated by haemorrhage or torsion. A typical sonographic appearance can be described as an unilocular sonolucent, thin-walled cystic mass in the ovary.

Corpus luteum cyst

Corpus luteum is formed from the graafian follicle within hours of ovulation. A fresh corpus luteum has an hypoechoic texture and measures less than 2 cm and has a thick wall with internal echoes. A persistent corpus luteum may enlarge and form a cyst. Corpus luteum may have a sonographically variable appearance which includes a solid echogenic area, multilocular mass or rarely that of a cavernous structure. Because of this variable appearance it may mimic a neoplastic lesion or sometimes an ectopic gestation. Visualisation of corpus luteum is difficult by abdominal scanning but has been made easy by transvaginal scanning. Doppler examination shows a typical low impedance waveform pattern.

Haemorrhagic cysts

Women with haemorrhagic cysts frequently present with sudden onset of pelvic pain. If sonography is done immediately after the onset of pain then it may show an echogenic appearance representing acute haemorrhage. When haemorrhage starts resolving it has a relatively complex appearance. Later on it has an appearance of a thin walled cyst with low level septae-like echoes floating within it. An acute haemorrhagic cyst simulates a solid mass. However on colour Doppler there is no intrinsic vascularity. These may occasionally be associated with haemoperitoneum.

Ovarian enlargements

These occur in the following conditions :

1. Polycystic ovarian disease
2. Ovarian torsion
3. Autoimmune oophoritis
4. Pelvic inflammatory disease

Polycystic ovarian disease (PCOD) has enlarged ovaries with small cystic areas scattered more commonly in the periphery in the subcapsular zone of ovary.

Ovarian torsion produces an enlarged oedematous ovary and may have small cysts in the periphery. These cysts are thought to be the result of circulatory impairment and secondary transudation of fluid into the peripherally located developing follicles. Torsion of the ovary may also have a solid appearance due to stromal oedema and vascular engorgement. On colour Doppler examination there is absent blood flow in the organ.

Other causes of an enlarged ovary include pelvic infection and autoimmune oophoritis.

Cystic masses

A simple unilocular cyst of ovary which is usually benign has a smooth thin outer wall with no internal echoes and a good internal transmission with acoustic enhancement.

Cystadenoma

Cystadenoma is the most common cystic ovarian tumor more commonly seen in postmenopausal women. These may contain a mucinous or serous substance. These are more often larger than 5 cm in size when diagnosed and some may have a benign unilocular appearance on sonography; while others have solid nodules, septation or complex elements within them. Transvaginal sonography is better in demonstrating wall nodularity and internal echoes.

Persistence of a cystic mass in the ovary beyond two menstrual cycles suggests a pathologic nature as opposed to a functional nature and warrants further workup or cyst aspiration and cytologic studies.

Pelvic cystic masses other than these include paraovarian cysts, peritoneal inclusion cysts, hydrosalpinges, tuboovarian abscesses, endometriomata, lymph nodes, etc. On transvaginal scanning one should always look for an extra-ovarian origin of any cystic mass.

Endometrioma

Endometriosis results from actively growing and functioning endometrial tissues in sites beyond the endometrial cavity.

Sonographic appearance of ovarian endometriosis can be variable. Early endometrial implants may be too small for transvaginal sonography to detect while large endometriomas have a typical appearance on sonography characterised by thick walls and uniform low level internal echoes. Gentle ballottment through the anterior abdominal wall during scanning may show movement of internal echoes suggesting the liquid nature of the mass. Colour Doppler shows absence of vascularity within the mass. Sonographic appearance sometimes may be indistinguishable from acute haemorrhagic cysts.

Tubo-ovarian abscesses

These are complex masses with multiple findings and associated often with dilated tortous fallopian tubes. Endothelium of the fallopian tubes may produce a bright echogenic border.

Cystic teratoma (dermoid)

As these are derived from all the three germ layers, most striking findings are from the elements of ectoderm, *i.e.*, hair, teeth, sebaceous material, etc. As most dermoids are asymtomatic these are discovered as incidental findings on routine examination. These may occasionally complicate as torsion or rupture. If ruptured then secondary chemical peritonitis may cause diffuse abdominal pain.

Sonographic appearance can be highly variable ranging from a solid appearance to cystic masses. Large fatty dermoids can be missed as they are mistaken for bowel loops. Layering of hair and fat may be visualised on transvaginal scanning. 10 to 20% of dermoids are bilateral and therefore a more careful evaluation of the contralateral ovary is indicated.

Solid masses of ovary

These include :

1. Benign ovarian tumors
2. Fibroma
3. Thecoma
4. Teratoma
5. Germ cell tumors
6. Malignant ovarian tumors

While evaluating ovarian malignancy both trans-abdominal and transvaginal scanning are necessary to detect the extension of the disease. Significant overlap in sonographic findings of ovarian tumors exists and therefore a pathologic diagnosis of ovarian tumours is not expected from a sonologist though in certain cases it may suggest a possibility of a certain type of pathology.

Summary

When an ovarian mass is detected by pelvic sonography, the following factors should be considered :

1. Size beyond 5 cm
2. Complex, cystic or solid appearance
3. Solid or nodular areas within the mass
4. Persistent over two menstrual cycles
5. Vascularity on colour Doppler

If any of the above mentioned factors are present then further immediate investigations are mandatory.

CHAPTER

14

Transvaginal Endosonography in the Assessment of Urinary Stress Incontinence

Shailesh Raina

Genuine Stress Urinary Incontinence may be defined as the involuntary loss of urine from the bladder due to an increase in intra-abdominal pressure.

The bladder neck may be displaced due to weakening of its supports, so that any increase in intra-abdominal pressure, as a result of, for example, coughing or sneezing leads to opening and descent of the bladder neck and urinary leakage[1].

These changes were originally described using lateral bead chain cystourethrography. With the advent of urodynamics, it became clear that the urethro-vesical angle was no more of great importance. The emphasis in the investigation of stress incontinence has changed to measuring the functional consequences of these anatomical changes, *i.e.*, alterations in intravesical and intraurethral pressure[2].

Urodynamic studies are currently the reference standard for the diagnosis of stress incontinence. They require established facilities and a specialist staff. The treatment for stress incontinence includes non-surgical and surgical procedures. Many surgical procedures have been proposed, however most surgeons now choose either a Burch colposuspension or a Stamey endoscopic sling procedure. It has been suggested that elevation of the bladder neck (an anatomical objective) is the primary requirement for a successful result.

Transvaginal endosonography

A single and convenient method to demonstrate the anatomy of the lower urinary tract is transvaginal endosonography. The technique is well accepted by patients as it is painless, carries no morbidity and permits the patient to view the examination concurrently. It may be used for the pre-operative, per-operative and post-operative assessment of women with stress incontinence. It has proved to be valuable in the diagnosis of both primary and recurrent stress incontinence and in the post-operative management of women with persistent symptoms.

Equipment

The commonly used transvaginal endoprobe is a B & K (Brüel & Kjaer) sector transducer type 8537 (Fig. 14.1). It has an external diameter of 20 millimetres and contains 7 MHz crystal mounted at 45 degrees to the long axis of the transducer. The size of the probe compares favourably to the more conventional methods of per-vaginal examination. The high frequency endoprobe scans through a sector of 112°, over a focal range of one to six centimeters.

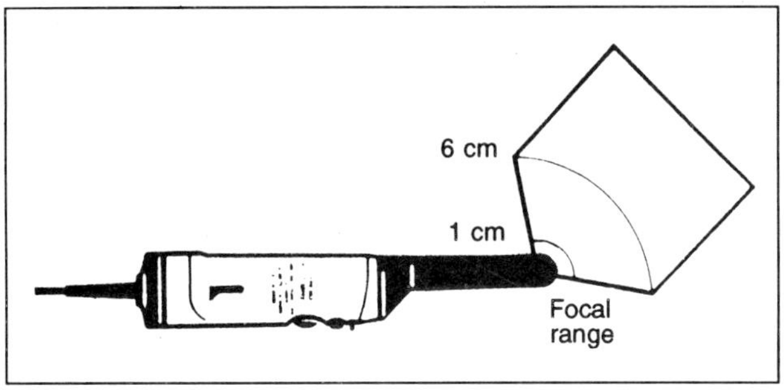

Fig. 14.1. Sector transducer type 8537 and its scanning plane.

This configuration permits the key landmarks of the inferior border of the symphysis pubis and the urethro-vesical junction to be consistently identified. The transducer is used in conjunction with the B & K ultrasound scanner type 1846. The attachment of a camera or video recorder would make it possible to document the examination. The compact dimension of the transvaginal endoprobe ensure that each examination is performed with minimal discomfort to the patient. In addition, the transducer is immersible in disinfecting solutions, thus minimising the risk of infection.

Technique

The patient is placed in the recumbent position with the hips and knees flexed. She is able to see the ultrasound images, and is able to explain her symptoms accurately. The bladder should be comfortably full. The transducer is lubricated with ultrasound gel and gently inserted in the vagina. The endoprobe is introduced horizontally. When scanning in the sagittal plane a direct image of the bladder neck, bladder base and proximal urethra is displayed, as well as the inferior border of the symphysis pubis (Fig. 14.2). The patient is asked to cough and perform a Valsalva manoeuvre so that the dynamic aspects of the examination may be observed. In subsequent scans the anatomical view is of a different format with the bladder to the left hand side

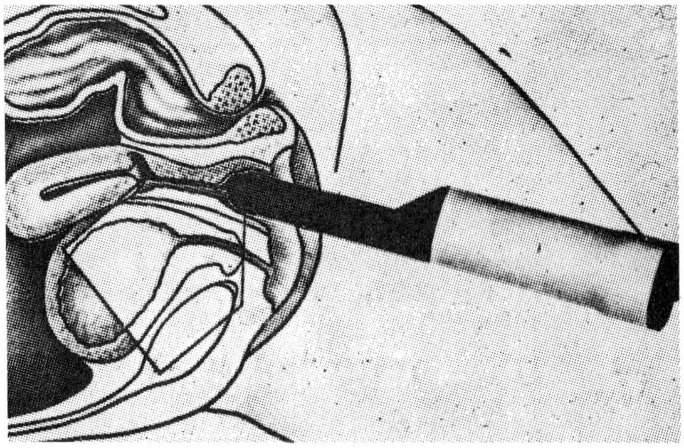

Fig. 14.2. The anatomy of the lower urinary tract as seen in the sagittal plane.

of the image. It is important to appreciate this change in the longitudinal axis of the patient, in order to understand the ultrasound images. The most important landmarks are the bladder neck and the inferior border of the symphysis pubis (Fig. 14.3). These are consistently seen in all the images. The position of the urethra cannot be consistently identified as, in many cases, a broad echo-free area is seen that includes the urethra and surrounding structures. A more precise position of the urethra may be seen following catheterisation of the patient. Since the crystal is mounted at 45 degrees, the longitudinal axis of the patient is the diagonal that extends from the top left corner of the image to the bottom right corner.

In a normal woman (nulliparous, with no symptoms), the bladder neck is well supported. The vertical height

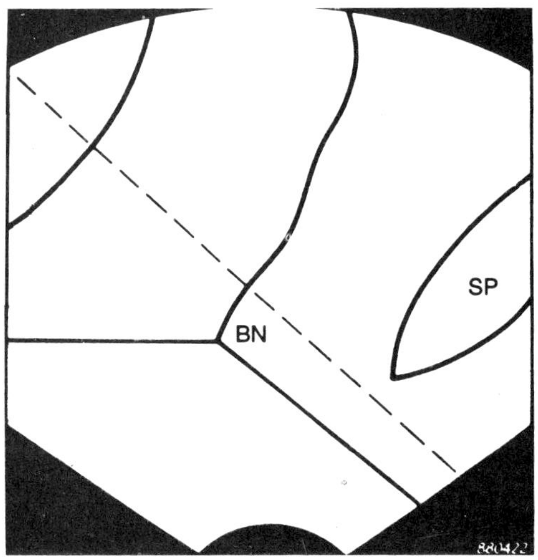

Fig. 14.3. Schematic diagram of structures in the lower pelvis that can be seen in the scanning plane. The longitudinal axis of the patient is indicated by the dotted line. BN — bladder neck; SP — symphysis pubis.

of the bladder neck, above the inferior border of the symphysis pubis is significantly greater than that of a woman with stress incontinence. There is no change in the bladder neck during a cough (Fig. 14.4).

In a woman with stress incontinence, there is a low position of the bladder neck in the resting phase, in relation to the inferior border of the symphysis pubis (Fig. 14.5).

Coughing will produce descent and opening of the bladder neck in a women with stress incontinence (Fig. 14.6).

Transvaginal endosonography is suitable for the per-operative assessment of patients. During a Burch colposuspension, where the bladder neck is supported by suturing the vaginal fornices to the ileo-pectineal ligament, transvaginal sonography can be performed to assess the accurate positioning of the sutures and elevation of the bladder neck[3] (Fig. 14.7).

The same is the case in a Stamey's procedure. The presence of a balloon catheter in the bladder facilitates the identification of the anatomical landmarks.

Post-operative assessment

Since many abdominal procedures for stress incontinence have an anatomical objective, this technique has been used for the assessment of surgical results. The post-operative configuration following a colposuspension is shown in Fig. 14.8.

The new elevated position of the bladder neck is clearly demonstrated.

The advantages of transvaginal endosonography in stress incontinence are that :

1. It is compact and convenient to use.
2. The anatomical view is both clearly and definitely identified.

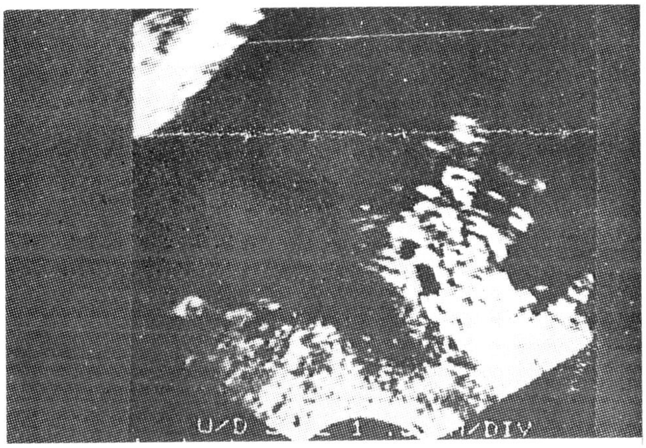

Fig. 14.4. Nulliparous woman with no stress incontinence. Bladder neck supported well above inferior border of symphysis pubis.

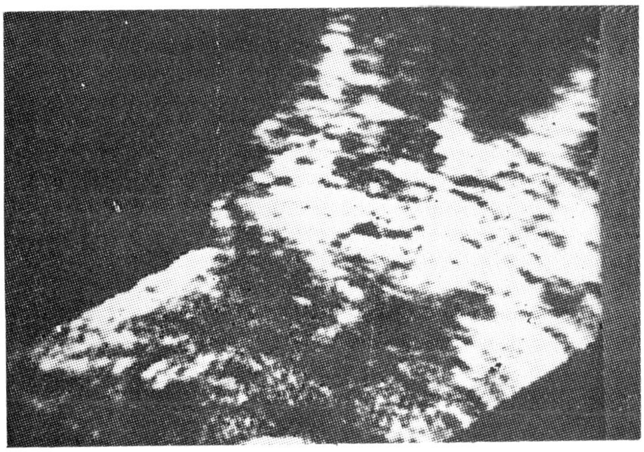

Fig. 14.5. A woman with stress incontinence. Note the relatively low position of the bladder neck.

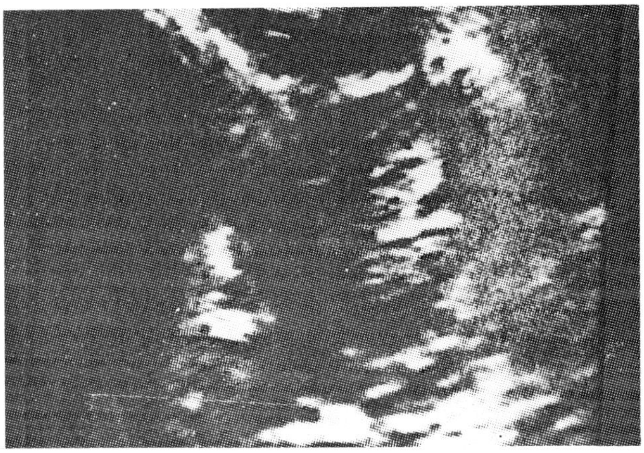

Fig. 14.6. Same patient as in Fig. 14.5. The patient has been asked to cough, which leads to opening and descent of the bladder neck.

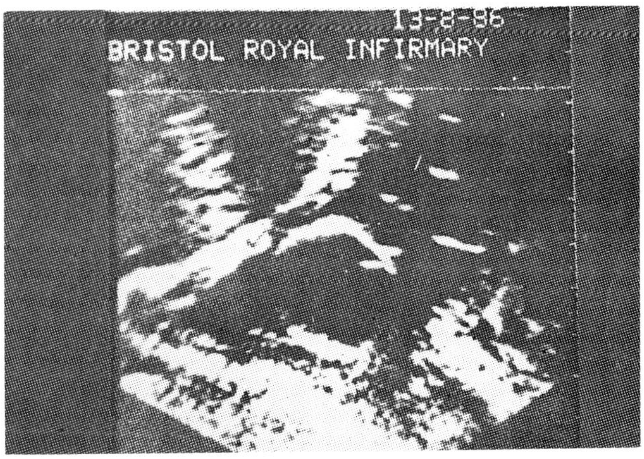

Fig. 14.7. Transvaginal endosonography used during colposuspension.

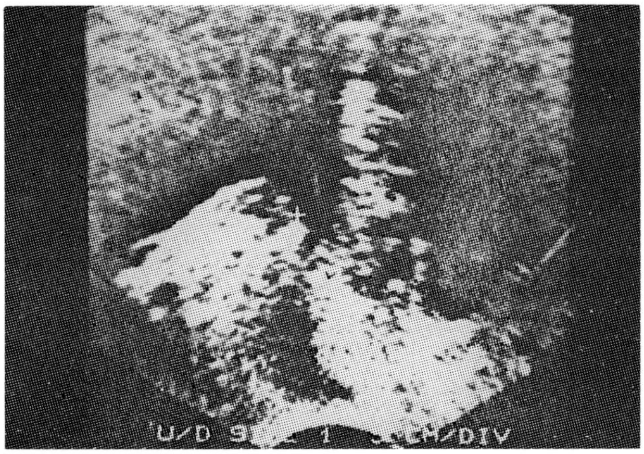

Fig. 14.8. A typical scan image following colposuspension.

3. The technique allows for both static and dynamic assessment.
4. The procedure is well accepted by patients.

The greatest disadvantage of transvaginal sonography is its inability to accurately diagnose urge incontinence. Thus transvaginal sonography cannot replace urodynamics. It is an extra useful tool for the diagnosis and workup of patients with stress incontinence.

Acknowledgements

I express my gratitude to Mr. P.J.B. Smith, Chm, F.R.C.S. — Consultant Urologist, Bristol Royal Infirmary, Bristol, UK, and Mr. Martin Quinn, M.R.C.O.G., who was my Gynaecological Registrar colleague during my tenure at the Royal Infirmary at Bristol.

REFERENCES

1. Hodgkinson CP. Recurrent stress incontinence. Am J Obstet Gynecol 1978; 132 : 844-6.
2. Hilton P. Urethral pressure measurements by micro-transducer : The results in symptom-free women and in those with genuine stress incontinence. Br J Obstet Gynaecol 1983; 90 : 919-21.
3. Quinn MJ. Transvaginal endosonography in the assessment of anatomical effects of colposuspension. Presented at the Royal College of Obstetricians and Gynaecologists, December 1987.

CHAPTER

15

Sonography in Gynaecologic Oncology

Mukund Joshi

Introduction

Transvaginal sonography (TVS), first described in 1969 by Kratochwil has come a long way and is today an established technique of imaging in obstetrics and gynaecology. Recent technical advances in TVS have greatly enhanced our ability to diagnose and characterize pelvic neoplasms[1].

Ultrasonography is useful in the preoperative staging of a neoplasm, evaluating post-operative residual disease, assessing recurrence and to follow the response of tumors to chemotherapy and radiotherapy. The introduction of colour flow imaging shows great promise. Several reports are now available that highlight its ability to differentiate between benign and malignant lesions[2,3,4]. The role of TVS in screening programmes to detect early ovarian cancers is gaining importance[5]. The usefulness of TVS in the evaluation of postmenopausal pelvis is now well established[6]. TVS is best used as a complimentary examination to transabdominal sonography (TAS)[7]. Combination of the two examinations gives better results and has had a greater impact on the diagnostic evaluation, management and follow up of pelvic malignancies. However, TVS is superior to TAS in delineating the internal structure of pelvic masses.

The role of ultrasonography in gynaecologic malignancy may be summarised as follows :

(i) Confirmation of the presence or absence of a pelvic mass.

(ii) Determination of the site of origin and the precise relation of the mass to other pelvic organs.

(iii) Evaluation of the size, echotexture and contour of the mass.

(iv) Delineation of ascites, lymphadenopathy and other features of malignancy[8].

The following discussion briefly outlines the role of ultrasonography, especially TVS, in the assessment of ovarian, fallopian tube, endometrial, uterine body and cervical malignancies. A mention has been made of trophoblastic disease and recurrent pelvic malignancies. The role of TVS in the evaluation of postmenopausal women, its utility in the screening programmes to detect early neoplasms and the role of colour flow imaging in the diagnosis of pelvic malignancies has been discussed.

Ovarian tumors

Ovarian malignancy is the leading cause of death for gynaecologic malignancies. The overall five year survival rate is 30-40%. The poor outcome is due to the late diagnosis as a result of lack of symptoms associated with early disease and the difficulty of detecting an increase in the ovarian size by clinical examination. Rodriguez *et al.*[9] have shown in their series the importance of TVS in visualising postmenopausal ovaries. However, Fleischer *et al.*[10] believe that 25-40% of postmenopausal ovaries are not visualised with ultrasonography. While TAS provides an overview of pelvic anatomy, TVS provides detail of the internal structure of the mass.

Staging

A simple and practical method of staging ovarian carcinoma is :

Stage I — Disease limited to the ovary.

Stage II — Extension to the surrounding pelvic structures.

Stage III — Spread in the abdominal cavity up to the diaphragm.

Stage IV — Hepatic metastases or disease beyond the diaphragm.

Tumors of the ovary may arise from one of the following components :

(i) Surface coelomic epithelium
 Serous cystadenocarcinoma
 Mucinous cystadenocarcinoma
 Ovarian carcinoma
(ii) Germ cell tumors
(iii) Sex cord stromal tumors
(iv) Primary lymphoma of the ovary
(v) Metastatic tumors
 Breast
 Bowel
 Endometrium
 Skin

The overall ultrasound findings in ovarian cancers may be summarised as :

(i) Solid, cystic or mixed mass

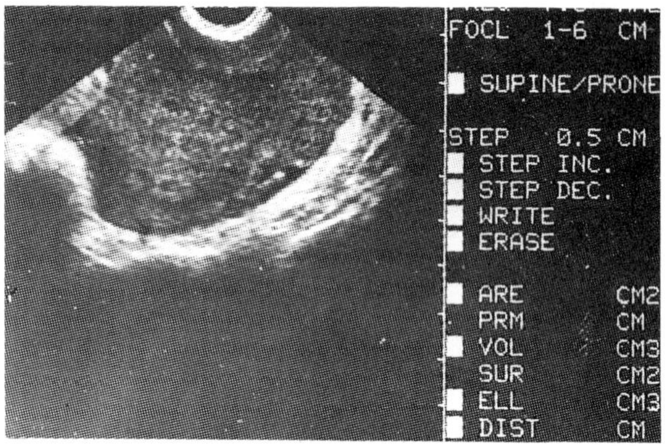

Fig. 15.1. Ovarian carcinoma. A solid echo-poor mass (right ovary).

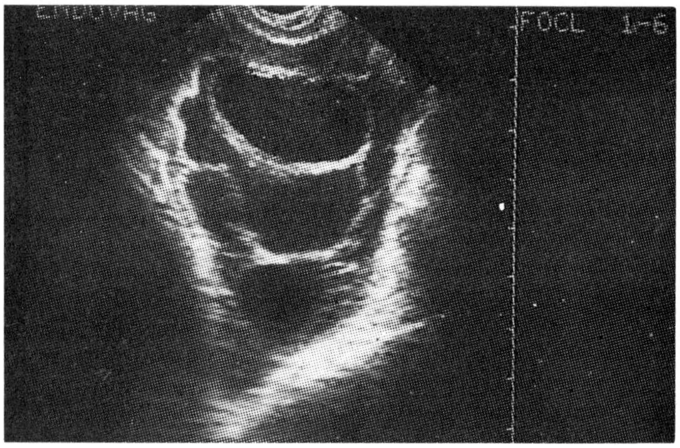

Fig. 15.2. Pseudomucinous cystadenocarcinoma. Multiple ovarian mass with low level internal echoes.

(ii) Presence of septae
(iii) Papillary projections
(iv) Daughter cysts
(v) Loculations
(vi) Large tumor size
(vii) Irregular external contour

However, the above features are often seen in benign lesions. Considerable overlap in the appearance of ovarian tumors is seen in day to day practice. Sonographic findings should not be expected to indicate a specific histologic diagnosis or the stage of the disease. Sonography can, however, suggest differential diagnosis by distinguishing predominantly cystic tumours from predominantly solid tumours and by demonstrating other characteristics of the mass. Demonstration of omental or peritoneal masses, hepatic metastases, ruptured capsule, pseudomyxoma peritonei, ascites or pleural effusion raise a high suspicion of the lesion being malignant[11]. When an ovarian mass in seen on sonography, factors which are associated with greater risk of malignancy are :

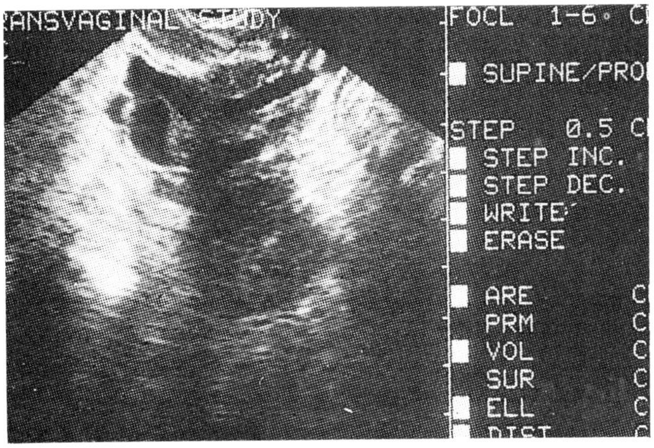

Fig. 15.3. Krukenberg's tumour. A known case of Ca breast showing a solid/cystic ovarian mass lesion.

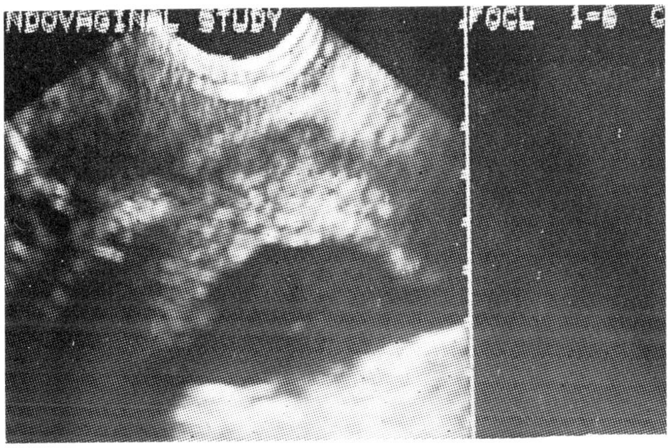

Fig. 15.4. Operated case of Ca ovary with ascites. TVS shows omental metastis.

1. A size larger than 5.0 cm[12]
2. A solid cystic complex mass[13,14]
3. Persistence over a period of time[15]

The importance of size of the mass as an independent factor has been debated and questioned since malignant masses are frequently 5.0 cm and cysts larger than 5.0 cm[16,17]. Purely cystic lesions have a low incidence of being malignant[18,19].

With the advent of TVS and colour flow imaging, it may now be possible to detect ovarian cancers before they have metastasized. Van Nagell *et al.*[20] have established characteristics of ovarian masses by TVS.

Serous cystadenocarcinoma is the most common malignant ovarian neoplasm. It is usually large and multilocular, containing papillary projections and solid nodules. Mucinous cystadenocarcinomas are the second most common tumours. They are usually very large and present as multiloculated cystic masses. Solid nodules and papillary projections are seen. Pseudomyxoma peritonei may result from spread of mucinous contents into the peritoneal cavity. Endometroid carcinoma constitutes 15% of all ovarian carcinomas. Typically, it is a cystic mass with solid elements. The sonographic appearance may be similar to an endometrioma. Granulosa cell tumors may be hormonally productive. In contrast to epithelial tumours, majority of granulosa cell tumours are stage I presentations, indicating their low malignant potential. They are generally solid, though they may show regions of degeneration. They may be multilocular or unilocular.

Metastatic carcinomas represent 10% of ovarian cancers. Those from the stomach are usually bilateral. Associated ascites is often seen.

Fallopian tube carcinoma

Adenocarcinoma of the fallopian tube is the rarest of gynaecologic malignancies. Their behaviour is similar to that of ovarian neoplasms. On the ultrasound study, a sausage-shaped solid adnexal mass with mixed echogenicity is observed[21]. However, the diagnosis is most often made on the surgical specimen.

Endometrial carcinoma

85% of endometrial carcinomas are postmenopausal. Endometrial carcinomas should be considered whenever the endometrium is abnormally thickened (8.0 mm) in postmenopausal women. The risk of endometrial carcinoma increases with the degree of endometrial thickening[22].

In addition to endometrial thickening sonographic findings of more advanced invasive endometrial cancer include mixed echogenicity of the myometrium and a lobular contour of the uterus. This indicates myometrial infiltration[23,24].

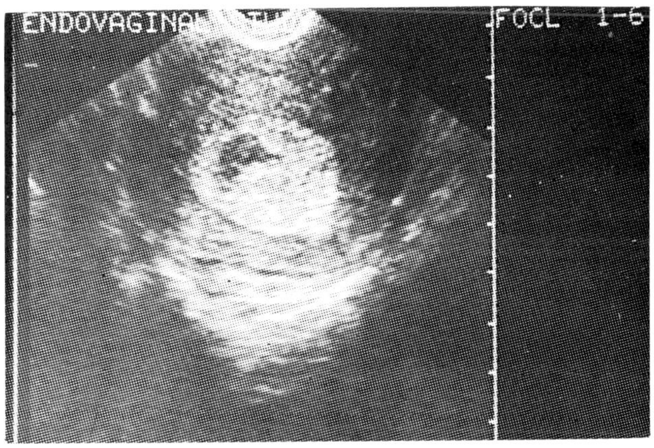

Fig. 15.5. Endometrial carcinoma in a postmenopausal patient with irregular thickening of the endometrium and fluid within the endometrial cavity. No myometrial invasion.

The other nonspecific sonographic findings include nonhomogeneous echogenicity of the endometrium and a polypoid mass or a small endometrial fluid collection[25].

Doppler evaluation has been helpful in distinguishing benign from malignant endometrial thickening[26]. It is found that in the normal postmenopausal women, (RI > 0.7) a high resistance flow pattern is seen. In comparison, low resistance patterns (RI < 0.7) may be seen in patients with endometrial carcinoma. It is suggested that one must perform Doppler ultrasound in all patients with an endometrial thickness of 8.0 mm. A high resistance pattern is reassuring of its benign nature. However one must be aware that in their recent study Bourne *et al.*[27] have shown a wide overlap between benign and malignant endometrial thickening.

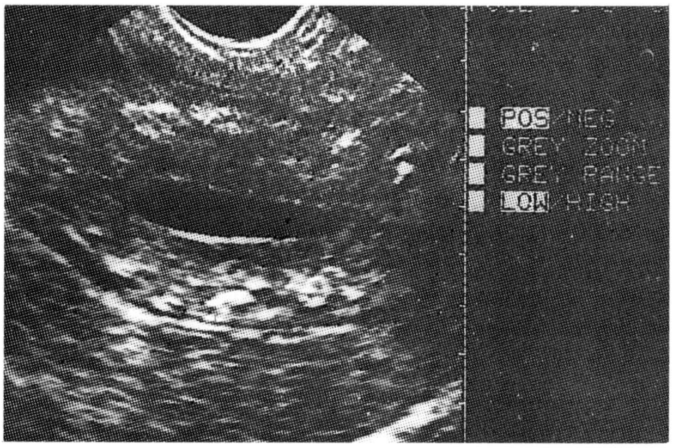

Fig. 15.6. Normal postmenopausal uterus. Vascular calcification in the myometrium. Thin endometrium. Small amount of fluid in the endometrial cavity — a normal finding.

Cervical carcinoma

Cervical carcinoma accounts for 15% of cancers in women. Assessment of tumor size and extent of invasion is crucial in planning treatment for carcinoma of cervix. TVS plays a major role in determining the maximum depth of invasion within the cervix and the adjoining tissues. To image the cervix with transvaginal technique, the probe must be pulled distally in the vagina. An enlarged cervix, a cervical mass or fluid collection in the endometrial cavity secondary to stenosis are the common ultrasound findings. TVS and more recently, transrectal sonography have been used in the staging of cervical cancer[28,29].

Trophoblastic disease

Sonographic appearance of molar pregnancy varies with the gestational age at which the study is

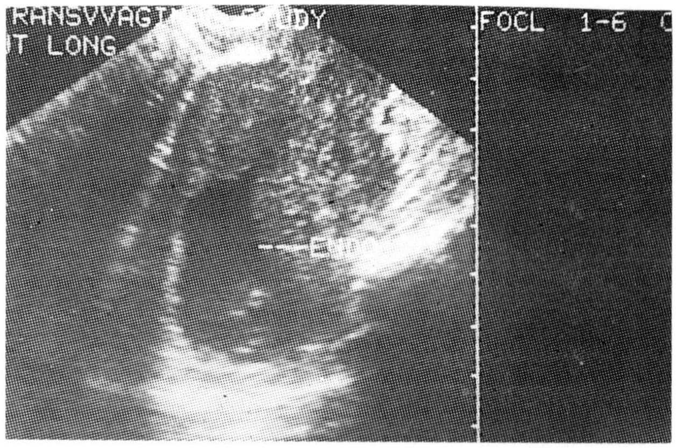

Fig. 15.7. Ca cervix with pyometra. Cervical solid mass lesion with fluid within the endometrial cavity. TVS shows echoes and debris within the fluid.

performed[30]. In the first trimester, it mimics a missed abortion. With advancing gestational age, multiple small cysts develop which increase in size over a period of time. TVS demonstrates not only the primary lesion but also myometrial invasion, thus assisting in clinical staging. Choriocarcinoma appears as an irregular echogenic tumor mass containing areas of necrosis and haemorrhage. Transvaginal colour flow studies are helpful in evaluating abnormal appearing areas of endometrium[31]. TVS is also useful to monitor tumor response to chemotherapy[32].

Recurrent gynaecologic malignancies

Gynaecologic neoplasms usually recur in the first two years. Most recurrences are located in the pelvis. Transvaginal and transrectal sonography are now being used to evaluate the therapeutic response to ovarian, uterine and cervical malignancies. Schoenfeld *et al.*[33] have used TVS to demonstrate vaginal vault recurrence.

TVS in postmenopausal women

Unexpected vaginal bleeding in a postmenopausal woman is always a cause of concern. The common causes for such bleeding include endometrial hyperplasia, polyps or endometrial carcinoma. The normal postmenopausal uterus is atrophic. The normal postmenopausal endometrium is also atrophic, appearing as a thin echogenic line. A sonographically measured endometrium of 8 mm or less is a common finding. A small amount of fluid of 2 cc within the endometrial cavity may be seen occasionally in an asymptomatic postmenopausal woman. However, endometrial fluid may be associated with a gynaecologic malignancy[34].

Increasing attention has been directed to postmenopausal women in an attempt to identify ovarian cancer at an earlier, treatable stage. The primary reason for doing TVS in the postmenopausal women is inadequate visualisation of the ovary on the TAS. The other indications are poor visualisation of the endometrial echoes, better characterization of a visualised TAS finding and a suboptimal TAS examination[8].

Ultrasound has been advocated as the method of choice for evaluation of ovaries in postmenopausal women, both, to visualise enlarged ovaries as well as to detect a possible mass lesion. TVS in particular is indicated in those women in whom ovaries are not adequately visualised by TAS.

Use of colour flow imaging has further enhanced the utility of TVS in detecting early ovarian neoplasms.

Screening

Screening for ovarian malignancy is a controversial subject especially in a country like India. This is because of our illiteracy and the lack of awareness of the significance of this dreadful disease. Also of importance is the problem of the undetectable nature and absence of symptoms in the early stages. The goal of these screening programmes should be the identification of ovarian tumors in ovaries that are not significantly enlarged. The recent developments of TVS, hormonal assays and measurements and other markers released from the ovaries have been of great help in the study of ovarian abnormalities.

Doppler

Colour flow imaging allows detailed depiction of the vessels supplying the uterus and the ovaries. Recent studies indicate that it may now be possible to differentiate between benign and malignant ovarian masses[35,36].

Colour flow studies detect blood flow in small low resistance vessels as are seen in neoplastic tissue. Pulsed Doppler studies can then quantify such colour flow. With colour flow studies, it is now possible to discover ovarian carcinoma at an early stage (stage 1 A). However this will need further observation. Only time will tell whether the diagnostic criteria used will be helpful since there is overlap of findings of different lesions. Colour flow imaging and TVS have shown great promise in identifying patients with endometrial carcinoma and differentiating between benign and malignant uterine neoplasms.

In brief, if a low resistance pattern is seen in an adnexal mass, it is abnormal and considered suspicious for a neoplasm. Although Doppler studies may be of value in detecting malignant lesions, there are still a number of benign adnexal processes including the normal corpus luteum that may demonstrate low resistance flow. Fleischer *et al.*[37] suggest that a pulsatility index (PI) of 1.0 indicates malignancy. The PI for benign lesions ranges from 0.7-0.4 and 0.4-1.9 for surgically proven malignancy.

Summary

TVS has significantly improved our ability to evaluate patients with pelvic and gynaecologic neoplasms. The most important contribution of TVS has been in the detection and characterization of pelvic masses in women who are not known to have a tumor.

Awareness of the typical sonographic and clinical features of pelvic tumors should further enhance the value of TVS in this evaluation. The development of colour flow imaging by the transvaginal probe is an excellent technical advance and there is good evidence to suggest that this imaging technique will be helpful in characterizing adnexal masses.

REFERENCES

1. Mendelson EB, Bohm-Velez M. Transvaginal sonography of pelvic neoplasms. Rad Clin of North Am 1992-30 : 703-5.
2. Bourne TH, Campbell S, Steer C. Transvaginal colour flow imaging : a possible new screening technique for ovarian cancer. BMJ 1989; 299 : 1367-9.
3. Kurjak A, Zalud I. Evaluation of adnexal masses with transvaginal color ultrasound. J Ultra Med 1991; 10 : 295-9.
4. Hata T, Hata K, Senoh D. Doppler assessment of tumor vascularity in gynecologic disorders. J Ultra Med 1989; 8 : 309-13.
5. Higgins RV, Van Negell JR, Donaldson E. Transvaginal sonography as a screening method for ovarian cancer. Gynecol Oncol 1989; 34 : 402-6.
6. Varner RE, Sparks JM, Cameron CD. Transvaginal sonography of the endometrium in postmenopausal women. Obstet Gynecol 1991; 78 : 195-9.
7. Coleman BG, Argen PH, Grumbach K. Transvaginal and transabdominal sonography. Prospective comparison. Radiology 1988; 168 : 639-43.
8. Arger Peter H. Transvaginal sonography in postmenopausal patients. Rad Clin North Am 1992; 30 : 759-63.
9. Rodriguez MH, Platt LD, Medearis AL. The use of transvaginal sonography for evaluation of postmenopausal ovarian size and morphology. Am J Obstet Gynecol 1988; 159 : 810-5.

10. Fleischer AC, McKee MS, Gordon AN. Transvaginal sonography of postmenopausal ovaries with pathologic correlation. J Ultra Med 1990; 9 : 637-42.
11. Moyle JW, Rochester D, Sider L. Sonography of ovarian tumors : Predictability of tumor type. AJR 1983; 141 : 985-9.
12. Sparks JM, Verger RE. Ovarian cancer screening. Obstet Gynecol 1991; 77 : 787-92.
13. Luxman D, Bergman A, Sagi J. The postmenopausal adnexal mass : correlation between ultrasonic and pathological findings. Obstet Gynecol 1991; 77 : 726-9.
14. Sassone AM, Timor-Tritsch TE, Artner A. Transvaginal sonographic characterization of ovarian disease, evaluation of a new scoring system to predict ovarian malignancy. Obstet Gynecol 1991; 78 : 70-5.
15. Hurwitz A, Fagel S, Zion I. The management of persistent clear pelvic cysts diagnosed by ultrasonography. Obstet Gynecol 1988; 72 : 320-6.
16. Granberg S, Norstrom A, Wikland M. Tumors in the lower pelvis as imaged by vaginal sonography. Gynecol Oncology 1990; 37 : 224-7.
17. Herrman UJ, Locher GN, Goldhirsch A. Sonographic patterns of ovarian tumors : prediction of malignancy. Obstet Gynecol 1987; 69 : 777-82.
18. Rulin MC, Preston AL. Adnexal masses in postmenopausal women. Obstet Gynecol 1987; 70 : 578-83.
19. Goldstein S, Subramanyam B, Synder F. The postmenopausal cystic adnexal mass. The potential role of ultrasound in conservative management. Obstet Gynecol 1989; 73 : 8-11.
20. Van Nagell JR Jr, Defriest PD, Puts PD. Ovarian cancer screening in asymptomatic postmenopausal women by transvaginal sonography. Cancer 1991; 68 : 458-62.
21. Meyer JS, Kim GS, Price HM. Ultrasound presentation of primary carcinoma of the fallopian tube. J Clin Ultrasound 1987; 15 : 132-6.
22. Varner ED, Sparks JM, Cameron CD. Transvaginal sonography of the endometrium in postmenopausal women. Obstet Gynecol 1991; 78 : 195-9.
23. Fleischer AC, Dudley BS, Entman SS. Myometrial invasion by endometrial carcinoma : Sonographic assessment. Radiology 1987; 162 : 307-12.
24. Gordon AN, Fleischer AC, Reed GW. Depth of myometrial invasion by endometrial cancer : Preoperative assessment by transvaginal ultrasonography. 1990; 39 : 321-5.
25. Luesley DM. Vaginal ultrasound and endometrial carcinoma. Lancet 1990; i : 256-61.
26. Bourne TH, Campbell S. Detection of endometrial cancer in postmenopausal women by transvaginal sonography and colour flow imaging. BMJ 1990; 301 : 369-72.
27. Bourne TH, Campbell S, Steer CV. Detection of endometrial cancer by transvaginal ultrasonography with colour flow imaging and blood flow analysis : A preliminary report. Gynecol Oncol 1991; 40 : 253-8.
28. Carter J, Carson LF, Elg S. Transvaginal sonography as an aid in the clinical staging of carcinoma of the cervix. J Clin Ultrasound 1991; 20 : 283-7.
29. Mage BJ, Locue JP, Swindell R. Tumor size as a prognostic factor in carcinoma of cervix : Assessment by transrectal ultrasound. Br J Radiol 1991; 64 : 812-7.
30. Munyer TP, Callen PW, Filly RA. Further observations on the sonographic spectrum of gestational trophoblastic disease. J Clin Ultrasound 1981; 9 : 349-53.
31. Desai RK, Desberg AL. Diagnosis of gestational trophoblastic disease : Value of endovaginal colour flow Doppler sonography. 1991; 157 : 787-92.
32. Schneider DF, Bukovsky I, Weinraub Z. Transvaginal ultrasound diagnosis and treatment follow up of invasive gestational trophoblastic disease. J Clin Ultrasound 1990; 18 : 110-7.
33. Schoenfeld A, Levai H, Hirsh M. Transvaginal sonography in postmenopausal woman. J Clin Ultrasound 1990; 18 : 350-7.
34. Chambers CB, Linis JS. Ultrasonographic evidence of uterine malignancy, postmenopausal uterus. AM J Obstet Gynecol 1986; 54 : 1194-9.
35. Fleischer AC, Rodgers WH, Rao BK. Assessment of ovarian tumor vascularity with transvaginal colour Doppler sonography. J Ult Med 1991; 10 : 563-6.
36. Fleischer AC, Rodgers WH, Kepple DM. Colour Doppler sonography of benign and malignant ovarian masses. Radiographics. 1992; 12 : 879-83.
37. Fleischer AC, Rodgers WH, Kepple DM. Colour Doppler sonography of ovarian masses. A multiparameter analysis. J Ultra Med 1993; 12 : 41-5.

CHAPTER

16

Transvaginal Sonography in the Diagnosis of Pelvic Inflammatory Disease

Shyam Baruah

Pelvic inflammatory disease in women is manifested as inflammation of the upper genital tract. The term embraces endometritis, salpingitis, and salpingo-oophoritis, together with spread to the peritoneum and along the paracolic gutters to cause the Fitzugh-Curtis syndrome of perihepatitis. It is virtually always due to ascending infection through the cavities of cervix, uterus and fallopian tubes; on histological examination the endometrium is always affected[1,2].

The clinical diagnosis of pelvic inflammatory disease (PID) can be incorrect in 35% cases. There is a strong case for performing laparoscopy to confirm the diagnosis[3]. By laparoscopy the fallopian tubes can be assessed for visual signs of salpingitis. Free fluid can be aspirated for bacterial examination and histological evidence obtained from fimbrial and endometrial biopsy[4,5]. Instead the most common approach is to treat first with a trial of antibiotics[6]. It is here that TVS has shown promising results, as a step prior to a trial of antibiotics. It has its use in identifying dilated fallopian tubes (Fig. 16.1)[7], detecting ovarian enlargement and ovarian thickening, and identifying small fluid collection in pelvic peritoneum[8] (Fig. 16.2). TVS has a role to identify a clinically detectable mass as a tubo-

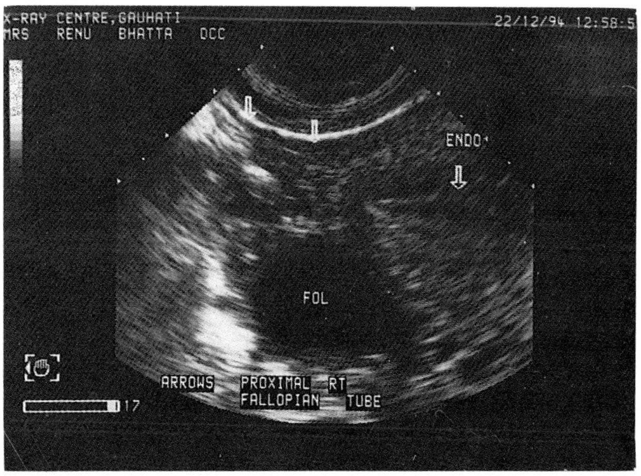

Fig. 16.1. Normal proximal fallopian tube as seen in TV scan.

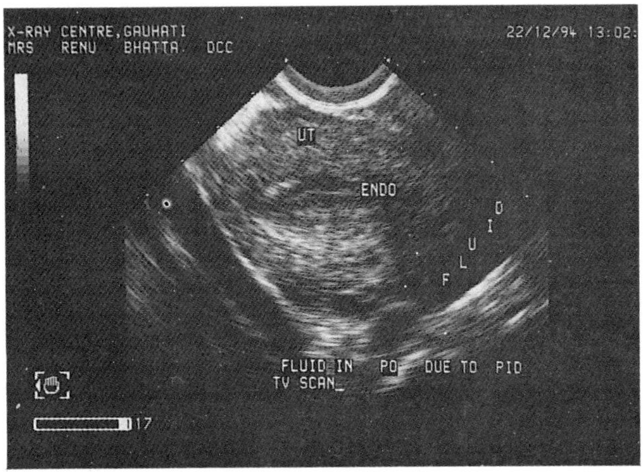

Fig. 16.2. Free fluid in POD in early PID.

ovarian abscess[6], and to guide the needle to aspirate the abscess[9].

TVS and endometritis

In our experience TVS detection of endometritis is by and large disappointing. In a study, only 25% of histologically proved endometritis showed nonspecific findings of increased uterine size, increased endometrial thickness (more than 12 mm) and either increased or decreased endometrial echogenicity in some cases. Uterine outline was indistinct due to periuterine exudates[10]. Finding of small endometrial fluid collection was occasionally present in acute endometritis[11]. In another study endometrial fluid collection was demonstrated in only 12% of endometritis[12].

TVS and salpingo-oophoritis

Early in the course of acute salpingitis TVS of pelvis may be entirely normal. The normal fallopian tube is narrow (1 mm to 4 mm) and mid and distal portion are not seen on TVS. The proximal portion of the tube with the round ligament is however consistently seen on TVS, and visualization of normal calibre tubes is enhanced if there is fluid surrounding tubes and in cul-de-sac. With erythema of tubes and early exudation on surface of tubes and ovaries, the outline of proximal tube and ovaries become indistinct. When exudates pour out from the fimbrial end, TVS can demonstrate early fluid collection in the periovarian region and cul-de-sac[12]; with spreading inflammation of pelvic peritoneum, such free fluid can get loculated higher at POD or around proximal tubes and ovaries and such demonstration of fluid pockets is a very useful TVS indicator of PID. Demonstration of fine echofloaters in fluid collection on high resolution TVS can suggest the seropurulent nature of the fluid[13]. As the infection ultimately spreads to ovaries, TVS can demonstrate enlarged globular ovaries with multiple cysts[14]. Fine echofloaters can be demonstrated in some of these cysts[12]. With subacute inflammation of fallopian tubes, the ostium may become occluded and the tube then fills up with serous fluid and pus. Acutely inflammed fallopian tubes become thick-walled and irregular and dilate and become convoluted (Figs. 16.3, 16.4 and 16.5). The tubes at this stage are consistently visualized on TVS. The tubes appear as a tubular structure (more than 4 mm) with a folded configuration. The wall of the structure represents the mucosa and is well-defined and echogenic[7] and small polypoidal nodules may be demonstrated projecting into the lumen[15]. Short linear

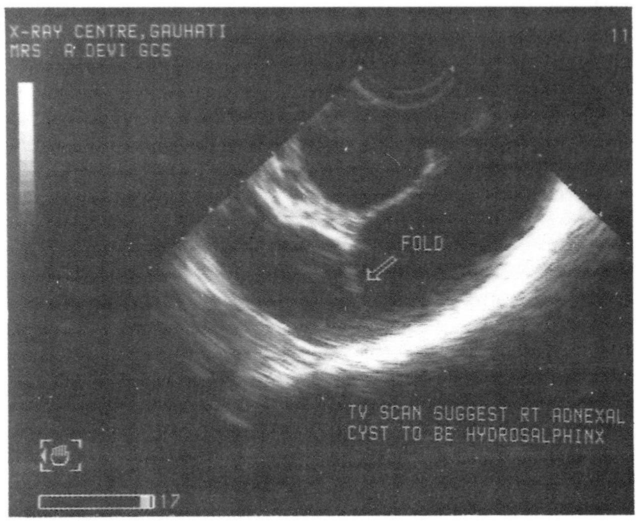

Fig. 16.3. Dilated fallopian tube due to hydrosalpinx as seen in TV scan.

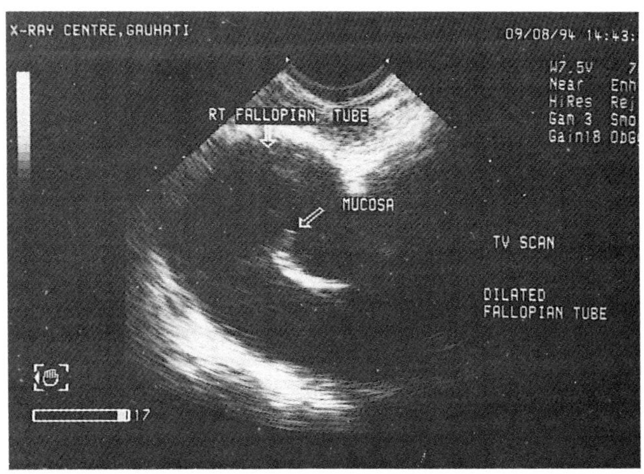

Fig. 16.4. Fallopian tube mucosal folds of a dilated fallopian tube.

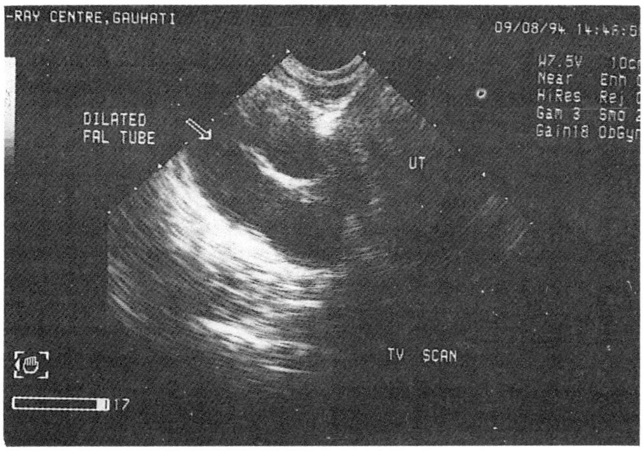

Fig. 16.5. Dilated fallopian tube and early fluid echoes suggesting a pyosalpinx in TV scan.

echoes protruding into the lumen is a feature that can be seen and is related to the wrinkled nature of the fallopian tube epithelium[7]. Colour flow Doppler may occasionally be necessary to distinguish pelvic varices from dilated fallopian tubes (Figs. 16.6A & B). Varicoid vessels generally extend more laterally towards the pelvic wall anterior to the iliopsoas bundle, and they tend to cross the midline with PID and often outline the posterior border of uterus. Pyosalpinx can be recognised on TVS as internal echoes within dilated fallopian tubes, and a fluid pus layer may sometimes be evident[16]. Anechoic fluid within a dilated tube suggests hydrosalpinx and correlates with chronic infection. With chronic infection and pelvic adhesions there is loss of motion of ovary on pressure with TVS probe; Ovary glide sign[17].

TVS and tubo-ovarian abscess

Progressive spillage of purulent exudate from the tube results in extensive inflammation, suppuration and adhesions and in advanced cases prevents identification of fallopian tube and ovaries as discrete structures by TVS. It commonly results in a complex mass and is seen on TVS as an hypoechoic adnexal mass with variable septations, irregular margins, scattered internal echoes and fluid debris level[18]. Tubo-ovarian mass can appear solid, when the contents represent complex fluid. Collection of gas is occasionally present. When performing TVS for diagnosis of tubo-ovarian abscess one must try to identify the fallopian tube and its mucosa and ovarian tissue within or near the mass. With TVS with high resolution probes it is often possible to do so even when margins of these structures are ill-defined[12]. The complex pelvic mass of a tubo-ovarian abscess on TVS may mimic benign and

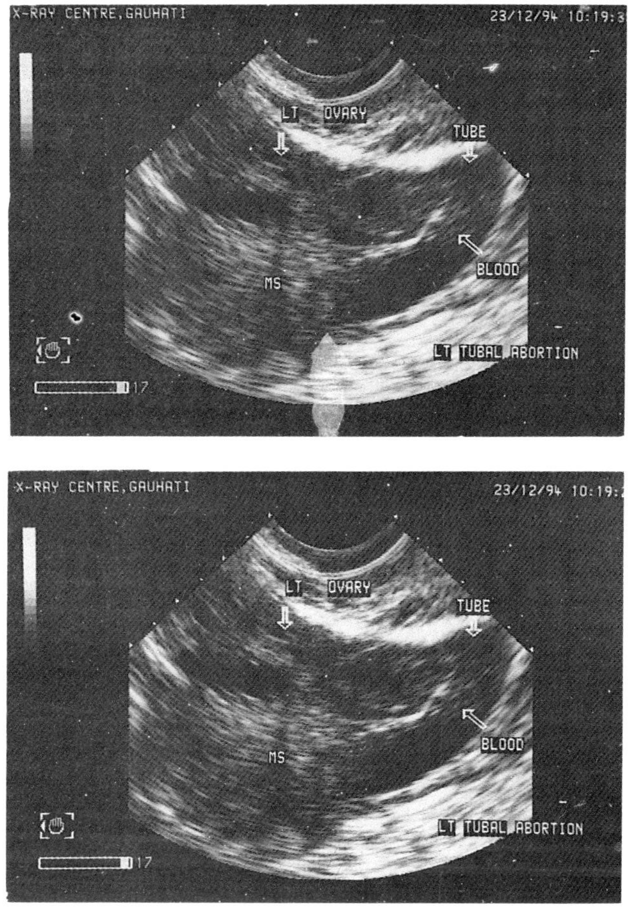

Fig. 16.6A & B. TV scan showing dilated tube and hematosalpinx.

malignant ovarian masses, endometriomas, and acute and chronic ectopic pregnancy. And in those cases where identification of fallopian tubes is not possible by TVS, a careful correlation of the sonographic findings with clinical examination and patient's history is essential before suggesting the correct diagnosis.

Transvaginal ultrasound-guided aspiration has been done to drain tubo-ovarian abscesses. Only light sedation is required and is recommended as alternative to open laparoscopy in the treatment of tubo-ovarian abscess[9]. Lastly serial TVS examination during the course of the disease is helpful in evaluating response to therapy, whether after antibiotics or after drainage.

REFERENCES

1. Westrom L. Incidence, prevalence and trends of acute pelvic inflammatory disease and its consequences in industrialized countries. Am J Obstet Gynecol 1980; 139 : 880-892.

2. Heinonen PK, Teisala K, Punnonen R, Miettenen A, Lehtinen M, Paavonen J. Anatomic sites of upper genital tract infection. Obstet Gynaecol 1985; 66 : 384-390.
3. Jacobson L, Westrom L. Objectivised diagnosis of acute pelvic inflammatory disease. Am J Obstet Gynecol 1984; 105 : 1088-98.
4. Mardh PA, Ripa T, Svensson L, Westrom L. Chlamydia trachomatis infection in patients acute salpingitis. N Engl L Med 1977; 296 : 1377-9.
5. Sellor J, Mathony J, Goldsmith C, Rath D, *et al.* The accuracy of clinical findings and laparoscopy in pelvic inflammatory disease. Am J Obstet Gynecol 1991; 164 : 113-120.
6. Lundborg WI, Wall JE, Mathers JE. Laparoscopy in evaluation of pelvic pain. Obstet Gynaecol 1973; 42 : 872-876.
7. Tessler FN, Perrella RR, Fleischer AC, *et al.* Endovaginal sonographic diagnosis of dilated fallopian tubes. AJR 1989; 153 : 523-525.
8. Lande IM, Hill MC, Cosco FE, Kator NN. Adnexal and cul-de-sac abnormalities : transvaginal sonography. Radiology 1988; 166 : 325-332.
9. Teisala K. Heinonen PK, Punnonen R. Transvaginal ultrasound in diagnosis and treatment of tubo-ovarian abscess. British Journal of Obstetrics and Gynaecology 1990; 97 : 178-180.
10. Patten RM, Vincent LM, Wolner Hanssen P, Thorpe E Jr. Pelvic inflammatory disease : endovaginal sonography with laparoscopic correlation. J Ultrasound Med 1990; 9 : 681-689.
11. Laing FC, Filly RA, Marks WM, Brown TW. Ultrasound demonstration endometrial fluid collection unassociated with pregnancy. Radiology 1980; 137 : 471-474.
12. Bulas I Dorothy, Ahstrom A. Promise, Sivit CJ, Blask ANR, M. O'Donnell R. Pelvic inflammatory disease in the adolescent : Comparison of transabdominal and transvaginal sonographic evaluation. Radiology 1992; 183 : 435-439.
13. Nyberg DA, Hughes MP, Mack LA. Extrauterine findings of ectopic pregnancy at transvaginal US : Importance of echogenic fluid. Radiology 1991; 178 : 823-826.
14. Lansdale RN, Roberts PF, Trowell JE. Autoimmune oophoritis associated with polycystic ovaries. Histopathology 1991; 19 : 77-81.
15. Spaulding LB, Gelman SR, Wood SD, *et al.* The role of ultrasonography in the management of endometritis/salpingitis/peritonitis. Obstet Gynaecol 1979; 53 : 442.
16. Laing FC, *et al.* Technical aspects of vaginal ultrasound. Semin ultrasound CT MR 1990; 2 : 4-11.
17. Timor-Tritsch IE, Rottem S, Lewit N. The fallopian tubes. In : Timor-Tritsch IE, Rottem S (editors). Transvaginal sonography. 2nd ed., Elsevier, New York, 1991.
18. Laing FC, Jeffrey RB Jr. The pelvis. In : Federle MP, Jeffrey RB Jr. (editors). CT and sonography of acute abdomen. Raven, New York, 1989.

CHAPTER

17

Transvaginal Sonography and the Postmenopausal Woman

Sukhpal Sawhney, Rajeev Jain, Alka Kriplani and Karuna Taneja

The superiority of transvaginal sonography (TVS), using high-frequency (5 or 7.5 MHz) transducers, in evaluation of the female pelvis has been established conclusively. Recently, Duplex Doppler and Colour Flow Imaging have been added to TVS in an attempt to further characterise endometrial and ovarian malignancies.

Menopause is an event in every normal woman's life. Problems faced by post-menopausal women are different from those faced by pre-menopausal women. One common clinical problem faced during the post-menopausal period is vaginal bleeding. During the post-menopausal period there is a significant increase in incidence of gynaecological neoplasms, especially endometrial and ovarian carcinomas.

While performing TVS in post-menopausal women, generous lubrication of the transducer must be used, to prevent difficulty or discomfort in insertion of the transducer, due to senile vaginitis. Vaginal sonography is safe and easy to perform and well accepted by patients.

The normal post-menopausal uterus

In the post-menopausal woman, the uterus is relatively small and atrophic, its exact size depending on the number of pregnancies and/or the amount and duration of hormonal supplements. Small leiomyomas, whether solid, cystic or calcified are frequently seen in the myometrium and should be of no concern, unless there is evidence of an increase in size. Adenomyosis may also present as myometrial cystic areas.

Symmetrical, curvilinear myometrial calcification is common and is suggestive of arcuate artery calcification[1]. Nabothian cysts in the cervix and small amounts of fluid in the Pouch of Douglas may be seen.

The normal post-menopausal endometrium, without any supplemental hormone therapy, is atrophic, appears as a thin echogenic line and measures less than 5 mm (in the sagittal plane) including both layers of endometrium, but excluding the periendometrial halo and any fluid within the endometrial cavity[1].

Small volumes (2 ml) of endometrial fluid can be a normal finding, specially in patients taking supplemental hormones[2]. In post-hysterectomy patients, the normal vaginal cuff can appear as a 'pseudo-mass' varying between 0.9 cm to 2.1 cm^3. Free fluid in the cul-de-sac can occasionally be seen in asymptomatic post-menopausal women; however large amounts of fluid, which may be clear or complex may suggest malignancy, hemorrhage or infection.

Normal post-menopausal endometrium

Disorders of the endometrium that occur in this period range from endometrial atrophy, polyps, endometrial hyperplasia, endometrial carcinoma and hormone replacement therapy. These lead to post-menopausal bleeding and necessitate invasive investigation.

While performing transvaginal sonography endometrial thickness should be measured on sagittal scans, at the thickest area of the endometrium from the outermost border on one side to the other side. The endometrial acoustic shadow and any alterations in the endometrial morphology should be noted.

Normal post-menopausal ovaries

In post-menopausal women, it may become difficult to identify the ovaries (specially, if the patient has had a previous hysterectomy), because the ovaries are small and atrophic, without the characteristic developing follicles. In the post-menopausal woman, an ovary should be considered abnormal if it is larger than 8 cm and its morphology gets altered to a heterogeneous, anechoic or hyperechoic pattern with alterations in its contours. Because normal ovarian size varies with hormonal status, and the number of years since menopause, some authors suggest that an ovarian volume twice that of the opposite side should be considered abnormal[4].

Abnormal uterine fluid collections

In the post-menopausal period intrauterine fluid collections are related to estrogen administration, cervical stenosis, cystic endometrial hyperplasia, endometrial polyps and malignancies. Even though most of these fluid collections are related to benign causes, cervical stenosis being one of the most frequent, endometrial fluid collections are an important pointer towards underlying endometrial and cervical malignancies[2] (Fig. 17.1).

Endometrial hyperplasia

Endometrial hyperplasia is abnormal proliferation of

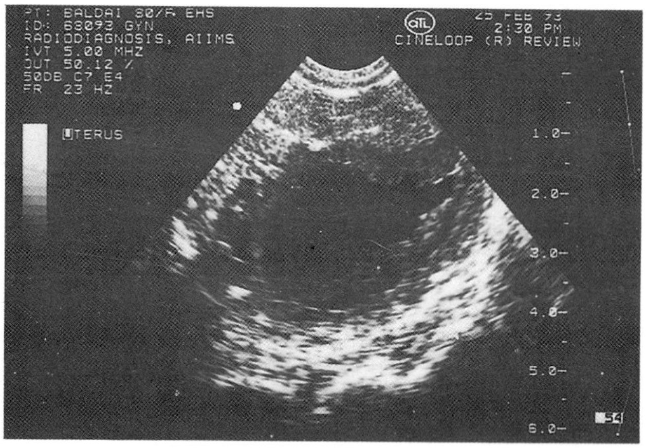

Fig. 17.1. TVS of the uterus shows a large intrauterine fluid collection with echogenic debris (suggestive of pyometra) with irregular endometrium. Histopathology of hysterectomy specimen revealed an endometrial carcinoma leading to cervical stenosis.

endometrial glands and stroma. Cystic hyperplasia is the benign variant. The adenomatous form of hyperplasia may be a precursor to endometrial carcinoma. Hyperplasia appears as thickened endometrium on sonography. When the endometrium has a homogeneous echotexture and the maximum diameter of the endometrium on sonography is 5 mm, a proliferative endometrium cannot be differentiated from hyperplastic endometrium or a superficial adenocarcinoma (Fig. 17.2).

Endometrial atrophy

Endometrial atrophy is a common finding in women with post-menopausal vaginal bleeding. Endometrial

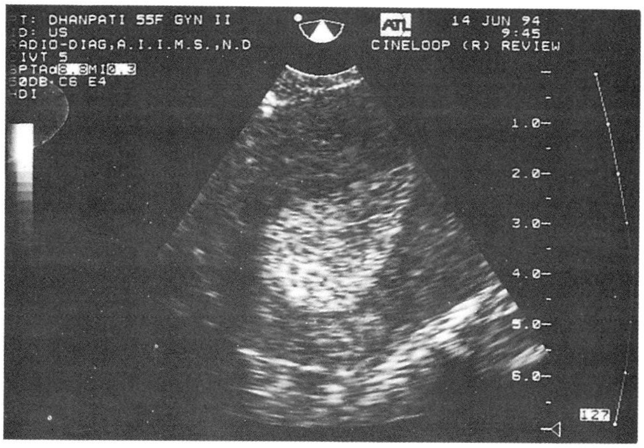

Fig. 17.2. Sagittal TVS reveals a benign hyperplasia of the endometrium measuring 2.4 cm in diameter with homogeneous hyperechoic pattern. The myometrium-endometrium interface is maintained.

thickness less than 5 mm is invariably associated with atrophy and it is suggested that endometrial curettage may not be necessary unless the endometrium is 8 mm or more in diameter.

Hormone replacement therapy

Endometrial diameters in post-menopausal women may be altered by hormone replacement therapy with estrogens and progestins. Sonography will demonstrate an atrophic endometrium that becomes a thickened secretory endometrium at the end of therapy.

Endometrial carcinoma (EC)

Approximately 10% of women with post-menopausal bleeding have endometrial carcinoma[5]. Therefore, it is important to assess the usefulness of TVS as a screening tool for early endometrial carcinoma and to lay down sonographic criteria that can help select women for further studies, *e.g.*, endometrial biopsy or magnetic resonance imaging.

Endometrial carcinoma typically demonstrates thickened endometrium of variable echogenicity, the range of thickness varying from 12-23 mm, though EC has been found in endometria as thin as 6-8 mm. A thickness of 4 mm or less has been found to have 97% sensitivity and 100% specificity for a normal endometrium with low estrogen stimulation. However, a thickness of 5-8 mm cannot be distinguished from hyperplastic endometrium, polyps or early carcinoma. When the endometrium measures more than 8 mm, one should consider the endometrium as abnormal[6]. These measurements can be used as a guide to further investigations, *e.g.*, endometrial biopsy.

The amount of myometrial invasion by endometrial carcinoma is estimated by measuring the distance from the lumen to the most distal interface thought to represent the tumor-myometrial interface and dividing that distance by the total thickness of uterine myometrium. Myometrial invasion is suspected if the ratio exceeds 30%[3].

Recently, the pulsatility index in uterine arteries (measured by Duplex and Colour Doppler studies) has been used to predict the presence of endometrial carcinoma. A value of 2.00 is a reasonable cutoff, with values more than 2.0 having a high predictability for normal endometrium with a high resistance flow. Indices of flow in intra-tumoral blood vessels may prove to be even more sensitive[7].

Ovarian masses

Various benign ovarian masses can be detected in post-menopausal women, such as cystadenomas, simple ovarian cysts, granulosa cell tumors, dermoids and fibromas. A high resistance flow pattern of the ovarian arteries on Doppler evaluation is also consistent with benignity. Dermoids appear as complex cystic masses, with echogenic nodules or areas of calcification or strands in it.

Ovarian carcinoma

Ovarian carcinoma is a leading cause of death in post-menopausal women. These often get diagnosed at a late stage because of lack of symptoms. TVS is excellent for screening the ovaries for early ovarian cancer — not only can it differentiate solid from cystic masses but can further characterise the mass by demonstrating presence of septae, debris, calcifications, nodules, etc. Ovarian cancers may arise from the germinal epithelium, germ cells or stromal cells.

When an ovarian mass is detected by pelvic sonography, factors associated with a greater risk of malignancy include

(a) size 5 cm

(b) a complex or solid appearance, and

(c) persistence over time[8].

An overlap of features exists in benign and malignant ovarian masses and no specific feature can characterise the histology of a mass. Ascites indicates advanced disease (Fig. 17.3). Transvaginal Colour Doppler Flow Imaging may be used to identify malignant ovarian masses and characterise early tumorogenesis. Vascularity is observed as flickering areas of colour in the tumor. The pulsatility index can be calculated according to the formula :

$$\text{Pulsatility index} = \frac{A - B}{\text{Mean}}$$

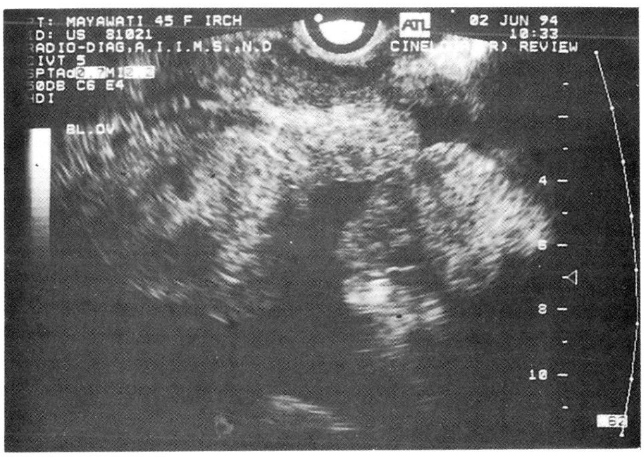

Fig. 17.3. Large, mixed, solid-cystic masses involving both ovaries with massive ascites. Shrunken atrophic uterus is seen between the ovaries.

where A = peak systolic Doppler shift frequency; B = peak diastolic velocity; and Mean = mean maximum Doppler shift frequency over the cardiac cycle[9].

Signs of ovarian malignancies on CDFI include low pulsatility, with some areas which demonstrate increased velocity and decreased impedance. Also the spectral waveform lacks a dicrotic notch in the diastolic phase.

Several studies have shown the sensitivity and specificity of TV-CDFI in differentiating benign from malignant tumors to range between 90-95 percent.

Some specific sonographic features have been seen in the following tumours :

Serous cystadenomas and cystadenocarcinomas. Serous ovarian tumours are the commonest malignant ovarian neoplasms. Cystadenomas are quite large by the time they are diagnosed, usually more than 5 cm. Sonographically, they are cystic and commonly unilocular. Rarely they may be septate with or without thick walls and tumour nodules may be seen.

Serous cystadenocarcinomas are commonly cystic, multilocular, thick-walled with nodules and papillary projections with some solid areas. About 30% are bilateral.

Mucinous cystadenomas and cystadenocarcinomas. Mucinous cystadenomas are large, multilocular cystic masses (some may be solid). Mucinous cystadenocarcinoma is a multiloculated cystic mass. Solid nodules and papillary projections may be seen. If the mucinous contents spill into the peritoneal cavity, pseudomyxoma peritonei can result.

Endometroid carcinoma. It is also a cystic mass and can have both solid and complex areas. Its contents are haemorrhagic.

Granulosa cell carcinoma. These tumours are derived from the sex cord elements of the ovary, and may be hormonally active. Over 40% of these tumours occur after menopause. Sonographically the tumours are predominantly solid (Fig. 17.4). Some cystic, necrotic or haemorrhagic areas may be present. Sometimes, the cystic variety can resemble cystadenomas.

Fallopian tube carcinoma. These tumours account for less than 1% of all gynaecologic malignancies. At sonography, a cystic adnexal mass away from the ovary in a post-menopausal woman can suggest the diagnosis.

Recurrences of gynaecologic malignancies

Gynaecological malignancies can recur following surgery, radiation and chemotherapy. A well-defined mass seen just above the vaginal cuff, or enlarged vaginal cuff should suggest recurrence (the antero-posterior diameter of the vaginal cuff ranges from 0.9 cm to 2.1 cm).

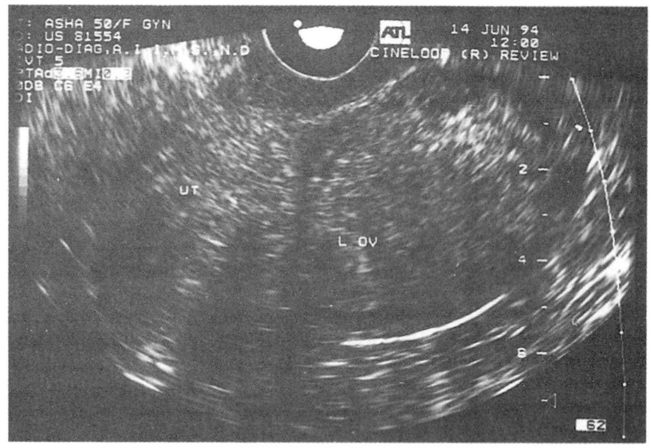

Fig. 17.4. Grossly enlarged left ovary replaced by large, solid, heterogeneous tumor. Uterus is seen separate from the mass.

Transvaginal sonographically-guided interventions

Transvaginal guidance helps in direct visualization and aspiration of ovarian cysts to help differentiate benign from malignant cysts.

Sonographic guidances can help drain pelvic abscesses and hydrosalpinx. Biopsy of adnexal and ovarian masses can also be performed easily.

TVS increases the confidence of detection of small lesions in the pelvis. Under TVS guidance, needles can be accurately placed into small ovarian, uterine or pouch of Douglas masses. Also, TVS guidance can be used for culdocentesis, drainage of pelvic abscesses, hydrosalpinges and other pelvic fluid collections. However, needle biopsy of localised ovarian masses is controversial, since there is a small but definite risk of tumour seeding along the needle tract, and subsequent recurrence, if the needle tract is not excised at the time of surgery.

Conclusions and future applications

Transvaginal sonography is an excellent tool for evaluating age related changes in the post-menopausal woman. It can accurately detect subtle changes in ovarian size and morphology, thereby enabling detection of early malignancies. Recent studies have shown transvaginal endometrial sonography to be useful in detecting endometrial abnormalities and also to predict which women with post-menopausal bleeding should have endometrial histologic assessment. TVS guidance is helpful for accurate placement of needles into masses for biopsy, or for drainage of abscesses and fluid collections.

TV-CDFI has an important role to play in differentiating benign versus malignant characteristics and in some cases it is helpful in detection of ovarian torsion.

REFERENCES

1. Nyberg DA, Hill LM, Bohm-Velez M, Mendelson EB, eds. Transvaginal ultrasound. Mosby Year Book Publishers, 1992.
2. Breckenridge JW, Kurz AB, Ritchie WGM, Macht EL. Postmenopausal uterine fluid collection : Indicator of carcinoma. AJR 1982; 139 : 529-534.
3. Schoenfeld A, Levavi H, Hirsch M, *et al.* Transvaginal sonography in post-menopausal women. JCU 1990; 18 : 350-358.
4. Goswamy RK, Campbell S, Royston J, *et al.* Ovarian size in post-menopausal women. Br Obstet Gynaecol 1988; 95 : 795-801.
5. Bourne T, Campbell S, Steer C, Whitehead MI, Collins WP. Transvaginal colour flow imaging : a possible new screening technique for ovarian cancer. Br Med J 1989; 299 : 1367-1370.
6. Varner RE, Sparks JM, Cameron CD, *et al.* Transvaginal sonography of the endometrium in postmenopausal women. Obstet Gynecol 1991; 78 : 195-199.
7. Bourne TH, Campbell S, Whitehead MI, *et al.* Detection of endometrial cancer in post-menopausal women by transvaginal sonography and colour flow imaging. Br Med J 1990; 301 : 369.
8. David NP, Ruben SC, Hoskins NJ, *et al.* Recurrence after negative second look laparotomy for ovarian cancer : analysis of risk factors. Am J Obstet Gynecol 1988; 159 : 1094-1098.
9. Fleischer AC, Emerson DS (Editors). Color Doppler sonography in obstetrics and gynecology. Churchill Livingstone, New York, 1993.

CHAPTER

18

Doppler in Reproductive Medicine

Gautam Allahbadia

Introduction

The most exciting and promising latest developments in the field of diagnostic and therapeutic ultrasonography in reproductive medicine are Doppler methods, transvaginal sonography and colour flow mapping. Transvaginal colour Doppler imaging has given the investigator a dramatic tool to study and observe the female reproductive system. The small distance between the probe and the pelvic structures supplies better resolution; and the empty bladder gives more patient comfort and convenience. The recent incorporation of colour Doppler processing in transvaginal probes has extended the scope of sonographic imaging from an anatomic to a physiological basis. Colour Doppler imaging involves detection of changes in phase and frequency in the incident and returned ultrasonic beam. This change in frequency and phase is primarily related to the flow of blood cells within blood vessels. Flow towards the transducer in encoded in shades of red, flow away in blue, and highest frequencies in white shades.

Discussion

Looking back over the evolution of the applications of the Doppler technique in infertility management, it is slowly becoming clear that what has been possible at any particular time has been determined by the capabilities of the instrumentation. As each technical innovation has emerged, investigators have explored the clinical usefulness of the new data that it has made available, and it is the value of the information and the practicality of the technique that have determined whether or not it has come into everyday practice. Thus, for all practical purposes, technology has led clinical application.

The main tools in the diagnosis of tubal disorders so far have been HSG and chromolaparoscopy. Apart from their obvious benefits, each of these methods has its risks. Patient's fear of anaesthesia, surgery or radiation exposure, combined with the need for stationary treatment and the objective risks of intervention have led to the recommendation that the examination of the tubal passage be given last priority in fertility diagnostics. This approach may lead to long periods of expensive attempts at treatment with ovulation-inducing drugs before the patient is finally referred to a hospital for tubal diagnosis. Since the 1980s, ultrasonography has been increasingly used to check for tubal patency[23,24,28]. In 1991 a process of contrast enhanced visualization of uterus and fallopian tubes combined with vaginosonography was introduced into the infertility diagnosis programme[25] (Figs. 18.1 and 18.2). In 1992, pulsed wave Doppler was used in

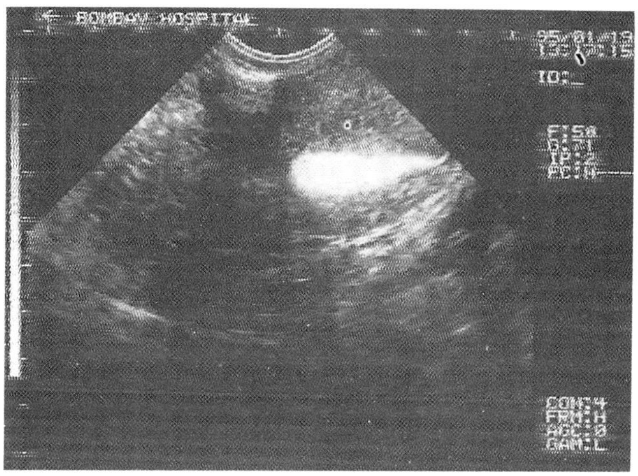

Fig. 18.1. Hysterosalpingo-contrast sonography. The uterine cavity and the intramural portion of the left fallopian tube visualised clearly during injection of the ultrasonic contrast medium.

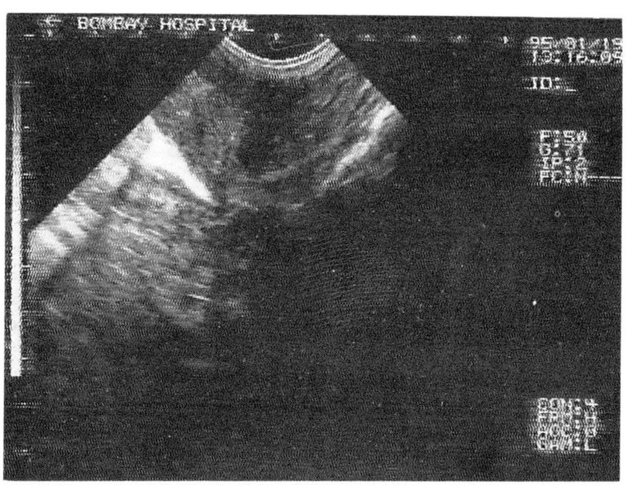

Fig. 18.2. Hysterosalpingo-contrast sonography. The entire length of the left tube now visualised clearly.

hysterosalpingo-contrast sonography as a supplement to grey scale imaging to improve tubal diagnosis[7]. In cases of patency, an audible, initially spitting, drawn out Doppler signal was obtained, and a broad band velocity signal was recorded simultaneously that correlated in time with the contrast injections and that decreased again slowly after the injection had stopped. The absence of this acoustic signal and of visual demonstration was interpreted as occlusion. In 1992, our own study was published in Fertility & Sterility where we assessed tubal patency with colour Doppler[2]. When microbubbles of saline enter the peritoneal cavity the turbulence is picked up by colour flow imaging as 'phasic colour indeterminance' or colour 'bruit' (Fig. 18.3 – Plate 5).

Preliminary work suggests a difference in the diastolic blood flow in benign versus malignant ovarian masses[34]. With malignant masses, there is typically a paucity of muscular lining of the tumour vessels. This finding, combined with increased arteriovenous shunting within the tumour, increases diastolic flow and results in low pulsatility indices[15]. Other applications of transvaginal colour may include detection of para-uterine vessels that should be avoided during needle aspirations[10]. Fine gauge needles and plastic catheters may not be well visualized by real time ultrasonic imaging under certain circumstances. This has prompted the use of various techniques to improve ultrasonic visualization, such as roughening the surface of needles or guidewires and using contrast material. In particular these methods have been used to improve the visualization. Kurohiji *et al.*[17] state that the addition of colour imaging permitted clear and distinct visualization of the needle shafts during motion. The colour coding of the needle motion marking corresponded to the direction of the motion in reference to the transducer.

Varicosity of veins of broad ligaments may cause ill-defined pelvic pain. Because the adnexa are often enlarged, the pelvic congestion is hardly distinguishable from real space occupying tumours. Transvaginal colour flow imaging is used not for the differential diagnosis of these rare cases but for in vivo 'tissue characterisation'. A 29 year old woman came to our OPD complaining of slight but diffuse lower abdominal pain. On initial pelvic examination the patient was believed to have a normal uterus and bilateral soft, plastic adnexal masses with moderately well-defined borders. Her lab tests were normal. A conventional transabdominal sonography indicated that "close to the normal uterus there are partly cystic, partly solid, bilateral adnexal masses with complex echo structure."

On transvaginal scanning we could confirm the finding of the abdominal scan. But colour flow mapping immediately showed that both the ovaries were normal in size and structure and that the cystic areas around them were dilated veins that showed prominent red and blue areas with expected continuous fluctuation. We believe that the routine application of this new diagnostic tool will enable us to determine the extent to which women with hydrosalpinges, pelvic adhesions, tumour-like conditions or benign tumours can be identified and saved unnecessary operations.

Torsion of one or more components of the adnexa is an emergency situation. The clinical picture varies from intermittent abdominal pain as a result of incomplete or recurrent partial torsion to that of an acute abdomen if the torsion is complete. The potential danger of adnexal torsion is the permanent destruction of the organs involved. Adnexal torsion of enlarged ovaries during early pregnancy is a serious complication of menotropin therapy (Figs. 18.4, 18.5 and 18.6 – all on Plate 5). Obstetricians caring for women conceiving with menotropin therapy must be aware of the possibility of adnexal torsion to allow for early diagnosis, treatment and ovarian conservation. Untwisting torsed necrotic adnexal tissue as a primary surgical procedure is a relatively new concept[21]. As there is currently no consensus on a management approach for adnexal torsion, treatment should be individualized on the basis of clinical circumstances. Because the clinical findings are nonspecific, delays in diagnosis and surgical management are common. Radiologic findings, including conventional ultrasonography, are also non-specific. The use of colour Doppler USG to detect the absence of blood flow to a torsed ovary was reported recently[33]. The ovary was untwisted, resulting in a return of normal colour and gradual reduction in ovarian volume. Intraoperative use of a Doppler probe confirmed return of blood flow to this ovary.

For the woman who is being treated for infertility, there is a small but real risk that the joyful achievement of pregnancy will turn into a nightmare of multiple foetuses, premature delivery and foetal demise. Sonographically-guided selective termination offers a way to improve the prospects of foetal survival in these 'premium' pregnancies. In our opinion, whether or not to perform selective termination is not a social decision, and the technique should be reserved for clinical situations in which the number of embryos per se threatens the outcome of the pregnancy. Virtually all the physicians now performing selective terminations leave 2 viable embryos. Three techniques have been employed for sonographically-guided, first trimester selective termination. The first to be described was the transcervical aspiration of gestational sacs[9]. A second technique involves transvaginal aspiration of the embryo leaving as much of the amniotic fluid as possible[27]. The most common method of selective termination employs transabdominal injection of potassium chloride into the embryonic thorax under real time sonographic guidance[4]. This technique is usually performed from 10 to 12 weeks after the LMP. In most of the series using gray scale USG, an ultrasound scan was performed the day after the procedure to confirm the death of the injected embryos. The procedure was repeated on the following day because of the persistence of embryonic life, despite initial signs of death. This was due to the poor quality of the ultrasound images after reduction. A recent paper has demonstrated the advantage of using colour Doppler for easy identification of cardiac motion and its disappearance after injection of KCl. This paper from Bombay Hospital has reported the first selective multifoetal reduction in septuplets using colour Doppler ultrasonography[8]. With the new technique of colour flow mapping, foetal demise can be confirmed on table at the same sitting thus eliminating the doubt of persistence of cardiac activity in injected foetuses and the possibility of a second procedure on the same patient. Because of the psychological and ethical drawbacks of embryo reduction, however, the main emphasis in limiting multiple gestations should be placed on improving the control of infertility therapies. Ending this section on an optimistic note we have recent reports on the physical and mental development of co-sibs surviving selective reduction of multifoetal pregnancies which emphasize that these babies are not handicapped and did not fall short of their matched controls in any way[5].

One area in which Doppler examination shows great promise is in the evaluation of the patient suspected of having an ectopic pregnancy. Nonspecific findings in cases of suspected ectopic pregnancy are more common in abdominal scans and often include a cystic adnexal mass. Because imaging alone provides only structural information, the examiner is usually unable to determine whether this mass represents an ectopic gestation or a luteal cyst. Only when imaging demonstrates an ectopic foetal heart within the adnexal mass can the diagnosis be made with certainty by this modality alone. When coupled with the structural information provided by the images, Doppler examination allows a specific diagnosis to be made in many cases. By detecting corpus luteal flow the possibility of pregnancy is established. By detecting extrauterine peritrophoblastic flow or ectopic foetal heart activity, the diagnosis is established. Doppler examination of the uterine contents can aid in differentiating between an abnormal intrauterine gestation and a pseudosac associated with an ectopic pregnancy. The echogenic rind around an intrauterine gestation, whether normal or abnormal, will demonstrate findings typical of the developing trophoblast. Colour flow imaging will demonstrate vascularity within this rind, while pulsed Doppler will yield low impedance disorganized signals with peak systolic frequencies around 2 to 4 kHz and diastolic frequencies in the range of 1 to 2.5 kHz[10]. In contrast examination of the area around a pseudosac will yield little or no signals reflecting the absence of surrounding trophoblastic tissue. A recent study compared the Doppler indices of blood flow in the uterine and spiral arteries and the corpus luteum in ectopic and intrauterine pregnancies[16]. Foetal heart activity was observed in all cases of IUP at 5 weeks of gestation. The mean uterine and spiral arterial RI decreased with the gestational age of IUPs but remained constant during EPs. The resistance index was similar in CL associated with both types of pregnancy. Transvaginal colour flow has superior accuracy, reproducibility and the ability to see small vessels. It has extraordinary value in the recognition of trophoblastic flow in complex adnexal masses in ectopic pregnancy[19].

Goswamy *et al.*[13] used transabdominal pulsed Doppler to obtain flow velocity waveforms from the uterine arteries during the midluteal phase of the ovarian cycle, and the preliminary results suggested that decreased uterine perfusion may be a cause of infertility. Tan *et al.*[32] confirmed his findings and stated that in addition, those subjects who demonstrate sustained diastolic flow arising from a well formed and functioning corpus luteum may promote successful implantation. The chance of being pregnant after embryo transfer (ET) has been studied with transvaginal colour flow imaging. Sterzik *et al.*[31] found that the uterine vascular impedance or the resistivity index (RI) on the day of oocyte retrieval was significantly lower in patients who subsequently became pregnant. Recent studies have all demonstrated an association between an increase in peripheral resistance of the uterine or the ovarian artery and a decrease in the pregnancy rate in patients undergoing assisted reproductive technologies. Flow velocity waveforms (Figs. 18.7 to 18.12) were examined in these patients on either the day of hCG administration, the day of egg retrieval or after embryo transfer. However this information lacks practical value because by this time the commitment to complete the cycle has already been made. Cassidenti *et al.*[6] from California prospectively

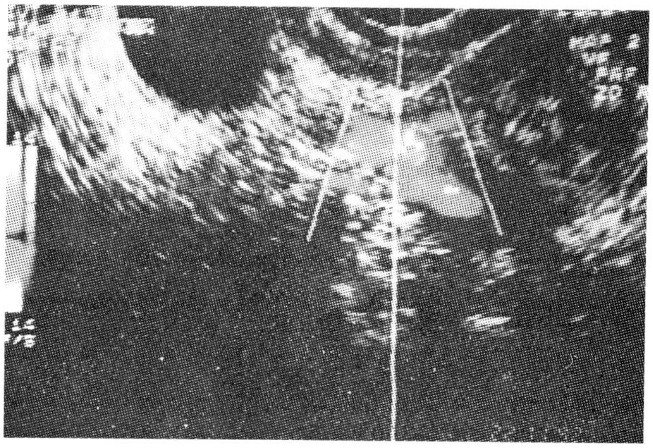

Fig. 18.7. The volume cursor outlining the uterine artery during transvaginal colour flow mapping.

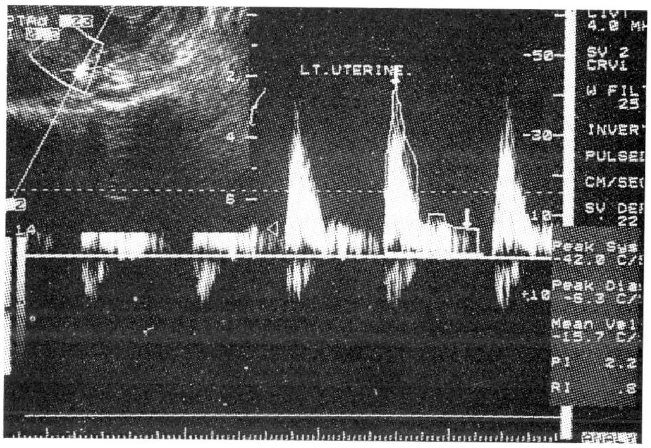

Fig. 18.8. Flow velocity waveforms and flow indices for the left uterine artery insonated for the same patient as in Fig. 18.4.

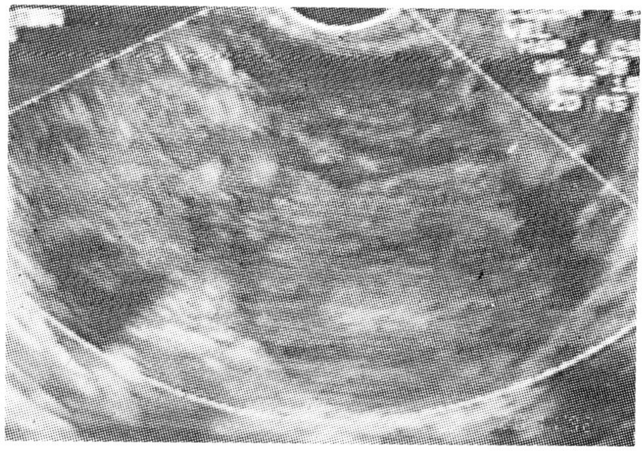

Fig. 18.9. The arcuate vasculature depicted clearly within the Doppler anatomic window using vaginal colour flow imaging.

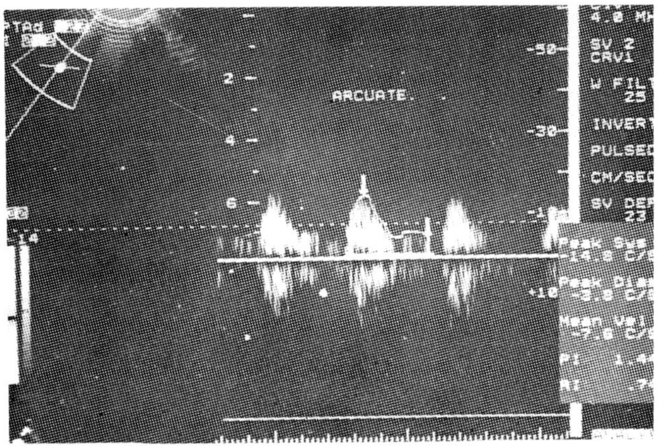

Fig. 18.10. The arcuate artery flow velocity waveforms and blood flow indices for the same patient as in Fig. 18.6.

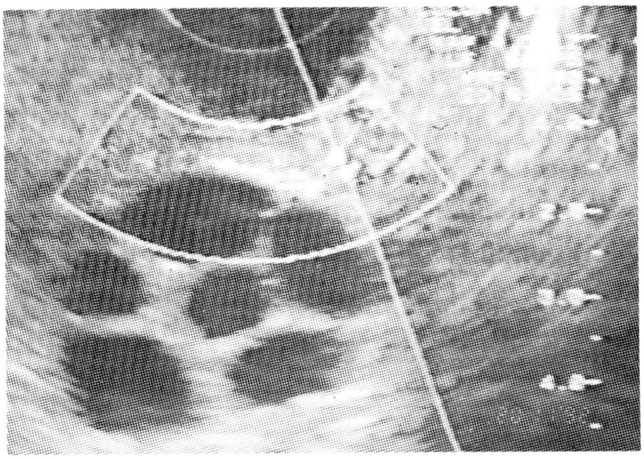

Fig. 18.11. The ovarian artery seen insonated using the 2 mm volume cursor.

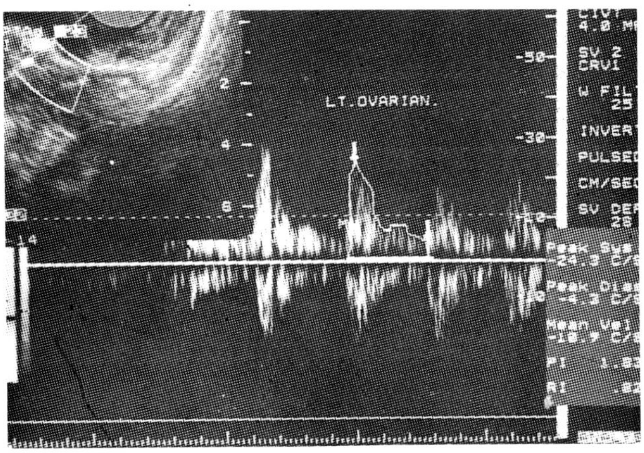

Fig. 18.12. The left ovarian flow velocity waveform and flow indices for the same patient as in Fig. 18.8.

studied 59 patients undergoing hypothalamic pituitary down regulation and ovarian stimulation for ART. Colour flow Doppler was used to determine the pulsatility index in the uterine vessels prior to down regulation, after down regulation with leuprolide acetate, and on the day of hCG administration. Their data suggest that no correlation is seen between early PI measurements and the subsequent pregnancy outcome. Therefore, early assessment of flow velocity waveforms is not useful in predicting success in patients undergoing ART. And therefore we come back to the periovulatory period and the secretory phase.

In a study from Australia the waveforms of vessels supplying the ovaries of 65 women on a IVF programme were studied at weekly intervals from 3 days after embryo transfer or 5 days after GIFT until confirmation of pregnancy or onset of menses[3]. There was a highly significant difference in the RI values between patients who became pregnant and those who did not; no patient who became pregnant had an RI greater than 0.5. A landmark study was published in 1992 from the Hallam Medical Center, London[30]. The aim of this group was to develop a technique to estimate uterine receptivity to decide whether or not cultured embryos should be transferred or frozen until the uterus is more receptive. All volunteers were scanned transvaginally with colour flow imaging approximately 30 minutes before embryo transfer. The mean PI of the left and right uterine arteries was calculated and used as a quantitative index of uterine receptivity. The results of this study show that optimal uterine receptivity for implantation of an embryo corresponds to a mean PI of 2 to 2.99. A mean PI of greater than 3.00 before the transfer of embryos could predict up to 35% of failures to become pregnant. This study has demonstrated that transvaginal blood flow imaging and the use of the PI could have an important role in medically assisted conception and might theoretically improve the pregnancy rate to almost 50% per embryo transfer. Conversely, this study has also identified a group of women with optimal uterine receptivity (PI 2 to 2.99) who are at high risk of developing a multiple pregnancy after embryo transfer.

Vaginal colour Doppler imaging may also have a role in assessing the development of adequate chorio-decidual vascularity. In abortions or nonviable pregnancies, there is initially reduced or absent diastolic flow followed occasionally by increased diastolic flow secondary to disrupted choriodecidual flow[10]. Identification of the normal low impedance luteal flow is particularly useful when assessing complications of early pregnancy. A functioning corpus luteum is necessary for the maintenance of pregnancy through most of the first trimester. Correspondingly luteal signals should be detectable in a viable pregnancy during this period. Their absence means either that the patient is not pregnant or that the pregnancy, whether normotopic or ectopic is not viable. Because the use of colour Doppler alone is associated with less intensities than when combined with pulsed Doppler, it is recommended that the use of pulsed Doppler be limited only after an optimal field of view is established by colour Doppler[10]. Monitoring of follicular growth and ovulation by ultrasonography is usually attempted from day 9 or 10 of a regular 28 day cycle. The dominant follicle continues to grow at a rate of 2 to 3 mm/day. With transvaginal colour Doppler, ovarian follicles differ from other anatomical structures. Follicular flow appears when the dominant follicle reaches 12 to 15 mm in diameter, and it may be a haemodynamic parameter of its growth, maturation and ovulation[18]. The waveform detected within an ovary varies with the functional activity of that ovary. An active ovary produces low amplitude, high impedance signals, whereas an active ovary produces more easily detected, low impedance signals. The ovary developing the dominant follicle initially demonstrates a high impedance pattern of flow. Thereafter impedance rapidly decreases and diastolic flow increases. If pregnancy does not occur, luteolysis occurs and the ovary returns to a high impedance pattern of flow. When pregnancy occurs, these cyclic changes in ovarian function cease. The active ovary that developed the dominant follicle must maintain a functioning corpus luteum for most of the first trimester in order for the pregnancy to remain viable. During this period, functional low impedance signals should be detectable from the ovary bearing the corpus luteum[18]. Knowledge of the normal cyclic changes in ovarian blood flow aids evaluation of the infertile patient. Normally the ovaries alternate in developing the dominant follicle. In some infertile patients, neither ovary may be undergoing normal cyclic change and consequently neither will demonstrate functional flow over several cycles. In other patients, only one ovary may be undergoing normal cyclic change. In this case, functional flow will be seen on that side every other cycle and will not be observed on the non-functional side in any cycle. In infertile patients with iatrogenically stimulated cycles, both ovaries typically develop follicles and ovulate. In these patients, low impedance functional flow is usually detected bilaterally. The presence of persistent luteal flow in these patients should not be misconstrued as representing an actual pregnancy. However, if no luteal flow is observed, pregnancy can be excluded.

Along with the research on blood flow patterns to predict implantation, workers have in recent times also attempted to identify endometrial factors that appear to be required for optimal uterine receptivity by the identification of ultrasonographic patterns of development and thickness. Smith *et al.*[29] have reported that no pregnancies occurred when the maximum endometrial thickness on the day of hCG administration was less than 5 mm. Glissant *et al.*[12] reported a significantly greater endometrial thickness in the periovulatory period in cycles that subsequently resulted in a pregnancy than in those that failed. Three sonographic patterns of periovulatory endometrium have been described[22]. A multilayered 'triple line' endometrium consists of prominent outer and central hyperechogenic lines and inner hypoechogenic or black regions. A intermediate isoechogenic pattern is characterized by the same reflectivity compared to the surrounding myometrium, with a non-prominent or absent central echogenic line. The third type is an entirely homogenous, hyperechogenic endometrium characterized by increased reflectivity compared to the myometrium and consequently appears brighter in its grey scale appearance. Here the central echogenic line is not visualized. Welker *et al.*[35] and Fleischer *et al.*[11] reported that a multilayered endometrium was present more frequently in those who conceived. Abae and Chapitis[1] prospectively examined the distribution of endometrial patterns as well as occurrence of thin endometrium during spontaneous and induced cycles utilizing clomiphene citrate and menotropins. Their data revealed that clomiphene citrate treatment yields thin endometrium. A prospective study assessing the endometrium in 218 IVF patients who achieved embryo transfer reveals that neither endometrial thickness not endometrial configuration appear to be reliable prognosticators for pregnancy in patients undergoing IVF[20]. Thus the search was on for a biophysical profile to predict pregnancy in advanced reproductive technology treatments. The first paper came from Pasadena, California[26]. Recent evidence if summed up has associated the success of Advanced Reproductive Technology Treatments (ART) with periovulatory ultrasonic endometrial thickness more than 8 mm, reflectivity appearance of a 'hypoechoic' halo and uterine vascular resistance (RI) less than 0.76. The presence or absence of these biophysical parameters were prospectively evaluated in 60 infertile women undergoing ovarian stimulation with leuprolide acetate and hMG for ART. Endometrial ultrasound thickness when more than 8 mm showed no discriminatory power to the establishment of a successful ART. The results of the ultrasonic reflectivity patterns yielded a test sensitivity and specificity of 73.5% and 70.3% respectively. The RI variable appears to be the most specific parameter for the prediction of pregnancies. The predicted probability of not establishing a pregnancy following ovulation induction with Lupron/hMG and ART procedure with fresh embryos was highly significant when all the uterine biophysical predictors were abnormal. Today we are at a stage where the assessment of the periovulatory biophysical predictors of pregnancy can be of paramount importance in the decision making process in reproductive medicine. But research still goes on to find better and more minimally invasive ultrasonic predictors of pregnancy. A group from France have studied the physiological modifications of Doppler signals of the medial thoracic artery along the human menstrual cycle[14]. Each phase of the cycle shows a characteristic pattern. The medial thoracic artery sustains physiologic modifications and the RI reduces along the menstrual cycle and rises in the menstrual phase.

Conclusion

The ability to assess utero-ovarian blood flow will have several applications in the assessment of women with fertility problems. Specifically, changes in ovarian and uterine perfusion during spontaneous or induced folliculogenesis can be assessed and thereby optimized so that embryo replacement is performed when most conducive to implantation. Pulsed Doppler examination and colour flow imaging are both forms of image directed Doppler ultrasound and are complementary to conventional grey scale ultrasound imaging. I am very sure that transvaginal colour Doppler imaging will play a major role in management decisions in reproductive medicine by the year 2000 AD.

REFERENCES

1. Abae M, Chapitis J. Sonographic assessment of endometrium in spontaneous and induced cycles. (Abstr. 0.021) Presented at the 48th Annual Meeting of the American Fertility Society, New Orleans, Louisiana. Published by the American Fertility Society, in the Program Supplement, pp S9, 1992.
2. Allahbadia GN. Fallopian tubes and ultrasonography : the Sion experience. Fertil Steril 1992; 58 : 901-7.
3. Baber RJ, McSweeney MB, Gill RW. Transvaginal pulsed Doppler ultrasound assessment of blood flow to the corpus luteum in IVF patients following embryo transfer. Br J Obstet Gynaecol 1988; 95 : 1226-30.
4. Berkowitz RL, Lynch L, Chitkara U. Selective reduction of multifetal pregnancies in the first trimester. N Eng J Med 1988; 318 : 1043-8.
5. Brandes JM, Itskovitz J, Scher A, Gershoni Baruch R. The physical and mental development of co-sibs surviving selective reduction of multifetal pregnancies. Hum Reprod 1990; 5 : 1014-7.
6. Cassidenti DL, Rosen GR, Yee B. Early assessment of uterine artery blood flow with color Doppler does not predict pregnancy outcome in patients undergoing ovarian hyperstimulation for IVF. (Abstr. 0.145) Presented at the 48th Annual Meeting of the American Fertility Society in the Program Supplement, pp S65, 1992.
7. Deichert U, Schlief R, Van de Sandt M, Daume E. Transvaginal hysterosalpingo-contrast sonography for the assessment of tubal patency with grey scale imaging and additional use of pulsed wave Doppler. Fertil Steril 1992; 57 : 62-7.
8. Desai SK, Allahbadia GN, Dalal A. Selective multifetal reduction in the first trimester using color Doppler. Hum Reprod 1993; 8 : 642-4.
9. Dumex Y, Oury JF. Method for first trimester selective abortion in multiple pregnancy. Contrib Gynecol Obstet 1986; 15 : 40-5.
10. Fleischer AC. Ultrasound imaging-2000 : assessment of utero-ovarian blood flow with transvaginal color Doppler sonography; potential clinical applications in infertility. Fertil Steril 1991; 55 : 684-91.
11. Fleischer AC, Herbert CM, Hill GA, Kepple DM. Transvaginal sonography of the endometrium during induced cycles. J Ultrasound Med 1991; 10 : 93-5.
12. Glissant A, De Mouzon J, Frydman R. Ultrasound study of the endometrium during in vitro fertilization cycles. Fertil Steril 1985; 44 : 786-90.
13. Goswamy RK, Williams G, Steptoe PC. Decreased uterine perfusion — a cause of infertility. Hum Reprod 1988; 3 : 955-9.
14. Guis F, Dautry RM, Fernandez H, Frydman R. Physiological modifications of Doppler signals in the study of medial thoracic artery. (Abstr. 0.085) Presented at the 48th Annual Meeting of the American Fertility Society, New Orleans, Louisiana. Published by the American Fertility Society, in the Program Supplement, pp S83, 1992.
15. Hata K, Makihara T, Takahashi K, Kitao M. Transvaginal color Doppler imaging for hemodynamic assessment of reproductive tract tumors. Int J Gynecol Obstet 1991; 36 : 301-8.
16. Jurkovic D, Bourne TH, Jauniaux E, Campbell S, Collins WP. Transvaginal color Doppler study of blood flow in ectopic pregnancies. Fertil Steril 1992; 57 : 68-73.
17. Kurohiji T, Sigel B, Justin J, Machi J. Motion marking in color Doppler ultrasound needle and catheter visualization. J Ultrasound Med 1990; 9 : 243-5.
18. Kurjak A, Kupesic-Urek S, Schulman S, Zalud I. Transvaginal color flow Doppler in the assessment of

ovarian and uterine blood flow in infertile women. Fertil Steril 1991; 56 : 870-5.

19. Kurjak A, Kupesic-Urek S. Infertility. In : Transvaginal color Doppler sonography. (ed) Kurjak A. Parthenon, London, England and Park Ridge, New Jersey, USA, 1991.
20. Noyes N, Berkeley A, Davis O. Endometrial thickness/ configuration does not appear to be a significant factor in embryo implantation. (Abstr 0.022) Presented at the 48th Annual Meeting of the American Fertility Society, New Orleans, Louisiana. Published by the American Fertility Society, in the Program Supplement, pp S10, 1992.
21. Oelsner K. Gesetzmalsige in der Torsion spirale torquiter ovarial tumorstiele. Zentralbl Gynakf 1992; 15 : 209-14.
22. Randall JM, Fisk NM, McTavish A. Transvaginal ultrasonic assessment of endometrial growth in spontaneous and hyperstimulated menstrual cycles. Br J Obstet Gynaecol 1989; 96 : 954-9.
23. Rasmussen F, Larsen C, Justesen P. Fallopian tube patency demonstrated at ultrasonography. Acta Radiologica Diagnosis 1986; 27 : 61-4.
24. Richman TS, Viscomi GN, DeCherney A. Fallopian tube patency assessed by ultrasound following fluid injection. Radiology 1984; 152 : 507-10.
25. Schlief R, Deichert U. Hysterosalpingo-contrast sonography of the uterus and fallopian tubes : Results of a clinical trial of a new contrast medium in 120 patients. Radiology 1991; 178 : 213-5.
26. Serafini P, Batzofin J. Peri-ovulatory uterine biophysical predictors of pregnancy in advanced reproductive technology treatments (ART). (Abstr 0.014) Presented at the 48th Annual Meeting of the American Fertility Society, New Orleans, Louisiana. Published by the American Fertility Society, in the Program Supplement, pp S6, 1992.
27. Shalev J, Frenkel Y, Goldenberg M, Lipitz S. Selective reduction in multiple gestations : pregnancy outcome after transvaginal and transabdominal needle-guided procedures. Fertil Steril 1989; 52 : 416-20.
28. Sharma RP. Fallopian tube patency by ultrasound scan. J Obstet Gynaecol India 1989; 39 : 700-1.
29. Smith B, Porter R, Ahuja K, Craft I. Ultrasonic assessment of endometrial changes in stimulated cycles in an IVF-ET program. J In Vitro Fert Embryo Transfer 1984; 1 : 233-8.
30. Steer CV, Campbell S, Tan SL. The use of transvaginal color flow imaging after in vitro fertilization to identify optimum uterine conditions before embryo transfer. Fertil Steril 1992; 57 : 372-6.
31. Sterzik K, Grab D, Sasse S. Doppler sonographic findings and their correlation with implantation in an IVF program. Fertil Steril 1989; 52 : 825-8.
32. Tan SL, Steer C, Mills C. Vaginal color Doppler assessment on the day of embryo transfer (ET) accurately predicts patients in an IVF programme with suboptimal uterine perfusion who fail to become pregnant. (Abstr 0.070) Presented at the 46th Annual Meeting of the American Fertility Society, Washington, D.C., Published by the American Fertility Society, in the Program Supplement, pp S30, 1990.
33. Voorhis BJV, Schwaiger J, Syrop CH, Chapler FK. Early diagnosis of ovarian torsion by color Doppler ultrasonography. Fertil Steril 1992; 58 : 215-7.
34. Weiner Z, Thaler I, Beck D. Differentiating malignant from benign ovarian tumours with transvaginal color flow imaging. Obstet Gynecol 1992; 79 : 159-62.
35. Welker B, Gembruch U, Diedrick K. Transvaginal sonography of the endometrium during ovum pickup in stimulated cycles for IVF. J Ultrasound Med 1989; 8 : 549-53.

CHAPTER

19

Transvaginal Colour Doppler in Gynaecology

Tom Bourne

Introduction

The use of ultrasonography in obstetrics and gynaecology has evolved rapidly since the pioneering work of Donald and the publication of his seminal paper in *The Lancet* during 1958. The introduction of gray-scale techniques enhanced the ability to identify different tissues on the basis of their texture. However, it was the introduction of the linear array real-time scanner in the mid-1970s that changed ultrasonography from being an 'eccentric art form' to a readily available and usable technique. In the midst of this activity, the parallel development of the transvaginal probe by Kratochwil went almost unnoticed by most gynecologists. However, the application of this technique has since had a major impact on many areas of gynaecological practice, and on the management of infertility in particular. By placing the probe closer to the area of interest, higher frequency ultrasound can be used and higher resolution images obtained. Transvaginal ultrasonography has now become routine in the assessment of many gynecological disorders[1-3]. Since the demonstration of transvaginal follicle aspiration, the use of this route has become standard practice for most invasive ultrasound-guided gynecological procedures[4]. The relatively new technical advance of transvaginal colour Doppler also promises to have a great impact. The introduction and use of transvaginal colour flow imaging has facilitated the study of vascular changes within the pelvis. The follicle and corpus luteum of the ovary and the endometrium of the uterus are the only areas in a normal adult body where angiogenesis (the development of new blood vessels) occurs to any significant extent. The same process occurs during the growth of carcinomas. The ability to recognize these early vascular changes with colour Doppler is facilitating the diagnosis of pelvic cancers as well as the assessment of normal and abnormal ovarian and uterine functions. It seems likely that this new technique will lead to a greater understanding of how vessel growth is involved in reproductive pathophysiology. The ability to monitor changes in vascularity may enable the development of methods to inhibit or enhance angiogenic activity in vivo.

This review will outline the principles of transvaginal colour Doppler and its practical use and discuss its current and possible future applications.

The technique

For some time research efforts have been directed towards developing techniques to observe vascular changes within the human pelvis. This work has concentrated on the use of Doppler ultrasound, and the principles and physics have been reviewed[5]. Whilst B-mode imaging has progressed to allow structures to be inspected in 'real time', up to now the use of pulsed or spectral Doppler has required a considerable length of time to select the point that best represents the vessel or area of tissue being investigated. The operator is limited by the fact that flow information is confined to the highly restricted pulsed Doppler range gate. As a result, sampling errors are not uncommon. These limitations have made the study of small vessels and minor vascular changes very difficult to carry out in a reproducible fashion. Colour Doppler may solve many of the problems. The B-mode image is divided into many pixels and by the use of multiple range gates the Doppler flow parameters for each of the pixels on the screen are demonstrated in 'real time'. The Doppler information is colour frequency-coded, *i.e.*, a converter assigns colour, based on the direction and variance of the detected frequency shifts. Red usually indicates flow towards the transfer, and the blue away. The brightness of the colour is proportional to the velocity of flow within the vessel, whilst turbulent flow may appear as various shades of green[6]. In this way regions of vascularization can be located anatomically as areas of colour. A pulsed Doppler range gate is placed over the area of interest to provide flow velocity waveforms which may be analyzed in a conventional fashion. This additional information is not achieved without some compromise. The maximum colour Doppler sensitivity is achieved at low frame rates, and is therefore prone to movement artifact. Attempts may be made to increase the frame rate by raising the minimum displayed Doppler shift frequency threshold, collecting fewer lines, or increasing the pixel size. Filling missing pixels by interpolation also adds to the amount of colour displayed. These ways of processing the image must be remembered when interpreting information displayed on screen, as the area of colour displayed may not be a totally accurate representation of the vascular area being interrogated. There is a tendency for manufacturers to try to make the images as attractive and thus commercial as possible, with little regard to how useful this extra colour might be clinically.

By placing the unit on a vaginal probe, other advantages are gained. There is the major practical advantage that a full bladder is not needed for the examination. A full bladder acts to displace the pelvic organs even further from the ultrasound source. Small blood vessels may also be compressed, leading to alterations in blood flow within them. Using the vaginal route means that an optimal angle of insonation is achieved for many of the pelvic vessels, especially the uterine arteries. Having the transducer placed closer to the tissues being studied permits the use of higher pulsed repetition frequencies. As a result, there are fewer limitations on the maximum Doppler shifted frequencies that can be measured without aliasing (the Nyquist limit). Whilst it is an elegant way of displaying Doppler information, at the present time it is not possible to quantify colour Doppler. It must be remembered that it acts to identify vessels such that a pulsed Doppler range gate can be used to obtain flow velocity waveforms. We therefore rely on the analysis of these frequency spectra for the collection of quantitative data. The conventional indices of resistance index (RI) and the pulsatility index (PI) are both thought to reflect changes in impedance to flow distal to the point of sampling[7,8]. In many cases these indices fail to show any differences when comparing physiological and pathological processes. In a study by Bower and Campbell[9], the presence or absence of a notch in the uterine artery waveform was far more predictive of future pregnancy outcome than the use of either the RI or PI. Similarly, we have been unable to define cut-off values to separate the RI and PI indices of early ovarian cancers, corpora lutea and preovulatory follicles (Table 19.1). Subtle differences in waveform shape and character are lost in the spectrum analysis. It is probable that this lost information is useful, and so new ways to analyze this Doppler information are needed.

The safety aspects of transvaginal colour Doppler must not be forgotten. In general the power output of colour Doppler units is not a cause for concern and for most units the spatial peak average intensity (SPTA) is of the order of 30 mW/cm^2. This is well within the highest limit recommended by the Food and Drug Administration (FDA) for use in obstetrics. There are, however, concerns regarding the use of the transvaginal pulsed Doppler units and a number of machines currently available have power outputs above the FDA

Table 19.1. Range of values for indices of intraovarian blood flow (King's College Hospital Ovarian Screening Clinic, 1991).

	Follicle (post-LH) (n = 12)		*Corpora lutea (n = 30)*		*Early invasive ovarian cancer (n = 7)*	
Variable	*Mean*	*Range*	*Mean*	*Range*	*Mean*	*Range*
Resistance index (RI)	0.48	0.36-0.58	0.43	0.28-0.54	0.46	0.33-0.78
Pulstility index (PI)	0.62	0.39-0.99	0.56	0.30-0.73	0.61	0.40-0.96
Velocity (cm/s)	26.1	14.3-45.2	41.2	16.1-73.4	44.0	35.6-57.5*

* n = 3

guidelines when used at high power settings. Such power outputs are not required to obtain good waveforms using transvaginal Doppler and the power should be reduced to the lowest level possible. The trend towards the display of power output levels on screen is to be recommended. The use of transvaginal colour Doppler should, if anything, lead to safety advantages when compared to the use of transvaginal pulsed Doppler alone. By reducing the time required to find and sample a vessel, the total exposure of the area of interest to ultrasound should be reduced.

Common practical difficulties

It is important to remember that any information obtained using transvaginal colour Doppler is of little value if the vessel sampled has been incorrectly identified. There are certainly published data claiming to relate to ovarian artery flow, when the waveforms shown are clearly iliac in origin. All of the major pelvic vessels have characteristic waveform 'signatures'; these have been confirmed in a study where a continuous wave Doppler probe was placed on the vessels in question at the time of laparotomy[10]. It is our experience that it is extremely difficult to measure blood flow in the ovarian artery. It is not clear whether this is because the angle of insonation is suboptimal, or because the blood flow velocity is very low, or a combination of both. In the absence of colour Doppler, it is common practice to move the pulsed Doppler range gate from the lateral ovarian surface medially along the infundibulo-pelvic ligament and through the ovarian stroma until flow velocity waveforms are obtained. The results often reflect a mixture of signals from the ovarian artery, the terminal branch of the uterine artery, and blood flow from within the ovary. Most reliable ovarian blood flow data refer to areas of intraovarian vascularity rather than the ovarian artery itself. When interrogating these vessels, the brightness point of colour must be sampled to obtain the highest velocity flows. The probe can then be angled very slightly to maximize the amplitude of the waveform. The first measurable waveform should not be accepted as being representative of blood flow within the tissue being studied. It is worth spending a little time to ensure that the vascular region with the highest velocity and lowest impedance has been sampled. In this way, highly reproducible measurements of both the RI, PI and velocity can be made. Often the identification of small subtle vascular areas within the ovary is made difficult by movement artifact. The proximity of the ovaries to the pulsatile iliac vessels makes this inevitable. With experience, it is possible to discriminate between artifact and areas of 'true' colour that represent blood flow. The vaginal approach provides an optimal angle of insonation for the uterine arteries. The main branch can be reliably identified lateral to the supravaginal portion of the cervix, where it is best seen in the longitudinal plane. Careful examination will usually demonstrate their tortuous path. Distally the radial arteries can be visualized, as can be the openings of the spiral arteries in pregnancy. In this way all points of the uterine circulation can be identified and sampled.

Potential uses

The interrelated effects of vascularization are illustrated in Fig. 19.1. It is clear that the growth of new vessels and the development of existing ones form a common thread throughout many areas of reproductive pathophysiology. In recent years, there has been an enormous increase in our knowledge of the factors that regulate this angiogenic activity[11]. It has been shown in a number of studies that ovarian tissue is capable of inducing angiogenesis[12]; the same effects on assays of angiogenesis can be observed in response to tissues from malignant tumors[12]. It is of particular interest that prostaglandins have also been shown to stimulate angiogenesis, and that the production of these substances by the ovary is increased by luteinizing hormone (LH)[14,15].

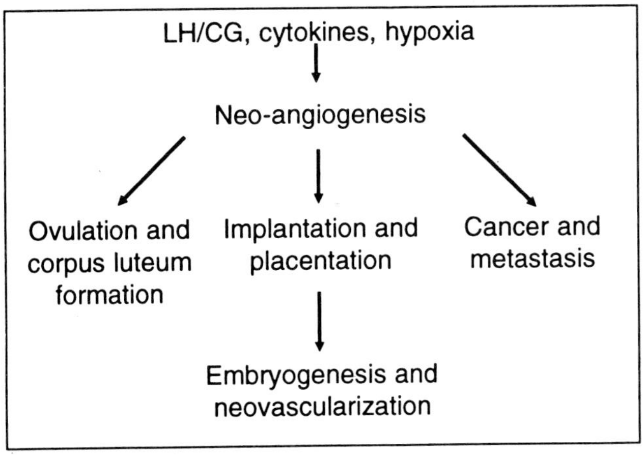

Fig. 19.1. The related effects of angiogenesis in reproductive pathophysiology.

Normal follicular and corpus luteum function depends on the development of a satisfactory blood supply. Malignant tumors exhibit the same reliance on new vessel formation. The detection of these vascular areas may be used as a criterion on which to judge the benign or malignant nature of an ovarian tumor. Furthermore, by altering these vascular responses, it may be conceivable to inhibit or enhance potential fertility, and the prospects of successful treatment for some types of carcinoma may be improved. Transvaginal colour Doppler can be used to identify areas of angiogenesis. There is therefore potential for the use of transvaginal colour Doppler as a way of identifying both pathological and physiological processes involving changes in tissue vascularity, as well as monitoring the effects of intervention.

Transvaginal colour Doppler also facilitates the study of major vessels. Arteries can be reliably identified and reproducible measurements made. The current major areas of use are in the fields of gynaecological oncology and infertility. Some of these potential applications are outlined below.

The normal pelvis and infertility

The ovary and ovulation

Normal ovarian morphology and function. The current status regarding the use of transvaginal colour Doppler in infertility has been discussed[16]. At the present time, there are no useful morphological markers of impending ovulation, although ultrasound has been used to monitor follicular growth and rupture as well as to observe the formation of the early corpus luteum[17]. Whilst the ability to detect follicular rupture is being used to develop practical self-tests for potential fertility, there is still a need for a technique that can predict (and possibly detect) the release or possible retention of a viable oocyte at the time of follicular rupture. Transvaginal colour Doppler has been used to monitor sequential changes in intrafollicular blood flow in the periovulatory period, and the data obtained related to defined biochemical indices. It is hoped that it will be possible to use information about ovarian blood flow both to predict ovulation and to investigate ovulatory dysfunction. Previous studies have shown that it is possible to assess ovarian blood flow during the normal menstrual cycle[18]. This study using trans-abdominal pulsed Doppler, showed significant changes in ovarian blood flow in the ovarian cycle. In particular, there was a marked drop in blood flow impedance within the ovary during the late follicular and luteal phases. Although the authors interpret their data as being from the ovarian artery, it is more likely that serial measurements of intraovarian flow have been recorded. Transvaginal pulsed Doppler has been used subsequently to record blood flow in the corpus luteum in in vitro fertilization (IVF) patients following embryo transfer[19]. In the absence of colour Doppler, the authors had to move the sample volume gate (of 3.5 mm) over the ovarian stroma until suitable waveforms were obtained. These waveforms are more likely to reflect intraovarian rather than ovarian artery blood flow. Impedance to blood flow was measured on days 3 and 10 following embryo transfer, and significantly higher impedance to flow was observed in the corpora lutea of women who failed to become pregnant. Using transvaginal colour Doppler, areas of vascularity can be clearly visualized on the follicular rim, or within or around the corpus luteum. Transvaginal colour Doppler has since been used to monitor intensively vascular events in the periovulatory follicle[20]. Colour Doppler facilitates the detection of small vascular areas in the ovarian stroma and follicular rim that are easy to miss when applying a pulsed Doppler range gate ‘blind’. In this study, the aim was to assess each patient every 3rd to 4th hour from the time of the serum LH surge up to the formation of the corpus luteum. Blood flow velocity waveforms from the follicular rim were first seen at the time of the LH surge (or estradiol peak). There is sequential increase in vascularity in the follicular rim from the time of the LH rise, at its peak, and finally just prior to follicular rupture and the formation of the corpus luteum. These observations represent the first report of the changes in intrafollicular vascularity over the periovulatory period in the human female. These data are supported by studies of ovarian blood flow and volume in laboratory animals[21], and the fact that red blood cells have been seen in the granulosa cell layer between the time of the LH peak and presumed ovulation[22]. A report of the vascular changes at the time of a presumed ovulation shows increased vascularity on the innermost rim of the follicle, and a coincident surge in blood flow velocity just prior to follicular rupture[23]. This may represent the dilatation of new vessels that have developed between the relatively vascular theca cell layer and the normally hypoxic granulosa cell layer of the follicle. Disruption of these vascular changes would have profound effects on the oxygen concentration across the follicular epithelium[24].

Ovulatory dysfunction. We have observed one case of drug-associated luteinized unruptured follicle (LUF); there was a reduction in vascularization and a failure of the blood flow velocity to peak in the immediate preovulatory period[25]. This is consistent with the view that the changes in oxygen tension within the follicle brought about by angiogenesis are necessary for normal ovulation to occur. Transvaginal colour Doppler may be used to monitor hormonal and other methods of increasing or decreasing intrafollicular blood flow. Steroids that inhibit angiogenesis in the presence of heparin have already been described[26]. If the process of ovulation could be inhibited independently of the main pathways of steroidogenesis, novel methods of contraception might be envisaged. Initial evidence suggests that transvaginal colour Doppler may be used to monitor progress towards these objectives. It is further hoped that this technique will facilitate the study of other aspects of ovarian function such as follicular recruitment and corpus luteum development and failure.

The uterus

The normal menstrual cycle. Transvaginal colour Doppler can be used reproducibly to obtain flow velocity waveforms from the uterine arteries at any time during the menstrual cycle[27]. It is apparent that there are complex relationships between the concentration of ovarian hormones in peripheral plasma and uterine artery blood flow parameters. Steer and colleagues[28] used transvaginal colour Doppler to study uterine artery blood flow in 23 healthy women. Fig. 19.2 shows the daily mean changes in pulsatility index within the uterine arteries relative to the mean concentration of plasma estradiol and progesterone. The overall trend suggests an increase in perfusion of the uterus during the course of the menstrual cycle. It is particularly interesting that the lowest blood flow impedance occurs during the time of peak luteal

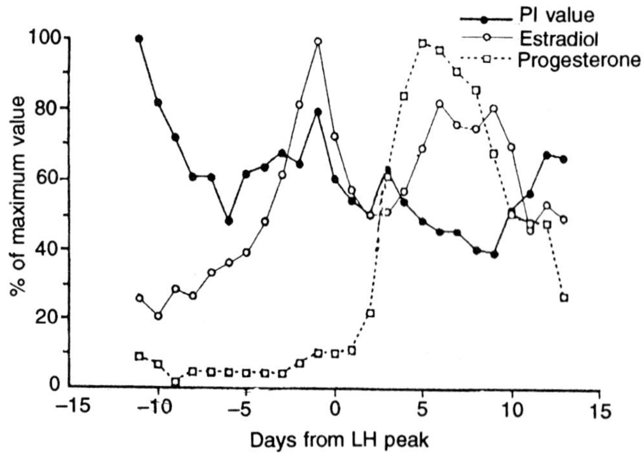

Fig. 19.2. Changes in the mean uterine artery pulsatility index during the ovarian cycle related to the mean concentrations of plasma estradiol and progesterone (Steer *et al.*[28]).

function, during when implantation is most likely to occur. Using transvaginal colour Doppler, it has therefore been possible to define normal uterine blood flow in the menstrual cycle.

Possible relevance to infertility. Goswamy and his colleagues (using transvaginal pulsed Doppler) have presented preliminary evidence that decreased uterine perfusion may be associated with infertility[29]. It has been suggested that one of the major reasons for the relatively low success rates for assisted reproduction techniques is the failure of embryos to implant. This has led to the transfer of up to four embryos in order to achieve a reasonable singleton pregnancy rate. However, the multiple pregnancy rate associated with such actions has major social and medical implications. A non-invasive assay of uterine receptivity would enable a clinician to cryopreserve embryos if uterine conditions were adverse, and to reduce the number of transferred embryos when conditions were optimal. Steer and colleagues have suggested that studies of uterine artery blood flow may be used to predict a hostile uterine environment prior to embryo transfer[30]. Women who failed to achieve a pregnancy in this study had significantly raised impedance to blood flow in their uterine arteries. There was a zero implantation rate associated with a mean uterine artery PI of greater then 3.0. According to these data, if this figure was used as the upper limit for the transfer of embryos, the sensitivity of the test for predicting an unreceptive uterus and thus failed implantation would be 35.2%, the specificity 100%, and the positive predictive value of a high-impedance blood flow result also 100%. If substantiated, these data may have important clinical implications. Those women with poor uterine perfusion could be advised that a pregnancy is unlikely in their current treatment cycle, and be advised to have their embryos cryopreserved for transfer at a later date. Colour Doppler may also be used to monitor ways of manipulating the uterine environment. Transvaginal colour Doppler measurements of uterine artery blood flow have the potential for use as a biological assay of uterine receptivity and may theoretically substantially improve the pregnancy rate per treatment cycle. Prospective controlled clinical trials based on these preliminary data are awaited with interest.

It is clear that changes in tissue vascularity are fundamental to many aspects of normal uterine and ovarian functions. The preliminary data with transvaginal colour Doppler suggest that it provides a relatively non-invasive tool for their detailed study. Prospective data are now needed to assess whether ways can be found to alter these vascular processes either to enhance or reduce the chance of a couple achieving a pregnancy.

Pregnancy

It is unclear as yet what role transvaginal colour Doppler will play in the study of pregnancy. The fact that it enables the operator reliably to identify the different branches of the uteroplacental circulation should enhance our ability to study the profound vascular changes that occur in the early stages of gestation.

Predicting pregnancy outcome

The assessment of uteroplacental blood flow has been suggested as an early screening test for the identification of pregnancies at increased risk of developing pregnancy-induced hypertension and growth retardation[31]. Using transvaginal colour Doppler, the main branch of the uterine artery can be reliably identified at its junction with the internal iliac artery. Analysis of waveforms from this point at 24/40 gestation has been shown to have a 75% sensitivity for the deduction of pregnancies that are going to suffer from proteinuric pregnancy-induced hypertension (PIH)[9]. Interestingly, it was found that the presence or absence of a 'notch' in the waveform was more predictive of poor pregnancy outcome than any of the indices of impedance to blood flow currently used. More recently, Jauniaux and colleagues[32] have demonstrated how the different branches of the uteroplacental circulation can be identified using transabdominal colour Doppler and characteristic flow velocity waveforms obtained. Sampling of these more distal points in the uterine circulation may prove to be a more useful predictor of potential fetal compromise than studies of the main branch of the uterine artery.

It has been shown previously that vaginal pulsed Doppler can be used to assess impedance to flow in the uterine arteries throughout pregnancy[33]. The use of transvaginal colour Doppler facilitates the identification of all branches of the maternal uterine circulation in early pregnancy[34]. In this way the point of sampling is more reproducible and the examination time required to obtain good quality flow velocity waveforms shortened. It is hoped that this will enable blood flow studies to be performed reliably earlier on in pregnancy around the time of trophoblast invasion. If poor uterine perfusion were recognized at an earlier stage, drug therapy such as aspirin might be used to try to improve placentation. However, a recent paper by Arduini and colleagues[35] was pessimistic about the use of measurements of uterine artery blood flow using Doppler ultrasonography to predict poor fetal outcome. Transvaginal colour Doppler was used to identify the arcuate and trophoblast vessels, the main uterine and the umbilical arteries in 282 pregnancies defined as normal and 48 pregnancies that were thought by the authors to be complicated either by gestational hypertension or growth retardation. Of the pregnancies thought to be abnormal, only four fell outside the normal ranges for any of the vessels assessed. The authors conclude that this information is unlikely to be of value in the identification of the 'at risk' pregnancy. However, this study has several limitations. First of all, the number of complicated pregnancies for each gestation is too small to make definite conclusions. In addition, the end-points of the study are unclear. How many of the hypertensive women were proteinuric? Moreover, a birth weight on the 10th centile does indicate a small baby but does not prove growth retardation. Once again, this study turns our attention to the question of flow velocity waveform analysis. It has been suggested that the presence or absence of a diastolic notch in the flow velocity waveform is more predictive than indices of impedance alone. By using the systolic/diastolic ratio, information available from the flow velocity waveforms may have been lost. Further data are therefore required to assess the full role of transvaginal colour Doppler in assessing the fetomaternal circulation to identify pregnancies in need of close monitoring.

The fetal circulation

Transvaginal colour Doppler is being used to make preliminary studies of the fetal circulation in the first trimester of pregnancy. Whilst much of the information derived from this work will not have any immediate clinical relevance, our knowledge of fetal physiology will be further advanced. Any transvaginal ultrasound study in early pregnancy is limited by fetal movement and positioning. Whilst recordings from fetal vessels can be made using pulsed Doppler, the use of colour Doppler reduces the examination time. This makes the study of fetal vessels at this gestation more practical and acts to reduce the fetal exposure to ultrasound. Recently, Wladimiroff and colleagues[36] have reported blood flow velocities from the atrioventricular valve and outflow tract in 30 pregnancies between 11 and 13 weeks' gestation. In a number of cases it was not possible to obtain acceptable flow velocity waveforms from the area of interest. Although they have yet to publish their data, the same group are also examining blood flow in the fetal internal carotid and middle cerebral arteries in the first trimester. There are anecdotal reports of other workers using transvaginal colour Doppler to confirm absent renal artery flow in pregnancies complicated by oligohydrammios[37]. Colour Doppler may help to facilitate such studies.

Ectopic pregnancy

The advent of relatively non-invasive approaches to the management of ectopic pregnancy[38] has led to the introduction of screening programs for this disorder[39]. The need for sensitive and specific tests to diagnose this condition is therefore greater than ever, and the availability of a technique other than serum human chorionic gonadotropin (hCG) estimation to monitor trophoblast activity would be of benefit. It is probable that transvaginal ultrasonography has facilitated the earlier and more accurate diagnosis of ectopic pregnancy. Whether transvaginal colour flow imaging is of any help in this context is not yet certain. Our experience is that, whilst it can be a useful adjunct, it is unlikely to change dramatically the diagnostic performance of ultrasound for this condition. Zalud and Kurjak[40] observed a significantly lower impedance to flow within the corpus luteum of women with ectopic pregnancies compared to intrauterine pregnancies of the same gestation. The mean RI for luteal blood flow in normotopic pregnancies was 0.53 compared to 0.48 for ectopic pregnancies. Although the difference in RI between the groups reached statistical significance, the practical application of using measurements of luteal blood flow to discriminate between intra- and extra-uterine pregnancies seems limited. Given a probable coefficient of variation in the assessment of RI of around 5-10%, the difference between the groups is easily obscured. Excluding what can be a lethal condition on the basis of an RI difference of 0.05 is unlikely ever to be considered a safe practice. In contrast, Jurkovic and colleagues[41] concluded that there were no significant hemodynamic differences either in the corpus luteum, uterine arteries or trophoblast when comparing intrauterine to ectopic pregnancies. The only significant difference was a reduction in blood flow velocity in the uterine arteries of women with ectopic pregnancies, perhaps suggesting an overall reduction in uterine blood supply. Whilst this difference was statistically significant and of academic interest, it has little if any clinical relevance. Although these data may suggest a limited diagnostic role for colour Doppler, this is not necessarily the case. Our impression is that the most clinically helpful role of colour Doppler in this context is in reliably identifying the side of the corpus luteum (on the same side as the ectopic pregnancy in over 85% of cases in our series) such that it can be used as a guide to direct the search for the ectopic gestational sac. Colour Doppler can also be used to delineate subtle vascular changes in the tube suggestive of the presence of trophoblast. Unfortunately, the low impedance blood flow pattern that can be observed in and around the corpus luteum is similar to that of the blood supply to the ectopic sac and can cause confusion. However, with care the vascular branches to both the corpus luteum and ectopic sac can be identified separately. It is this capability that can be particularly helpful in trying to make a definitive diagnosis in the presence of an adnexal mass. Vessels are often seen at the periphery of the ectopic sac and are usually confined to one segment of the trophoblast ring. Reports showing the presence of low impedance flow on the side of most ectopics are not surprising given the ipsilateral presence of the corpus luteum in most cases. The blood supply to the ectopic sac must be demonstrated as separate from that to the ovary for its recognition to be diagnostically useful. Those of us familiar with the technique of transvaginal colour Doppler find that it enhances our ability to make a definitive diagnosis of ectopic pregnancy. However, at this time there are limited data from well designed trials to demonstrate a significant benefit from the use of colour Doppler for the diagnosis of this condition. Good comparative data are needed to establish the precise role of colour Doppler in this context. There is also the possibility that the technique may be used to monitor treatment. It has yet to be established whether an apparent decrease in the vascular supply to an ectopic sac is an indication of poor viability and hence whether it can be used to form the basis of criteria to select patients for observation alone, or local non-invasive treatment.

Ovarian malignancy

Background

Ovarian cancer remains the most common cause of death from gynaecological malignancy. About 5000 women in England and Wales and 22000 in the United States of America develop the disease each year[42,43]. In the early stages of the disease there are few characteristic symptoms or signs and as a result the majority of women with this disease present at stage III or IV[44] when palliation is often the only realistic management strategy. The overall 5-year survival rate of 30%[45] is a reflection of the limited impact that new approaches to treatment have had on mortality from this disease. Conversely, the 5-year survival rate for women with stage 1 ovarian cancer may be over 90%[46]. In view of the depressing results relating to the treatment of late-stage disease, attempts are being made to develop effective screening procedures for early cancers in asymptomatic women. Once a test with suitable sensitivity and specificity for early-stage disease has been identified, a randomized trial will need to be carried out to determine whether earlier diagnosis and treatment will improve the prognosis for substantially more women. The problems associated with ovarian cancer screening have been reviewed[47,48].

Cancer screening

The use of ultrasonography to screen for ovarian cancer was first proposed by Campbell and colleagues in 1982[49]. Subsequently, in a large prospective trail, transvaginal ultrasound was used to screen over 5000 women for the presence or absence of ovarian pathology[50]. This study suggests that, whilst conventional transabdominal ultrasound is a sensitive technique for the detection of small cystic lesions suggestive of cancer, it is difficult to discriminate between malignant and benign cystic lesions on the basis of B-mode imaging alone. There are now preliminary reports on the use of higher-resolution transvaginal ultrasound to screen asymptomatic women for ovarian cancer both in low-[51] and high-risk populations[52]. The consensus view is that transvaginal ultrasonography is a sensitive first-stage screening test and will detect nearly all cystic ovarian lesions suggestive of carcinoma. What is needed is a second-stage test that will discriminate between benign and malignant cysts. Colour Doppler may fulfill this role, being used after an ovarian morphological abnormality has first been detected using B-mode imaging. Changes in tissue vascularity, mediated by angiogenic factors, are associated with the early stages of ovarian oncogenesis. Recent studies with transgenic mice have shown that, for at least one type of cancer, angiogenesis occurs during the transition from hyperplasia to neoplasia[53]. An inhibitor of angiogenesis has also been found that is produced by cells when they are capable of expressing an active cancer suppressing gene[54]. This evidence suggests that angiogenesis may well be an obligate event in the earliest stages of ovarian carcinoma. In animal models Doppler techniques have been used to identify areas of altered vascularization within tumors as small as 50 mg. In this study, vascular morphology was further evaluated by digital angiography. This technique demonstrated coincidence between the site of high-velocity low-impedance signals and the presence of arteriovenous anastomoses[55]. Initial experience with the use of colour Doppler was limited to tumors other than the ovary[56].

Preliminary data suggest that it may be possible to detect the vascular changes associated with early ovarian cancers using colour Doppler. In malignant lesions, blood flow can be demonstrated throughout diastole, probably reflecting a decrease in impedance to flow distal to the point of sampling. A possible explanation for this is that the new vessels associated with carcinoma have limited vascular tone due to the absence of the tunica media, and as a result they form low-impedance shunts. It is hoped that it will be possible to characterize benign and malignant lesions on the basis of their vascularity and in so doing reduce the false-positive rate of an ultrasound-based screening program. We have used transvaginal colour Doppler to examine 30 women with no apparent pelvic pathology and 18 women with ovarian tumors[57]. All cases of invasive cancer showed evidence of neovascularization with low-impedance blood flow. One serous cystadenoma of borderline malignancy did not demonstrate an abdominal blood flow pattern and there was one false-positive test result (a benign teratoma). Two of the invasive cancers were at stage 1a, suggesting that this technique can detect ovarian cancer when it is still confined within the capsule of the ovary. These results were supported by the work of Kurjak and co-workers[58], who studied infertile women with normal pelvic morphology and patients with known pelvic masses. Low-impedance intratumoral flow was seen in four cases of unstaged primary ovarian cancer; the resistance index was used as an index of impedance to flow and was below 0.40 in all cases. There was one false-positive result (a granulosa cell tumor) amongst the 15 benign cystic lesions that were studied. Hata and colleagues studied eight cases of ovarian cancer, and the mean RI value of the tumors was 0.503 ± 0.216[59]. It is of interest that this group was unable to discriminate between the blood flow of a corpus luteum cyst, an endometrioid ovarian cyst and carcinoma. The same authors point out that in one case flow velocity waveforms from the internal iliac artery were mistaken for those from within the ovary, a common and important source of error. More recently, Kurjak and colleagues have presented data on the colour Doppler findings in 624 benign and 56 malignant ovarian masses. Presumed neovascularization was demonstrated in six out of seven stage 1 primary ovarian cancers, and in 48 of 49 of the other malignant lesions in the study[60]. In all of the cases where neovascularization was seen, the RI value was again less than 0.40. The authors regard on RI value of 0.40 as a significant cut-off, values below this being thought to have a high predictive values for carcinoma. However, the data of Hata and colleagues[59] suggest that we have yet to determine the value that defines normal and abnormal blood flow within the ovary. Data from our own clinic are supportive of this view (Table 19.1) and demonstrate a clear overlap between the blood flow within normal physiological ovarian cystic lesions and carcinomas[61]. The use of an arbitrary cut-off value of 0.40 seems likely to result in a number of both false-positive and negative results. In our series of seven cases of stage 1 ovarian carcinomas, neovascularization was seen in all cases of invasive carcinoma. The details of each case as well as their RI values are shown in Table 19.2[61]. Clearly, more data are needed to define ways of discriminating between malignant conditions and some benign processes on the basis of flow velocity waveform analysis.

Potential limitations

Whilst it is not unreasonable to be optimistic, we must remember that there are potential limitations. For women in whom ovarian activity has ceased, there are no physiological events occurring within the ovary that may lead to altered vascularity. In our ovarian cancer screening program, there have been no false-positive results from postmenopausal women. In premenopausal women this is not the case. Similar processes of angiogenesis, and thus very similar indices of impedance to blood flow are seen from within the developing corpus luteum and the preovulatory follicle as are seen in early cancer. The appearance of altered vasculature within the follicle has been directly related to defined biochemical indices such as the LH surge and peak[20].

The identification of the β core fragment of hCG as a tumor marker in the urine of women with ovarian cancer may reflect a degree of angiogenic activity from these related hormones[62,63]. Great care must, therefore, be taken to exclude vascular changes that are secondary to normal physiological events. Vascular information derived from the ovary must be viewed critically and related to the patient's ovarian cycle, and any abnormal findings subjected to a repeat scan. There is probably quite a narrow window within any ovarian cycle during which there will be a complete absence of angiogenic activity. Accordingly, for the purposes of ovarian cancer screening, we currently examine premenopausal patients between days 3 and 11 of their cycle. If such a policy is adhered to, the majority of physiological

Table 19.2. The detection of early ovarian cancer by transvaginal ultrasonography with colour flow imaging and blood flow analysis (King's College Hospital Ovarian Screening Unit, 1991)

Case number	*Age (years)*	*Menopausal status*	*Histological classification*	*FIGO stage*	*Test result*	*RI*
1	63	art+	borderline serous cystadenocarcinoma	1a	negative*	0.96
2	54	pre	endometrioid cystadenocarcinoma	1a	positive	0.68
3	46	pre	borderline endometrioid cystadenocarcinoma	1a	positive	0.34
4	52	post	serous cystadenocarcinoma	1a	positive	0.37
5	52	post	serous cystadenocarcinoma	1b	positive	0.38
6	53	post	endometrioid cystadenocarcinoma	1c	positive	0.58
7	37	pre	serous cystadenocarcinoma	1c	positive	0.33

+ Artificially postmenopausal following hysterectomy

* Woman had one scan only

lesions will be identified and false-positive test results avoided. The uncritical enthusiasm of some authors for transvaginal colour Doppler is to be deprecated and is unhelpful to those of us who believe that this technique will improve our ability to diagnose early ovarian carcinoma. A recent unsigned *Lancet* editorial states that transvaginal colour Doppler can be used to detect ovarian cancer before it is otherwise discernible, and that it should be utilized to characterize the nature of cystic ovarian lesions in pregnancy[64]. There are little data to support the former statement and none to support the latter. These problems have been discussed[65].

Future prospects

Despite these possible pitfalls, transvaginal colour Doppler has already been shown to reduce the false-positive rate of an ultrasound-based screening program. When applied to cystic ovarian masses detected in a screening program for women with a family history of ovarian cancer, the odds of finding a cancer amongst women referred for surgery were reduced from about 1 : 15 to 1 : 5[65]. Knowledge of the lesions likely to cause false-positive results with colour Doppler suggests that similar figures will be obtained when screening the general population. It has often been said that, for a screening test for ovarian cancer to be credible, it would have to achieve a positive predictive value of better than 10% (an odds ratio of about 1 : 10). A combination of transvaginal sonography and colour flow imaging satisfies this criterion. Any worries about colour Doppler findings in physiological lesions must be seen in the context of the technique being used as a second-stage test, its use being limited to persistent ovarian masses. Hence any mass found at screening would be subjected to a repeat scan at an interval at which time colour Doppler would be performed. In this way most physiological lesions will have regressed. The fact, that all cases of invasive stage 1 ovarian cancer examined with transvaginal colour Doppler in our series showed evidence of neovascularization, gives cause for optimism about the sensitivity of the test for early-stage disease. That colour Doppler can detect vascular changes in the ovary around the time of ovulation suggests that, if the development of new vessels is an obligate event in the earliest stages of ovarian cancer, colour Doppler will be able to demonstrate them. However, even in a high-risk population, the prevalence of the disease means that about 300 women need to be screened in order to detect one case of early ovarian cancer. To examine the sensitivity and specificity of colour Doppler as a second-stage test in an ovarian cancer screening program will require large-scale screening trials in order to have enough clinical material with which to work. A prospective randomized trial is now required to satisfy this requirement, as well as to answer the large question of whether screening and hence early treatment will reduce the currently high mortality rate from this disease.

Benign and malignant disorders of the uterus

Endometrial cancer

About 33,000 new cases of endometrial cancer are reported in the United States each year. Uterine bleeding is the most frequent initial sign of this disease, and at present demands invasive investigation (*i.e.*, endometrial biopsy). However, less than 10% of women with postmenopausal bleeding have endometrial cancer. A less invasive technique than diagnostic biopsy that also has a high detection rate and low false-positive rate would be of value. If this test could detect cancers at an early stage in asymptomatic women, then the number of women cured by surgery alone might be increased, and the morbidity and mortality from the disease reduced. These would be particularly relevant for women at increased risk of developing endometrial abnormalities, such as those taking unopposed estrogens or tamoxifen therapy[66]. It has been proposed that tamoxifen be given to apparently healthy women at increased risk of breast cancer[67]. It may be necessary to monitor the endometrium of such patients at regular intervals. There are now good data to suggest that the measurements of endometrial thickness made using transvaginal ultrasonography can have both high positive and negative predictive values for malignancy. An endometrium that measures greater than 8.0 mm from one myometrial endometrial interface to another is highly likely to be associated with significant endometrial pathology[68]. There is, however, a significant false-positive rate. The characteristic flow velocity waveforms that can be obtained from the uterine artery have been described[10]. Recent reports have suggested that transvaginal colour Doppler can be used reproducibly to measure impedance to blood flow in the uterine arteries[68,69]. The uterine arteries can be identified in the longitudinal plane slightly lateral to the supravaginal portion of the cervix. Colour Doppler enables the main branch of the vessels to be reliably identified and then sampled using pulsed Doppler. This should be carried out once the probe has been angled to obtain the maximum colour intensity from the vessel in question. Using the pulsatility index, a one-way analysis of variance of replicate data from 20 women gave a coefficient of variation of about 10% for both uterine arteries[70]. We recently reported the impedance to blood flow in the uterine arteries and the endometrial thickness in women with postmenopausal bleeding both with and without cancer, as well as women taking hormone replacement therapy and those thought to have a normal uterus taking no drug therapy[70]. Data from this study suggest that, in the presence of malignant tissue, the impedance to blood flow within the uterine artery is reduced significantly when compared to control groups. By using colour Doppler whilst maintaining sensitivity, the false-positive rate of the ultrasound-based test is reduced. If colour Doppler is used to interrogate the endometrium in such cases, angiogenesis can be demonstrated as areas of colour superimposed on the B-mode grey-scale image and the sensitivity of the technique enhanced. An interesting observation in this study was that there was a marked reduction in blood flow impedance within the uterine arteries of women taking hormone replacement therapy. Other workers have also reported vascular changes in the presence of uterine cancer using colour Doppler. In one report, two cases of endometrial cancer were examined. RI values from the periphery of the endometrial echo were 0.26 and 0.31, respectively[58]. Hata and colleagues[59] examined ten women with endometrial cancer and found areas of low-impedance blood flow in all cases (PI 0.535 ± 0.158); in patients with uterine myomata the intra-tumoral blood flow impedance was 0.679 ± 0.131. Our experience of uterine fibroids is that they are characterized by low-impedance but high-velocity blood flow. Attempts have been made to characterize uterine tumors using transvaginal colour Doppler[71]. Intratumoral blood flow was looked for in 191 benign and 17 malignant uterine tumors. The RI value was 0.58 ± 0.12 SD for cases of uterine myomata and 0.34 ± 0.03 in cases of endometrial carcinoma. The authors conclude that transvaginal colour Doppler can be used to help discriminate between benign and malignant uterine tumors and that an intratumoral RI value of < 0.40 should be regarded as malignant and between 0.40 and 0.50 as suspicious. In general the ultrasound appearances of myomata and endometrial carcinoma are distinct and quite different. To what extent colour Doppler will ever be necessary to discriminate between the two is uncertain. The observation in the same report that a uterine sarcoma (RI 0.31) had significantly lower-impedance blood flow than benign myomata may have more practical clinical implications.

Management of fibroids

Impedance to blood flow within the uterine arteries has been assessed in women taking a gonadotropin-releasing hormone agonist for the treatment of uterine myomata[72]. Transvaginal colour Doppler permits the accurate measurement of blood flow within myomata rather than just the uterine arteries. There is, therefore, the potential to monitor the response of myomata to a trial of medical therapy and in some cases optimize the timing of surgery.

Hormone replacement therapy

Following the observation that there was a decreased PI in the uterine arteries of women taking hormone replacement therapy, attempts have been made to quantify this effect. In a subsequent study, estrogen was shown to reduce impedance to blood flow in the uterine artery by 50%[73]. If extrapolated to the general vasculature, this would have important implications with regard to the cardioprotective effect of estrogen replacement therapy. The changes in uterine artery impedance occurred rapidly. A protein related to the estradiol receptor has been identified in the intima of major vessels[74], and it is possible that estrogens affect arterial status through a conventional sex hormone receptor mechanism. The addition of progestogens appears partially to reverse this drop in impedance, although not to pretreatment levels[75]. This takes effect within 36 hours of starting progestogen therapy, suggesting that the mechanism is also receptor-mediated (M.S. Marsh and T.H. Bourne, unpublished data). A particularly interesting observation in this study was that the response to exogenous estrogens was proportional to the number of years since the menopause. If this is confirmed, there may be cardiovascular benefit from estrogen administration even in very elderly women, as they may still show a significant vascular response to therapy. Selecting progestogens that have the least effect on the vasodilation brought about by estrogen therapy may be of great importance if the beneficial effects of hormone replacement therapy are to be maximized. Such a choice may be investigated with the use of transvaginal colour Doppler. These data were later supported by that of de Ziegler[76]. In six women with either idiopathic premature ovarian failure or ovarian failure secondary to chemotherapy, uterine artery blood flow was assessed before and during estrogen therapy. The PI before treatment was 5.2 ± 0.4 (mean ± SEM), dropping to 1.3 ± 0.3 when taking exogenous estrogens. Studies of other vessels have shown similar changes in response to estrogen therapy[77]. Doppler echography of the aorta has demonstrated that estrogens increase both stroke volume and flow acceleration. These are thought to reflect a combination of inotropism and vasodilatation. Changes in uterine artery response to exogenous estrogens seem to act as a model for what is happening in the general vasculature. Transvaginal colour Doppler can, therefore, be used to assess the effect of drugs on the circulation and on the uterine arteries in particular.

Future developments

New approaches to the assessment of blood flow are being investigated. The use of volume flow measurements is one possibility, but obtaining this information from small pulsating vessels seems rather optimistic. Volume flow is the product of mean velocity and vessel area, thus any errors in the measurements of vessel diameter will be multiplied. Attempts to quantify the information generated by colour Doppler have been disappointing, but it may be possible to estimate the number of pixels that are excited using the digitized memory of the scanner. The new colour velocity imaging scanners may have a role to play. Colour velocity imaging uses the data contained in the gray-scale B-mode image scan lines to determine the velocity of blood flow[78,79]. The potential advantages of colour velocity imaging include both quantitation of flow and tissue motion assessment both at lower power outputs. The relative importance of this new technology awaits evaluation in clinical trials.

Conclusions

Transvaginal colour Doppler promises to play a major role in obstetrics and gynecology over the next decade. The development of the follicle and corpus luteum as well as cancers depends on the parallel development of adequate blood supplies. The ability to study these processes and the factors that may enhance or inhibit them using a non-invasive technique, offers a new opportunity to researchers. The practical clinical role of colour Doppler is not yet clear. However, it seems certain to improve our ability to diagnose and thus treat gynaecological malignancies, early pregnancy complications and infertility secondary to ovarian and uterine dysfunction. Transvaginal colour Doppler has great potential, but we must be certain of its precise clinical role before it is allowed to move from being an exciting research tool into routine clinical practice.

Acknowledgements

Financial support for the ovarian screening clinic at King's College Hospital is provided by the Cancer Research Campaign (CRC) and the Imperial Cancer Research Fund (ICRF). I am grateful to Keymed Ltd. (Southend, UK) and to the ALOKA Co. Ltd. (Tokyo, Japan) for the use of their ultrasound equipment.

REFERENCES

1. Timor-Tritsch IE, Yeh MN, Peisner DB, Lesser KB, Shavik TA. The use of transvaginal sonography in the diagnosis of ectopic pregnancy. Am J Obstet Gynecol 1989; 161 : 157-60.
2. Gramberg S, Friberg LG, Norstrum A. Endovaginal ultrasound scanning of women with postmenopausal bleeding. J Ultrasound Med 1988; 7 : 256-9.
3. Gramberg S, Norstrum A, Wikland M. Tumors in the lower pelvis as imaged by transvaginal sonography. Gynecol Oncol 1990; 37 : 224-9.
4. Timor-Tritsch IE, Peisner DB, Monteagudo A. Puncture procedures utilizing transvaginal ultrasonic guidance. Ultrasound Obstet Gynecol 1991; 1 : 144-50.
5. Wells PNT. Review article : Doppler ultrasound in medical diagnosis. Br J Radiol 1989; 62 : 399-420.
6. Omoto R, Kasai C. Physics and instrumentation of Doppler color flow mapping. Echocardiography; a Review of Cardiovascular Ultrasound 1987; 4 : 467-83.
7. Thompson RS, Trudinger BJ, Cook CM. Doppler ultrasound waveform indices : A/B ratio, pulsatility index and Pourcelot ratio. Br J Obstet Gynaecol 1988; 95 : 581-8.
8. Trudinger BJ, Thompson RS. Do velocity indices measure resistance? Ultrasound Obstet Gynaecol 1991; 3 : 160-1.
9. Bewer S, Campbell S. The study of uterine artery blood flow to predict IUGR and pregnancy induced hypertension. Proceedings of the International Perinatal Doppler Society, Los Angeles, June, 1990.
10. Taylor KJW, Burns PN, Wells PNT, Conway DI, Hull MGR. Ultrasound Doppler flow studies of the ovarian and uterine arteries. Br J Obstet Gynaecol 1985; 92 : 240-6.
11. Holkman J, Klagsbrun M. Angiogenic factors. Science 1987; 235 : 442-7.
12. Koos RD, LeMaire WJ. Factors that may regulate the growth and regression of blood vessels in the ovary. Sem Reprod Endocrinol 1983; 1 : 295-307.
13. Folkman J, Cotran R. Relation of vascular proliferation to tumor growth. Int Rev Exp Pathol 1976; 16 : 207-48.
14. Ben Ezra D. Neovasculogenic ability of prostaglandins,

growth factors and synthetic chemoattractants. Am J Ophthalmol 1978; 86 : 455-61.

15. LeMaire WJ, Clarke MR, Marsh JM. Biochemical mechanism of ovulation. In Halez HSF. (ed.) Hum Ovulation, Amsterdam : Elsevier/North Holland pp. 187-200, 1979.
16. Fleischer AC. Ultrasound imaging-2000 : assessment of utero-ovarian blood flow with transvaginal color Doppler sonography, potential clinical applications in infertility. Fertil Steril 1991; 55 : 684-91.
17. Queenan JT, O'Brien GD, Bains LM, Simpson J, Collins WP, Campbell S. Ultrasound scanning of ovaries to detect ovulation in women. Fertil Steril 1980; 34 : 99-105.
18. Hata K, Hata T, Senoh D, Makihara K, Aoki S, Takaniya O, Kitao M. Change in ovarian arterial compliance during the human menstrual cycle by Doppler ultrasound. Br J Obstet Gynaecol 1990; 97 : 163-6.
19. Baber RJ, McSweeny MB, Gill RW, Porter RN, Picker RH, Warren PS, Kossoff G, Saunders DM. Trans-vaginal pulsed Doppler ultrasound assessment of blood flow to the corpus luteum in IVF patients following embryo transfer. Br J Obstet Gynaecol 1988; 95 : 1226-30.
20. Collins W, Jurkovic D, Bourne T, Kurjak A, Campbell S. Ovarian morphology, endocrine function and intra-follicular blood flow during the periovulatory period, Hum Reprod 1991; 6 : 319-24.
21. Tanaka N, Espey LL, Okamura H. Increase in ovarian blood volume during ovulation in the gonadotropin-primed immature rat. Biol Reprod 1989; 40 : 762-8.
22. Bomsel-Helmreich O, Gougeon A, Thebault A, Salarelli D, Milgrom E, Frydman R, Papiernik E. Healthy and atretic human follicles in the procovulatory phase : differences in evolution of follicular morphology and steroid content of follicular fluid. J Clin Endocrinol Metab 1979; 48 : 86-94.
23. Bourne TH, Jurkovic D, Waterstone J, Campbell S, Collins WP. Intrafollicular blood flow during human ovulation. Ultrasound Obstet Gynecol 1991; 1 : 53-9.
24. Gosden RG, Byatt-Smith JG. Oxygen concentration across the ovarian follicular epithelium : model, predictions and implications. Hum Reprod J 1986; 1 : 65-8.
25. Bourne TH, Reynolds K, Waterstone J, Okokou H, Jurkovic D, Campbell S, Collins WP. Paracetamol associated with luteinized unruptured follicle syndrome : effects on intrafollicular blood flow. Ultrasound Obstet Gynaecol, in press, 1991.
26. Ingber DE, Madri JA, Folkman J. A possible mechanism for inhibition of angiogenesis by angiostatic steroids, induction of capillary basement membrane dissolution. Endocrinology 1986; 19 : 1768-75.
27. Scholtes MCW, Wladimiroff JW, Van Rijen JJJM, Hop WCJ. Uterine and ovarian flow velocity waveforms in the normal menstrual cycle : a transvaginal Doppler study. Fertil Steril 1989; 52 : 981-5.
28. Steer CV, Campbell S, Pampiglione J, Kingsland C, Mason BA, Collins WP. Transvaginal color flow imaging of the uterine arteries during the ovarian and menstrual cycles. Hum Reprod 1990; 5 : 391-5.
29. Goswamy RK, Williams G, Steptoe PC. Decreased uterine perfusion a cause of infertility. Hum Reprod 1988; 3 : 955-9.
30. Steer CV, Mills CL, Campbell S. Vaginal colour Doppler assessment on the day of embryo transfer (ET) accurately predicts patients in an in vitro fertilisation programme with suboptimal uterine perfusion who fail to become pregnant. Ultrasound Obstet Gynaecol 1991; 1 : (Suppl) 1-79.
31. Campbell S, Pearce JMF, Hackett G, Cohen-Overbook TE, Hernandez C. Qualitative assessment of utero-placental blood flow : early screening test for high-risk pregnancies. Obstet Gynaecol 1968; 68; 649-53.
32. Jauniaux E, Jurkovic D, Campbell S, Kurjak A, Hustin J. Investigation of placental circulations by color Doppler ultrasonography. Am J Obstet Gynaecol 1991; 64 : 486-8.
33. Deutinger J, Rudelstorfer R, Bernaschek G. Vagino-sonographic velocimetry of both main uterine arteries by visual recognition and pulsed Doppler method during pregnancy. Am J Obstet Gynecol 1988; 159 : 1072-6.
34. Durkovic D, Jauniaux J. Kurjak A, Hustin J, Campbell S, Nicolaides K. Transvaginal color Doppler of the uteroplacental circulation in early pregnancy. Obstet Gynecol 1991; 27 : 365-9.
35. Arduini D, Rizzo G, Romanini C. Doppler ultra-sonography in early pregnancy does not predict adverse pregnancy outcome. Ultrasound Obstet Gynaecol 1991; 1 : 180-5.
36. Wladimiroff JW, Huisman TWA, Stewart PA. Fetal cardiac flow velocities in the late 1st trimester of pregnancy : a transvaginal Doppler study. J Am Coll Cardiol 1991; 17 : 1357-9.
37. Twining P. Second-trimester oligohydrammios, the combined approach : transvaginal and transabdominal colour flow Doppler. Br J Radiol 1991; 64 : 662-3.
38. Feichtinger W, Kemeter P. Conservative treatment of ectopic pregnancy by transvaginal aspiration under sonographic control and methotrexate injection. Lancet 1987; i : 381-2.
39. Popp LW, Mettler L, Weisner D, Mecke H, Freys I, Senm K. Ectopic pregnancy treatment using pelviscopic or vaginosonographically-guided intrachorionic injection of methotrexate and POR 8. Ultrasound Obstet Gynecol 1991; 1 : 136-43.
40. Zalud I, Kurjak A. The assessment of luteal blood flow

in pregnant and non-pregnant women by transvaginal colour Doppler. J Perinat Med 1990; 18 : 215-7.

41. Lukovic D, Bourne TH, Jauniaux E, Campbell S, Collins WP. The use of transvaginal colour Doppler in the diagnosis of ectopic pregnancy. Fertil Steril 1991 (in press).
41. Office of Population Censuses and Surveys Cancer Statistics : Registrations, England and Wales 1984 (London : HMSO), 1988.
43. Silverberg E, Boring CC, Squires TS. Cancer statistics 1990. CA, 1990; 40 : 9-23.
44. Shepherd JH. Revised FIGO staging for gynaecological cancer. Br J Obstet Gynecol 1989; 96 : 889-92.
45. Kottmeier H. (ed) Annual Report on the Results of Treatment in Gynaecological Cancer, Vol. 18. (Stockholm : FIGO), 1982.
46. Young RC, Walton LA, Ellenberg SS. Homeskey HD, Wilhanks GD, Decker DG, Miller A, Park R, Major Jnr E. Adjuvant therapy in stage I and Stage II epithelial ovarian cancer — results of two prospective randomised trials. N Engl J Med 1990; 332 : 1021-7.
47. Bourne TH, Reynolds K, Campbell S. Ovarian cancer screening, Eur J Cancer 1991; 27 : 655-9.
48. Cuckle HS, Wald NJ. The evaluation of screening tests for ovarian cancer. In Sharp F, Mason WP. Leake RE. (eds) Ovarian Cancer : Biological and Therapeutic Challenges, (Cambridge : Chapman and Hall Medical) pp. 229-39, 1990.
49. Campbell S, Goessens J, Goswamy R, Whitehead MJ. Real-time ultrasonography for determination of ovarian morphology and volume — a possible new screening test for early ovarian cancer? Lancet, 1982; i : 425-6.
50. Campbell S, Bhan V, Royston P, Whitehead MI, Collins WP. Transabdominal ultrasound screening for early ovarian cancer. Br Med J 1989; 299 : 1363-7.
51. Van Nagell JR, Higgins RV, Donaldson ES, Gallion HH, Powell DE, Pavlik FJ, Woods CH, Thompson EA. Transvaginal sonography as a screening method for ovarian cancer : a report of the first 1000 cases screened. Cancer 1990; 65 : 573-7.
52. Bourne TH, Campbell S, Whitehead MI, Collins WP. Ultrasound screening for sporadic and familial early ovarian cancer. J Ultrasound Med 1991; 10 : S43.
53. Folkman J, Watson J, Lugber D, Hanahan D. Induction of angiogenesis during the transition from hyperplasia to neoplasia. Nature (London), 1989; 339 : 58-61.
54. Rastincjad F, Pelverini PJ, Bouck NP. Regulation of the activity of a new inhibitor of angiogenesis by a cancer suppresser gene. Cell 1985; 56 : 345-55.
55. Ramos J, Fernandez IA, Morse SS, Fortune KI, Taylor KJW. Detection of neovascular signals in a 3 day Walker rat carcinoma by CW Doppler ultrasound. Ultrasound Med Biol 1988; 14 : 123-6.
56. Shinamoto K, Sakuma S, Ishigaki T, Makino N. Intratumoral blood flow : evaluation with colour Doppler echography. Radiology 1987; 165 : 683-5.
57. Bourne TH, Campbell S, Steer CV, Whitehead MI, Collins WP. Transvaginal colour flow imaging : a possible new screening technique for ovarian cancer, Br Med J 1989; 299 : 1367-70.
58. Kurjak A, Zalud J, Jurkovic D, Alfrovie Z, Miljan M. Transvaginal color flow Doppler for the assessment of pelvic cricunation. Act Obstet Gynecol Sound 1989; 33 : 131-5.
59. Hata K, Makihara K, Hata T, Takahanshi K, Kitao M. Transvaginal color Doppler imaging for haemodynamic assessment of tumors in the reproductive tract. Int. J Gynecol Obstet 1991 (in press).
60. Kurjak A, Zalud I. Early detection of ovarian cancer by transvaginal color Doppler. J Ultrasound Med 1991; 10 : S57.
61. Campbell S, Bourne TH, Reynolds K, Hampson J, Royston P, Whitehead MI, Collins WP. Role of color Doppler in an ultrasound based screening program. In Sharp F, Mason WP, Leake RE. (eds) Ovarian Cancer : Biological and Therapeutic Challenges, Vol. II. (Cambridge : Chapman and Hall Medical), 1991.
62. Cole LA, Joo-Hyun N, Chambers JT, Schwartz PE. Urinary gonadotropin fragment, a new tumor marker, H. Differentiating benign from a malignant pelvic mass. Gynecol Oncol 1990; 36 : 391-4.
63. Koos RD. Potential relevance of angiogenic factors to ovarian physiology. Sem Reprod Endocrinol 1989; 7 : 29-40.
64. Editorial. First catch your deer. Lancet, 1990; ii : 147-9.
65. Campbell S, Bourne TH, Collins WP. Screening for ovarian cancer (letter), Lancet, 1990; ii : 436.
66. Hardell I. Tamoxifen as a risk factor for carcinoma of the corpus uteri. Lancet 1989; i : 126-31.
67. Rowles TJ, Hardy SE, Ashley SF, Farrington GM, Cosgrove D, Davey JB, Dowsett M, McKinna JA, Nash AG, Sinneti HD, Tilyer CR, Treleaven JG. A pilot trial to evaluate the acute toxicity and feasibility of tamoxifen for prevention of breast cancer. Br J Cancer 1989; 60 : 126-31.
68. Osners R, Volksen M, Schauer A. Vaginosonography for early detection of endometrial carcinoma. Lancet 1990; i : 1569-71.
69. Bourne TH, Campbell S, Whitehead ML, Royston F, Steer CV, Collins WP. Detection of endometrial cancer in postmenopausal women by transvaginal ultrasonography and colour flow imaging. Br Med J 1990; 301 : 369-71.
70. Bourne TH, Campbell S, Steer CV, Royston P, Whitehead MI, Collins WP. Detection of endometrial cancer by transvaginal ultrasonography with color flow imaging and blood flow analysis : a preliminary report. Gynecol Oncol 1991; 40 : 253-9.
71. Kurjak A, Zalud L. The characterization of uterine

tumors by transvaginal color Doppler. Ultrasound Obstet Gynecol 1991; 1 : 50-2.

72. Matta WBM, Stabile J, Shaw RW, Campbell S. Doppler assessment of uterine blood flow changes in patients with fibroids receiving the gonadotropin-releasing hormone agonist buserelin. Fertil Steril 1988; 49 : 1083-5.
73. Bourne TH, Hillard T, Whitehead MI, Crook D, Campbell S. Evidence for a rapid effect of estrogens on the arterial status of postmenopausal women. Lancet 1990; 335 : 1470-1.
74. Fadwick MI, Whitehead MI, Coffer A, King RJB. Demonstration of estrogen receptor related protein in female issues. In Studd JWW, Whitehead MI. (eds) The Menopause, (Oxford : Blackwell), pp. 226-33, 1989.
75. Bourne TH, Hillard T, Whitehead M, Campbell S, Conns WP. Transvaginal ultrasonography with color flow imaging to monitor hormone replacement therapy in postmenopausal women. Br J Radiol 1991; 64 : 657-9.
76. De Ziegler D, Bessis R, Frydman R. Vascular resistance of uterine arteries : physiological effect of eradiol and progerone. Fertil Steril 1991; 55 : 775-9.
77. Fines A, Fisman EZ, Levo Y, Averbuch M, Lidor A. Drofy Y, Finklestiein A, Hetman-Peri M, Moshkowitz M, Ben-Ari E, Ayalon D. The effects of hormone replacement therapy in normal postmenopausal women; measurements of Doppler-derived parameters of aortic flow. Am J Obstet Gynecol 1991; 164 : 806-12.
78. Boncfous O, Presque P. Time domain formulation of pulse Doppler ultrasound and blood velocity elimination by cross correlation. Ultrasonic Imaging 1986; 8 : 73-85.
79. Tegeler CH, Krenkau HW, Hitchings LP. Color velocity imaging : introduction to a new ultrasound technology. J Neuroimag 1991; 1 : 85-90.

CHAPTER

20

Role of Transvaginal Colour Doppler for Tubal Patency

Gautam Allahbadia

Introduction

The incidence of tubal sterility is on the rise because of an increasing prevalence of salpingitis, ectopic pregnancies and surgical interventions on the pelvic organs[1]. The main tools in the diagnosis of tubal disorders so far have been hysterosalpingography (HSG) and chromolaparoscopy. Each of these methods carries a risk of complications. Chromolaparoscopy requires anaesthesia and the surgical intervention carries a 1-2% risk of complications, such as infections or injury of the intestine or blood vessels[2]. Radiographic HSG involves radiation exposure and is also contra-indicated in patients with idiosyncrasies to X-ray contrast agents[3]. Also, inherent risks of ionising radiation on the oocyte which may result in congenital malformations if conception were to take place in the investigation cycle cannot be excluded. Ultrasound scan does not require general anaesthesia or carry the risks outlined above. The technique has received wide acceptance by both technologists and physicians alike and has established itself as a definitive diagnostic test in many clinical situations. Previously, attempts have been made with the institution of sterile dextran, hyskon and antibiotic solutions under ultrasound scan guidance and tubal patency was deduced indirectly from the finding of increasing fluid in the cul-de-sac[4-6]. The results have been unsatisfactory. The aim of a prospective study from Bombay[7] using colour Doppler sonography and normal saline was to demonstrate the diagnostic efficacy of colour Doppler in assessing fallopian tube patency as compared to HSG and laparoscopic chromopertubation. When the results of TVCD were compared with those of HSG and chromolaparoscopy, there was a 92.5% agreement, that is, there was patency or occlusion of the fallopian tubes. In addition TVCD can demonstrate all the soft tissues and their vascularity as well as mobility. The colour signals generated by the air bubbles make it possible to demonstrate tubal patency on both sides separately. Vaginal colour Doppler offers a much better resolution with the advantage of lesser volume of normal saline being utilised. Tubal patency can be demonstrated in the presence of anatomical complications and requires only a small quantity of normal saline[7].

Procedure

A detailed history was taken and the nature and duration of infertility noted. After performing the other routine investigations for infertility, the patency of fallopian tubes was checked using TVCD in the preovulatory phase of the menstrual cycle. After an informed consent, the patient is given Inj. Atropine 0.6 mg, Inj. Diazepam 10 mg and Inj. Fortwin 15 mg IM and an 8F Foley catheter or an HSG cannula was inserted into the uterine cavity, the bulb inflated with 1.5-2.5 ml of saline and a routine pelvic scanning is performed. The uterus was used as a landmark for depiction of other adnexal structures. The Doppler window was then narrowed down to an area between the left ovary and the left cornual region of the uterus. 5-10 ml of sterile normal saline was next injected through the Foley catheter. Direction of flow into and out of the fallopian tubes was observed with TVCD. At the end of the procedure, the Foley bulb was deflated and the catheter removed.

Before the advent of TVCD into our infertility diagnosis program, we were using abdominal colour Doppler sonography (Figs. 20.1 to 20.3 – all on Plate 6) where a Leech-Wilkinson cannula can be used instead of the intrauterine catheter.

A patent fallopian tube was diagnosed when colour flow signals were recorded during pertubation of normal saline for at least ten seconds. When no fluid was seen to enter the peritoneal cavity, tubal occlusion was diagnosed. The same procedure was repeated on the right side. Each tube could be assessed separately and the free spill from each tube was depicted with a characteristic colour bruit showing phasic indeterminate colour assignment (Figs. 20.4 to 20.6 – all on Plate 6, and 20.7 and 20.8 – both on Plate 7). The patients were allowed to rest for about an hour and a half and then sent home on a seven day course of ampicillin and metronidazole. The entire procedure can be recorded on a videocassette and preserved by the patient as permanent documentation of her tubal status.

Discussion

Patency of the tubes was the earliest, and until recent decades, the only aspect of the tubal function that was studied and evaluated. The beginning of this century was marked by the development of diagnostic procedures for tubal patency and pathology with the introduction of HSG, tubal pertubation and laparoscopic chromopertubation. Radiological studies complement endoscopic investigations as each provides information, albeit with a varying degree of accuracy, on one or more segments of the oviduct, and each can also be used to confirm the findings of the other. Sonography as a tool for checking the patency of fallopian tubes was an expected development in the giant strides of progress the field of gynaecology was taking[7-9].

The advent of duplex Doppler techniques in the late 1970s opened up a new field of sonographic investigation namely, the direct recording of peripheral, abdominal and cardiac blood flow, albeit limited to a relatively small sample volume. Normal and abnormal flow characteristics were defined by duplex Doppler techniques setting the stage for clinical acceptance of a new generation of sonographic imaging devices, namely, colour Doppler units capable of displaying regional physiologic and pathophysiologic arterial and venous flow in the familiar anatomic format of a gray scale sonographic image[10].

An important finding from our experience using TVCD revealed a much better resolution and image of the free spill with only 10 ml of normal saline sufficing for testing the patency on both sides as compared to the 20-40 ml required for abdominal colour Doppler testing. Further, in case of a bilateral blockage, the reflux of normal saline was picked up clearly in the stem of the Foley catheter. An area of criticism would be that the site of blockage in the fallopian tube could not be clearly defined even on TVCD. TVCD can be used in an office setting, which makes it more convenient for both the patient and physician. Difficulty in making a diagnosis of tubal occlusion arises in patients with dilated hydrosalpinges because flow through the dilated fallopian tube may simulate spillage on the Doppler ultrasonography screen[11]. The limitation of this modality compared with conventional standard studies (HSG, laparoscopy) seems to be the impaired diagnostic value if no tubal flow can be demonstrated[12]. In addition, tubal architecture is not demonstrated with TVCD as it is with HSG. However, a recent study has shown that this information is not useful in preoperative salpingoplasty procedures[13]. Although the mucosal folds can be outlined by HSG, the co-relation between radiological studies and endoscopy in the assessment of tubal mucosa is poor. Investigators[14] have used scanning electron microscopy on microbiopsy specimens to demonstrate that in infertile patients with apparently normal tubes on HSG and laparoscopy, there were lesions of the mucosa, such as flattening of the folds, loss of cilia and alteration of cilial pattern. They considered these lesions to be a major cause of infertility and of failure of tubal reconstructive surgery.

Radionuclide hysterosalpingography has been recently described to evaluate the functional capability of the tubal mucosa[15]. Further work is required, but the initial impression is that radionuclide hysterosalpingography (RN-HSG) could be used in combination with other tests of tubal morphology to detect a possible cause of unexplained infertility when the tubes are patent and apparently normal. Another important advance that might overtake everything else in tubal diagnosis is positive contrast sonography of the fallopian tubes (HyCoSy), which is covered in another chapter in this textbook. We have some experience with this new modality (Figs. 20.9 to 20.14) and until it becomes established TVCD could be considered as a

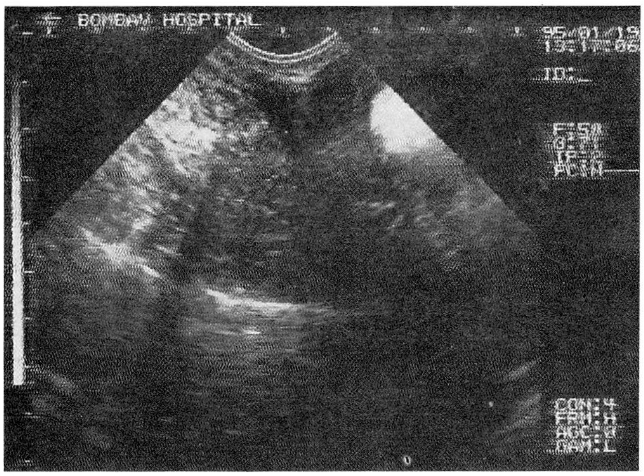

Fig. 20.11. HyCoSy. Distended uterine cavity with right cornual region with no spill seen in a case with bilateral cornual block.

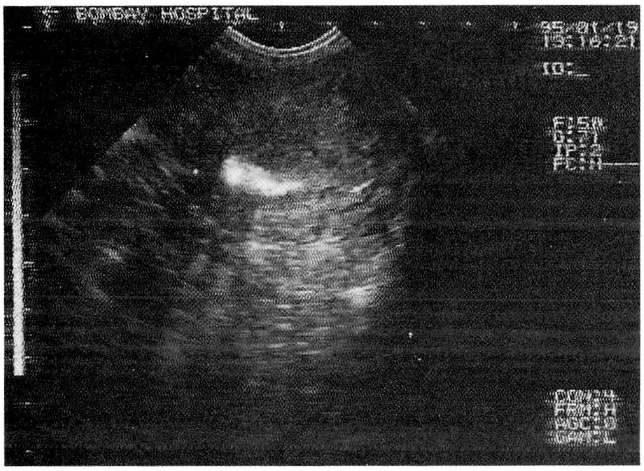

Fig. 20.9. HyCoSy. Uterine cavity and intramural portion of the left tube seen here.

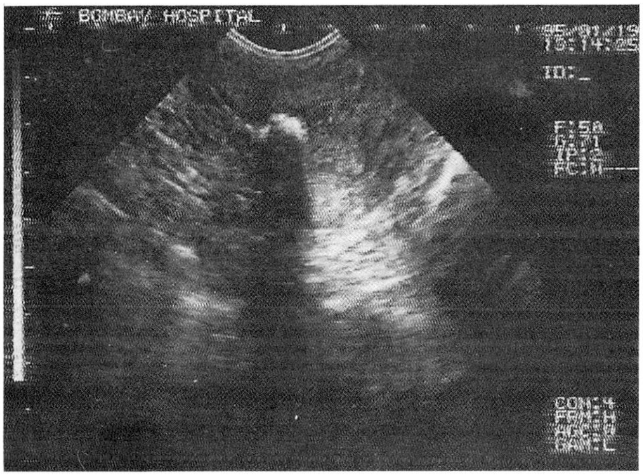

Fig. 20.12. HyCoSy. Uterine cavity with intramural and isthmic portion of right tube seen.

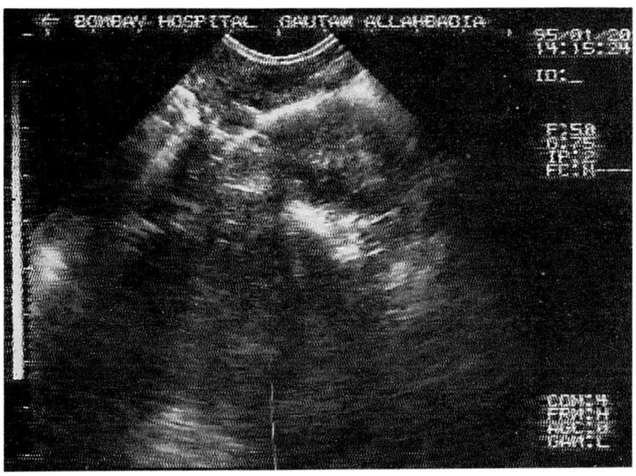

Fig. 20.10. HyCoSy. Intramural portion, isthmic portion, ampullary portion as well as exit of contrast from the left fallopian tube seen here.

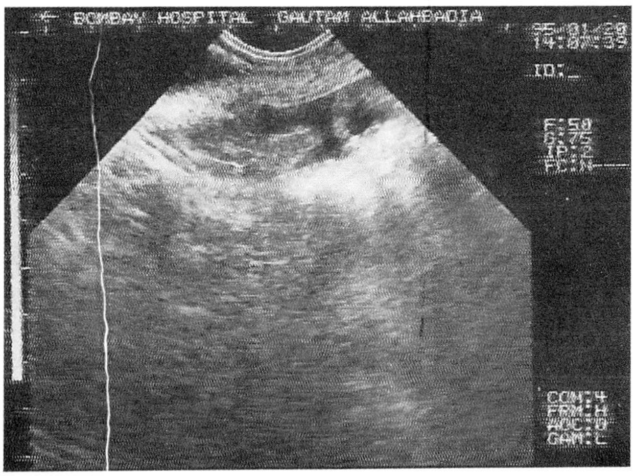

Fig. 20.13. HyCoSy. Fimbrial end of the left tube seen surrounded by saline and contrast at the end of the procedure.

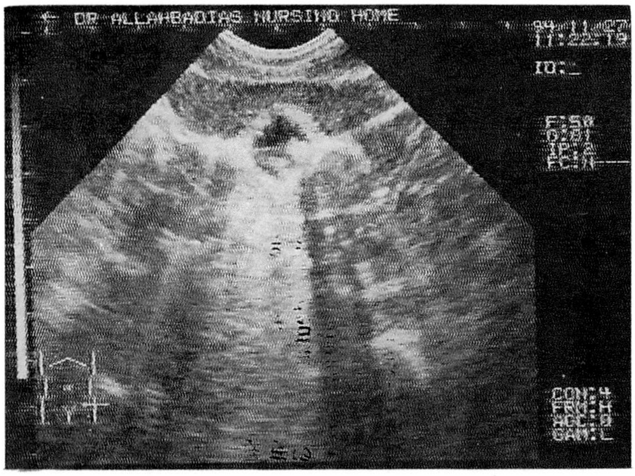

Fig. 20.14. HyCoSy. Transverse view of intrauterine Foley bulb with bilateral intramural and isthmic portions of fallopian tubes seen outlined with Echovist.

standard screening tool for tubal diagnosis. Keeping all the above-mentioned recent advances in mind, the author proposes that TVCD for evaluating fallopian tube patency be used as a basic screening test followed by either RN-HSG or salpingoscopy if there is bilateral free spill. If the colour bruit showing phasic colour indeterminance is not seen on one or both sides, then the entire gamut of investigations should be done for the tubal factor.

REFERENCES

1. Gomel V, Filmar S. Arrested tubal pregnancy. Fertil Steril 1987; 48 : 1043-7.
2. Gerhard I, Kasonovic A, Runnebaum B. Bedetung und moglichkeiten der tubendiagnostik bei der sterilitats-beratung. Geburtschilfe Frauenheilkld 1978; 38 : 805-15.
3. Sanfilipo JS, Yussman MA, Smith O. HSG in the evaluation of infertility : a six year review. Fertil Steril 1978; 30 : 636-43.
4. Sharma RP. Fallopian tube patency by ultrasound scan. Obstet Gynaecol India 1989; 39 : 700-01.
5. Richman TS, Viscomi GN, DeCherney A, Polan ML, Alcebo LO. Fallopian tubal patency assessed by ultrasound following fluid injection. Radiology 1984; 152 : 507-10.
6. Deichert U, Van de Sandt M, Daume E. Die vaginale hysterokontrastsonographie in ersatz oder erganzung zur differential diagnostichen hysterosalpingographie und chromolaparoscopie. Ultraschall Klin Prax 1987; 1 (suppl) : 48-51.
7. Allahbadia GN. Colour coded duplex sonography for the assessment of fallopian tube patency. Ann Acad Med 1994; 23 : 98-101.
8. Allahbadia GN, Nalawade YV, Patkar VD, Niyogi GM, Shah PK. The Sion test. Aust NZ J Obstet Gynaecol 1992; 32 : 67-70.
9. Allahbadia GN, G, Nalawade Y, Panjwani M, Vaidya P, Merchant S. The Sion procedure. J Obstet Gynaecol India 1992; 42 : 814-18.
10. Merrit CRB. Doppler flow colour imaging. J Clin Ultrasound. 1987; 15 : 591-97.
11. Peters AJ, Coulam CB. Hysterosalpingography with colour Doppler ultrasonography. Am J Obstet Gynaecol 1991; 164 : 1530-4.
12. Schlief R, Deichert U. Hysterosalpingocontrast sonography of the uterus & fallopian tubes : Results of a clinical trial of a new contrast medium in 120 patients. Radiology 1991; 178 : 213-15.
13. Groff TR, Edelstein JA, Schenken RS. Hysterosalpingography in the preoperative evaluation of tubal anastomosis candidates. Fertil Steril 1990; 53 : 417-20.
14. Brosens IA, Vasquez G. Fimbrial microbiopsy. J Reprod Med 1976; 16 : 171-8.
15. Brundin J, Dahlborn M, Ahlberg Ahre E, Lundberg HJ. Radionuclide hysterosalpingography for measurement of human oviductal function. Int J Obstet Gynecol 1989; 28 : 53-9.

CHAPTER

21

Transvaginal Colour Doppler Sonography in the First Trimester of Pregnancy

Nilesh Shah and Geeta Shah

Introduction

Colour Doppler sonography is a recent technological innovation which allows real-time sonographic visualization and evaluation of vascular structures both within and surrounding the pelvic organs. These imaging capabilities have only recently been incorporated into a transvaginal probe. This configuration affords detailed delineation of the vascular tree within and around the uterus and ovaries.

Colour Doppler sonography or colour flow mapping combines the physiologic information obtained by Doppler assessment of vessels with anatomic depiction of the location of blood flow within or adjacent to a particular organ[1] (Fig. 21.1 – Plate 7). Colour Doppler sonography assigns a colour to the frequency shift detected; red colour indicates flow toward the transducer, while blue indicates flow away from the transducer[2].

Arterial and venous blood flow to the arteries of choriodecidua can be seen from the fifth week of an intrauterine pregnancy. In addition, colour identification of the embryonic heart and major vessels can be seen by six weeks onwards (Fig. 21.2 – Plate 7). Initial work indicates that colour signal within the choriodecidua can be detected even before an embryo can be seen within the chorionic sac and that systolic velocities within the spiral arteries increase during the first 10 weeks[3]. With development of placental vascularity, significant diastolic flow within the spiral arteries can be documented. This is a sign that the spiral arteries that supply oxygenated blood are losing their muscular coating, permitting more passive flow[4].

Since the major vessels of the embryo and early fetus can be easily identified by transvaginal colour Doppler sonography, which includes the aorta and umbilical vessels; typically there is absent diastolic flow to the aorta, intracranial and umbilical arteries throughout the first trimester. During the 10th week, the renal arteries and the aortic bifurcation into the common iliac arteries can be identified[5].

Transvaginal colour Doppler sonography can also evaluate the low lying or placenta praevia or the possibility of placental vessel invasion of the myometrium (placenta percreta, accreta)[6].

Due to potential bio-effects, colour Doppler examination in normal early intrauterine pregnancies should be done with caution. The intensities used for transvaginal colour Doppler range from 52-60 mW/cm^2 spatial peak temporal average (SPTA) which is below the limit currently recommended by the FDA of 94 mW/cm^2 for fetal evaluation. The use of pulsed Doppler with colour Doppler increases the intensities up to 70-80 mW/cm^2. Hence examination time should be kept to a minimum and the low power setting should be used[1].

Transvaginal colour Doppler imaging in abnormal first trimester

Intrauterine pregnancies

Several etiologic mechanisms have been suggested for early pregnancy failure : abnormal chromosomal structure, poor implantation, and faulty vascularization with poor blood flow[7].

A higher rate of colour detection was found in gestations defined as anembryonic, as compared to those defined as missed abortions[4]. 64% of the anembryonic pregnancies showed flow as compared to 12% of missed abortions. Although this absence of flow in missed abortions could be a secondary phenomenon, it may indicate that circulatory problems can cause this type of early pregnancy failure. On the other hand, these preliminary data may indicate that a blighted ovum possibly develops owing to an embryonic factor and, at least early in this process, the uteroplacental circulation appears to be normal by the results of this study[4].

Chromosomal abnormalities occur with a higher frequency in the pregnancy failures classified as *blighted ova*[7]. All embryos with abnormal karyotypes had blood flow detected by colour Doppler imaging. Evaluation of spectral waveforms from these vessels demonstrated flow that was within the normal calculated range, emphasizing that early in the abortion process the circulation is still normal[3]. The S/D ratios and RI values calculated from waveforms obtained after colour detection in abnormal gestations were not significantly different from those obtained from normal intrauterine pregnancies at the same gestational ages[8,9].

This is an indication that we may be able to use this technique to distinguish between early failures due to circulation abnormalities, as is probably the case in most missed abortions, and failures of embryonic origin causing the anembryonic gestation, with initial normal uteroplacental circulation.

Ectopic pregnancy (Fig. 21.3 – Plate 7)

Since the process of placentation in the uterus or in the tube is the same, the vascular and flow patterns that occur during placentation localize the products of conception. The characteristics of placental (peritrophoblastic) flow are high velocity and low impedance. The high velocity probably results from the large pressure gradient (around 60 mm Hg) between the maternal arteries and the intervillous space. Placental flow, in either the uterus or the tube has a velocity of approximately 20-24 cm/sec and low impedance (RI = 0.375 ± 0.2). Hence presence of a peritrophoblastic type of a flow seen in the adnexal region, with an empty uterus, is highly suggestive of an ectopic pregnancy[3,10].

It is important to differentiate placental flow (20-40 cm/sec) from luteal flow (less than 20 cm/sec). Since ovarian ectopics are very rare (less than 1%), low impedance ovarian flow is due to luteal flow change.

Colour Doppler can differentiate an ectopic pregnancy pseudo sac from an incomplete abortion. The former will not show any detectable flow, whereas the latter will show a peritrophoblastic type of a flow.

REFERENCES

1. Kurjak A, Zalud I, Alfirevic Z. The assessment of abnormal pelvic blood flow by transvaginal color and pulsed Doppler. Ultrasound Med Biol 1990; 16 : 437-9.
2. Maulik D. Basic principles of Doppler ultrasound as applied in obstetrics. Clin Obstet Gynecol 1989; 32 : 628-30.
3. Stabil I, Grudzinskas J, Campbell S. Doppler ultrasonographic evaluation of abnormal pregnancies in the first trimester. J Clin Ultrasound 1990; 18 : 497-9.
4. Jaffe R, Warsof SL. Transvaginal color Doppler imaging in the assessment of utero-placental blood flow in the normal first trimester pregnancy. Am J Obstet Gynecol 1991; 164 : 781-6.
5. Schulman JH, Winter D, Farmakides G. Pregnancy surveillance with uterine-umbilical Doppler. Am J Obstet Gynecol 1989; 160 : 192-4.
6. Brosens IA. Morphological changes in the utero-placental bed in pregnancy hypertension. Clin Obstet Gynecol 1977; 4 : 573-5.
7. Pritchard JA, MacDonald PC, Gant N (eds.). Abortion In Williams Obstetrics, 17th edition, Norfolk, CT, Appleton-Century-Crofts, pp. 467-9, 1985.

8. Trudinger BJ, Giles WB, Cook CM. Utero-placental blood flow velocity-time waveforms in normal and complicated pregnancy. Br J Obstet Gynecol 1985; 92 : 39-43.
9. Stuart B, Drumn J, Fitzgerald DE. Fetal blood flow velocity waveforms in normal pregnancy. Br J Obstet Gynecol 1980; 87 : 780-4.
10. Goldstein SR. Early detection of pathologic pregnancy by transvaginal sonography. J Clin Ultrasound 1990; 18 : 262-5.

CHAPTER

22

Transvaginal Colour Doppler in Infertility

Chander Lulla

Transvaginal colour Doppler study in the assessment of uterine and ovarian blood flow

Ultrasonography, specifically the transvaginal approach, allows highly detailed anatomic exploration of the pelvic organs. Endovaginal colour doppler is an exciting innovation of great importance for the infertile patient. The newly developed colour Doppler sensitivity and pulsed-wave Doppler on normal pelvic vessels has made it possible to study the physiology of blood flow to the pelvic organs. Increased angiogenesis is considered to be a precursor for morphological changes that are observed during the menstrual cycle.

Ovarian circulation

With increasing estrogen during the follicular phase there is associated increased blood flow to the ovaries.

The description of changes in blood flow in the ovarian arteries in humans has been made possible by the development of high resolution transvaginal ultrasonography, particularly, Doppler imaging and colour flow mapping.

Normal menstrual cycle

Both ovarian arteries take origin from the aorta and reach the ovaries through the infundibulo-pelvic ligaments. After giving off small branches that penetrate the ovarian stroma, they anastamose with distal vessels of the ascending branches of the uterine arteries. The clearest Doppler signals can be obtained in the ovarian artery just before it reaches the ovarian hilus (Fig. 22.1 – Plate 7). This vascular position also corresponds most closely to the general ovarian impedance. Flow can also be elucidated from within ovarian tissue.

The functional ovary reveals cyclical changes in blood flow patterns. In the initial phase of the cycle there is high impedance blood flow pattern (low or absent diastolic flow) (Fig. 22.2 – Plate 8). The ovary which will develop the dominant follicle begins to show increasing diastolic flow (low impedance pattern)

(Fig. 22.3 – Plate 8). Differences in ovarian blood flow between the ovulatory and non-ovulatory sides can be recognized early in the cycle (Fig. 22.4 – Plate 8). The dominant ovary may be recognised earlier with colour flow imaging than with other present methods.

Around periovulatory period of the cycle the diastolic flow increases markedly indicating that ovulation is imminent. This low impedance, intra-ovarian vascularity increases with both ovulation and corpus luteum development (Fig. 22.5 – Plate 8) and usually resolves by the 24th day of the menstrual cycle (Fig. 22.6 – Plate 8).

If pregnancy occurs, the low impedance luteal activity persists throughout the first trimester (Fig. 22.7 – Plate 8).

Thus colour Doppler may help to elucidate the pathophysiology of luteal phase defects or early pregnancy loss.

The mechanism of ovarian blood flow changes has a hormonal basis; the hormonal relationships have been demonstrated in various animal species.

A poor ovarian blood flow may be responsible for poor quality ova and failure in rupture of the follicle resulting in a luteinised ruptured follicle syndrome (Fig. 22.8 – Plate 9).

Ovulation induction and other assisted reproductive technologies

Prediction of the probability of success in assisted reproductive procedures [IVF, gamete intrafallopian transfer (GIFT)] was the first clinical demonstration of the importance of Doppler flow studies in pelvic vessels. The increased use of assisted reproduction techniques for the treatment of infertility requires advanced imaging capabilities as well as functional analysis. Laboratory methods, such as endocrine assays for the reproductively active hormones or histologic examination of uterine biopsy specimens, are routinely used but are inconvenient, expensive, and results are not immediately available. Two-dimensional ultrasonographic imaging and transvaginal Doppler (particularly with the addition of colour flow mapping) permits rapid, noninvasive visualization and immediate conclusions.

Ovarian artery blood flow velocities differ between fertile and infertile women. In fertile women, a clear drop in RIs has been demonstrated before ovulation (Fig. 22.9 – Plate 9).

Doppler studies in animal models have demonstrated that ovarian blood flow increases significantly in female rabbits within 1 hour after human chorionic gonadotropin (hCG) administration and then gradually decreases. Histopathologic examination of peri-follicular and ovarian stromal vessels has been used to demonstrate vasodilation corresponding to the observed blood flow changes.

Deutinger and coworkers studied 38 patients from their IVF program. All patients were treated with GnRH agonists to suppress ovarian function before follicular stimulation with administration of hCG in accordance with standard ovulation induction protocols. Doppler measurements were performed daily on both ovarian arteries. A marked increase in diastolic flow velocity was observed toward the middle of the ovulation induction cycle, before follicular puncture for ovum harvesting. Decreased pulsatility indices, a sign of decreased resistance to flow, continued after follicle puncture. Resistance to flow was significantly lower in patients defined as high responders, that is, with high estradiol levels (higher than 200 pg per follicle greater than 15 mm) on the day of hCG administration, than in those defined as low responders. Fleischer reported that stimulated ovaries exhibit higher flow velocities, and the pulsatility index and RI depend on the number of follicles induced in each cycle.

Ovarian stimulation by pergonal or clomid causes bilateral increased flow in the ovaries (Fig. 22.10 – Plate 9). Correlation between vascular flow and ovarian hormonal response is probable, but requires further evaluation. Serial colour Doppler evaluation therefore can help in better timing the hCG administration in cases of E_2/USG mismatch or utero-ovarian mismatch and therefore may help improve the results of IVF/GIFT procedures. Early prediction of hyperstimulation may be possible with premature disproportionately increasing vascularity of the ovary.

Uterine circulation

The bilateral uterine arteries originate from the anterior division of the internal iliac arteries. On reaching the uterus, they divide into ascending and descending branches. After penetrating the myometrium, the arteries divide further into arcuate arteries that course within the uterine walls (Fig. 22.11 – Plate 9). In the arcuate arteries, blood flows in a direction parallel to the surface. The radial arteries arise perpendicular to the arcuate arteries and are, therefore, directed towards the uterine cavity. Radial arteries give rise to basal and spiral arteries. The latter are under hormonal influence and are the uterine vessels affected most by cyclic changes.

The first report of the use of Doppler ultrasonography in gynaecologic practice appeared in 1985. Several possible criteria could be evaluated :

1. Presence or absence of blood flow or determination of its direction.
2. Presence of enhanced blood flow in a solid mass as an indication of neovascularization associated with malignancy as described previously in the breast.
3. Quantification of blood flow and characterization of downstream impedance.
4. Quantification of changes associated with hormonal modifications, whether during the menstrual cycle or throughout pregnancy, in particular, evaluation of the ovarian and uterine circulations.
5. Actual blood flow rate analysis. In the same report, Taylor and coworkers demonstrated that different vessels have specific waveforms (Vessel signatures).

Doppler signals can be obtained from several areas of the uterus, but are optimal in the main uterine arteries lateral to the cervix and lower uterine segment, that is, roughly at the level of the internal os. The first Doppler studies of uterine blood flow were performed with transabdominal ultrasonography during pregnancy. Later, the method was applied for gynaecologic purposes. Transvaginal continuous wave Doppler imaging was described initially, followed by pulsed Doppler imaging, and then colour-coded Doppler.

Uterine blood flow is regulated by many factors, primarily the levels of the reproductively active steroid hormones. Estrogens dilate uterine vasculature and augment blood flow to the uterus, whereas progesterone has the opposite effect. In non-pregnant, oopherectomized sheep, estrogens were demonstrated to be vasodilators of the uterine vasculature, with 17 estradiol being the most potent. In guinea pigs, estrogen action increased the diameter of mesometrial arteries, whereas progesterone reduced their diameter. In gilts, progesterone increased in vivo contractility of the uterine arteries in response to neural stimulation. Estrogens decreased arterial contractility and, therefore, facilitated a marked increase in uterine blood flow. Similar findings have been described in other animals. Demonstrable increases in uterine weight or uterine blood flow parallel peak estradiol levels.

Estrogen and progesterone receptors are present in human uterine arteries. Cyclic variations in the levels of these receptors have been observed in normal endometrial tissue and within uterine fibroids. The receptor content of arterial walls is highest just before ovulation. Uterine blood flow closely follows these changes. In this regard, Doppler ultrasonography has been used to describe changes in the resistance of the uterine arteries secondary to hormone administration in rats. These physiologic changes have long been known, and Doppler ultrasonography is a logical approach to study uterine vascularity.

Nevertheless, changes in blood flow characteristics in uterine vessels during spontaneous cycle have been depicted in several studies performed in humans. Goswamy and Steptoe used a modified systolic/diastolic ratio (S/D) and modified resistance index (RI) to characterise uterine perfusion and changes thereof during the menstrual cycle. They demonstrated that the RI and the S/D ratio fell with the rise in estrogen level during the early follicular phase (Fig. 22.12 – Plate 9), then rose in the periovulatory period (Fig. 22.13 – Plate 9) parallel to the preovulatory progesterone levels. These changes indicated increased uterine perfusion in the follicular phase (Fig. 22.14 – Plate 10) with lower perfusion in the periovulatory period (Fig. 22.15 – Plate 10). A secondary increase in the luteal phase was also closely related to changes in hormone levels. The changes in the impedance of uterine arterial vessels during the ovarian and menstrual cycles have been further detailed. The pulsatility index was found to fall from a mean of 3.8 in early follicular phase to 3.0 in late follicular phase. A further decrease to 2.5 was observed in the luteal phase.

The changes in Doppler measurements observed in the uterine vessels are dose-dependent and are present regardless of the source of estrogen, whether it be endogenous or exogenous. Differences are not found in the uterine arteries when ovulatory and non-ovulatory sides were compared. Other important factors are patient's age, previous pelvic surgery, presence of endometriosis, administration of gonadotropic-releasing hormone agonists, and the presence of a pregnancy or uterine tumors.

Ovulation induction and assisted reproductive technologies

Many changes occur in the endometrium in response to hormonal manipulation. These changes consist of variation in endometrial thickness, changes in peristaltic activity, and blood flow changes similar to those occurring in nonstimulated cycles. The RI as measured in the uterine artery is relatively low in patients before gonadotropin stimulation for the in vitro fertilization (IVF). With continuous exogenous gonadotropin administration, there is a gradual increase in the indices until the day of follicle aspiration and a subsequent rapid decline throughout the luteal phase. These changes coincide closely with variations in circulating estrogen levels.

Specifically, in a study of endometrial receptivity in an IVF and embryo transfer (ET) program, poor uterine perfusion (Fig. 22.16 – Plate 10) was postulated to be a cause for failure of embryo implantation. The quality of ova, sperm, embryo, and endometrium all are crucial for implantation, both in natural cycles or in IVF/ET programs. Assessment of endometrial quality is a necessary component of the infertility work-up. Endometrial biopsy so far has been the only objective way of directly evaluating the endometrium, but ultrasonographic investigation (in particular, transvaginal colour Doppler ultrasonography) can now furnish much more information on function as well as morphology of the endometrium. Many pregnancies fail to develop even when endometrial characteristics are adequate. One presumption is that this is because the blastocyst fails to implant in the endometrium. Recently, Goswamy and coworkers described decreased uterine perfusion as a possible cause of infertility. Our investigators have shown that improved pregnancy rates seem to be correlated with enhanced blood flow in uterine vessels. Changes in uterine blood flow are not completely related to hormone levels, and some IVF patients with high levels of estrogens do not have adequate uterine flow indices. Among 20 IVF patients studied in a particular study with transvaginal Doppler ultrasonography the worst factors in terms of pregnancy rate, not unexpectedly, were low estradiol levels and a lack of increase in blood flow between the beginning of the cycle and the day of embryo transfer.

Contrary to what has been shown in the ovarian arteries, that is differences between the ovulatory and contralateral side, flow indices in both uterine arteries behave similarly during the cycle regardless of location of the luteal cyst.

It follows that the best combination of factors for the establishment of pregnancy are high estradiol levels and improved blood flow. It may then be speculated that, in the presence of elevated estradiol, unimproved velocimetry and lack of implantation are secondary to reduced levels of hormone receptors in the uterus or uterine vessels or are the poor response of the receptors to the hormone. Vascular flow changes may thus provide additional information on uterine receptivity when deciding to perform or withhold embryo transfer.

Women with blood flow characteristics indicative of a better-than-expected uterine environment may be at higher risk of implantation of transferred embryos and, therefore, at higher risk of a multiple pregnancy. In a study of 82 patients, uterine receptivity, uterine blood flow impedance (lower impedance = better flow = better receptivity). Ideal values of pulsatility index were between 2.00 and 2.99 with a pregnancy rate of 47% (17 of 36 patients) but a high multiple pregnancy rate of 47% (8 of 17 patients).

Colour Doppler HSG can be used to study the patency of the fallopian tubes noninvasively, without radiation and use of contrast material. Normal saline is injected via the cowins cannula and its passage is observed as colour flow signals passing from the tubes into the peritoneal cavity (Fig. 22.17 – Plate 10).

In conclusion transvaginal colour Doppler has provided new insights into the physiology of changes occuring in menstrual cycle and will play an important role in the future management of the infertile patient.

PART II

Infertility

CHAPTER

23

Induction of Ovulation with Clomiphene Citrate

R.K. Sharma

Historical background

Interestingly clomiphene citrate was initially investigated for its antifertility properties. In 1960, its antigonadotropic and infertility-promoting action in rats was investigated[1]. Further studies revealed that clomiphene was clinically an effective inducer of ovulation in certain amenorrhoeic and anovulatory women. Kistner and Smith carried out first clinical trials of ovulation induction with MER-25, a close structural analogue of clomiphene[2]. Greenblatt *et al.*[3] reported the successful induction of ovulation with clomiphene (MRL-41) in 78% of 36 patients with secondary amenorrhoea.

Chemistry

2-[P-(2-chloro-1,2-diphenyl vinyl) phenoxy] triethylamine dihydrogen citrate, is an orally active, nonsteroidal agent distantly related to diethylstilbestrol and chlorotrianisene (Tace). Clomiphene is a racemic mixture of its 2 stereochemical isomers, originally

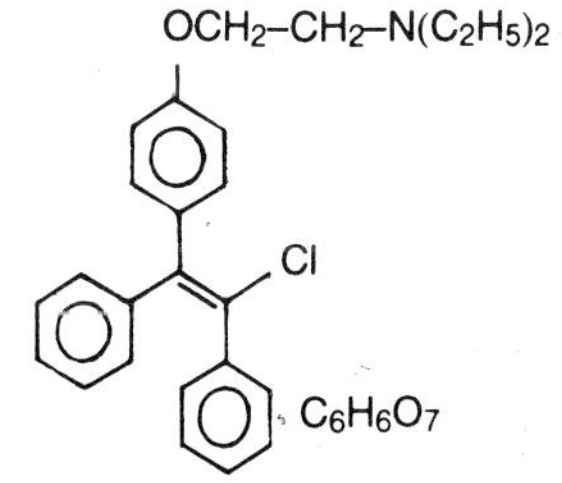

cis-zuclomiphene citrate

defined as the cis and trans isomers. These have been now relabelled as zuclomiphene and enclomiphene respectively[4]. Clomiphene is available as 50 mg tablets, containing 38% of the active zuclomiphene form.

Mode of action

Clomiphene citrate is capable of interacting with estrogen receptor-binding protein like native estrogens[5]. But it is known for its propensity to prolong nuclear receptor occupancy[6-8]. Indeed, it may occupy nuclear receptor sites for weeks at a time, as compared with native estrogens capable of clearing the cell within 24 hours.

When exposed to clomiphene, the hypothalamic-pituitary axis cannot perceive or act upon the true endogenous estrogens. This activates the neuro-endocrine mechanism of GnRH release. FSH and LH pulse frequency (but not amplitude) is increased, suggesting enhanced GnRH pulse frequency[9,10]. Miyake *et al.*[11] found in experiments utilizing hypo-thalamic in vitro preparations that clomiphene increases GnRH secretion in the presence of estradiol.

During the period of clomiphene administration, there is an immediate increase in FSH, which usually drops by day 4 or 5 of CC administration. The increase in LH begins somewhat more slowly and continues throughout the entire course of CC, decreasing a day or two after discontinuation. The ovulation that occurs after clomiphene citrate therapy is a result of the morphological and hormonal changes produced by the growing follicles. Clomiphene does not directly stimulate ovulation, but it supports a sequence of events that are physiologic features of a normal cycle.

The effectiveness of the drug, however, may not be due to its ability to cause an appropriate GnRH discharge.

Clomiphene has been found to exert estrogenic effect on the pituitary and directly stimulate the gonadotropin release, independently of its action on GnRH[12]. This direct estrogenic action may consist in part of sensitization of the gonadotroph to the action of GnRH.

Effect of clomiphene on the ovary appears to be estrogenic by enhancing FSH stimulation of LH receptors in granulosa cells[13].

In uterus, cervix and vagina, clomiphene acts primarily as an antiestrogen, potentially important actions affecting implantation and early embryonic development[14].

The mixed agonist and antagonist actions of clomiphene vary from species to species and from tissue to tissue.

Clomiphene does not display progestational, cortico-tropic, androgenic, or anti-androgenic properties.

Metabolism of clomiphene citrate

In humans, studies with ^{14}C-labeled clomiphene citrate, disclosed that it is readily absorbed from the gut, metabolised in the liver and it is excreted primarily in the feces[15-17]. Half-life is estimated to be 5 days suggesting finite residual drug concentrations until and possibly beyond mid-cycle. The role of the residual clomiphene at midcycle in the ovulatory agenda remains uncertain. In vitro, clomiphene inhibits progesterone production by luteal granulosa cells in a fashion that suggests that clomiphene, by virtue of its anti-estrogenic action, interferes with the induction of LH receptors[19]. This inhibition is reversed by Human Chorionic Gonadotropin (hCG).

Anti-estrogenic effects on the cervix and endometrium

The discrepancy between the ovulation rate (85%) and the pregnancy rate (43%) in women receiving clomiphene citrate treatment can be explained by the detrimental effect caused by its competition for estrogen receptors[20]. Despite the relatively high levels of estrogens in the circulation there is decreased amount of mucus, Spinnbarkeit and ferning due to antiestrogen effect of clomiphene. However, in some patients on CC, the elevated estrogen levels, 5 to 10 times higher than in normal cycles, may mask the antiestrogenic effects of CC on the cervix and uterus[21]. In these the cervical mucus does not exhibit any depressed effect.

Selection of patients

Over the years an increasing number of indications for clomiphene use have evolved. Anovulation of varied etiologies responds well to clomiphene. Patients with hypothalamic dysfunction, polycystic ovaries, post-pill amenorrhoea and adrenal androgen hyperfunction are good candidates for clomiphene therapy. Patients who have an inadequate reserve of pituitary gonadotropins and are deficient of estrogen usually do not respond to clomiphene[22]. Prior to use of substitutional gonado-tropin therapy in these patients, however, a limited trial of clomiphene treatment is wise, since it may occasionally yield surprisingly satisfactory results.

Patients with polycystic ovaries are very sensitive to clomiphene therapy and respond with a high percentage of ovulation[23]. Induction of ovulation often occurs in these patients with less than the usual starting dose. Whether the already elevated LH levels seen in this condition contribute to this sensitivity is unclear.

Although patients with galatorrhea are responsive to clomiphene induction of ovulation[24], they are more refractory to treatment. It is possible that prolactin, acting at either the hypothalamic-pituitary level[25] or directly upon the ovary[26], may function as an inhibitor of ovulation. L-dopa or bromocriptine should be used both to inhibit lactation and to induce ovulation[27,28].

Clomiphene citrate has also been suggested as therapy for luteal phase defects in selected patients. It is observed that certain types of luteal phase defects are the result of poor FSH stimulation of the follicle during folliculogenesis[30]. Or, a poor LH surge in the face of normal preovulatory FSH levels may also lead to abnormal luteinization[31]. Although the occasional central defect responsible for luteal phase inadequacy is correctable by clomiphene, Jones[29] recommended substitutional progesterone therapy as a generally more successful approach to this problem. Clomiphene does not prolong the luteal phase (as progesterone supplementation does). This is an important advantage of clomiphene, avoiding the anxiety and heightened monthly emotional response of infertile couples.

The administration of clomiphene to normally ovulating women is definitely not recommended, since these patients are at high risk for ovarian hyperstimulation. However, in those who are candidates for donor insemination, regulation of ovulation with clomiphene helps, as, not infrequently, because of the emotional stress of the procedure, previously regularly ovulating women develop erratic, unpredictable cycles[32]. The use of clomiphene permits predictable timing of ovulation and a more effective scheduling of insemination. Clomiphene is also indicated for oligo-ovulators, who, because of the infrequency of their ovulation, are unable to establish a pregnancy. The use of the drugs for induction of ovulation does not improve the quality of the ovum, and the chance of pregnancy is not improved in women who ovulate regularly and spontaneously.

In the devout orthodox Jewish couples, intercourse is prohibited in the presence of menstrual flow and for 7 days following its conclusion. In some women the menstrual flow is prolonged or the follicular phase is shortened, so that coitus does not take place until after ovulation. In these cases, the ovulation can be delayed to a more appropriate time by starting clomiphene later, usually on day 7 or 8 of the cycle. Ovulation can be expected in the interval 5-10 days after the last date of medication. This has its own limitations as administration of clomiphene, beyond day 9, may have no effect.

Clomiphene therapy should not be used for initiation of cyclicity in the oligoamenorrhoeic patients who do not seek fertility. The effectiveness of the clomiphene is restricted to the cycle in which it is used and it does not induce cyclicity following the conclusion of treatment. Secondly, by increasing the LH stimulation of ovarian steroid production, the clinical problem of acne and hirsuitism may increase.

Age, per se, is not a selection criteria for treatment, since arbitrary limits can wrongly influence treatment decisions. Ovarian responsiveness, especially in women older than 35, can be predicted on the basis of gonadotropin response to CC stimulation. An augmented FSH response to CC (compared to LH response) is found to be associated with a diminished ovarian reserve, probably because of reduced capacity of the ovary to secrete inhibin[33].

Dosage schedules

At present there is no clinical or laboratory parameter which can predict the dose of clomiphene necessary to achieve ovulation. Androgens and estrogens levels do not show any correlation with the dose of clomiphene which causes ovulation[34].

Although, there is a significant correlation between body-weight and the dose of clomiphene required for ovulation[34,35], one must adhere to the usual regime, because the weight cannot be used to predict prospectively the correct ovulatory dose. Some obese patients ovulate at the same low dose which achieves ovulation in thin women. Clomiphene is not stored in adipose tissue, and the increased dose often required in obese women is more likely due to higher androgen levels, producing more resistant hypothalamic-pituitary-ovarian axis.

The usual starting dose is 50 mg administered daily for 5 days beginning on the 5th day of the cycle. If the patient does not ovulate at this dose after two or three cycles, in subsequent cycles the dosage can be increased in increments of 50 mg per day for each of the 5 days. Alternatively, it is possible to increase the length of the time that clomiphene is given each cycle, that is from, 5 to 7 or even to 10 days[36].

Some patients of Stein-Leventhal are very sensitive to clomiphene. In them 2 or 3 days of therapy may be sufficient to induce ovulation. A full 5 day course of clomiphene may result in hyperstimulation.

The dosage of clomiphene citrate to induce ovulation should be titrated to the response of the patient. Dosage up to 250 mg per day for 5 days have been used, however, without any apparent increase in the side-effects[36,37]. The risk of complications in any patients given her minimal ovulatory dose does not appear to increase with the dose[36]. Majority of patients ovulate in response to a dose of 50 or 100 mg per day. There is a diminishing return in the percentage of positive responses at the higher dose levels[36]. If ovulation with an apparently satisfactory luteal phase has occurred at a lower dose, there appears to be no rationale or advantage in increasing the dosage of clomiphene in subsequent cycles and, in fact, there may be some risk[38].

Provided that other causes of infertility have been excluded, there is no arbitrary limit on the number of cycles a patient may take clomiphene. Pregnancy has been reported during the 29th cycle of treatment with clomiphene[39]. However, 4 to 6 months' effort at conception is indicated prior to any further intervention. Most of the clomiphene citrate associated pregnancies[20] are anticipated within the first 6 ovulatory cycles.

Intercourse every other day for 1 week beginning 4 days after the last day of clomiphene administration ensures optimal timing for conception.

Beginning clomiphene on the 5th day has been arrived at empirically. The clomiphene-induced increase in gonadotropins during days 5-9 occurs at a time when the selection of dominant follicle is taking place. Beginning clomiphene earlier than 5th day of cycle, stimulates multiple follicular maturation resulting in a greater incidence of multiple gestation. In in vitro fertilization program, clomiphene is administered earlier in order to obtain more than one oocyte. Better ovulation rates have been documented starting clomiphene on days 3, 4 or 5 of the cycle, compared to days 2 and 6[40].

Monitoring

In the first cycle, estrogenic mucus response and the normality of corpus luteal function is documented. Basal body temperature chart is maintained to aid in interpretation and scheduling of tests. Patient is evaluated for side-effects like residual ovarian enlargement after every cycle of treatment. Cysts within reasonable size range (3-6 cm) do not require a rest from treatment; they do not respond to further stimulation[41].

If an inadequate luteal phase is detected (temperature elevation less than 11 days duration) the amount of clomiphene is increased to the next dose level. If the patient is already on the maximal dosage, human chorionic gonadotropin (hCG) is added. Biphasic changes are taken as an indication of ovulation and success. Maintenance of the temperature elevation beyond the expected time of menses is the earliest practical indication of success and pregnancy.

When the BBT chart is inconclusive or when the patient does not become pregnant despite a period of normal ovulation, an endometrial biopsy to document the adequacy of luteal phase is indicated. Luteinized unruptured follicles can be detected by ultrasonographic monitoring.

In inadequate luteal phase, if an increase in dosage of clomiphene fails, then either progesterone supplementation or treatment with hMG is instituted. As the luteal phase defect is due to the result of antiestrogenic action of clomiphene on endometrial receptor levels, progesterone treatment would be ineffective. Hence, hMG is preferred over the progesterone in these cases. When androgens are elevated, suppression with dexamethasone should be tried in combination with clomiphene before proceeding to hMG.

Those patients who fail to ovulate at the maximal dose levels or when at that level, a short luteal phase is detected, then hCG is given to improve the midcycle LH surge, in the dose of 10,000 I.U. as a single intramuscular injection on the 7th day after clomiphene when follicular maturation is maximum as detected by measurement of blood estradiol levels or estimation of follicular size (18-20 mm diameter) by ultrasonography.

Results

In a large retrospective study, MacGregor and associates[35] reported a 70% to 80% ovulatory rate in most patients receiving clomiphene therapy. Pregnancy rates range from 15-60% in various studies. This large discrepancy between ovulation and pregnancy rates in patients treated with clomiphene has been variously explained. Ovulation is commonly diagnosed on the basis of the thermal shift in the BBT. The elevation in BBT may be the result of a direct action of clomiphene on regulatory centres within the hypothalamus, rather than a consequence of ovulation[42].

Follicular luteinization, and hence a thermogenic response, without ovum release may also take place[43]. The intracortical ovulation with ovum entrapment within the ovary may rarely occur and mimic true ovulation in terms of thermal shift and progesterone increase[42].

Inadequate cervical mucus, causing a cervical-seminal factor in infertility may develop in patients on clomiphene therapy. Luteal phase defects in clomiphene cycles may also prevent pregnancy.

It is possible that the abnormal milieu induced by clomiphene may in some way interfere with normal tubal function resulting either in failure of transport of the ovum or a accelerated transit time within the fallopian tube[42].

Side-effects

Side-effects of clomiphene citrate do not appear to be dose related occuring more frequently at the 50 mg dose. Patients requiring the high doses are probably less sensitive to the drug. The most common problems are vasomotor flushes (10%), abdominal distention, bloating, pain or soreness (5.5%), breast discomfort (2%) nausea and vomiting (2.2%), visual symptoms (1.5%), headache (1.3%) and dryness or loss of hair (0.3%).

Visual symptoms like blurring of vision, scotoma or abnormal perception disappear upon discontinuation of the therapy within a few days, but may take 1 or 2 weeks.

Significant ovarian enlargement is associated with larger periods of treatment, and is infrequent (5%) with the usual 5 days course. Maximal enlargement of the ovary usually occurs several days after discontinuing the clomiphene (due to increase in gonadotropins). If the patient is symptomatic, pelvic examination, intercourse and undue physical exertion should be avoided as the enlarged ovaries are very fragile. Ovarian enlargement disappears rapidly and only rarely is a subsequent treatment cycle delayed.

Following therapy with clomiphene citrate increased risk of multiple births is reported. Although there have been reports of congenital disorders like neural tube defects or Down's syndrome in infants born to women treated with clomiphene, the role of the drug in the causation of these defects has not been established and the incidence reported is similar to that in women with other types of infertility problems[44].

There are reports suggesting an association between follicular stimulation with clomiphene citrate and the development of ovarian cancer[45-47].

Contra-indications

Clomiphene citrate is contra-indicated in patients with liver disease or a history of liver dysfunction, endometrial carcinoma, ovarian failure or ovarian cyst (other than polycystic ovary), undiagnosed abnormal uterine bleeding and during pregnancy.

Clomiphene failure

Clomiphene failure can be either failure to ovulate or failure to conceive. 10-20% of women fail to conceive with the highest dose of clomiphene even with added hCG. In these cases it should be ensured that galactorrhoea or hyperprolactinemia is not overlooked. After 6-9 months of clomiphene therapy, and in the absence of any other infertility factors one can proceed to the following :

(i) Addition of corticosteroid

Patients with hirsuitism and high circulating androgens are more resistant to clomiphene. Dexamethasone 0.5 mg at bed-time to blunt the night time peak of ACTH, is added to decrease the adrenal contribution of circulating androgens, which decreases the androgen level in the follicular microenvironment[48,49]. The dexamethasone is maintained daily until pregnancy is confirmed. Clomiphene is again titrated starting with 50 mg/day and increased in stepwise fashion as required.

(ii) Extended clomiphene treatment

250 mg of clomiphene for 8 days followed by 10,000 I.U. hCG 6 days later[50] or increasing dose of clomiphene every 5 days, with some patients receiving up to 25 days of consecutive treatment, the last 5 days at 250 mg daily[51] have been tried. In those patients who responded, measurement of gonadotropins revealed sustained elevation of FSH. Estrogen monitoring with discontinuation of clomiphene is essential when an increase in estrogen is detected. A simple approach is to extend the duration of clomiphene therapy until a follicle of 18 mm diameter (on ultrasound) is detected, then administer hCG. However, Pergonal is preferred in these cases rather than extended clomiphene with a few results.

(iii) Addition of bromocriptine

Use of bromocriptine in cases of clomiphene failure with normal prolactin and no galactorrhoea is controversial. Though clinical response is sometimes impressive but the effectiveness of this therapy has not been established by controlled studies.

(iv) Addition of hMG

Clomiphene during recruitment and selection increases the FSH level which is further maintained by hMG thus ensuring proper follicular growth. This method has found wide acceptance in in vitro fertilization programs and some acceptance in 'Clomiphene-failure' patients prior to putting them through an hMG protocol. CC-hMG protocol reduces the necessary hMG requirement by 50%[52]. Kistner[53] found a pregnancy rate of 28% and Robertson[54] reported a pregnancy rate of 49%. In the latter study a high level of hyperstimulation, as evidenced by two triplets and three quadruplets have been reported[54]. CC-hMG combination is helpful in in vitro fertilization programs where the main aim is to obtain multiplicity of eggs.

(v) Addition of tamoxifen

In the induction of ovulation and luteal phase defect

addition of tamoxifen has been found to be more effective than clomiphene alone[55,56]. It increases the progesterone level, midcycle estradiol peak and the midluteal glycogen content of endometrium.

Summary

The availability of clomiphene citrate has revolutionized the care of the anovulatory, infertile patients. In general the side-effects of clomiphene therapy are not serious. By observing certain simple safeguards and precautions, one can safely induce ovulation in a high percentage of well-chosen women. With attention to other aspects of the infertility evaluation and the occasional adverse milieu caused by clomiphene itself, a respectable pregnancy rate can be achieved.

REFERENCES

1. Holtkamp DE, Greslin JG, Root CA, Lerner LJ. Gonadotropin inhibiting and anti-fecundity effects of clomiphene. Pro Soc Exp Biol Med 1960; 105 : 197-198.
2. Kistner RW, Smith OW. Observations on use of non-steroidal estrogen antagonist : MER 25II. Effects in endometrial hyperplasia and Stein-leventhal syndrome. Fertil Steril 1961; 12 : 121-122.
3. Greenblatt RB, Barfield WE, Jungct EC, Roy AW. Induction of ovulation with MRL-41. JAMA 1961; 178 : 101-103.
4. Ernst S, Hite G, Cantrell JS, Richardson A Jr, Benson HD. Stereochemistry of geometric isomers of clomiphene : A correction of the literature and a re-examination of structure-activity relationships. J Pharm Sci 1976; 65 : 148-150.
5. Clark JH, Markaverich, BM. The agonistic and antagonistic properties of clomiphene review. Pharmacol Ther 1982; 15 : 467-469.
6. Clark JH, Peck EJ Jr. Oestrogen receptors and antagonism of steroid hormone action. Nature 1974; 251 : 446-450.
7. Clark JH, Peck EJ Jr. Estrogen-receptor binding : Relationship to estrogen-induced responses. J Toxicol Environ Health 1976; 1 : 561-562.
8. Adashi EY, Hsueh AJW, Yen SSC: Alterations induced by clomiphene in the concentrations of oestrogen receptors in the uterus, pituitary gland and hypothalamus of female rats. J Endocrinol 1980; 87 : 383-387.
9. Kerin JF, Liu JH, Phillipou G, Yen SSC: Evidence for a hypothalamic site of action of clomiphene citrate in women. J Clin Endocrinol Metab 1985; 61 : 265-268.
10. Judd SJ, Alderman J, Bowden J, Michailov L. Evidence against the involvement of opiate neurons in mediating the effect of clomiphene citrate on gonadotropin-releasing hormone neurons. Fertil Steril 1987; 47 : 574-576.
11. Miyake A, Tasaka K, Sakumoto T, Kawamura Y, Nagahara Y, Aono T. Clomiphene citrate induces luteinizing hormone release through hypothalamic leuteinizing hormone-releasing hormone in vitro. Acta Endocrinol 1983; 103 : 289-290.
12. Adashi EY. Clomiphene citrate-initiated ovulation : A clinical update. Seminars Reprod Endocrinol 1986; 4 : 255-260.
13. Oelsner G, Barnea ER, Mullen MV, Mikkelson TJ, Tarlatzis BC, Naftolin F, DeCherney AH. Simultaneous measurements of clomiphene citrate in plasma and follicular fluid in women undergoing IVF & ET Program. American Fertility Society, Abstract 1986; 39.
14. Birkenfeld A, Beier HM, Schenker JG. The effect of clomiphene citrate on early embryonic development, endometrium and implantation. Human Reprod 1986; 1 : 387-390.
15. Schreiber E, Johnson JE, Plotz EJ, Wiener M. Studies with ^{14}C-labeled clomiphene citrate. Clin Res 1966; 15 : 287-289.
16. Holtkamp DE, Staples RE, Gresline JG, Davis RH. Pharmacodynamics of clomiphene in animals. Excerpta Med Int Congr Ser 1966; 133 : 68-70.
17. Clomiphene citrate (clamid), The William S. Merrell Company, Clin Pharmacol Ther 1967; 8 : 891-894.
18. Terakawa N, Shimizu I, Tsutsumi H, Aono T, Matsumoto K. A possible role of clomiphene citrate in the control of pre-ovulatory LH surge during induction of ovulation. Acta Endocrinol 1985; 190 : 58-60.
19. Lavy G, Fazio D, Polan ML. Human chorionic gonadotropin reverses the inhibitory effect of clomiphene citrate on progesterone production by granulosa-luteal cells obtained following different ovarian stimulation protocols. Program, American Fertility Society, Abstract 1986 : 40.
20. Gyster M, March CM, Mishell DR. A decade's experience with an individualized clomiphene treatment regimen including its effects on the post-coital test. Fertil Steril 1982; 37 : 161-167.
21. Topper R, Lunenfeld B, Shalev J, *et al.* The effect of clomiphene citrate and tamoxifen on the cervical mucus. Acta Obstet Gynaecol Scand 1988; 67 : 311-314.
22. Jones GS, de Moraes-Ruehsen MD. Clomiphene citrate for improvement of ovarian function. Am J Obstet Gynaecol 1967; 99 : 814-816.
23. Jayez JA. Selection of patients for clomiphene citrate therapy. Obstet Gynaecol 1976; 47 : 671-674.
24. Gambrell RD, Greenblatt RB, Mahesh VB. Post-pill

and pill related amenorrhoea-galactorrhoea. Am J. Obstet Gynecol 1971; 110 : 838-840.

25. Le Mair WJ, Shapiro AG, Riggall F, Yang NST. Temporary pituitary insensitivity to stimulation by synthetic LRF during the post-partum period. J Clin Endocrinol Metab 1974; 38 : 916-918.
26. McNatty KP, McNeilly AS. A possible role for prolactin in control of steroid secretion by the human Graafian follicle. Nature 1974; 250 : 653-655.
27. Turkington RW. Inhibition of prolactin secretion and successful therapy of the Forbes-Albright syndrome with L-dopa. J Clin Endocrinol Metab 1972; 34 : 306-308.
28. Varga L, Wenner R, Del Pozo E. Treatment of galactorrhoea amenorrhoea syndrome with Br-ergo-cryptine (CB154): Restoration of ovulatory function and fertility. Am J Obstet Gynecol 1973; 117 : 75-78.
29. Jones GS. The luteal phase defect. Fertil Steril 1976; 27 : 351-353.
30. Strott CA, Cargille CM, Ross GT, Lipsett MB. The short luteal phase. J Clin Endocrinol Metab 1970; 30 : 246-248.
31. Jones GS, Madrigal-Castro V. Hormonal findings in association with abnormal corpus luteum function in the human; the luteal phase defect. Fertil Steril 1970; 21 : 1-3.
32. Beck WW Jr, Barrett ATM. Adjunctive therapy to the woman in couples undergoing artificial insemination (abstr.). Fertil Steril 1978; 29 : 254-256.
33. Navot D, Rosenwaks Z, Marglioth EJ. Prognostic assessment of female fecundity. Lancet 1987; 8560 : 645-47.
34. Lobo RA, Gysler M, March CM, Goebelsmann U, Mishell DR Jr. Chemical and laboratory predictors of clomiphene response, Fertil Steril 1982; 37 : 168-70.
35. MacGreger AH. Further clinical experience with clomiphene citrate. Fertil Steril 1968; 19 : 616-68.
36. Adams R, Mishell DR, Israel R. Treatment of refractory anovulation with increased dosage and prolonged duration of cyclic clomiphene citrate. Obstet Gynaecol 1972; 39 : 562-565.
37. Rust LA, Israel R, Mishell DR. An individualized graduated therapeutic regime for clomiphene citrate. Am J Obstet Gynaecol 1974; 120 : 785-787.
38. Kistner RW. Induction of ovulation with clomiphene citrate. In : Progress in infertility, Second edition, edited by SJ Behrman, RW Kistner. Boston, Little, Brown and Co. 1975; 509.
39. March CM, Israel R, Mishell DR. Pregnancy following 29 cycles of clomiphene citrate therapy, a case report. Am J Obstet Gynecol 1976; 124 : 209-11.
40. Ruby M, Wu CH, Dein RA. The therapy initiation day and the outcome of clomiphene and short cause menotropin induction of ovulation. Program, American Fertility Society, Abstract 1986; 187.
41. Clinical Gynaecologic Endocrinology and Infertility, Fourth edition, edited by Leon Speroff, Robert H. Glass and Nathan G. Kase, p-590.
42. Whitelaw MJ, Kalman CF, Grams LR. The significance of the high ovulation rate versus the low pregnancy rate with clamid. Am J Obstet Gynecol 1970; 107 : 865-68.
43. Kase N. Mroueh A, Olsen L. Clamid therapy for anovulatory infertility. Am J Obstet Gynecol 1967; 98 : 1037-40.
44. Rosa F. Ovulation-induction and neural tube defects. Lancet 1990; 336 : 1327-1330.
45. Fishel S, Jackson P. Follicular stimulation for high tech pregnancies; are we playing it safe. Br Med J 1989; 299 : 309-311.
46. Kulkarni R, McGarry JM. Follicular stimulation and ovarian cancer. Br Med J 1989; 299 : 740-742.
47. Diett J. Ovulation and ovarian cancer. Lancet 1991; 338 : 445-446.
48. Lobo RA, Paul W, March CM, Granger L, Kletzkey OA. Clomiphene and dexamethasone in women unresponsive to clomiphene alone. Obstet Gynaecol, 1987; 60 : 497-500.
49. Daly DC, Walters CA, Soto-Albers CE, Tohan N, Riddick DH. A randomized study of dexamethasone in ovulation induction with clomiphene citrate. Fertil Steril 1984; 41 : 844-846.
50. Lobo RA, Granger LR, Davajan V, Mishell DR Jr. An extended regimen of clomiphene citrate in women unresponsive to standard therapy. Fertil Steril 1982; 37 : 762-765.
51. O'Herlihy C, Pepperell RJ, Brown JB, Smith MA, Sandri L, McBain JC. Incremental clomiphene therapy : A new method for treating persistent anovulation. Obstet Gynaecol 1981; 58 : 535-539.
52. March CM, Tredway DR, Mishell DR. Effect of clomiphene citrate upon amount and duration of human menopausal gonadotropin therapy. Am J Obstet Gynecol 1976; 125 : 699-700.
53. Kistner RW. Sequential use of clomiphene citrate and human menopausal gonadotropin in ovulation induction. Fertil Steril 1976; 27 : 72-75.
54. Robertson S, Birrel W, Grant A. Fewer multiple pregnancies using clomiphene/human gonadotropin sequence. Fertil Steril, 1977; 28 : 294-296.
55. Suginami H, Kitagawa H, Nikahashi N, Yano K, Matsubara K. A clomiphene citrate and tamoxifen citrate combination therapy : a novel therapy for ovulation induction. Fertil Steril, 1993; 59 : 976-979.
56. Fukushima T, Tajima C, Fukuma K, Maeyema M. Tamoxifen in the treatment of infertility associated with luteal phase deficiency. Fertil Steril 1982; 37 : 755-759.

CHAPTER

24

The New Frontiers in Ovulation Induction

Sadhana Desai

Ovulation is the result of balanced and coordinated effects of hypothalamic gonadotropin releasing hormones, pituitary gonadotropins, ovarian estrogens and follicular response. Any derangement of the above factors can result in ovarian dysfunction. The availability of ovulation induction medications and development of radioimmunoassays has allowed reproductive physiology to unravel many secrets of normal and abnormal menstrual cycles.

In the past the knowledge of reproductive endocrinology came from a search for a means to control population but since 1978 much of this new knowledge has come from science and technology developed in relation to in vitro fertilization. Today we can not only make anovulatory women ovulate but we can also make ovulatory women produce more than one egg as and when we want.

Ovulation induction in modern infertility management is therefore carried out not only in women having ovulation disorders but also in infertile women requiring assisted reproduction and in women with unexplained infertility and women requiring intrauterine insemination.

Several ovulation inducing or cycle regulating drugs are available and each one of them can be used in various dose levels for different treatment schemes. A decision has to be taken as to the type of therapy each patient should receive. The treatment will be reasonably successful only if the decision is 'correct'. In the past few years there is a new thinking for induction of ovulation by availability of recombinant h-FSH and a third generation GnRH antagonist Nal-Lys (Antide)[1].

Normal physiology of ovulation

In women there seem to be about 10-20 small antral follicles at the time of luteal regression in the previous cycle. From this pool a single follicle is selected for development in next cycle and rest of the follicles undergo regression. FSH appears to play a crucial role in this selection process[2,3]. Healthy follicles destined to undergo maturation process contain detectable amounts of FSH with higher concentration of oestradiol than follicles destined to undergo atresia. Once selected, the chosen follicle ensures suppression of the rest of the follicles by a rising level of oestradiol and inhibin secreted by the dominant follicle which cause suppression of FSH during the follicular phase of the ovarian cycle. High intrafollicular concentration of oestradiol in the dominant follicle enhances the responsiveness of granulosa cells to the action of FSH even though it is low in the follicular phase[4].

In the early follicular phase of a natural cycle, the concentration of LH rises as the suppressive effect of progesterone is removed following regression of the corpus luteum. The number of LH pulses increases from one in every 4-6 hours during the luteal phase to one per hour during the mid follicular phase. Each pulse of LH stimulates the secretion of androstenedione and testosterone by the thecal cells of the follicle. These are then converted to oestradiol by the granulosa cells.

The availability of recombinant gonadotropins for follicular stimulation provides new opportunities for new directions in folliculogenesis. The potential exists for examination of whether follicular recruitment may be persisted by recombinant FSH administration in the late luteal phase of an ovarian cycle. Moreover augmentation of selection of codominant follicles for IVF may be possible from recombinant human FSH without the side effects of LH[5]. This may be used for women with polycystic ovary syndrome.

What is recombinant FSH?[6–9]

α and β genes have been isolated from follicle stimulating hormone (FSH). The genes are inserted into a single vector so that expression is directed by two juxtaposed transcription units. The DNA has subsequently been transferred to the chinese hamster ovary cells and transferred cell clones have been isolated. The cells produced consistently recombinant FSH; highly purified FSH free of any LH effect. It does not contain any other protein contamination as present in FSH isolated from urine of menopausal women. It has the same biological property as natural FSH. Both natural and recombinant h-FSH preparations are composed of populations of molecules which have identical peptide sequences. They have minor difference in the glycosylated composition such as 'sialic acid'. Satisfactory trials have been already completed to assess and compare :

1. Pharmacological process of RhFSH with urinary h-FSH preparation to stimulate multiple follicular development.
2. Safety of RhFSH with that of urinary h-FSH.
3. Tolerance of subcutaneous administration of RhFSH with that of intramuscular administration of urinary h-FSH.

Advantages of RhFSH[10–15]

1. An improved batch to batch consistency.
2. High purity allowing chemical characteristics for qualitative control and product specification purpose.
3. High purity allowing subcutaneous administration.
4. Complete absence of LH.
5. Potential for designing new preparations with altered pharmacokinetic characteristics.
6. Urinary collection is avoided.

These advantages are likely to lead in the future towards replacement of urinary gonadotropin preparations by recombinant products.

GnRH analogue and GnRH antagonist[16,17]

Use of GnRH agonist as adjuvant therapy with gonadotropins for controlled ovarian hyperstimulation is now standard clinical practice. These drugs are employed for two principal reasons :

1. Prevention of untimely endogenous LH surge.
2. To gain some degree of control over and when oocytes retrieval must be performed.

Advantages and disadvantages of GnRH analogues[18–20]

Advantages :

1. Less cycle cancellation.
2. Less untimely LH surge.
3. Less poor response.
4. More flexible schedule.
5. More oocyte recovery.
6. Higher pregnancy rate.

Disadvantages :

1. More hMG.
2. More expensive.
3. More inconvenience.
4. ? embryo quality.

The recent development of potential third generation GnRH antagonist Nal-Lys (Antide) free from the marked histamine release effects that stymied earlier compounds may provide attractive alternative methods and allow more greater degree of flexibility in patient scheduling. GnRH antagonists have distinct advantages over GnRH analogues as they provide all the benefits of GnRH analogue without bothersome flare-up phase prior to suppression. GnRH antagonist may for the first time also allow control of gonado- tropin secretion in natural cycles making unstimulated IVF a practical reality.

Potential advantages of GnRH antagonist over currently used GnRH agonist

1. Immediate suppression of gonadotropin secretion and thereby ovarian function.
2. Possibility of suppression without initial flare-up effect.
3. Blockage of LH surge without nullifying FSH/LH secretion thereby reducing total number of exogenous gonadotropin doses needed.
4. Concurrent administration of GnRH pulses during GnRH antagonist suppression may be employed for controlled restoration of ovulation.
5. Greater degree of flexibility in stimulation regimes.

GnRH antagonists can be used at the onset of menstruation for cycle control for a variable period, then stopped with the onset of hMG stimulation and reinstituted at 12 mm follicular size until hCG administered. It can also be used only starting at 12 mm follicular size. Either method will reduce the duration of pituitary suppression from the usual three weeks to less than one week[21]. However, large randomised studies will be required to determine whether these approaches can achieve all the benefits of GnRH agonist/hMG stimulation.

Further uses of GnRH antagonists are for normal women attempting to conceive but having lower fecundity in cycles with higher follicular phase LH, and women with PCOD undergoing ovulation induction with hMG. A better quality of oocytes may be obtained with the use of GnRH antagonists by suppression effect of LH in the follicular phase in these women.

REFERENCES

1. Schmidt F, Sundaram K. [Ac-D-Nal (2), 4FD-Phe, D Trp, D-Arg] - LHRH, a potent antagonist of LHRH, produces transient edema and behavioral changes in rats. Contraception. 1984; 29 : 283-7.
2. Zeleznik AJ, Kubik CJ. Ovarian responses in macaques to pulsatile infusion of follicle-stimulating hormone (FSH) and luteinizing hormone (LH) : increased sensitivity of the maturing follicle to FSH. Endocrinol 1986; 119 : 2025-32.
3. Hiller SG. Paracrine control of follicular oestrogen synthesis. Sem Reprod Endocrinol 1991; 9 : 332-40.
4. Abdulwahid NA, Adams J. Gonadotropin control of follicular development. Clin Endocrinol 1985; 23 : 613-26.
5. Germond M, Desole S. Successful in vitro fertilization and embryo transfer after treatment with recombinant human FSH. Lancet 1992; i : 1170-1.
6. Chappel S. Kelton C. Expression of human gonadotropins by recombinant DNA methods. In : Genazzani AR, Petraglia F. (eds) Hormones in gynecological endocrinology, pp 179-84, 1992.
7. Deboer W, Mannaerts B. Recombinant human follicle stimulating hormone and its biochemical and biological characteristics. Crommelin DJA, Schellekens H. (eds) From clone to clinic, pp 253-9, 1990.
8. Mannaerts B, De Leeuw R. Comparative in vitro and in vivo studies on the biological characteristics of recombinant human follicle-stimulating hormone. Endocrinol 1991; 129 : 2623-9.
9. The Proceedings of a Symposium held at the 8th Annual Meeting of ESHRE — the European Society of Human Reproduction and Embryology — The Hague, The Netherlands, pp 6-7, July 1992.
10. Hillier SG. Ovarian manipulation with pure gonadotropins. J Endocrinol 1990; 127 : 1-4.
11. Gemzell CA, Diczfalusy E. Human Pituitary follicle-stimulating hormone. I. Clinical effect of a partly purified preparation. Ciba Foundation Colloquia Endocrinol 1960; 13 : 191-5.
12. The Proceedings of the 8th World Congress on IVF and Assisted Reproduction held at Kyoto, Japan in September, 1993. (Press). Van Wezenbeek P, Olijve W. Recombinant Follicle Stimulating Hormone I. Construction, Selection and Characterization of a Cell Line. From Clone to Clinic, pp 245-51, 1990.
13. Shoham Z, Insler V. Induction of follicular growth using recombinant human follicle-stimulating hormone in two volunteer women with hypogonadotropic hypogonadism. Fertil Steril 1993; 59 : 738-42.
14. Steven WJ, Lamberts I. Human recombinant follicle-stimulating hormone induces growth of preovulatory follicles without concomitant increase in androgen and estrogen biosynthesis in a woman with isolated gonadotropin deficiency. J Clin Endocrinol Metab 1987; 74 : 1471-3.
15. Devroey P, Mannaerts B. First established pregnancy and birth after ovarian stimulation with recombinant human follicle stimulating hormone (Org 32488). Hum Reprod 1993; 8 : 863-5.

16. Davis MR, Veldhuis JD. Sustained inhibitory actions of a potent antagonist of gonadotropin-releasing hormone in postmenopausal women. J Clin Endocrinol Metab 1987; 64 : 1268-74.

17. Leal JA, Gordon K. Probing studies on multiple dose effects of Antide (Nal-Lys) GnRH antagonist in ovariectomized monkeys. Contraception (in press), 1990.

18. Danforth DR, Gordon K. Extended presence of Antide (Nal-Lys GnRH antagonist) in circulation : Prolonged duration of gonadotropin inhibition may derive from Antide binding to serum proteins. J Clin Endocrinol Metab 1990; 70 : 554-6.

19. Danforth D, Williams R. Development of an in vitro bioassay for GnRH antagonists : Measurement of circulating Nal-Lys GnRH antagonist levels to examine the mechanism of its long action. 22nd Annual Meeting of the Society for the Study of Reproduction. Abstr 364, 1989.

20. Pavlou SN, Wakefield GB. Suppression of pituitary-gonadal function by a potent new luteinizing hormone-releasing hormone antagonist in normal men. J Clin Endocrinol Metab 1987; 64 : 631-6.

21. Mais V, Kazer RR. The dependency of folliculogenesis and corpus luteum function on pulsatile gonadotropin secretion in cycling women using a GnRH antagonist as probe. J Clin Endocrinol Metab 1986; 62 : 1250-5.

CHAPTER

25

Gonadotropin Therapy : Current Concepts

R.K. Bhathena

Gonadotropin therapy has been extensively used for more than two decades for the induction of ovulation in ovulatory disorders where more simple and safer alternative methods have failed. In recent years, gonadotropin preparations have also been utilized for multiple follicular development in assisted reproduction.

Selection of patients

Since some hypothalamic-pituitary disorders can now be treated specifically to induce ovulation (for instance, correction of weight loss or emotional disorders, or of hyperprolactinaemia), gonadotropin therapy can ideally be utilized for the following groups of patients :

(i) Hypothalamic-pituitary failure (WHO Group I) : These women have primary or secondary amenorrhoea, low levels of endogenous gonadotropins, and lack of endogenous oestrogenic activity.

(ii) Hypothalamic-pituitary dysfunction (WHO Group II) : These women have anovulation with menstrual disorders, with normal levels of endogenous gonadotropins, and evidence of endogenous oestrogenic activity.

A majority of these patients have polycystic ovarian disease (who have been "clomiphene-failures"). One of the greatest practical problems is maturation of too many follicles. The original follicular state of the ovaries influences the selection and control of gonadotropin therapy.

(iii) In recent years, gonadotropin therapy has also been used in long-standing cases of unexplained infertility, and luteal phase defect, but most of all for controlled superovulation in assisted reproduction.

Principles of gonadotropin therapy

The response to gonadotropin therapy depends on the number of antral follicles that are ready[1]. In cases of

PCOD, the starting dose should be 75 IU of purified FSH daily. In other cases, larger doses (150 IU of purified FSH) may be safely used. It is important to determine the state of the ovaries because a number of women may have polycystic ovaries without significant hirsutism or obesity.

In 1978, Brown demonstrated the importance of increasing the levels of follicle stimulating hormone only in modest amounts (less than 30 per cent) to stimulate folliculogenesis[2]. While exceptionally large dose increments may be appropriate (for instance, an older woman being prepared for IVF), in women with polycystic ovaries the dose should not be increased by more than 37.5 IU or 75 IU of purified FSH, and not until the previous smaller dose has been ineffective for a period of at least 7-10 days.

Purified FSH or hMG? Regan has demonstrated that excessive LH in the follicular phase decreases the chance of obtaining a pregnancy. In her series, women with a high LH (more than 10 IU in the early or mid-follicular phase) had a significantly lower pregnancy rate (65 per cent) than women with a normal LH (less than 10 IU) (88 per cent)[3]. Also, from the women who conceived, those with the high LH had a much higher miscarriage rate (65 per cent) than the women who miscarried in the normal LH group (12 per cent)[3]. Excessive LH also increases the risk of the ovarian hyperstimulation syndrome[1]. Administration of purified FSH may help to correct the LH : FSH imbalance. On the other hand, it can be argued that hMG seems to contribute only a negligible increase in LH. However, even after pituitary down-regulation, there is sufficient endogenous LH to require only exogenous purified FSH to obtain ovulation. For these reasons, the author prefers to use purified FSH in almost all cases requiring gonadotropin therapy, with or without down-regulation of the pituitary (the only exception being women with hypothalamic hypogonadism belonging to WHO Group I).

Even if the ovarian response has been favourable, the chance of conception (in the absence of other adverse factors) is only about 20-25 per cent per cycle, but that chance remains the same for numerous cycles[1]. Treatment should therefore be offered as many times as possible, to obtain a pregnancy.

Monitoring of gonadotropin therapy

There are considerable variations in the response of the ovaries to exogenous gonadotropins. It is therefore illogical to set a uniform dose regimen. The dose needs to be individually adjusted, depending on the ovarian response. Hence there is a need for meticulous monitoring of the ovarian cycle with ultrasonography and with biochemistry.

Ultrasonographic monitoring

Transvaginal ultrasonographic monitoring may be started five or six days after commencing gonadotropin therapy, and performed almost daily. There is a need to confirm the presence of a single or more growing follicles. If no growing follicles are seen, the gonadotropin dose may be increased after 7-10 days.

The dominant follicle is generally ovoid in shape, and the mean follicular diameter is calculated from the follicular measurements carried out in 3 perpendicular planes. When the dominant follicles reach a size of at least 17-18 mm, and the endometrium has a thickness of 10 mm or more and a double layered (outer echogenic and inner hypoechoic) pattern, the ovulating dose of hCG (5,000-10,000 IU) may be given.

If there are more than four or five large growing follicles, multiple pregnancies may occur if the hCG injection is not withheld.

The intermediate follicles, ranging from 12 mm to 15 mm, have a significant role in the development of ovarian hyperstimulation. It may be prudent to withhold the hCG injection if there are more than eight such follicles.

Monitoring oestradiol secretion

Monitoring with serum oestradiol may be started five or six days after commencing gonadotropin therapy. The assays may be repeated initially frequently, and then daily. When gonadotropin therapy is effective, the baseline oestrogen is enhanced.

Serum oestradiol levels reflect total follicular function. They do not give information on the number and size of the follicles.

If the pre-ovulatory serum oestradiol is over 4000 pmol per l, the hCG injection should be withheld, and the couple advised against intercourse for 4-5 days.

Serum luteinizing hormone

A serum LH assay requested around day 8 suggesting a high LH level (more than 10 IU/l) would mean a decreased chance of conception, and would be a strong predictive test for an increased risk of miscarriage, if pregnancy occurs.

Serum progesterone

Adequacy of the ovulatory response needs to be assessed by higher mid-luteal serum progesterone levels (more than 40 nmol/l) than in unstimulated cycles (more than 30 nmol/l) because of the contribution from the subsidiary follicles stimulated by exogenous gonadotropins.

Results with gonadotropin therapy

The pregnancy rate in patients with hypothalamic-pituitary failure (WHO Group I) is significantly higher (more than 80 per cent within 6 cycles) than in patients with hypothalamic-pituitary dysfunction (WHO Group II) (around 35 per cent within 6 cycles), suggesting that ovulation induction may generally be more difficult in patients with variable endogenous gonadotropin pulsatility. Premature luteinization may also be contributing to the lower pregnancy rate in WHO Group II patients.

The cumulative pregnancy rate is generally higher in younger women.

Potential problems with gonadotropin therapy

Ovarian hyperstimulation syndrome

Hyperstimulation reaction occurs when the ovaries respond with a vast overproduction of intermediate follicles, and, after administration of injection hCG, develop follicular cysts and corpus luteum cysts. Close clinical, biochemical and ultrasonographic observations are most useful in preventing or reducing hyperstimulation.

In cases where pituitary down-regulation was employed prior to exogenous gonadotropin therapy, when hyperstimulation is anticipated, exogenous gonadotropin therapy should be discontinued, but GnRH-agonist treatment continued to assist follicular regression.

In moderate or severe hyperstimulation, the treatment should be directed to prevent hypovolaemia which may lead to haemoconcentration, decreased renal perfusion, and, ultimately hypovolaemic shock. A solution of albumin (50 gm) in normal saline (1000 ml) is effective in reducing hyperstimulation. Very occasionally, fluid may need to be drained (with ultrasonographic guidance) from the abdominal and pleural cavities to alleviate symptoms.

Multiple pregnancy

The incidence of multiple births has increased after gonadotropin therapy. The majority of multiple births are twins.

Early pregnancy loss

The early pregnancy loss rate after the use of gonadotropins (20-30 per cent) is significantly greater than the rate of spontaneous abortion occurring in spontaneous pregnancies in a normal population (12-15 per cent). Since high follicular phase LH levels are known to significantly increase the early pregnancy loss rate[3], it may be appropriate to use purified FSH after pituitary down-regulation, to reduce early pregnancy wastage.

Premature luteinization

Premature luteinization precludes successful fertilization. These patients would benefit from pituitary down-regulation followed by purified FSH therapy.

Recent advances

Normegon

Organon (U.K.) has recently introduced a human menopausal gonadotropin injection containing FSH and LH in a proportion of 3 : 1. Careful research would be needed to establish any additional advantage of this combination.

Metrodin High Purity (Metrodin HP)

In 1993, Serono (U.K.) introduced Metrodin High Purity containing follicle stimulating hormone purified from the urine of post-menopausal women.

Traditional gonadotropin preparations have a protein content consisting of only 2 per cent FSH and 98 per cent uncontrolled extraneous urinary proteins [uromodulin, gammaglobulin (IgG), and epidermal growth factor], which are biologically active. With state-of-the-art purification technology, these extraneous proteins are removed, to provide more than 95 per cent purified FSH. Batch-to-batch consistency is a potential advantage. The greatest benefit is that this purity allows subcutaneous injections which can be self-administered to make the fertility treatment more convenient and less disruptive, while retaining privacy. Metrodin HP has a lower risk of adverse reactions at the site of the injection.

Serono (U.K.) has introduced patient care kits for patients wishing to self-administer Metrodin High Purity and Profasi by the subcutaneous route. The kit provides all the necessary equipment required for self-administration, as also instructions in leaflet and video form, and the option of using an autoinjector.

The results of a recent multinational clinical trial using Metrodin HP demonstrate that subcutaneous injections of Metrodin HP can be self-administered without compromising efficacy or safety[4].

Recombinant human FSH (Gonal-F)

Recombinant hFSH (Gonal-F) (Serono Laboratories, Switzerland) is produced by genetically engineered mammalian cells (Chinese hamster ovary cells) in which the genes encoding for the hFSH subunits have been inserted. Gonal-F does not contain LH activity.

The results of a recent multinational collaborative study using Gonal-F suggest that recombinant hFSH produced in vitro appears to be as effective and safe and well tolerated as natural hFSH extracted from post-menopausal urine[5]. Recombinant hFSH alone is effective to stimulate ovarian follicular development and steroidogenesis in women pretreated with a GnRH-agonist despite complete LH suppression. This preparation has improved batch-to-batch consistency, and the high purity allows subcutaneous self-administration. These observations clearly suggest that recombinant hFSH will, in the near future, replace urinary FSH in fertility clinics.

REFERENCES

1. Hull, M.G.R. Gonadotropin therapy in anovulatory infertility. Proceedings of an Infertility Meeting, The Royal Baths Assembly Rooms, Harrogate, UK, 1991; 56-69.
2. Brown, J.B. Pituitary control of ovarian function — concepts derived from gonadotropin therapy. Aus NZ J Obstet Gynaecol, 1978; 18 : 47-54.
3. Regan L. The luteinizing hormone hypothesis — high follicular phase luteinizing hormone : lessons from assisted conception and anovulatory infertility. Proceedings of an Infertility Meeting, The Royal Baths Assembly Rooms, Harrogate, UK, 1991; 29-38.
4. Barri PN, Brinsden PR, Cittadini E *et al.* Preliminary results of a multinational clinical trial using a high purified urinary human FSH preparation, Metrodin HP, combined with a GnRH-agonist in patients undergoing IVF/ET. Proceedings of a symposium held at the eighth annual meeting of ESHRE, The Hague, Netherlands, 1992; 11-22.
5. Loumaye E, Alvarez S, Barlow D *et al.* Clinical experience with recombinant human FSH (Gonal-F) : a collaborative study in IVF/ET. Proceedings of a symposium held at the eighth annual meeting of ESHRE, The Hague, Netherlands, 1992; 27-38.

CHAPTER

26

The Changing Roles of FSH and LH in Ovulation Induction

Bruno Lunenfeld

Introduction

The ovulatory cycle is governed by an elaborate neuro-endocrine system involving the brain, adenohypophysis and ovaries and is regulated by complex feedback systems. Internal and external environmental cues are relayed by synaptic transmission to hypothalamic neurons which process and transform the neural input into a neurosecretory endocrine outflow. The GnRH neurons, acting as chemoeffector cells liberate their product (GnRH) in a pulsatile fashion into the perivascular space of the pituitary portal system and thence to the anterior pituitary gonadotrophs that regulate the pituitary production of gonadotropins. During the last few years it has become evident that besides the complicated endocrine system also autocrine and paracrine processes take part in the complex regulation of ovarian events. Important elements in this regulatory function are played by the opioid system, serotoninergic pathways, GnRH, FSH, LH, prolactin and sex steroids as well as by many peptide growth promoting, differentiating and inhibitory substances.

For some of these peptides there is now evidence for synthesis within the ovary, evidence for specific granulosa cell membrane receptors and evidence for biological action within the ovary.

In this presentation we will attempt to delineate the different roles of each of these regulatory elements in folliculogenesis and ovulation.

The gonadotropin 'independent' follicular recruitment phase

About 3 months prior to ovulation, 30-300 follicles are recruited for growth and development. This initial recruitment of follicles and the early replication of granulosa cells can take place independent of gonadotropic hormones. Animal experiments demonstrated that follicular development up to the antrum stage was gonadotropin independent[1,2].

Lunenfeld and Eshkol[3] showed that in gonadotropin deprived prepubertal mice, follicular development could proceed up to the preantral stage.

In women, it has been suggested by Gougeon[4] that it may take about 10 weeks for an oocyte surrounded by a single layer of granulosa cells (primordial follicle) to develop into an antral follicle capable of gonadotropic responsiveness.

In the primate model the gonadotropin independent part of folliculogenesis is most probably controlled by genetic components and modulated by a number of growth factors. Whereas several hundred primordial follicles probably start to grow, 90% will degenerate and no more than about 30 precursor follicles are likely to become gonadotropin dependent and be present at the beginning of the menstrual cycle.

Of the cluster of about 30 remaining follicles, under physiological conditions, and under optimal FSH and LH stimulation few will be selected for further growth and development. Usually only one will mature, reach dominance and ovulate. The others will undergo atresia, or luteinization.

A predominantly intrafollicular estrogenic milieu will permit and favour follicular growth and development, an intrafollicular androgenic milieu is associated with follicular degeneration and atresia.

In the primate model the gonadotropin dependent folliculogenesis proceeds by the following steps :

Rescue of a follicular cohort

As follicles enter the gonadotropin-sensitive phase, it becomes apparent that a specific frequency and amplitude of GnRH pulses are necessary to assure the proper gonadotropin milieu. FSH binds almost exclusively to the large N terminal extracellular segment of a 'seven arm' trans-membrane receptor on the granulosa cells, induces their multiplication and stimulates biochemical processes mediated through cAMP. The LH receptor on thecal cells is also composed of a large N terminal extracellular segment responsible for hormone binding and constituted of repeated leucine-rich motifs. It is followed by a segment spanning seven times the membrane, characteristic of G-protein couples receptors, and by a short C-terminal domain[5]. LH binding to this receptor stimulates thecal cell development and androgen production. The rescue of a follicular cohort from further degeneration is dependent on a rise of FSH to predetermined threshold level. A physiological raised FSH level during the late luteal phase and early follicular phase will rescue one or more of the approximately 20-40 follicles which have sufficient intact FSH receptors on their granulosa cells and have become gonadotropin dependent. The higher the FSH level the more follicles will be rescued from degeneration and will continue to grow and develop. If at that time FSH levels are below the threshold level, the developing follicles will degenerate[6,7].

Follicular selection

FSH reaches most or all the follicles within the ovary, but only a minority respond with growth, development and ovulation. The selectivity of gonadotropin action requires local regulatory mechanism which may serve to enhance, amplify or decrease FSH action in certain follicles. The ovarian IGF-1 system has emerged as one plausible mechanism to fulfill this role. Studies in support of this hypothesis have shown that each of the ovarian cell types examined possesses an IGF-1 response system including IGF receptors and an intracellular transduction mechanism[8-12]. Acting through this system the IGFs can promote either replication or differentiation of ovarian cells. IGF-1 receptors possess an integral intracellular tyrosine kinase moiety that is activated upon the binding of its specific ligand to the extracellular domain of the receptor. Activation of the tyrosine kinase initiates an intracellular tyrosine phosphorylation/ dephosphorylation cascade leading to the effects of IGF-1. Human granulosa cells most probably incapable of producing IGF-1 are highly effective in producing IGF binding proteins[13]. These will compete for free IGF-1 (mainly produced by the liver under growth hormone stimulation) and regulate the amount of free IGF-1 available to the follicular cells.

It is postulated that the rescue of follicles from degeneration by FSH is achieved by reducing 'androgenicity' and by maintaining a predominant estrogenic milieu. Initially this is accomplished by FSH indirectly through stimulating local production of activin (a potent inhibitor of androgen synthesis in small follicles), and later directly by metabolizing LH induced thecal androgens to estrogens through stimulation of the aromatizing process in the granulosa cells. The aromatizing process in the granulosa cells can also be stimulated by IGF-1. While evaluating the intracellular signalling mechanisms of FSH and IGF-1 we found[13] that both increased estradiol (E2) production in granulosa cells from androstenedione by about 600%, but only addition of FSH led also to a concomitant rise in cAMP. Specific tyrosine kinase inhibitors (tyrphostins) blocked the effects of both FSH and IGF-1 on E2 production without altering FSH induced cAMP accumulation. Since also vanadate a tyrosine phosphate inhibitor caused significant E2 increase, it can be postulated that by activating either the soluble or receptor-bound forms of tyrosine kinase, E2 production is increased. These findings support a pivotal role for a tyrosine phosphorylation event distal to cAMP production, in the intracellular signalling mechanism of both FSH and IGF-1 effect on aromatase activity. Since an intrafollicular estrogenic milieu is of vital importance for follicular survival two alternative pathways for estrogen production seem to exist.

Sufficient amounts of FSH and IGF-1 will ensure and maintain a predominant intrafollicular estrogenic milieu, favouring follicular development and maturation. An excess of free IGF-1 may over-amplify gonadotropin action as noted in PCOD or in the ovarian hyperstimulation syndrome.

Sub-threshold levels of FSH, abnormal levels of free IGF-1, decreased levels of IGF binding proteins, or excess of LH will favour androgenicity within the follicle resulting in degeneration (atresia).

Thus it can be postulated that the fate of a follicle will depend on its threshold requirement of FSH and the degree of androgenicity within the follicle.

The selection process is completed during the early follicular phases (usually within the first seven days of the cycle). From a clinical oriented point of view it can be postulated that administering, at this stage of the cycle, FSH at a dose which will increase serum levels above the threshold will directly or indirectly increase the estrogenic milieu and prevent atresia. The administration of a gonadotropin preparation with a high LH or LH like content, may increase intrafollicular androgenicity and induce atresia.

Follicular dominance

Following its selection the dominant follicle grows and matures at a higher rate than the other follicles due to its increased sensitivity to FSH. Moreover by producing estrogen as well as inhibins the dominant follicle regulates to a certain extent gonadotropin secretion which enables its final maturation on the one hand and inhibits further development of other follicles of the same cohort on the other hand[6]. (Thus administering FSH at a dose which will increase serum levels above the threshold will allow more follicles to gain dominance and this may result in the final development of multiple dominant follicles capable of ovulating, resulting in multiple corpora lutea and possible multiple pregnancies.)

It thus became evident that by using the threshold principle, which has already been advocated in the mid-sixties[14-17], it is possible to regulate to a certain extent the number of follicles which will ultimately reach dominance and ovulate. Low dose FSH step up protocols could thus decrease the occurrence of hyperstimulation and multiple pregnancies not only in PCOD patients.

The dominant follicle at the proper time causes the occurrence of the estrogen provoked LH surge and subsequently ovulates and is transformed into a functional corpus luteum.

Excessive LH at this stage can cause premature luteinization of the dominant follicle(s) as expressed by an untimely increase in progesterone[7].

The fate of the oocyte in the dominant follicle

The continuation of the meiotic process of the oocyte in the pre-antral follicle is inhibited by a meiosis-inhibiting system. At this stage the chromosomes of the oocyte are arrested in the prophase stage of meiosis. Only when the meiosis-inhibiting system is inhibited in the maturing follicle directly or indirectly by the pre-ovulatory rising LH, will the first meiotic division be completed, and the first polar body expulsed. In this stage the egg is very sensitive, and if it will not be fertilized by a sperm, within 48-72 hours the second meiotic division will not occur and the egg will die. This ensures at ovulation the release of a mature egg at the appropriate time[18]. Timely maturation of the oocyte is essential if fertilization and the development of an embryo are to occur. Premature reactivation of meiosis caused by high basal concentrations of LH may lead to karyotypic abnormalities and death of the embryo and fetus.

It has been suggested that a high concentration of LH through the follicular phase allows the developing oocyte to mature prematurely[19] producing at ovulation an oocyte that is physiologically aged. Such oocytes may have a decreased capacity to fertilize, if they fertilize they are unlikely to implant, and if they implant their survival rate is decreased and early abortion will result[7].

From work involving women having IVF several authors have reported that high concentration of LH in the few days before oocytes are collected were associated with reduced rates of fertilization and conception[20-22]. The above results were confirmed by McFaul *et al.*[23]. These authors suggest that exposure of the maturing oocyte to high levels of LH during follicular development is detrimental to fertilization and conception.

They also demonstrated that, if conception is

achieved in a cycle in which the oocyte is prematurely exposed to elevated LH, there is a significantly higher probability that an early abortion will result. This situation occurs according to McFaul *et al.*[23] in patients diagnosed as Polycystic Ovarian Disease (PCOD), where ovulation rates following ovulation induction are high but pregnancy rate low.

In a very elegant paper Regan *et al.*[24] demonstrated that when ovulation induction was attempted in patients with LH levels below 10 IU/l, 88% conceived and only 15% aborted. However in patients with elevated LH level the conception rate was only 67% and of these 65% ended in miscarriage.

Johnson and Pearce[25] support this concept and conclude that pituitary suppression by GnRH analogues before induction of ovulation (reducing LH levels) reduces the risk of spontaneous abortion in women with PCOD and primary recurrent spontaneous abortion following induction of ovulation. Spontaneous abortion occurred in 11 of 20 women given clomiphene citrate, compared with only 2 of 20 who had pituitary suppression with buserilin followed by administration of pure FSH.

The adverse effect of an excess of LH in mid and late follicular phase can also be observed when attempting to induce ovulation with Clomiphene citrate (CC)[26]. When measuring FSH and LH in anovulatory women with no detectable features of PCOD undergoing ovulation induction with CC one can note two hormonal patterns. One group exhibits an excessive LH secretion and in the second group the LH/FSH ratio never exceeds 1.7. Not a single clinical pregnancy occurred in the group which responded with an excessive LH response. Further more the estrogen secretion pattern in this group was reminiscent of that seen in PCOD patients. All the pregnancies occurred in the group of patients who did not exhibit an excessive LH response. These observations indicate that also an iatrogenically induced excess of LH in mid and late follicular phase can adversely affect the outcome of the treatment cycle. Furthermore this study[26] indicates that determination of FSH and LH one or two days following termination of CC administration may help to select patients either for continuation of CC therapy, or (those with excessive LH) for FSH therapy.

It can thus be concluded that the different stages of follicular development may have different FSH threshold levels and that FSH is the fundamental gonadotropic hormone during the early and late follicular phase. Basal levels of LH for the supply of androgen precursor are necessary for the functional development of the follicle and its estrogen production. In the total absence of LH, thecal cell proliferation will be impaired and androgen and estrogen production will be lacking[3]. This situation may occur in some of the 1.2% infertile patients pertaining to WHO Group I.

In all patients with hypothalamic pituitary dysfunction WHO II, or in patients downregulated with GnRH analogues, pure FSH can stimulate follicular development as effectively as hMG. This has been proven beyond doubt since induction of ovulation followed by conception could be induced in GnRHa downregulated patients with recombinant FSH devoid of any LH or LH-like activity[27,28].

The above findings have prompted many investigators and clinicians to re-design protocols for ovulation and superovulation induction which safeguard against elevated LH levels. These include administration of agents to reduce endogenous LH secretion and the use of predominantly FSH containing preparations. This was made possible by the development of affinity purification processes which opened the door for large scale production of FSH (Metrodin). This technology utilized polyvalent antibodies, which yielded a relatively biological pure FSH product containing less than 1 IU of LH activity.

Recent technological advances made it possible to replace polyvalent antibodies with highly specific monoclonal antibodies. Whereas the production of 'Metrodin' was essentially a 'passive process', in which LH was separate from bulk material and FSH together with urinary proteins were collected and lyophylized for use, the 'third generation product' Metrodin HP production is a more direct process. In this procedure highly specific monoclonal antibodies to FSH selectively bind the FSH molecules in the hMG bulk material as they pass through the affinity column. The unbound urinary protein along with the LH pass through the column and are removed. The column then contains pure FSH. This is extracted from the column as a highly purified product devoid of both LH and contaminating urinary proteins.

As a result of this improved processing, this FSH preparation (Metrodin HP) contains less than 0.1 IU of LH activity and less than 5% of unidentified urinary proteins. The specific activity of the FSH has been increased, from approximately 100-150 IU/mg of protein for 'Metrodin' to about 9,000 IU/mg protein for 'Metrodin HP'. The purity is also increased from 1-2% in Metrodin to 95% in Metrodin HP. Due to its enhanced purity the total amount of injected protein is very small and therefore Metrodin HP is suitable for subcutaneous administration. Batch to batch variability is practically eliminated and the product lends itself to detailed analysis by physico-chemical methods in addition to the classical in vivo bioassay. This purified preparation also permits to assess the pharmacodynamics and pharmacokinetics of FSH.

The technical developments which have led to the production of highly purified FSH (Metrodin HP) and a deeper understanding of the pharmacodynamics and pharmacokinetics of these preparations, have all made it possible to re-design ovulation inducing protocols (for example, low dose regimens, low dose increments, subcutaneous injection route).

These new protocols may prove to be more efficient and may result in fewer multiple pregnancies, a lower abortion rate and an even lower risk of hyperstimulation.

With the use of highly purified FSH preparation, a re-evaluation may be necessary of the role of estrogen as a marker of ovulation induction. Now that highly purified urinary FSH preparations with about 9,000 IU FSH/mg protein are becoming accessible, we have to ask ourselves if it is ethically admissible to continue to use earlier preparations with 100-200 IU FSH/mg protein, containing 95% co-purified urinary proteins. The highly purified urinary preparations will surely replace within the next two years all commercially available hMG preparations as well as Metrodin.

REFERENCES

1. Greep RO. Histology, histochemistry and ultrastructure of adult ovary. In : The Ovary (eds.) Grady HG, Smith DE. William & Wilkins, Baltimore; pp. 48-56, 1963.
2. Herz R. Pituitary independence of the prepubertal development of the ovary of the rat and rabbit and its pertinence to hypo-ovarism in women. In : The Ovary (eds.) Grady HG, Smith DE. William & Wilkins, Baltimore; pp. 56-61, 1963.
3. Lunenfeld B, Eshkol A. Immunology of follicle stimulating hormone and luteinizing hormone. Vitamins and Hormones 1970; 27 : 131-59.
4. Gougeon A. Origin and growth of the preovulatory follicles(s) in spontaneous and stimulated cycles. In : Human in vivo fertilization, Inserm Symposium No. 24, (eds.) Testard J, Friedman R. Elsevier Science Publishers, Amsterdam; pp. 7-23, 1985.
5. Milgrom E. International symposium on ovarian function, Jerusalem, 1993. (Unpublished)
6. Glasier AF, Baird DT, Hillier SG. FSH and the control of follicular growth. J Steroid Biochem 1989; 32 : 167-70.
7. Lunenfeld B. Stimulation de l'ovulation : une nouvelle approche basee sur de donnees physiologiques et clinicques recentes : Perspectives d'avenir. Contracept Fertil Sex 1993; 21 (suppl 4) : 1-7.
8. Adashi EY, Carol H, Resnick A, D'Ercole J, Svoboda EM, Van Wyk JJ. Insulin-like growth factors as intraovarian regulator of granulosa cell growth and function. Endocr Rev 1985; 6 : 400-10.
9. Adashi EY, Resnick A, Svoboda EM, Van Wyk JJ. Somatomedin C synergizes with FSH in the acquisition of projection biosynthetic capacity by cultured rat granulosa cells. Endocrinology 1985; 116 : 2135-42.
10. Adashi EY, Resnick A, Svoboda EM, Van Wyk JJ. Somatomedin C enhances induction of LH receptors by FSH in cultured rat granulosa cells. Endocrinology 1985; 116 : 2369-75.
11. Adashi EY, Resnick CE, Hernandez ER. The ovarian IGF-1 system as a paradigm for putative intra-ovarian regulators. In : Neuroendocrine regulation of reproduction, Serono Symposia, (eds.) Yen SSC, Vale WW. Massachusetts, USA : Norwell, pp. 185-94, 1990.
12. Ericson GF, Garzo VG, Magoffin DA. Insulin-like growth factor-I regulates aromatase activity in human granulosa and granulosa luteal cells. J Clin Endocrinol Metab 1989; 69 : 716-24.
13. Costrici N, Lunenfeld B, Pariente C. Activation of aromatase in human granulosa cells by both FSH and insulin-like growth factor-1 involves tyrisine phosphorylation, 1993. (Unpublished)
14. Townsend SL, Brown JB, Johnstone JW, Adey FD, Evans JH, Taft HP. Induction of ovulation. J Obstet Gynaecol Br Commonw 1966; 73 : 529-42.
15. Insler V, Lunenfeld B. Application of human gonadotropins for induction of ovulation. In : Human Reproduction, (eds.) Campos da Paz A, Hasegava T, Notake Y, Hayashi M. Igaku Shoin, Tokyo : pp. 25-38, 1974.
16. Lunenfeld B. Treatment of anovulation by human gonadotropins. Internat J Obstet Gynecol 1963; 1 : 153-8.
17. Brown JB. Gonadotropins. In : Infertility : male and female, (eds.) Insler V, Lunenfeld B. Churchill Livingstone, London : pp. 359-96, 1986.
18. Tsafriri A, Pomerantz SH. Oocyte maturation inhibitor. J Clin Endocrinol Metab 1986; 15 : 157-70.
19. Homburg R, Armar NA, Eshel A, Adams J, Jacobs HS. Influence of serum luteinizing hormone concentration on ovulation, conception and early pregnancy loss in polycystic ovary syndrome. Br Med J 1988; 297 : 1024-6.
20. Stanger JD, Yovitch JL. Reduced in vitro fertilization of human oocytes from patients with raised basal luteinising hormone levels during the follicular phase. Br J Obstet Gynaecol 1985; 92 : 385-90.
21. Howles CM, Macnamee MC, Edwards RG, Goswamy R, Steptoe PC. Effect of high tonic levels of luteinising hormone on outcome of in vitro fertilisation. Endocrinology 1986; 2 : 521-33.

22. Punnonen R, Ashorn R, Vilja P, Heinonen K, Kunjansuu E, Tuohimaa P. Spontaneous luteinizing hormone surge and cleavage of in vitro fertilized embryos. Fertil Steril 1988; 49 : 479-81.
23. McFaul PB, Traub AI, Thompson W. Premature luteinization and ovulation induction using human menopausal gonadotropins or pure follicle stimulating hormone in patients with polycystic ovary syndrome. Acta Eur Fertil 1989; 20 : 157-62.
24. Regan L, Gwen EJ, Jacobs HS. Hypersecretion of LH and spontaneous miscarriage : A field study. J Endocrinol 1989; 123 : 21-2.
25. Johnson P, Pearce JM. Recurrent spontaneous abortion and polycystic ovarian disease : Comparison of two regimens to induce ovulation. Br Med J 1990; 300 : 154-5.
26. Shoham Z, Borenstein R, Lunenfeld B, Pariente C. Hormonal profiles following CC therapy in conception and nonconception cycles. Clin Endocrinol 1990; 33 : 271-8.
27. Germond M, Dessole S, Senn A, Loumaye E, Howles C, Beltrami V. Successful in vitro fertilization and embryo transfer after treatment with recombinant human FSH. Lancet 1992; ii : 1170-1.
28. Devroe P, Van Steirteghem A, Mannaerts B, Coelingh Bennink K. Successful in vitro fertilization and embryo transfer after treatment with recombinant human FSH. Lancet 1992; ii : 1171-2.

CHAPTER

27

Role of the Postcoital Test in Contemporary Infertility Management

R.K. Sharma

Sperm transport in the female appears to be very complex and probably involves mechanism for accumulation and preservation of sperm as well as for their transport to the site of fertilization in synchrony with the arrival of oocyte[1]. Normal, midcycle mucus facilitates the passage of normal, motile spermatozoa, and it acts as a filter, restricting entry of morphologically abnormal spermatozoa[2]. The cervical crypts fill with mucus and provide storage for viable sperms, to be gradually released to the uterus and the fallopian tubes. The first stage of capacitation may also occur in the crypts[3].

A cervical factor accounts for 5 to 10% of infertility[4]. For more than a century PCT, also known as the Simms-Huhner test, has been considered valuable in examination of the sperm-mucus interaction in vivo. There is controversy regarding the clinical value of the PCT in predicting fertility[5,6,7], but there is general agreement that the test is indicated early in the workup of the infertile couple.

Method

The PCT should be performed close to ovulation as predicted by BBT, change in cervical mucus, LH surge, or ultrasound. The couple is instructed to abstain from intercourse for 48 hours before the test. After wiping the external os, the mucus is obtained with a polyp forceps or aspirated with a tuberculin syringe or 16 gauge angiocath. Because sperm distribution is uniform throughout the cervical canal, there is no need for selective sampling[8,9]. Grossly the quantity, colour and viscosity are assessed. The mucus should be clear and abundant. Spinnbarkeit is assessed when obtaining the specimen from the cervix or by stretching it between the slide and coverslip and measuring the length of CM before it breaks. Eight to ten cm is normal[9]. The microscopic examination assesses fern pattern, cellularity, debris, WBC, number and motility of spermatozoa. Cellular elements and an atypical fern pattern indicate a possible underlying chronic cervicitis. Treatment with a course of doxycycline may improve subsequent PCT[8].

The number of motile sperms considered adequate remains debatable[9,10]. Several authors have published definition of a normal PCT[9,10,11,12].

1. 7 motile sperms progressing purposefully.
2. ≥ 10 sperms per hpf when 50% show purposeful motility.
3. ≥ 10 sperms per hpf with directional motility.
4. > 20 sperms per hpf.
5. A single sperm per hpf.

According to Speroff[1], the majority use 5 motile sperms per hpf.

Another unresolved issue, which deserves attention, is the timing of the PCT in relation to coitus. Many physicians carry out the test 2 to 8 hours after coitus, and often at 2 hours or less. There is little biological justification for this approach. Huhner stated that the test that bears his name should be performed as soon as possible after coitus[11]. He gave no reason. Southam & Buxton[14] wrote, "Perhaps the spermatozoa in the CM at the time of the PCT are those without sufficient strength to progress further, whereas those with high velocity had progressed beyond the cervix." However, they offered no proof for this statement. Treadway[15] suggested that PCT be performed 2.5 hours after coitus because he found this to be the time when most sperms were found.

Most of the current, authoritative reviews of infertility fail to resolve this issue. In the latest edition of 'Progress in Infertility', there is no chapter on the cervical factor. In a chapter reviewing infertility, the PCT is mentioned, but the time after coitus when the test is performed is not specified. Conversely, in the second edition of 'Progress in Infertility', Davajan & Nakamma[16] recommended 2-hour interval because it was "reasonable".

Leaving for the moment the question of a physiologic rationale, one could ask for whom is the 2 to 4 hours test "reasonable and practical". Certainly not for the patients. The 2-hour test requires that intercourse takes place in the morning. Though this may be reasonable time for some couples to "make love", perform the act according to a precise schedule that may conflict with the daily routines and professional commitments of one or both partners. If a time interval for this test is being chosen solely on the basis of reasonableness and practicality, it certainly would be more comfortable for the couple to have intercourse "at bedtime", but not at a prescribed hour, on the evening before the day of testing. The appointment for the PCT could be made for any time in the working day that is mutually convenient for physician and patient. Greater flexibility in timing of the PCT (*i.e.*, 10-16 hours after coitus) will lead to wider application of the test as well as more informative test results.

However, beyond reasonableness and practicality, there are also physiologic reasons for delaying the PCT. There is good evidence that the human cervical mucus serves as a reservoir for sperm. There is a significant relationship between sperm survival for 48 hours in CM and conception in donor artificial insemination cycles[17]. There is little change in motility of normal sperm after 48 hours in CM[18] and the sperm recovered from the mucus at this time can penetrate the human zona pellucida and fuse with zona free hamster oocyte[19]. It is likely that conception depends in part on the ability of sperm to survive in cervical mucus and maintain function there. The oocyte is probably fertilizable for < 24 hours. When the sperms are able to survive in the CM for 24 hours or more it is logical that the chances of conception will be greater. As Treadway[15] pointed out, most PCTs will be positive at 2.5 hours. But, significant information may be lost when sperm survival at larger intervals is not observed. Many times PCT is adequate at 2 hours, but unsatisfactory after a longer interval. These include cases of male and female factor infertility, some related to antisperm antibodies and some to non-immunological causes.

Both for physiologic reasons, and for the emotional comfort of the patients, it is recommended that physicians adopt a more rational and flexible approach to PCT and take advantage of the clinical information that may be gained from observation of sperm longevity in the cervix.

Prognostic value of PCT

The PCT provides assessment of coital technique. Jette & Glass[9] examined the relation of the quality of CM to subsequent pregnancy and found a PR of 53.8% and 37% for good and repeatedly poor mucus, respectively. A previous study reported 43% and 14.5% respectively (Jette *et al.*)[9]. Clear, watery CM without WBC was good; and thick, tenacious cloudy mucus, loaded with WBC was poor. Some authors support the view that a good PCT implies a good PR, whereas others report no correlation between PCT results and pregnancy in fertile couples or infertile couples[4,9,21]. Several studies report no difference in PR with 1 to 5 sperms/hpf compared with 11-20 sperms/hpf[4]. In addition, the association of postcoital motility with pregnancy has not been shown to be statistically significant[21]. Although a correlation between the concentration of sperms in the semen and the number of spermatozoa in

Table 27.1. Etiologies of abnormal sperm-mucus interaction[20]

Female related causes	*Male related causes*
1. Inappropriate timing	1. Deposition problems
2. Ovulatory disorders	(a) Impotence
(a) Anovulation	(b) Retrograde ejaculation
(b) Subtle anomalies of ovulatory process	(c) Hypospadias
3. Deposition problems	2. Semen abnormalities
(a) Dysparennia	(a) Low concentration
(b) Prolapse	(b) Low motility
(c) Congenital and anatomical anomalies	(c) High percentage of abnormal forms
4. Anatomic and organic causes	(d) High volume (> 8 ml)
(a) Amputation or deep conization of cervix	(e) Low volume (< 1 ml)
(b) Tumours : polyps, leiomyomas	(f) Non-liquefying semen
(c) Severe stenosis	3. Antisperm antibodies in serum or seminal plasma
(d) Endocervicitis	
5. Hostile cervical mucus	
(a) ↑ Viscosity	
(b) ↑ Cellularity (infection)	
(c) Acid mucus	
(d) Presence of sperm antibodies	
(e) Drugs — nicotine in cigarette smokers	

cervical mucus has been found (over 20 sperms per hpf has been associated with counts > 20 × 10^6/ml)[23]. A semen analysis is still necessary to evaluate morphology[9].

Next, does an abnormal PCT indicate that sperm did not reach its destination, the ovum? Apparently not, because peritoneal aspirates, obtained via the laparoscope up to 28 hours after the abnormal PCT have revealed sperm in the cul-de-sac[5]. One author has proposed use of endometrial aspiration to more accurately determine that sperm has entered the uterine cavity[3].

Nevertheless, the PCT is valuable in assessing coital technique, cervical mucus and antisperm antibodies. If the PCT reveals good mucus but no sperm or only immobile sperm, the use of spermicidal lubricants (K-Y Jelly, Surgilube) must be ruled out[1]. Vegetable oil is not spermicidal and can be used if lubricant is necessary for intercourse. Hostile CM may be secondary to inappropriate timing of the PCT, hyporesponsiveness of the cervix to E_2, inadequate E_2 level, vaginal or cervical infections, acid mucus, or presence of sperm antibodies. Several PCTs, serum E and P, or the LH surge kit can be used to improve timing. Exposure to diethyl stilbesterol in utero or before cervical surgery can affect CM production[24]. Disorders of folliculogenesis produce inadequate E level leading to poor mucus. In addition, CC can have an anti E effect on CM. Supplementary E_2 in the late follicular phase may improve the PCT results.

In the presence of acidic CM, Ansari *et al.*[25] showed that the PCT results improved if the mucus is alkalized by douching with sodium bicarbonate (1 tablespoon/ quart of H_2O) 30-60 minutes before intercourse. Possible mechanisms of action of soda bicarb. include : (1) alteration of vaginal pH; (2) alteration of cervical pH; (3) alteration of CM electrolytes; (4) removal of excess vaginal discharge; and (5) reduction of pathogenic organisms[25]. Douching with tap water alone did not yield favourable results[25].

The presence of white blood cells in the CM may implicate an underlying infection. The importance of microbial colonization for sperm-mucus interaction and the benefit of antimicrobial therapy in asymptomatic patients in controversial mycoplasma are microorganisms of the size of large viruses having no cell wall[26]. Two types recovered from the genital tract are mycoplasma homines and mycoplasma urealyticum, formerly T-mycoplasma[26]. Ureaplasma was first considered as a cause of infertility. Several studies reported a greater prevalence of genital mycoplasma in cervical mucus and semen of infertile couples than fertile couples[1,25,26]. Some have reported decreased sperm quality associated with poor motility and increased abnormal morphology associated with genital ureaplasma[25,26]. Upon successful treatment of ureaplasma urealyticum, the same authors found improved motility and decrease in certain abnormal morphology. Other studies report no significant influence of genital mycoplasma on sperm quality or sperm mucus interaction in infertile couples[27,28,29]. In addition, genital mycoplasma colonization has been found in up to 50% of normal males[29]. However, several studies report increased conception after eradication of ureaplasma[25]. Although the correlation of genital mycoplasma with male or female unexplained infertility remain debatable, a positive culture of genital mycoplasma warrants treatment with a course of Doxycycline and delay of invasive procedure until the organism is eradicated.

Sperm antibody testing may play a role in the

infertility investigation if the PCT reveals no sperm or non-motile sperm without explanation or shaking sperm with good mucus[1].

The PCT plays an integral role in the evaluation of sperm-mucus interaction in infertile couple. A good PCT is reassuring. Spermatozoa unable to penetrate preovulatory CM are generally also unable to fertilize human oocytes[30,31]. Various studies have looked at hormonal patterns in infertile women with abnormal PCTs[32,33] as well as evaluating daily plasma levels of gonadotropins and steroids in CC therapy[34]. Premature luteinization as defined by an elevated progesterone level at the time of an appropriately timed PCT, in both unstimulated and CC-stimulated cycles, could explain poor CM. Frances *et al.*[35] showed that good CM scores on PCT. PCTs prospectively timed to follow the day of spontaneous LH surge detection were always associated with P levels < 2.5 ng/ml. In contrast, those patients' cycles having poor CM were accompanied by either low or high P levels. Levels of $P \geq 2.5$ ng/ml at the time of anticipated ovulation may help to distinguish between poor CM quality attributable to premature luteinization and inadequate folliculogenesis. They found high percentage of cycles in the CC group with poor CM and high P levels suggest that premature luteinization challenges the purported anti E effect of CC on CM. Therefore, a P level drawn at the time of a poor PCT, particularly in cycles stimulated by CC, can signal premature luteinization as the etiology of sub-optimal mucus. Alternately this may suggest the failure of LH surge kits to consistently predict ovulation in women on CC. In turn, premature luteinization would justify alteration in the CC ovulation induction regimen and would obviate the addition of E to ameliorate the mucus.

With regard to fertility prognosis, in vitro testing of sperm-mucus interaction by means of the SCMPT has been shown to be superior to PCT.

W. Eggert *et al.*[36,37] recommend mixed antiglobulin reaction (MAR test) as a valuable adjunct to sperm-mucus interaction testing to detect immunological causes of impaired sperm function test.

Conclusion

The postcoital test which has stood the test of time for almost a century should be done early in the workup of the infertile couple. A positive, well-timed postcoital test gives the assurance about coital technique, cervical mucus and semen factors and a negative PCT gives direction for further investigations.

REFERENCES

1. Overstreet JW, Katz DF, Cross NL. Sperm transport and capacitation. *In* Gynaecology and Obstetrics, Vol. V, Reproductive Endocrinology, Infertility and Genetics, Edited by L. Speroff, J.L. Simpson. Philadelphia, Harper and Row, 1988, Chap 45, p 1.
2. Gonzales J, Jazequel F. Influence of the quality of the cervical mucus on sperm penetration : Comparison of the morphologic features of spermatozoa in 101 post-coital tests with those in the semen of the husband. Fertil Steril, 1985; 44 : 796-797.
3. Roland M. Pitfalls of the postcoital test. Int J Fertil, 1985; 30 : 29-31.
4. Dodson MC, Joshi PN. Male factor infertility and the gynaecologist. Am J Gynecol Health, 1989; 3 : 9-11.
5. Asch RH. Laparoscopic recovery of sperm from peritoneal fluid in patients with negative or poor Simms-Huhner test. Fertil Steril, 1976; 27 : 1111-1112.
6. Stone SC. Peritoneal recovery of sperm in patients with infertility associated with inadequate cervical mucus. Fertil Steril, 1983; 40 : 802-805.
7. Templeton AA, Mortimer D. Laparoscopic sperm recovery in infertile women. Br J Obstet Gynaecol, 1980; 87 : 1129-1130.
8. Eggert-Kruse W, Hofmann H, Gerhard J, Bilke A, Ruhnebaum B, Petzoldt D. Effects of antimicrobial therapy in sperm-mucus interaction. Hum Reprod, 1988; 3 : 861-864.
9. Jette NT, Glass RH. Prognostic value of the postcoital test. Fertil Steril, 1972; 23 : 29-32.
10. Galle PC, McRae MA, Colliver JA, Alexander JS. Sperm washing and intrauterine insemination for cervical factor, oligospermia, immunologic infertility and unexplained infertile couples. Fertil Steril, 1984; 41 : 703-706.
11. Huhner M. Sterility in male and female and its treatment. New York, Robman; 1943.
12. World Health Organization : WHO laboratory manual for the examination of human semen and semen cervical mucus interaction. 2nd edition. Cambridge, The Press Syndicate of the University of Cambridge, 1987, p 27.
13. Moghissi KS. Cervical mucus changes and ovulation prediction and detection. J Reprod Med, 1986; 31 : 748-750.
14. Southam A, Buxton L. Seventy postcoital tests made during the conception cycles. Fertil Steril, 1956; 7 : 133-136.
15. Treadway DT, Settlage DF, Nakamura RM, Motoshima M, Umezaki CU, Mishell JR. Significance of timing of postcoital evaluation of cervical mucus. Am J obstet Gynecol, 1975; 121 : 387-390.
16. Davajan V, Nakamma RM. The cervical factor. *In*

Progress in Infertility, 2nd edition, Edited by SJ Behraman, RW Kistner, Boston, Little Brown 1975, p 17.

17. Hanson FW, Overstreet JW, Katz DF. A study of the relationship of motile sperm numbers in cervical mucus 48 hours after artificial insemination with subsequent fertility. Am J Obstet Gynecol 1982; 143 : 85-88.
18. Hanson FW, Overstreet JW. The interaction of human spermatozoa with cervical mucus in vivo. Am J Obstet Gynecol 1981; 140 : 173-175.
19. Gould JE, Overstreet JW, Hanson FW. Assessment of human sperm function after recovery from the female reproductive tract. Biol Reprod, 1984; 31 : 888-890.
20. Moghissi K. Cervical and uterine factors in infertility. Obstet Gynecol Clin North Am, 1987; 14 : 893-895.
21. Collin JA, SOY, Wilson EH, Wrixon W, Casper RF. The PCT as a predictor of pregnancy among 355 infertile couples. Fertil Steril, 1984; 41 : 703-705.
22. Bronson RA, Cooper GW, Rosenfeld DL. Autoimmunity to spermatozoa : Effect in sperm penetration of cervical mucus as reflected by PC Testing. Fertil Steril, 1984; 41 : 609-612.
23. Daling JR, Muellar BA, Weiss N, Moore DE, Spadoni LR, Soderstrom RM, Stadel BV. Postcoital test abnormalities in relation to contraceptive use. Int J Fertil, 1987; 32 : 436-440.
24. Corson SL. Ovulation prediction in the treatment of infertility. J Reprod Med, 1986; 31 (suppl) : 739-740.
25. Ansari AH, Gould KG, Ansari VM. Sodium bicarbonate douching for improvement of the postcoital test. Fertil Steril, 1980; 53 : 608-610.
26. Friberg J. Mycoplasmas and ureaplasmas in infertility and abortion. Fertil Steril, 1980; 33 : 351-354.
27. Cassell GH, Younger JB, Brown MB, Blackwell RE, Davis JK, Marriott P, Stagno S. Microbiologic study of infertile women at the time of diagnostic laparoscopy — association of ureaplasma urealyticum with a defined sub-population. N England J Med, 1983; 308 : 502-505.
28. Eggert-Kruse W, Gerhard I, Hofmann H, Runnebaum B, Petzoldt D, Influence of microbial colonization in sperm-mucus interaction in vivo and in vitro. Human Reprod, 1987; 2 : 301-303.
29. Soffer Y, Ron ELR, Golan A, Herman A, Caspi E, Smraz. Male genital mycoplasma and chlamydia trachomatis culture : its relationship with accessory gland function, sperm quality and autoimmunity. Fertil, 1987; 48 : 337-340.
30. Hellstrom WJ, Schachter J, Sweet RL, McClure RD. Is there a role for chlamydia trachomatis and genital mycoplasma in male infertility. Fertil Steril, 1987; 48 : 337-340.
31. Megory E, Zuckerman H, Shoham 2, Lunenfeld B. Infections and male infertility. Obstet Gynaecol Surv, 1987; 42 : 283-285.
32. Hull MGR, McLeod FN, Joyce DN, Ray BD, McDermott A. Human in vitro fertilization, in vivo sperm penetration of cervical mucus and unexplained infertility. Lancet, 1984; 1 : 245-250.
33. Roumen F, Doesburg WH, Rolland R. Hormonal patterns in infertile women with a deficient PCT. Fertil Steril, 1982; 38 : 42-45.
34. Wu CH. Plasma hormones in clomiphene citrate therapy. Obstet Gynecol, 1977; 49 : 443-445.
35. Frances H, Taney, Richard V Grazi, Gerson Weiss, Cecilia L Schmidt. Detection of premature luteinization with serum progesterone levels at the time of the PCT. Fertil Steril, 1991; 55 : 513-515.
36. Eggert-Kruse W, Gerhard I, Tilegen W and Runnebaum B. Clinical significance of crossed in vitro sperm-cervical mucus penetration test in infertility investigation. Fertil Steril, 1989; 52 : 1032-1040.
37. Eggert-Kruse W, A HofsäB, E Henry, W Tilegen, I Gerhard and B Runnebaum. Relationship between antisperm antibodies and sperm-mucus interaction in vitro and in vivo. Human Reprod, 1991; 6 : 267-276.

CHAPTER

28

A Critical Appraisal of Endometriosis Associated Subfertility : To Treat or Not to Treat

Mehroo Hansotia

This article reviews the rapidly increasing information on the aetiopathogenesis of endometriosis-associated subfertility, the relevance of the revised AFS classification in infertility practice and the various modalities of treatment with their efficacy in terms of achieving pregnancy. The observational study conducted among infertile women treated with IVF-ET at our Fertility Clinic, Bombay with an aim of identifying the prognostic variables which may lead to success (pregnancy) or failure (no pregnancy), establishing the relative importance of these variables and developing a quantitative model to predict the outcome of treatment is reviewed with particular reference to results in endometriosis. Although newer methods of management continue to evolve, it appears that patients with minimal to mild endometriosis may best be managed by expectant treatment, while more aggressive management results in higher pregnancy rates in moderate and severe disease.

Ever since Sampson first coined its name in 1921, endometriosis still remains a mysterious, poorly understood disease of the female reproductive system. It is characterised by the ectopic growth of the endometrium and typically affects women during the reproductive period, limiting their fertility and impairing their health.

Incidence and prevalence

Endometriosis may be accompanied by reduced cycle fecundity or subfertility. The true incidence of endometriosis is difficult to determine, since it varies between studies depending on the patient population assessed. Thus it is found in 2-5% of women undergoing voluntary sterilization, in 10-15% of those who have a laparoscopy for gynaecological symptoms and in 30-40% of those undergoing laparoscopy for infertility. The prevalence of endometriosis seems to be increasing during recent years, which could either be due to the more frequent use of diagnostic laparoscopy or a true increase as more and more women postpone pregnancy and have fewer children, to actively pursue independent careers. Thus more women have a greater number of menstrual cycles during their life span due to an earlier age at menarche, fewer pregnancies and a later onset of menopause than their counterparts of yesteryears.

Pathophysiology of endometriosis

Various theories[1] have been postulated to explain the disease process. These include :

- Transplantation theory (Sampson)
- Theory of coelomic metaplasia (Meyer and Iwanoff)
- Induction theory (Levander)
- Retrograde menstruation (Sampson)
- Peritoneal irritation
- Luteinised Unruptured Follicle Syndrome (Brosens)

On the basis of the above theories, the following scenario on the development of endometriosis can now be postulated.

Retrograde menstruation transports shed endometrial fragments to ectopic locations. Here the implantation or rejection of such fragments is controlled by cell mediated immunity. In women with a deficient cell mediated immunity implantation of ectopic endometrial fragments give origin to endometriosis. Such an immune deficiency could be both qualitative and quantitative in nature, resulting in the variable age of onset, extent and kinetics of endometriosis and could be transmitted genetically. Autoantibody production would be a secondary phenomenon in response to the ectopic endometrial growth.

Morphologic evolution

It appears that the initial lesions in endometriosis are clear fluid-filled papules. Local peritoneal inflammation converts these clear papules into red spots. The retention of haemosiderin in these lesions leads to the formation of black, burnt matchstick areas. When these lesions occur in the ovary, endometriomas may result. Adhesions in the subovarian fossa may become extensive eventually leading to a frozen pelvis.

Recently, subtle forms of endometriosis are being recognised. These include circular peritoneal defects, spider nodules, non-pigmented forms and brim nodules. These lesions appear to be more active and are thus of greater significance in infertile patients with endometriosis.

Pathogenesis of subfertility in endometriosis

Deficient folliculogenesis, corpus luteum insufficiency, ovulatory dysfunction, the luteinised unruptured follicle syndrome all contribute to the ovarian factor for infertility in patients with endometriosis. The expanding endometriomas tend to crush functional ovarian tissue and may impair ovulation and hence conception.

Increased levels of prostaglandins in the cul-de-sac peritoneal fluid affect tubal peristalsis, ovum pickup and sperm transport. Macrophages phagocytose sperm and produce gamete hostility. These could lead to functional infertility.

Ovum pick up and transport is affected by distorted tubo-ovarian relationships in advanced endometriosis.

The endometrium too is hostile to the conceptus. Early loss of ovum and impairment of implantation leads to infertility. Decreased coital frequency due to dyspareunia is also an important factor leading to infertility.

Luteinised Unruptured Follicle Syndrome (LUF)

Brosens[1] has postulated that the LUF could be an antecedent to endometriosis. During ovulation, prostaglandins and other chemical substances are released into the peritoneal cavity. These substances do not allow the endometrial fragments to implant on the peritoneal surface.

In LUFS there is no follicular rupture which may allow endometrial fragments to get implanted easily. LUFS is seen in 20% of infertile patients with endometriosis, while 98% of LUFS are found in patients with endometriosis.

Endocrine disturbances reported with endometriosis such as a delayed rise in progesterone concentration after the LH surge, low preovulatory LH receptor content in the granulosa cells and low steroid hormone levels in the peritoneal fluid during the luteal phase as well as the absence of the ovulatory stigma all indicate a luteinisation of the graafian follicles without rupture. The lack of a preovulatory peak in follicular fluid type IV collagenolytic activity in patients with endometriosis also supports disturbance in the mechanism of follicular rupture in this disease.

Ovum capture inhibitor

An experimental study carried out by Yano *et al.*[2] showed that the peritoneal fluid of patients with endometriosis prevented ovum pick up and transport.

Fimbriae pick up the oocyte cumulus complex but not the immature oocyte. It also picks up loose connective tissue but not dense connective tissue. The evidence suggests that fimbriae recognise intercellular matrix as the first step of ovum capture and transport.

The current study clearly demonstrated the presence of a factor inhibitory to in vitro ovum capture by the oviductal fimbriae (OCI) in endometriosis peritoneal fluid. They report the OCI is a water soluble macromolecule that inhibits the fimbrial recognition of cumulus oophorus by forming net-like aggregates on the surface of the fimbriae. Characterisation and identification of OCI would provide us with a fascinating new concept about the aetiology of endometriosis-associated infertility and in the management of infertile patients with endometriosis.

Endometriosis and spontaneous abortion

There is a high incidence of abortions reported in patients with untreated endometriosis possibly because of the associated corpus luteum insufficiency, the presence of circulating anti-endometrium antibodies[3] and the production of prostaglandins by endometriotic foci[4] that cause uterine contractility sufficient to disrupt pregnancy and produce abortion. Medical or surgical therapy by removing or reducing the endometriotic lesions might reduce autoantibody production.

Endometriosis and IVF

Pregnancy rates[5] are lower in women with stage IV endometriosis due to poor development of follicles, reduced number of oocytes obtained, lower fertilization rates, reduced number of embryos transferred, poor luteal function and an unsuitable uterine environment for the development of early embryos.

The fewer oocytes obtained could be because of a suboptimal response to ovarian stimulation or a technical difficulty in gaining access to the ovaries.

Diagnosis of endometriosis

Endometriosis should always be considered in patients with worsening dysmenorrhoea, dyspareunia, pelvic pain and infertility, these being considered the four cardinal symptoms. Characteristic physical findings include pelvic tenderness, adnexal masses and fixed retroversions. The presence of uterosacral nodularity is almost pathognomonic, particularly when elicited during menstruation. Confirming the clinical diagnosis before instituting treatment is essential since the differential diagnosis of endometriosis includes any cause of pelvic pain or adnexal masses during reproductive years.

The diagnosis of endometriosis being primarily visual, laparoscopy is mandatory for diagnosis. It is best performed perimenstrually when the lesions are most easily visualised. A systematic laparoscopic inspection must always include a second puncture probe for manipulation to allow thorough assessment.

The typical vesicular, puckered black lesions result from tissue bleeding and retention of blood pigments. However the subtle, non-pigmented endometriotic lesions are now considered to be far more common and clinically significant. It is hence important for the endoscopist to be familiar with their varied appearances. Non-pigmented lesions can be enhanced to ease diagnosis by the thermocolour test which endocoagulates the peritoneum, causing a brownish discolouration of subtle lesions and a blanching of normal peritoneum. One can use concentrated methylene blue to selectively stain and identify non-pigmented lesions.

The revised American Fertility Society classification (1985) is the most widely used system for the documentation and staging of the disease. Various feature of endometriosis are assigned points, the total score being translated into four ranges, from minimal to severe disease. The main pitfall of staging is that while the pigmented lesions are more visually obvious but less active, the significant deeply infiltrating lesions may show a minimally affected surface peritoneum. Biopsies could help confirm the diagnosis but are sometimes misleading.

Chronic salpingitis and endometriosis involving extra pelvic sites is not represented and incompletely resected or unresectable endometriosis is not taken into account.

Ultrasound is useful in diagnosing ovarian endometriomas. These show smooth walls with well defined borders, liquid contents but finely dotted, the last particular may indicate the presence of blood in it and ensures the diagnosis. Endometriosis should also be suspected with any persistent ovarian cyst.

The role of biological markers such as CA-125 and antiendometriosis antibodies in the diagnosis is as yet tentative, but may ultimately be used for screening or to monitor the disease during therapy.

Management of endometriosis

The three main modalities of treatment are expectant management, medical therapy and surgical treatment.

In order to decide how to select patients for medical or surgical treatment, first the following relevant questions should be addressed. Should endometriosis be treated? If so, how should it be treated? Can endometriosis be treated at all?

If a disease is symptomatic the severity of symptoms determines the need for treatment. Analgesics, anti-ovulatory drugs and surgery are of proven value in patients who require treatment for pain or in those in whom distortion of tubo-ovarian spatial relationships constitute an indisputable cause of infertility.

The reasons for treating asymptomatic endometriosis in subfertile patients are twofold, either the actual asymptomatic stage of the disease has been proven to be causally related to existing subfertility (which is not true) or the disease is progressive, will eventually lead to destruction of the reproductive organs of their inter-relationship, and will cause subfertility in that way. Based on the literature we have no hard data to support treating asymptomatic endometriosis in sub-fertility patients with a view to curing their inability to conceive.

However there is evidence in literature that in some patients the disease may be progressive; it deteriorates if not treated. Thomas and Cooke[6] found endometriosis to be progressive in 47% of the patients in whom they performed a second look laparoscopy after 6 months of placebo treatment, while the disease regressed or even disappeared completely during placebo treatment in 53%.

Jansen and Russell[7] found in 6 patients with observation, but no treatment, non-pigmented early endometriosis progressing to the more classical pigmented form within the course of 6-24 months; thus confirming the existence of a biologic continuum between non-pigmented and pigmented endometriotic lesions.

Redwine[8] disclosed an age related evolution in the colour appearance of endometriosis from clear papules only (mean age 21.5 ± 3.5 yrs) via red lesions (26.3 ± 5.4 yrs) to the classical blue black powder burn lesions (31.9 ± 7.5 yrs). The finding that no factor, including the actual severity of the disease at laparoscopy, can accurately predict spontaneous improvement or deterioration in a given endometriosis patient led Thomas and Cooke to the recommendation that asymptomatic disease should always be treated.

Expectant management is indicated if the patient is asymptomatic and while investigating and treating other more obvious causes of infertility. A simple laparoscopic or ultrasound-guided aspiration of peritoneal fluid with hydrotubation have been reported to result in significant pregnancy rates of 53% in mild and 21% in moderate endometriosis[9].

Medical treatment acts by inhibiting cyclical endometrial changes, leading to the eventual atrophy and resorption of ectopic endometrium. Therapy aims at either inducing pseudopregnancy using progestogens or pseudomenopause using danazol or gonadotropin-releasing hormone agonists.

Histologic features associated with hormonal responsiveness of ectopic endometrium have been described by Metzger *et al.*[10]. The unpredictable response of endometriotic implants to cyclic endogenous hormones and hormonal therapy may be related to the architectural relationships between the cellular elements found in normal endometrium. Implants that have a greater amount of stroma and the presence of surface epithelium are more responsive while fibrosis, endometriomas and foci of haemorrhage also indicate a poorer response. Danazol induces an inhibition of the hypothalamic pituitary-ovarian axis and is the only drug actually approved by the US FDA for treating endometriosis. Danazol is administered in a dose of 12 mg/kg/day, that approximates to 600-800 mg in three or four divided doses daily for 6 to 9 months. Androgenic manifestations which are dose related are the major disadvantages of danazol therapy.

Seibel and coworkers[11] have been the first in 1982 to report the results of a randomized study into the effect of danazol versus no treatment upon minimal endometriosis. They reported the results in an extended follow up period in 1989 and virtually found the same results. The cumulative pregnancy rate was 37.2 ± 8.4% in the danazol group and 57.4 ± 10.4% in the untreated group. This study showed for the first time that danazol is no more effective than no treatment at all in reversing the subfertility seen in patients with minimal endometriosis. Progestational agents while better tolerated have the disadvantage of frequent breakthrough bleeding. Medroxyprogesterone acetate is either administered orally 30 mg per day for 90 days or intramuscularly 50 mg weekly or 100 mg every second week. Alternatively dehydrogestrone 20-30 mg daily or gestrinone 2.5 mg two or three times a week are used for 6 months.

Thomas and Cooke[12] reported the first double blind randomised placebo controlled trial of any treatment of endometriosis. The 12 month cumulative conception rate in asymptomatic endometriosis patients treated with gestrinone was 25% and in those given placebo 20%. This study was not able to show that either treatment or elimination of the disease affected future fertility which questions a causal role of asymptomatic endometriosis in subfertility.

In 1988 Telimaa[13] reported a prospective placebo controlled study of 49 patients, randomly allocated to receive either danazol or high dose medroxy progesterone acetate (MPA) or placebo for 6 months. The follow up time was 30 months. The cumulative pregnancy rate of 33% in the danazol group, 42% in the MPA group and 46% in the placebo treated group did not significantly differ from each other. The mean time interval to pregnancy was 17.7 ± 8.4 months in the danazol group, 18.9 months in the MPA group and 10 ± 5.8 months in the placebo treated group. Telimaa concludes that if subfertility is the main complaint associated with endometriosis, danazol or MPA has no therapeutic value. On the contrary, hormonal therapy with these drugs appeared to delay fecundation in this study.

Gonadotropin releasing hormone agonist analogues are superior to danazol in their ability to suppress ovarian function. Supraphysiological release of an LHRH-agonist leads to a reversible downregulation of the pituitary ovarian axis. There are two types of responses :

1. Slow but sufficient decrease
2. Initial fall with intermittent peak

Nafarelin in two doses of 200 μg or buserlin in three doses of 300 μg administered daily as intranasal sprays or lupron depot injected intramuscularly for 6 injections over 20 weeks all achieve therapeutic suppression. While the temporary hypoestrogenic side effects are common, it is the metabolic derangements that are of concern. Subcutaneous route has a better response; pregnancy rate after completion of therapy is 33%.

A randomised controlled study describing the effects of buserelin versus placebo on fertility of patients with minimal and mild endometriosis, shows that there is no significant difference between the treatment and control groups. The 1 and 2 year actuarial overall pregnancy rates were similar in the two groups; 30% and 37% for the GnRh and the control group respectively after 1 year, and 61% respectively after 2 years. The authors[14] conclude that treatment with GnRH agonists is unlikely to have a marked influence on the reproductive outcome of infertile women with minimal or mild endometriosis.

Medical therapy is mainly used to treat the earlier stages of disease causing infertility. Interestingly recent studies have shown no difference in pregnancy rates with progestogens, danazol or expectant therapy in mild and moderate endometriosis[15]. This may justify a period of observation before instituting medical or surgical therapy.

Surgical therapy aims at cytoreduction of ectopic endometrium, restoration of normal tubal anatomy, removal of ovarian endometriomas and an interruption of sensory afferent pathways to counter pain. Operative laparoscopy using unipolar or bipolar electrocautery is effective for cauterising implants, lysing adhesions and treating ovarian endometriomas with a 50% pregnancy rate in infertility[16]. It is reported that simple drainage of ovarian endometriomas is as effective as excision, stripping or laser vapourization of the lining in treating the disease[17].

Laser laparoscopic surgery with either the CO_2 or KTP/YAG lasers is highly precise in vapourising endometriosis with minimal damage to underlying and surrounding tissues. Sutton[18] reported pregnancies in 80% of infertile patients with endometriosis. Laser uterine nerve ablation aims to destroy the sensory afferent nerve fibres by vapourising the uterosacral ligaments at the cervix, with significant improvement in pain due to endometriosis reported in 86%[18]. Conservative laparotomy is now being increasingly marginalised by the advent of operative laparoscopy and is mainly indicated when a simultaneous micro-surgical tubal repair is required.

Combined therapy uses both the medical and surgical modalities for cumulative benefit. Preoperative medical therapy, long advocated for facilitating surgery, has the disadvantage of decreasing visible endometriotic lesions. In my opinion since a visual diagnosis is necessary to effect surgery the preoperative shrinkage of lesions appears to be self-defeating.

Postoperative therapy however eradicates residual disease and prevents implantation of disease spill at surgery. Since medical therapy has the maximal histological effect within 2 months there seems little benefit extending such therapy beyond 3 months.

Various treatment protocols evolved over 12 years were evaluated by Rajan[19] in 517 cases. The pregnancy rates in this series increased from 25% with conservative laparotomy alone to 51% with combined therapy, using operative laparoscopy with pre- and postoperative danazol.

Alternative treatment options

These include artificial reproductive techniques and immunomodulators of the main constituents in the peritoneal cavity. In our series[20] 17% of patients (8/46) had success with IVF (Table 28.1).

IVF-ET is indicated with severe tubal distortion while GIFT is an appropriate alternative in the earlier stages with apparently normal tubes. There is also a potential for managing severe disease not amenable to conservative therapy, by bilateral salpingo-oophorectomy while retaining the uterus to allow IVF-ET with donor oocytes or embryos.

Table 28.1. Success rate of IVF by indication (Fertility Clinic) Univariate analysis

Indication	*n*	*Success*	*Rate*
Failed induction	23	8	35%
Tubal/genital TB	227	52	23%
Male factor	44	10	23%
Endometriosis	46	8	17%
Failed AID	7	1	14%
Unexplained	56	6	11%
Total	403	85	21%

(Hansotia — March 1993)[20]

Conflicting results have been reported regarding results of ART in endometriosis patients. Yovich and coworkers[21] reported poorer oocyte quality in 30 patients with severe endometriosis as compared to 28 women whose subfertility was solely caused by tubal disease. Tummon and collaborators[22] showed live birth rates not reduced in 240 IVF cycles in 124 women with advanced degrees of endometriosis and no other cause of subfertility. Workers[23] have found better embryo quality and less abortions if patients with severe endometriosis undergoing IVF have been pretreated with GnRH analogues, as compared to patients with comparable degrees of endometriosis who had not been pretreated.

Finally one group[24] has studied the effect of modulating the peritoneal immune system, specifically peritoneal macrophages. They showed that intra-peritoneal transfer of hyperactivated macrophages, but not of basal state macrophages into syngenetic mice, significantly inhibited fertilization. This fertility lowering effect of activated macrophages was reversed by periovulatory administration of pentoxyfylline, a methylxanthine derivative which has been shown to inhibit macrophage activation of inflammatory mediators.

Assessment of therapy

Several criteria have been employed to assess the result of endometriosis therapy, the disappearance of symptoms (predominantly pain), the change in plasma levels of marker substances (*e.g.*, CA 125), the change of aspects of the endometriotic lesions at second look laparoscopy and the pregnancy rate during the follow up period. Very often the visible number of implants decrease during danazol therapy, but increase again rapidly after the end of therapy, and so does the cumulative diameter of the implants. This finding supports Brosens[1] conclusions that the peritoneal implant is a small lesion which sometimes cannot even be recognised at laparoscopy but may be seen on laparoscopy by the presence of sequelae of endometriotic activity such as secretion, haemorrhage, inflammatory reaction and fibrosis.

The second look laparoscopy to evaluate effectiveness is commonly performed during the last week of ovarian suppression therapy, unfairly comparing the moist, active pretreatment pelvis, with the dry, inactive pelvis during suppression. It is hence recommended that second look laparoscopy be performed in the follicular phase of a spontaneous menstrual cycle after cessation of medical therapy. Pregnancy rates are the ultimate test in evaluating therapy for infertility. Olive and Haney[25] assessing data on conceptions following various treatments, compiled pregnancy rates cited below from various sources (Table 28.2).

It may be concluded from Table 28.2 that treating mild endometriosis to enhance fertility may be futile given the comparable results without treatment; surgery may impede the long-term development of this progressive disease. The more severe stages are associated with lower pregnancy rates and are more likely to need and respond to surgery in view of the distorted peritoneal relationships. Finally the conception rates were found to be better with preoperative danazol treatment.

Table 28.2[25].

Category of disease	*Pregnancy rate*
Mild endometriosis	
No treatment	50.3%
Danazol alone	37.6%
Conservative surgery	60.7%
Laparoscopic surgery	52.9%
Moderate endometriosis	
Conservative surgery	50.0%
Laparoscopic surgery	41.0%
Danazol followed by surgery	66.6%
Severe endometriosis	
Conservative surgery	39.2%
Laser laparoscopy	46.6%
Danazol followed by surgery	50.0%

REFERENCES

1. Brosens IA. New concepts in pelvic endometriosis. Contr Gynaecol Obstet 1989; 17 : 36-43.
2. Yano K, Suginami H, Matsuura S. An ovum capture inhibitor present in endometriosis peritoneal fluid. Adv Fertil Steril 1987; 5 : 41-7.
3. Williamson HO, Youman CD, Nancy SA, Garvin AJ, Rust PF, Funenberg HH. Autoimmunity to endometriosis and ovary in endometriosis. Clin Exp Immunol 1987; 50 : 259-63.
4. Drake TS, O'Brien WF, Ramwell PW, Metz SA. Peritoneal fluid thromboxane B2 & 6 keto-prostaglandin FI alpha in endometriosis. Am J Obstet Gynecol 1987; 140 : 401-6.
5. Richardson PA, Blackledge DG, Turner SR, Matson PL, Yovich JL. Severe endometriosis and pregnancy following IVF-ET. Adv Fertil Steril, 1987; 5 : 91-5.
6. Thomas EJ, Cooke ID. Successful treatment of asymptomatic endometriosis — does it benefit infertile women? Br Med J 1987; 294 : 1117-9.
7. Jansen RPS, Russel P. Non-pigmented endometriosis — clinical laparoscopic and pathologic definition. Am J Obstet Gynecol 1986; 155 : 1154-9.
8. Redwine DB. Age related evolution in colour appearance of endometriosis. Fertil Steril 1987; 48 : 1062-3.
9. Haney AF, Muscato JJ, Weinberg JB. Peritoneal fluid cell populations in infertile patients. Fertil Steril 1981; 5 : 696-9.
10. Metzger DA, Szpak CA, Haney AF. Histologic features associated with hormonal responsiveness of ectopic endometrium. Fertil Steril 1993; 59 : 83-5.
11. Seibel MM, Berger MJ, Weinstrom FG, Taymour ML. The effectiveness of Danazol on subsequent fertility minimal endometriosis. Fertil Steril 1982; 47 : 502-3.
12. Thomas EJ, Cooke ID. Impact of gestinone on the course of asymptomatic endometriosis. Br Med J 1987; 294 : 272-4.
13. Telimaa S. Danazol and medroxy-progesterone acetate inefficacious in the treatment of endometriosis. Fertil Steril 1988; 50 : 872-5.
14. Fedele L. Parazzini F. Buserelin acetate versus expectant management in the treatment of infertility associated with minimal or mild endometriosis : A randomised clinical trial. Am J Obstet Gynecol 1992; 166 : 1345-50.
15. Hull M. Should early endometriosis always be treated? Fertil Steril 1987; 53 : 156-7.
16. Murphy A. Laparoscopic cautery in endometriosis related infertility. Fertil Steril 1991; 55 : 246-9.
17. Adamson D, Hurd SJ, Pasta DJ, Rodriquez BD. Laparoscopic endometriosis treatment — Is it better? Fertil Steril 1993; 59 : 1-3.
18. Sutton C, Hill D. Laser laparoscopy in the treatment of endometriosis. Br J Obstet Gynaecol 1991; 97 : 187-9.
19. Rajan R. Danazol, surgical pelviscopy and conservative surgery in endometriosis and infertility. J Obstet Gynaecol India 1991; 41 : 34-7.
20. Hansotia MD. Endometriosis & IVF, March 1993 (Unpublished observations).
21. Yovich JL, Matson PL, Richardson PA, Hillard C. Hormone profiles and embryo quality in women with severe endometriosis treated by IVF/ET. Fertil Steril 1988; 50 : 308-13.
22. Tummon TS, Colwell KA. Endometriosis associated infertility correlates with IVF success. J IVF Embryo Transfer 1991; 8 : 149-53.
23. Olive DL, Franklin RR, Gratkins LV. Association between endometriosis and spontaneous abortions in patients with endometriosis. Obstet Gynecol 1982; 57 : 509-12.
24. Steinleitner A, Lambert H, Roy S. Immunomodulation with pentoxyfylline abrogates macrophage medicated infertility in an in vivo model, a paradigm for a novel approach to the treatment of endometriosis associated subfertility. Fertil Steril 1989; 55 : 26-31.
25. Olive DL, Haney AF. Comparative pregnancy rates with different modalities of management of endometriosis. Fertil Steril 1986; 52 : 253-7.

CHAPTER

29

Unexplained Infertility

B.N. Chakravarty

Broadly speaking, all infertile couples can be placed in one of three categories following routine investigations. The results of investigation may reveal single defect in one of the partners, multiple defects in one of the partners, multiple defects in one or both partners and no defect in either partner. The last group is customarily designated as the group of unexplained infertility. The minimal investigations required to make such a diagnosis must include histological, biophysical and biochemical confirmation of ovulation, hysterosalpingography, laparoscopy and semen analysis. The diagnostic and prognostic usefulness of postcoital test is doubtful and hence this test is not considered while identifying a case of unexplained infertility.

The incidence of unexplained infertility will obviously depend on the extent of investigation which is possible in a particular set-up. The incidence is usually quoted as 10 per cent of all infertile couples; with the help of additional screening parameters the incidence could be reduced to 3.5 per cent[1].

It is surprising as to why normal sexually active couples remain infertile in spite of attempting to conceive for at least two years. Using cumulative life table projections on the observed pregnancy rate in this untreated and presumably discouraged group, it has been observed that a couple with primary unexplained infertility has a 36.2 per cent chance of conceiving over a seven year period[2]. Nonetheless, their infertility rate is significantly lower than in the population as a whole.

In addition, apparently unexplained infertility may be due to unrecognized early pregnancy wastage with or without disturbance of menstrual rhythm[3].

The author[3] states that ovulation on or after the 15th day of the cycle predisposed to an increase in the number of bad oocytes and consequently unrecognised early pregnancy wastage is certainly provocative and requires collaboration.

There are four main areas which are currently being investigated to understand some of the etiological factors of unexplained infertility. These are : occult defects of the oocytes, occult defects of the spermatozoa, occult endometriosis and luteinised unruptured follicle syndrome. Luteal phase defect may have some role; but cervical and seminal infection with ureaplasma or chlamydia and antisperm antibodies in maternal serum are unconfirmed etiological factors of unexplained infertility.

Functional defect of oocytes may be an important cause of unexplained infertility. In IVF programmes several investigators have reported a lower fertilisation rate (35-40%) in unexplained infertility patients when compared with those suffering from tubo-peritoneal factor (60 to 75%)[4]. Failure of fertilisation in cases of unexplained infertility may be due to functional defects of oocytes at different sites. It has been hypothesized that failure could be due to defective zona pellucida protein-3 (ZP 3). Thus either the sperm-egg attachment or the acrosome reaction process are impaired. Another possible explanation for the failure of fertilization may be the formation of anti-ZP antibodies which may block the receptor site on the ZP, thus interfering with sperm-egg interaction. However, the role of these antibodies in unexplained infertility is not yet fully determined since the activation process of the intra-cellular decondensing factor may include sperm DNA depolymerisation and the second pronucleus formation. It may be that defect in this step of fertilisation may result in lack of syngamy and arrest of further cleavage. Differentiation between zona pellucida defects and those occuring in the ooplasm is theoretically possible by using the procedure of micro-injection of spermatozoa bypassing the zona pellucida.

The true prevalence of this group is undoubtedly more than 4 per cent of couples with unexplained infertility. But before the defect in the oocyte is established, final proof of husband's sperm competence should be established by ovum donation procedure in vitro.

Like defective oocytes, there should be defective spermatozoa as well which may be responsible for some cases of unexplained infertility. Apart from numerical count, sperm morphology and velocity, there are other factors either in the seminal plasma or on the surface of sperms which play a significant role in the fertilisable capacity of the spermatozoa. Antigen on the sperm surface may produce antibodies in the female genital tract or on the surface of zona leading to immunological infertility. Various biochemical constituents of seminal plasma like carnitine, Zn, fructose, vesiculase, etc., play important accessory roles in sperm function. Even when these parameters are normal, it is difficult to predetermine whether or not the apparently normal looking sperm will be able to fertilise the oocyte. Establishment of pregnancy was the only yardstick to determine this specific sperm efficiency. Sperm-zona free hamster oocyte penetration test was used to determine this type of human sperm function in vitro. But the results were unpredictable and at times confusing.

IVF has opened up the window of opportunity in this area. IVF has made it possible to determine sperm oocyte interaction in the humans and now animals are not required. This observation has stimulated further research on an ill-understood mechanism of human sperm capacitation, sperm-oocyte interaction and the intricate process involved in zona penetration. This knowledge is likely to explain many aspects of the so called 'Unexplained Male Infertility'.

Those who work in IVF laboratories are quite familiar with the observation that the sperms which were normal in all standard parameters are unable to penetrate the zona and fertilise the oocytes. In order to understand why such apparently normal spermatozoa cannot fertilise, it is important to know more subtle biochemical processes that are required for successful fertilisation.

At its anterior portion, the sperm head is surrounded by a membrane-limited vesicle, the acrosome. The acrosome contains enzymes that are necessary for the penetration of the spermatozoon through the cumulus layers surrounding the oocyte. The best studied acrosomal enzymes are acrosin (a proteinase that causes lysis of the zona pellucida) and hyaluronidase (causes lysis of the cumulus oophorous matrix). Acrosin is primarily present in an inactive from, called proacrosin.

Ejaculated spermatozoa are unable to fertilise the oocyte unless they undergo an activation process, called capacitation. Capacitation occurs during the transport of the spermatozoa through the female genital tract and causes the biochemical alteration of the anterior sperm head membranes. This change allows the acrosome reaction to occur when the spermatozoa reaches the zona pellucida. The acrosome reaction results in the removal of the outer acrosomal membrane and surrounding plasma membrane as well as the acrosomal matrix. This in turn causes the localised release of the acrosomal enzymes, including acrosin which disintegrates and allows a passage in front of the spermatozoon through the zona pellucida.

A series of biochemical events occur within the acrosomal compartment through protein phosphorylation, involving intracellular changes in ionic and osmotic components, eventually leading to the fusion and disappearance of the outer acrosomal membrane and the plasma membrane. In addition proacrosin (precursor of acrosin) is converted to acrosin. Acrosin causes the dispersal of acrosomal matrix (within the acrosomal compartment) and finally acrosin is liberated. All these events carefully control the acrosome reaction and release of the acrosomal contents (particularly acrosin) at the correct place and time. This is known as 'Acrosome Reaction'. An inability of the spermatozoon to undergo any one of these processes may prevent or decrease its ability to fertilise. Such defects are not usually detected by routine semen analysis. Therefore, even though the semen parameters are normal by average standard, the cause of infertility will remain unexplained if such defects in the spermatozoa exist which are not detected by ordinary laboratory procedures.

Luteinized Unruptured Follicle (LUF) syndrome

The LUF syndrome is the absence of ovulation in women with apparently normal ovulatory cycles as judged by BBT charts, increased peripheral progesterone in the luteal phase and secretory endometrium by biopsy. Several methods have been proposed to diagnose LUF.

1. Absence of an ovulatory stigma at laparoscopy : This method is impractical and highly inaccurate because of rapid epithelialization of the stigma site and occasional difficulty in visualization of the entire ovarian surface.
2. Peritoneal fluid E_2 and P determinations : It has been proposed that higher concentrations of E_2 and P are found in the peritoneal fluid of women with an ovulatory stigma at laparoscopy than in women without an ovulatory stigma[5]. This method is also impractical and has a high incidence of false positive and false negative results.
3. Ultrasonography : Several studies[6,7] have pointed to the value of serial ultrasonography in the diagnosis of the LUF syndrome. The diagnosis is made when the dominant follicle fails to collapse despite indirect evidence of ovulation (BBT chart, high P levels). This method is simple to perform but has not been correlated with peritoneal fluid sampling of steroid levels and the presence/absence of an ovulatory stigma by laparoscopy.

The incidence, frequency, and repetition of the LUF syndrome in fertile and infertile women are controversial. The value of serial ultrasound in diagnosing the condition in women with unexplained infertility has not been established[8]. In one diagnostic study[9] using serial ultrasonography, 40 of 600 cycles in 27 of 270 infertile patients were found to have the condition. Correlation with serum hormone levels revealed significantly lower mean LH peak levels in midcycle and lower midluteal P levels in the LUF cycles than in control cycles.

Occult endometriosis

The term refers to the presence of pelvic endometriosis despite a lack of visualisation of endometrial implants by laparoscopy. In one study[10] using scanning electron microscopy, foci of endometriosis were identified in 25% of random biopsies of normal epithelium in patients with unexplained infertility. Several theories have been suggested, including macrophage-mediated autoimmune response; increased prostaglandins in peritoneal fluids; association with the LUF syndrome; association with hyperprolactinaemia and luteal phase defects; presence of constituents in peritoneal fluid that may impair sperm/oocyte interaction and early embryonic developments; and recent observations of increased concentrations of interleukin-1 in peritoneal fluid in infertile women with early stages of endometriosis[11].

Luteal phase defect

The cause of luteal phase inadequacy still remains obscure. However, there is no doubt that it may follow poor follicular development and is seen commonly in subjects having ovulation induced with clomiphene citrate, bromocriptine or pituitary gonadotropins. All these subjects have abnormal gonadotropin and/or prolactin levels, the luteal phase abnormality may be due to these or to the excessive ovarian steroid hormone secretion which often occurs due to hyperstimulation with these agents. There is some evidence that high oestrogen levels may be luteolytic[12].

Prolactin plays some role on corpus luteum function. High and low levels are both detrimental for normal corpus luteum function[13]. Bromocriptine has been used in the treatment of unexplained infertility and the authors[14] have achieved an overall pregnancy rate of 40 per cent. In one oligoprolactinaemic woman chlorpromazine was used to make her euprolactinaemic and pregnancy could be achieved[15].

Ureaplasma infections

Although the incidence of ureaplasma infections (in cervical mucus and/or seminal plasma) is higher in infertile couples than in fertile ones, several studies[16,17] have found no difference in the pregnancy rates of treated and untreated infertile couples. Therefore, a definitive role for ureaplasma infections in infertile couples have not been established.

Management

The management is mostly empirical so long as the etiology of infertility remains unexplained. Except for assisted conception, it is difficult to evaluate the efficacy of treatment as pregnancy may occur as a direct consequence of or in spite of the treatment offered. Pregnancy may also be observed simply due to the passage of time and the effect of one particular therapy may be spurious.

The drugs generally used to treat a case of unexplained infertility are clomiphene citrate, ethinyl oestradiol, bromocriptine and danazol.

Clomiphene citrate is used in a dose of 50 mg daily or twice daily from D_3 to D_7. The beneficial effect of clomiphene may originate from an improvement of follicular development with increased oestrogen secretion, improved corpus luteum function consequent upon the improved follicular development or the stimulation of multiple rather than a single ovulation. Use of clomiphene citrate appears to be paradoxical because the same drug may lead to corpus luteum inadequacy and inadequate production of cervical mucus. But the rationale of use of clomiphene citrate is based on increased production of FSH by pituitary and consequently elevated levels of oestradiol by follicles.

Bromocriptine in a dose of 2.5 mg daily is given in the luteal phase in cases where the level of prolactin is high normal or shows modest elevation. Elevation of prolactin will suppress corpus luteum function and presuming that high normal levels of prolactin may adversely affect corpus luteum adequacy, bromocriptine has been advocated for treating cases of unexplained infertility with encouraging results.

Ethinyl oestradiol is given in a dose of 0.01 mg daily from D_5 to D_{10} with the idea of increasing the quality and quantity of preovulatory cervical mucous in order to help sperm penetrability. This drug is also used in combination with clomiphene citrate to counteract the anti-oestrogenic effect of clomiphene. Low dose danazol (100 mg daily) is used to treat asymptomatic or occult endometriosis. A 35% pregnancy rate has been achieved in patients with unexplained infertility following a three month course of this treatment[18].

Intrauterine insemination (IUI) has been advocated in cases where defect in the cervical mucus is suspected or post-coital test is found negative. We have tried this method and compared the results with Timed Vaginal Intercourse (TI) following strict monitoring of ovulation with or without HCG induction. In cases of unexplained infertility the pregnancy rates were 18 per cent and 16 per cent respectively following IUI and TI which is not statistically significant.

Gamete Intra Fallopian Transfer (GIFT) has been suggested with the idea that unexplained infertility may be due to failure of ovum pick up by the fallopian tube or due to ovum entrapment syndrome (LUF). Further, sperm washing may eliminate the seminal antigens which often is quoted as one of the factors of unexplained infertility. The results of GIFT have been reported to be encouraging though not specifically for unexplained infertility. The results of GIFT may be better for oligospermia, cervical mucus defect or unilateral tubal block. In our experience, for unexplained infertility IUI and GIFT produce the same results. This is because we follow the same protocol for monitoring folliculogenesis and ovulation and technique of semen preparation is same in IUI as is followed in GIFT. GIFT is far more expensive and invasive than IUI.

IVF, and sometimes GIFT and IVF have been suggested for unexplained infertility specially when repeated attempts with IUI have failed. Certainly the results with IVF for unexplained infertility have not been very much encouraging but in IVF, the sperm-ovum interaction in vitro can be demonstrated and the inherent defects in the gametes, often responsible for unexplained infertility, can be identified.

REFERENCES

1. Drake T, Tredway D, Buchanan G, Lakaki N, Daane T. Obstet & Gynecol 1977; 50 : 644-8.
2. McBain JC, Pepperell RJ. The infertile couple (ed) Pepperell RJ. Churchill Livingstone, Edinburgh, London, pp 164-72, 1980.
3. Hertig AJ. Progress in infertility (eds) Behram SJ and Kistner RW. Little Brown & Co., Boston pp 435-52, 1975.
4. Simon EY, Laufer N. Fertil Steril 1992; 58 (i) : 24-7.
5. Koninckx PR, Dc Moor P, Brosens IA. Br J Obstet Gynecol 1980; 87 : 929-31.
6. Coulam LB, Hill LM, Breckle R. Fertil Steril 1982; 37 : 524-8.
7. Liukkonen S, Koskimies AL, Tenhunen A, Ylostalo P. Fertil Steril 1984; 43 : 62-5.
8. Daly DL, Soto-Albors C, Walters C. Fertil Steril 1985; 43 : 62-4.
9. Hamilton CJ, Wetzels LC, Evers JLH, Hoogland HJ, Muijjens A, Dehaan J. Fertil Steril 1985; 43 : 541-4.
10. Murphy AA, Green WR, Bobbie D, De La Cruz ZL, Rook JA. Fertil Steril 1986; 46 : 522-4.

11. Fakih H, Baggett B, Holtz G. Fertil Steril 1987; 47 : 213-6.
12. Stouffer RL, Nixon WE, Hodgen GD. Endocrinol 1977; 101 : 1157-9.
13. McNatty KP, Sawers RS, McNeilly AS. Nature 1974; 250 : 653-6.
14. Lenton EA, West GA, Cooke ID. Fertil Steril 1977; 28 : 913-7.
15. Chakravarty BN, Gupta N, Ghosh DS, Chattopadhyay S. J. Obstet Gynaecol India 1985; 35 : 762-9.
16. Harrison RF, Blades M, Delouvois J, Hurley R. Lancet (i) 1075; 605 : 222-6.
17. Hinton RA, Edgell LM, Andrews BE, Br J Obstet Gynecol 1979; 85 : 379-81.
18. Chakravarty BN, Ghosh DS, Chattopadhyay S. J. Obstet Gynaecol India 1986; 36 : 385-8.

CHAPTER

30

Use of Micronised Progesterone in Luteal Phase Support

Rajam Jaishankar

Luteal phase deficiency is encountered both in normal[1,2] and stimulated cycles[3,4,5]. Use of specially micronised natural progesterone in such cycles provide adequate substitution.

Luteal phase deficiency can occur during spontaneous cycles and related to insufficiency of corpus luteum. Of course, stimulated cycles show an impaired luteal phase especially true with GnRH analogues as well as hMG. Therapy includes use of human chorionic gonadotropin and progesterone, perhaps progesterone supplements may alleviate the effect of hyper-estrogenism and induce a beneficial advanced endometrial maturation.

Though corpus luteum deficiency is not limited to one hormone, *i.e.*, progesterone, 17-β-oestradiol, 17-OH progesterone can be decreased along with others. It is difficult to assess their precise role.

Synthetic progestins have different biological effects compared to those of natural progesterone.

Micronised progesterone is easy to use and effective.

Materials and method

Synthetic progestins have different biological effects compared to those of natural progesterone.

Progesterone is a hormone of ubiquitous origin. It transforms the proliferative estrogen dependent endometrium into secretory endometrium. Progesterone is a nesting hormone and competes with active androgens by fixation to the cytoplasmic receptor of androgen dependent target organs.

Progesterone is the antagonist of aldosterone on a level with its specific renal receptors.

Micronisation means particles of 20 μ and 10 μ as against crystallized P which has particles of 100 microns.

Fig. 30.1 shows that micronisation to 10 microns obtained three hours after administration of the drug

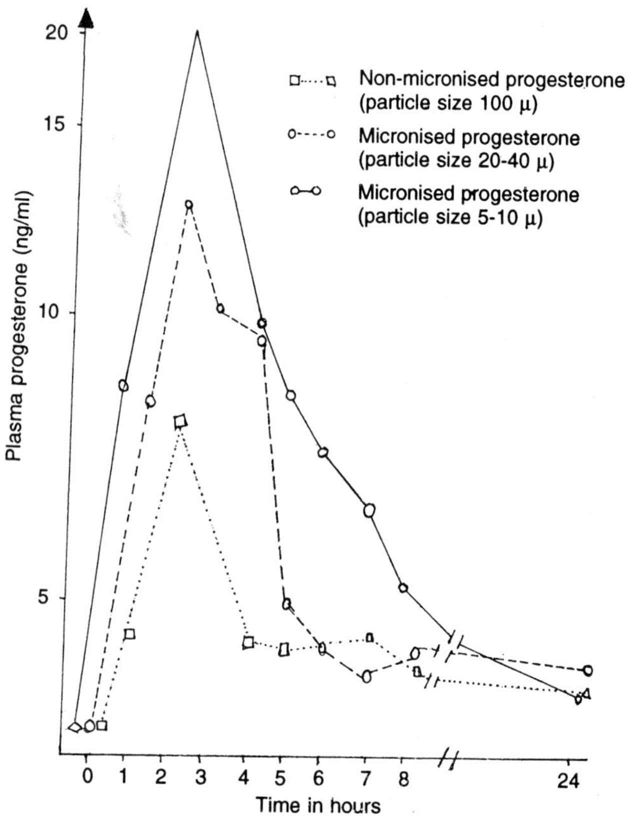

Fig. 30.1. Mean plasma progesterone levels in women after oral administration of 200 mg of progesterone.

concentration which are three times superior to those obtained with crystalline progesterone.

Pharmacokinetics

Oral route

Absorption : Micronised progesterone is absorbed by the gut. The progesterone plasma levels rise during the first hour of the treatment and the highest plasma rates are noted after 1 to 3 hours of administration.

The pharmacokinetic studies carried out on volunteers show that after the simultaneous ingestion of 2 capsules, the plasma progesterone results increased to a mean of 0.13 ng/ml to 4.25 ng/ml after 1 hour, 11.75 ng/ml after 2 hours, 8.37 ng/ml after 4 hours, 2.00 ng/ml after 6 hours then 1.64 ng/ml after 8 hours.

In view of the tissue retention time of the hormones, it would appear necessary to divide the posology into two intakes spaced by about 12 hours, to obtain impregnation throughout.

Perceptible individual variations exist, however the same person keeps the same pharmacokinetics characteristics for several months which permits good individual adaptation to the dosage.

Metabolism : In the plasma, the main metabolites are 20α-hydroxy-Δ4α-pregnanolone and 5α-dihydro-progesterone.

The urinary elimination is observed for 95% in the form of glycuroconjugated metabolites mainly 3α-5-pregnanediol (pregnandiol). These plasma and urinary metabolites β are similar to those found during the physiological secretion of the corpus luteum.

Vaginal route

Absorption : Progesterone administered vaginally has an optimal therapeutic effect since it induces rapid high plasma levels of progesterone after one hour.

The optimal plasma concentration of progesterone is reached within 2 to 6 hours after the applications remain at an average concentration of 9.7 ng/ml over 24 hours, after administration, with a dose of 100 mg, in the morning and in the evening. This mean recommended dose therefore induces steady physiological plasma concentrations of progesterone, similar to those observed during the luteal phase of normal ovulatory cycle. The weak inter-individual variations of the progesterone levels enable one to anticipate the reactions expected with a standard dose.

With the doses superior to 200 mg daily, the progesterone concentrations are similar to those of the first trimester of pregnancy.

Metabolism : Plasma levels of 5β-pregnanolone do not increase. Urinary elimination is mainly observed in the form of 3α,5β-pregnanediol (pregnandiol) as is revealed by its progressive increase in concentration (142 ng/ml maximal concentration at 6 hours).

Analysis of therapeutic efficiency was made in dysovulation, premenstrual tensions, and luteal phase defects. The micronised progesterone (Utrogestan, Besins Iscovesco, Paris) was administered in dose of 2-8 capsules per day (average 2-3 capsules). Duration of therapy was either between 10th to 25th day or from 17th to 27th day and stimulated cycles throughout first 3 months of pregnancy. General tolerance, endometrial tolerance, metabolic tolerance (plasma lipids) were evaluated — systemic effects, *e.g.*, thermogenic effect, was assessed. Likewise plasma progesterone levels were assessed.

Conclusions[6]

The best efficacy was found with 3 capsules of Utrogestan per day. Best tolerance and efficacy were obtained with administration during 10 days between

17th and 27th day. Continuation of therapy at 3 capsules per day during first three months of pregnancy is beneficial in stimulated cycles. Similar beneficial effect is reported with Utrogestan along with Oestradiol in hormonal replacement regimes during in vitro fertilisation-donated oocytes (IVF-OD programmes[7]).

REFERENCES

1. McNeely MJ, Soules MR. The diagnosis of luteal phase deficiency — a critical review. Fertil Steril 1988; 50.
2. Jones GS. Corpus luteum composition and function. Fertil Steril 1990; 54 : 21.
3. Porter RW, Smith J, Craft IL, Abdul Wahid WA, Jacobs AS. Induction of ovulation for in vitro fertilisation using busevetin and gonadotropins. Lancet, ii; 1984 : 284.
4. Wildt T, Dietrich K, van der H, Al Hasani S, Hubner H, Klalsen R. Ovarian hyperstimulation for in vitro fertilisation in combination with human menopausal gonadotropins. Hum Reprod 1986; 1 : 15.
5. Smitz J, Devroey P, Braekmans P, Camus M, Khan I, Staessen C, van Waesberghe L, Wisanto A, van Steirteghem AC. Management of failed cycles in IVF/GIFT programme with combination of GnRH analogue and hMG. Human Reprod 1987; 2 : 309.
6. Data on file clinical studies with Utrogestan. Besins Iscovesco/Chemech Laboratories Ltd., 4, K.H. Road, Madras 600034, India.
7. P Devroey, J Smitz, C Bourgain, A van Steirteghem. Only micronised progesterone is needed to substitute luteal phase in stimulated cycles. Contracept, Fert Sex 1992; 20 : 7.
8. D de Ziegler, R Frydman, P Bouchard. Hormonal replacement for recipients of egg donation — an insight into endometrial action of progesterone (P). Contracept Fert Sex 1992; 20 : 8.

CHAPTER

31

Modern Trends in Management of Elderly Infertile Women

Sulochana Gunasheela

Introduction

We are in a period when women are increasingly delaying childbirth until their thirties, a period of their lives when fertility is decreasing rapidly and during which the risk of congenital abnormalities in potential offspring is rising. The increasing frequency of pregnancy wastage associated with maternal age points to errors in meiosis of aging oocytes. Other age related causes of declining fertility include uterine ageing, which may result in inhibition or delay in implantation. Currently there is a controversy as to whether ageing of oocytes or endometrial inadequacy or both are responsible for age related decline in fertility. There is also an increased risk of acquiring tubal disease, pelvic infection, endometriosis and fibroids. Besides there are important and specific risks related to pregnancies in older women such as increased incidence of hypertension, preeclampsia, diabetes mellitus, premature rupture of membranes, etc.

Modern methods of management of elderly infertile women include superovulation along with intrauterine insemination (IUI) or Assisted Reproductive Techniques (ART). Pregnancy rates obtained are comparable to those obtained in younger women but the spontaneous abortion rate is much higher. In elderly women with premature ovarian failure, ovulation may be induced by gonadotropin suppression followed by administration of gonadotropins to induce ovulation. However the success rate with this method is low (2.2%). Transfer of oocytes or embryos donated by younger women to elderly infertile women, especially those with premature ovarian failure, result in clinical pregnancy and take home baby rates similar to their younger counterparts. In an ongoing ART programme at GIRR we have observed that pregnancy rates decreased with increasing age. We have also obtained pregnancies in amenorrhoeic women as well as in perimenopausal women with oocyte donation thus showing that the drawbacks of both oocyte and endometrial aging can be overcome.

Discussion

It is well known that there has been a steady increase in the number of women wanting to start their family after the age of 30, in the western industrialised world and among the more emancipated communities of the eastern world as well. In USA only 10% of births occurred between the ages of 30-44 in 1970. A decade later this figure doubled to 20%. The highest increase was in the early thirties age group but there was also a highly significant increase in those aged above 40[1]. Several factors influence this delay; their education, career, ambitions, narrowing down on choice of marriage partner and increasing ability to control their own fertility. Thus women prefer to fulfill their ambitions and establish financial stability before starting their families. There is also a considerable increase in the number of divorces with subsequent marriages, thus resulting in women trying for pregnancy at a later age.

Prolonged postponement of the first pregnancy however carries with it a significant disadvantage : as women grow older it becomes more and more difficult for them to become pregnant. The decline in natural fertility becomes noticeable over the age of 30. Fertility is at its maximum at the age of 24, when the average time taken for a planned pregnancy is about 2 months, compared with 4 months between the ages of 35 and 45[1]. However advancement in technology has given hope of delivering reproductive potential to most types of infertility. Most couples have less cause to worry about their infertility than they would have to 10 years ago, since they now have the security of knowing that help is at their doorstep.

Currently a controversy is raging as to whether age related decrease in fertility of the female is caused by diminishing oocyte quality, uterine endometrial inadequacy or both. To address these issues several studies have been carried out.

Results of artificial insemination in 2193 nulliparous women with azoospermic husbands were analysed by Schwartz *et al.*[2] in an attempt to study female fecundity as a function of age. This study showed that a decrease in fecundity was slight but significant after 30 years of age and marked after 35 years. The probability of success of AID for 12 cycles which was about 73% for women under 31, dropped to 61% for those between 31 to 35 and 54% for those over 35. Van Noord-Zaadstra *et al.*[3] conducted a similar study on the fecundity and outcome of pregnancy in 571 women who entered a donor insemination programme. They too observed a declining fecundity in women above 31 years. The likelihood of having a healthy infant declined by 3.5% yearly after age 30 and a woman aged 35 had about half the chance of having a healthy infant as did one aged 25 years. The increased incidence of spontaneous abortions after age 35 was attributed not only to an increased incidence of chromosomally abnormal conceptuses but also to an increased risk of abortion of chromosomally normal embryos.

There is a marked decline in the number of available oocytes with age. While the number of oocytes at birth is about 733,000 the same between the age of 25 to 31 decreases to 62,500 and between 39 to 45 there is further decrease to 10,900. The relationship between the incidence of chromosomal trisomy and other cytogenetic abnormalities with maternal age is well known[4]. The estimated rate of all clinically significant cytogenetic abnormalities rises from about 2 per 1000 at the youngest maternal ages to about 2.6 per 1000 at age 30, 5.6 per 1000 at age 35, 15.8 per 1000 at age 40 and 53.7 per 1000 at age 45. An increased incidence of ovulatory dysfunction due to ageing of the hypo-thalamo pituitary ovarian axis has been reported by De Cherney and Berkowitz[5]. Thus one of the most important causes of diminished fertility has been traced to ageing of the ova.

Other causes of age related decrease in fertility include an increase in the incidence of gynaecological disease such as endometriosis, uterine fibroids and pelvic inflammatory disease. Deciliation of the fallopian tubal endothelium is also believed to occur with age, resulting in decreased efficiency of tubal transport. A reduction in the vascular perfusion of the uterus has also been shown by ultrasound Doppler studies[6].

Further in women who do conceive, there are considerable problems with management of pregnancies due to increased incidence of hypertension and preeclampsia, diabetes mellitus, prematurity, dysmaturity and premature rupture of membranes causing high perinatal mortality rate[7].

Uterine ageing can be due to several factors :

1. The number of pinopodes in the uterine epithelium may be drastically decreased leading to inhibition or delay in implantation[8]. The function of these pinopodes is to pump out uterine fluid during implantation so that the embryos can adhere tightly to the epithelium, thus facilitating implantation.
2. Studies on older experimental animals show that fertility may decrease because of diminished number of recruited follicles, decreased fertilization rate and a uterine environment which

hinders implantation. Furthermore the uterus becomes fibrous, microvilli density at endometrial level is decreased, vascular supply is poorer and the ability to synthesize prostaglandins is reduced[9].

3. Reactive oxygen species (peroxide and free oxygen radicals) produced in the reproductive tract of older women, is also thought to inhibit implantation. Maly *et al.*[10] have shown that mononuclear cells from women who fail to implant their transferred embryos produce an increase in reactive oxygen species as compared to those women who successfully implanted their embryos.

Since advancement of age exponentially decreases the chances of pregnancy and subsequent healthy children, the question of early treatment of these elderly women is inevitably raised. It is inappropriate to advise women above the age of 30 to wait for natural conception in a period of their life during which their fertility is rapidly decreasing and risk of congenital abnormalities in potential offspring is rising.

Modes of treatment

Superovulation alone may be quite sufficient to achieve regular ovulation and pregnancy in women who are in their late thirties and early forties. Simple agents such as clomiphene citrate with or without human menopausal gonadotropins (hMG) may achieve pregnancies. There is evidence that the superovulation together with high intrauterine insemination with processed husband's sperm can achieve pregnancy rates of about 15% per treatment cycle[11].

Induction of ovulation in menopausal women

It is said that 1% of all women of reproductive age undergo premature menopause and surely women around the age of 40 are very likely to have a high gonadotropic profile indicating a state of incipient ovarian failure. Sporadic conception has been recorded when such patients were on estrogen replacement or on oral contraceptives. Ovulation can be accomplished by first suppressing pituitary gonadotropins with estrogen followed by ovarian stimulation with human menopausal gonadotropins.

Check *et al.*[12] studied 100 women with hypergonadotropic amenorrhoea (FSH and LH 35 IU/l) who were estrogen deficient (Serum E2 25 pg/ml). Another criteria was that all these women had a period of amenorrhoea of at least 12 months with failure of withdrawal menses despite treatment with medroxy progesterone acetate (10 mg per day for 10 days).

The treatment regime was as follows :

Patients were treated for a minimum of two weeks with Ethinyl Estradiol (EE2), 0.05 mg per day. EE2 was chosen because this estrogen has very little cross reactivity with serum 17-B estradiol. The idea of giving EE2 for 2 weeks prior to starting gonadotropin therapy was to reduce the levels of FSH and LH, thus withdrawing the down regulatory effect of elevated gonadotropins on LH and FSH receptors and restoring the sensitivity of the remaining follicles. EE2 might also enhance response to gonadotropin by direct effect on the receptors. At the end of 2 weeks the serum FSH and LH reduced to normal range. hMG was started at 150 IU/day and the dose increased depending upon serum E2 level checked after 5 days of therapy. If endogenous E2 was less than 35 pg/ml the dosage of hMG was increased to 225 or 300 IU/day (3 to 4 amps) and serum E2 repeated. Failure of increase in serum E2 above 50 pg/ml despite increasing hMG dose to 5 amps/day indicated cancellation of therapy for that cycle.

Pelvic sonography and serum E2 level were employed to monitor follicular maturation. If the patient attained a follicle with a minimum diameter of 17 mm with a serum E2 of at least 200 pg/ml, hMG was discontinued and 10000 IU of human chorionic gonadotropin (hCG) was given. EE2 was continued along with hMG injection till the day of hCG administration. The results given by Check *et al.* after this therapy are very impressive. 91 patients underwent 311 cycles of ovulation induction. Ovulation was achieved in 68 out of 361 cycles of induction (19%). There were 19 pregnancies (5.2%) and the take home baby rate was 2.2% (8/361). 10 patients aborted and there was one stillbirth. The high abortion rate is probably attributed to chromosomal abnormalities occurring in older patients than the protracted use of estrogen causing an abnormal endometrium or luteal phase defect. These workers also attempted suppression of gonadotropins by GnRH agonist, leuprolide acetate, 1 mg/day subcutaneously. Of the 9 women treated, only 3 women ovulated but there were no pregnancies.

Assisted Reproductive Technology (A.R.T.)

There is no place for tubal operative procedures for treatment of tubal factor in women over 40. Since they may reach menopause by the time they can achieve a spontaneous pregnancy, women with tubal factor, endometriosis, even if mild, and relative male infertility may be encouraged to proceed directly to I.V.F.

Romeu *et al.*[13] of the Jones Institute of Reproductive Medicine reported their results of I.V.F. treatment on 29 patients of age 40 and above, who were stimulated with gonadotropins for multiple follicular development for I.V.F., in comparison with 1068 stimulated cycles in women below 40. There were no statistically significant differences in serum estradiol, progesterone, number of oocytes harvested, fertilized or transferred between the two groups. Oocytes with fractured zona constituted 12.4% of the total collected oocytes in patients above 40 and atresia was noted in 8.9% of oocytes. This number was significantly higher than in the younger age group and probably reflected changes in oocyte quality due to impending ovarian deficiency. There were 15 pregnancies in the above 40 group, for a pregnancy rate of 23.4% per cycle and 29.4% for transfer. The ongoing pregnancy rate (12%) was low and total abortion rate (60%) was higher in patients above 40 in comparison with those below 40 years.

Padilla and Garcia[14] studied the effect of maternal age and number of I.V.F. procedures on pregnancy outcome in 512 patients who underwent 1101 oocyte retrievals for I.V.F. Ongoing pregnancy rate per embryo transfer for patients below 30 years was 26% as compared with 9% for patients aged 37 years. Patients 40 and above had a 50% miscarriage rate compared with 29% in patients below 40. The response to ovarian hyperstimulation and IVF in 25 women above 35 years of age was compared to a control group of 48 women below 35 by Segal and Casper[15]. They too observed no difference in the number of oocytes and embryos between the two groups. However conception rates were markedly lower in the older women (4%) as compared to an overall pregnancy rate of 12% per cycle in the younger age group.

These results agree with the concept of decreased fecundity and higher incidence of miscarriage in the higher age group. The reason for low developmental potential of embryos in these older women appears to be due to production of chromosomally abnormal gametes caused by errors of meiosis in the already depleted pool of oocytes. Impaired receptivity of the endometrium resulting in reduced implantation is also a possibility.

Oocyte donation

Application of oocyte donation technology has proven to be the best method of extending the reproductive potential in women above 40 years who are peri-menopausal, postmenopausal or those who respond poorly to follicular stimulation. With time the uterus will presumably become ineffective as it ages like all other tissues. This process however could be delayed and it could retain its implantation ability, providing a broad window of 10 to 20 years for implantation after the menopause.

The IVF treatment of women with ovarian failure employing donated eggs demonstrates the feasibility of pharmacological induction of endometrial maturation. Hormone treatment triggers growth and proliferation of a dormant endometrium followed by timed secretory transformation. In the first human pregnancy originating from a donated egg, which was reported in 1984[16], an artificial endometrial cycle was created by administration of oral estradiol valerate and natural progesterone in a sequential manner. An effort was made to mimic the hormonal dynamics of the normal 28 day ovulatory cycle as closely as possible. They had a regime of gradually increasing the dosage of estradiol valerate given orally as 2 mg tabs. They proposed the dose of 2 mg per day (1 tab. of Progynova) from day 1 to 5 followed by 2 mg b.d. from day 6 to 9 and 2 mg t.i.d. from day 10 onwards till the day of oocyte pick up in the donor. The dose was then reduced to 2 mg per day for the next 14 days, when serum β-hCG was estimated. 50 mg progesterone was given in the form of vaginal pessaries for two days commencing from the day of oocyte pick up and then increased to 100 mg/day until hCG estimation. If pregnancy was confirmed estrogen and progesterone administration were continued until the luteoplacental shift occurred. This would be indicated by the rising levels of E2 and P despite the exogenous administration of fixed doses of these hormones. The level of estradiol rises earlier (7-9 weeks) than that of progesterone (9-15 weeks). Hence the exogenous administration of estrogen is stopped by about the 10th week of gestation while progesterone administration is continued till 14 to 18 weeks gestation.

The basic concept of this treatment protocol has been widely accepted and successfully applied by several others. However difficulties in synchronisation between the donor and recipient cycles soon emerged. Thus the fixed 14 days proliferative phase was abandoned and replaced by variable periods of estrogen priming ranging from 6 to 35 days. A study by Navot *et al.*[17] elucidated the nature of endometrial response to exogenous ovarian steroid stimulation. They demonstrated that a brief estrogen priming of only 6 days duration as well as prolonged treatment of up to 5 weeks were equally effective in promoting adequate endometrial proliferation. However the pregnancy rate was higher in those treated with a longer duration of estrogen.

In lieu of estradiol valerate (Progynova), various other estrogen preparations such as micronized estradiol (Estrace), conjugated equine estrogens (Premarin), transdermal estradiol, etc., have been used successfully for induction of endometrial proliferation. It is important that the type of estrogen administered is measurable in any standard immunoassay.

The most easily available donors are women being superovulated for the purpose of assisted conception. Supernumerary oocytes from these women have been inseminated by sperm of the recipients' husbands. However such oocytes have become a rare commodity since the introduction of cryopreservation. Hence one has to look for voluntary donors comprising of friends, relatives, siblings or needy women willing to undergo the procedure for a remuneration. All donors must be screened for genetic and familial disease as well as for CMV and HIV.

Navot *et al.*[17] have also shown that the window of Embryo Transfer (ET) extends from day 1 of progesterone administration (designated day 15) to day 6 of progesterone administration (day 20), with the maximum number of viable pregnancies being obtained when embryo transfers were done on days 16, 17 or 18, *i.e.*, days 2 to 4 of progesterone administration.

Edwards *et al.*[18] examined pregnancy rates in two embryo transfer programmes in relation to embryo quality and type of menstrual cycle. Women who had regular cycles received their own fresh embryos either in the stimulated cycle or on the third day of progesterone therapy in an artificial cycle. Amenorrhoeic women received donated oocytes fertilized in vitro by their husbands' sperm. In both programmes pregnancy rates were higher in previously amenorrhoeic women above 40 (25%) compared with 10% or less for cyclic patients in the same age group. Oocyte quality as determined by age of oocyte donor and growth of embryos in culture did not contribute to the difference. They therefore suggested that a uterus that has not been subjected to regular menstrual cycles was probably a favourable factor and hence a period of induced amenorrhoea might be beneficial for infertile women.

In an investigation of the pregnancy potential of menopausal women over 40 by use of donor eggs, Pantos *et al.*[19] established 41 clinical pregnancies in 134 recipient cycles. The 30.6% pregnancy rate per embryo transfer remained constant for the age groups 40-43, 44-47 and 48 and above. The oldest woman to deliver was 54 years old. Navot *et al.*[20] investigated ovum donation in 35 infertile women aged 40 and above who had failed at attempts at conception with their own oocytes. Oocytes were donated by 29 young individuals (mean age 33.4) undergoing IVF. The rate of implantation for embryo transfer was higher (14.7%) with donated oocytes than with self oocytes (3.3%). Rates for clinical pregnancies and delivery did not differ between donors and recipients. These data suggest that age related decline in female fertility is attributable to oocyte quality and is correctable by oocyte donation.

G.I.R.R. experience

In an ongoing research in reproductive technology (RRT) programme at our centre which includes GIFT, ZIFT and IVF-ET procedures, we retrospectively studied reproductive performance of 166 women versus age. 54 women were below 30 years (mean age 25.7), 102 were in the age group 30-39 (mean age 34) and 10 were 40 and above (mean age 41). The average gonadotropic hormone requirement increased with age with a concomitant decrease in the number of follicles and hence oocytes. Although the fertilization rates were comparable in all three groups, the clinical pregnancy rate decreased from 19% in the below 30 age group to 14% in the 30-39 age group while no pregnancies were achieved in patients 40 and above.

Women with primary amenorrhoea (hypergonadotropic) and elderly women who were poor responders, perimenopausal or postmenopausal were taken up for ART with oocyte donation. Our hormone replacement regime consisted of oral estradiol valerate (Progynova) to the recipient about 5 days prior to ovarian stimulation of the prospective donor. The dose of Progynova was gradually increased from an initial administration of 2 mg per day until the thickness of the endometrium was at least 7-8 mm with a serum estradiol of at least 200 pg/ml (preferably a supraphysiological level of 350 to 400 pg/ml). Instead of Progynova, Premarin was used in few cases administered at an initial dose of 1.25 mg/day and increased accordingly to achieve optimal thickness of endometrium and serum estradiol. The maximum dose of Progynova or Premarin administered was continued until serum β-hCG was estimated to detect pregnancy. In most cases a prior trial cycle was carried out. Progesterone injections were commenced from the day prior to or the day of oocyte pick up in the donor. The initial dose was usually 25 mg followed by 50 mg the next day and then increased to 100 mg/day until the day of serum β-hCG estimation.

Six patients in the study were below 30 years, 14 women 30-39 years and 7 were 40 and above. Donation was by young anonymous donors or by siblings. The age of donors did not exceed 32. Two pregnancies, both in patients with primary amenorrhoea and streak ovaries, were achieved in the below 30 age group, one in the 30-39 age group and one in the above 40 age group. The pregnancies in the latter groups were achieved in a perimenopausal and a poor responder respectively. Although the number of cases done is small it nevertheless shows the feasibility of achieving pregnancies in amenorrhoeic agonadal women as well as in patients with incipient ovarian failure.

The question whether older infertile women especially those over 40 should be actively encouraged to have treatment by ART is controversial. Many recommend that women over 40 should not be offered treatment, but should be strongly advised to accept their infertility status. Careful counselling is mandatory giving realistic assessment of clinical status and an approximate estimate of their failure and success. Certain groups of child activists strongly believe that the psychological barriers between parents and the baby, due to age disparity can result in unhappy childhood for the offspring. However many women will not settle down to this mode of rejection and may want at least one attempt in order to have the satisfaction of having tried all available methods.

REFERENCES

1. Adams MM, Oakley GP, Marks JS. Maternal age and births in the 1980s. JAMA 1982; 247 : 493-5.
2. Schwartz D, Mayaux MJ, Federation CECOS. Female fecundity as a function of age. N. Engl J Med 1982; 306 : 404-6.
3. Van Noord-Zaadstra BM, Looman CWN, Alsbach H, Habbema JDF, Te Velde ER, Karbaat J. Delayed child bearing : Effect of age on fecundity and outcome of pregnancy. Br Med J 1991; 302 : 1361-5.
4. Hook EB. Rates of chromosome abnormalities at different maternal ages. Obstet Gynecol 1981; 58 : 282-5.
5. De Cherney AH, Berkowitz GS. Female fecundity and age. N. Engl J Med 1982; 306 : 424-6.
6. Goswamy RK, Williams G, Steptoe PC. Decreased uterine perfusion : a cause of infertility. Hum Reprod 1988; 3 : 955-9.
7. Hansen JP. Older maternal age and pregnancy outcome : A review of the literature. Obstet Gynecol Surv 1986; 41 : 726-41.
8. Martel D, Monier MN, Roche D, Psychoyos A. Hormonal dependence of pinopode formation at the uterine luminal surface. Hum Reprod 1991; 6 : 597-603.
9. Gosden RG. Maternal age : a major factor affecting the prospects and outcome of pregnancy. Ann NY Acad Sci 1984; 442 : 45-57.
10. Maly EE, Sterzik K, Henderson D, De Weck AI. Enhancement of mononuclear cell oxidative burst by early post-transfer sera from unsuccessful human embryo transfer patients. Hum Reprod 1990; 5 : 342-4.
11. Brinsden P. Assisted conception for the elderly infertile patient in Proceedings of the First International Scientific Meeting of the Royal College of Obstetricians and Gynaecologists, Singapore, World Scientific, 1990; 178-82.
12. Check JH, Nowroozi T, Chase, JS, Nazari A, Shapse D, Vaze M. Ovulation induction and pregnancies in 100 consecutive women with hypergonadotropic amenorrhoea. Fertil Steril 1990; 53 : 811-6.
13. Romeu A, Muasher SJ, Acosta AA. Results of IVF attempts in women 40 years of age and older : the Norfolk experience. Fertil Steril 1987; 47 : 130-6.
14. Padilla SL, Garcia JE. Effect of maternal age and number of IVF procedures on pregnancy outcome. Fertil Steril 1989; 52 : 270-3.
15. Segal S, Casper RF. The response to ovarian hyperstimulation and IVF in women older than 35 years. Hum Reprod 1990; 5 : 255-7.
16. Lutjen PJ, Trounson AO, Leeton FJ, Wood C, Renou P, Chan LK. The establishment and maintenance of pregnancy using IVF and embryo donation in a patient with primary ovarian failure. Nature 1984; 307 : 174-6.
17. Navot D, Bergh PA, Williams M. An insight into early reproductive processes through the in vivo model of ovum donation. J Clin Endocrinol Metab 1991; 72 : 408-14.
18. Edwards RG, Morcos S, Macnamee M, Balmaceda JP, Walters DE, Asch R. High fecundity of amenorrhoeic women in embryo transfer programmes. Lancet 1991; ii : 292-4.
19. Pantos K. Meimeti-Damianaki T, Vaxevanoglou T, Kapetanakis E. Oocyte donation in menopausal women aged over 40 years. Hum Reprod 1993; 8 : 488-91.
20. Navot D, Bergh PA, Williams M. Poor oocyte quality rather than implantation failure as a cause of age related decline in female fertility. Lancet 1991; i : 1375-7.

CHAPTER

32

Current Trends in Infertility Management : Endocrine, Autoimmune and Male Factors

Brij Saxena, Mukul Singh and Benny Bartoov

In spite of the availability of sophisticated diagnostic methods, fertility drugs and assisted reproductive techniques, the average 'take home baby' rate among infertile couples has not exceeded 15-20%. Similarly the enigma of unexplained infertility as well as unexplained fertility also remains to be elucidated. Obviously, yet unrecognized factors, play an important role in the regulation of human reproduction. For example, further understanding of the endocrine regulation of luteal-placental shift[1], autoimmune disease[2] and male factor, is required. Because of the plurality of the sperm, the semen analysis in males has remained in the constraints of light microscopy. Recently, ultramorphological studies of sperm, using scanning (SEM) and transmission electron microscopy (TEM), have revealed ultrastructural defects in the sperm which have been directly related to sperm malfunction in infertile males[3].

In this presentation we shall discuss the following factors, which have not been fully elucidated, and may be linked with infertility.

1. (a) Interaction of human chorionic gonadotropin (hCG) and prolactin (PRL) receptors in the regulation of luteal placental shift.
   (b) Role of human chorionic gonadotropin (hCG) and prolactin (PRL) in thyroid dysfunction in early pregnancy loss.
2. Autoimmune factors : antibodies to gonadotropin receptor.
3. Aesthenoteratozoospermia — Ultramorphological sperm defects.

In a normal conceived cycle, an estradiol (E_2) induced increase in PRL during luteal phase facilitates the binding of hCG to the luteal cell receptors. There is a temporal relationship between PRL and hCG binding to their receptors, to regulate the optimum production of progesterone (Fig. 32.1). Prolactin autoregulates both its own receptors and heteroregulates hCG receptors in the gonadal cells[4]. For example, the down regulation of hCG receptors is followed by those of PRL receptors. During recovery

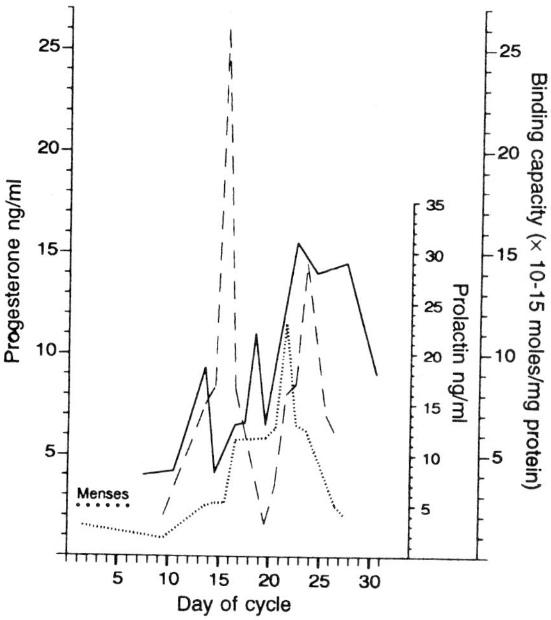

Fig. 32.1. Temporal relationship of serum prolactin (_____) and LH-receptor binding to the ovary (.....) with serum progesterone (- - - -) during the luteal phase.

phase, the PRL receptors are regenerated prior to those of hCG. These observations further underscore a luteotrophic role of the prolactin in the maintenance of corpus luteum function.

During the luteal-placental shift and until term during pregnancy, an increase in E_2 is accompanied with the increase in the synthesis and release of prolactin. Prolactin in normal levels is luteotrophic. Administration of prolactin to hypoprolactinemic patients decreases the amount of hCG required to prolong the short luteal phase. At higher levels PRL acts as a luteolytic agent, and may cause early abortion, either spontaneous or induced, which is accompanied by a striking increase in basal levels of prolactin. Stress and prolonged sensory stimulation can also stimulate an increased output of PRL, which may be responsible for early pregnancy loss[5].

The importance of PRL in the maintenance of normal pregnancy is further borne out from a study of 12 pregnancies[6], in which the initial serum hCG levels were subnormal and indicated threatened abortion. Three of the 12 patients delivered term babies. The hCG titers remained subnormal throughout the pregnancy, while serum E_2, progesterone and PRL levels in these three patients remained normal. One of the 12 patients aborted in week 25 of gestation. The serum hCG and PRL in this patient were subnormal while serum E_2 and P were, however, normal. The normal level of E_2 (which is responsible for the release of PRL) indicates that hypoprolactinemia or lack of the ability to synthesize or release prolactin by the pituitary may be responsible for the pregnancy loss. Eight of the 12 patients aborted prior to 100 days of gestation. In these patients the serum E_2, PRL and hCG were subnormal, whereas the P levels were normal. Therefore, in patients who have subnormal serum hCG titers, serum E_2 and PRL may provide a prognostic index of impending spontaneous abortion. Availability of recombinant prolactin will provide the therapeutic support in the maintenance of early pregnancy (Table 32.1).

Prolactin and hCG also play an important role during perimplantation and early pregnancy in patients with thyroid dysfunction and infertility. Early pregnancy is at risk in 40% of patients with hyperemesis gravidarum, free thyroxin (T_4) is elevated and TSH is suppressed with symptoms of thyrotoxicosis due to the thyroid stimulating activity (TSA) of circulating hCG, since the alpha-subunit is shared with hCG and TSH[7] and the cDNA sequence of TSH and hCG receptors have extensive homology. Alpha-subunit of the glycoprotein hormones is implicated in the receptor binding. Kimura *et al.*[8] found TSA activity of hCG in the sera of hyperemesis patients, by significantly high cAMP release from FRTL-5 cells, which could be abolished by treatment with anti-hCG-antibody. In patients with Hashimoto's syndrome the antibodies against the TSH-receptor cause elevated TSH and sometimes in prolactin levels. Such patients require close observation

Table 32.1. Twelve patients with low serum hCG titers throughout pregnancy

No. of patients	*Serum hCG*	*Serum E_2*	*Serum hPRL*	*Serum P*	*Outcome*
3	Subnormal*	Normal**	Normal**	Normal**	Term delivery
1	Subnormal*	Normal**	Subnormal*	Normal**	Spontaneous abortion at 25 week
8	Subnormal*	Subnormal*	Subnormal*	Overlap with normal range	Spontaneous abortion prior to 100 days' gestation

* Subnormal : Hormonal level is below mean minus 1 S.D. as calculated for 15 normal controls for each hormone.

** Normal : Hormonal level is in the range of ± 1 S.D. as represented for each hormone.

of their thyroid function during synthroid replacement therapy, if they are candidates for IVF, to prevent early pregnancy loss, due to gestational thyrotoxicosis.

The foregoing is illustrated in a case history of a 38-year-old female with a history of infertility. Physical and gynaecologic examinations as well as endocrine workup were within normal limits. Histosalpingography revealed tubal patency. The patient was free of gynaecological infection. Antinuclear and antimitochondrial antibodies were negative. Karyotype and male factor were normal. However, she complained of joint pain, lethargy, and non-specific health problems, which prompted a thyroid function workup. The patient had no physical signs of thyroid disorder. Thyroid profile revealed high serum TSH (9.4-10.8 mIU/ml). Anti-TSH-receptor antibodies were positive, and led to the diagnosis of Hashimoto syndrome. PRL levels were in high normal range of 15-27 ng/ml. With a synthroid dose of 112 μg per day the TSH levels were maintained at normal level. The patient became euthyroid and felt better. During her next cycle she missed her period and waited for more than two weeks to report to the clinic when she developed emesis and suspected pregnancy. The pregnancy test was positive. A sonogram revealed two implantation sites. However, β-hCG and hCG levels being 2300 and 4800 mIU, were subnormal for the duration of the pregnancy. Serum PRL levels were, however, elevated (33.7-58 ng/ml) for the duration of the pregnancy. Progesterone levels during the subsequent weeks were also subnormal being 7.5 ng and 10.7 mg/ml which declined further to 5.9 mg/ml and indicated missed abortion. She was advised to use progesterone suppositories and was evaluated for thyroid function. TSH was suppressed (0-0.1 mU/ml) and T_4 was high (16.7-19.1 mg/dl), which may be due to thyroid stimulating activity (TSA) of hCG. Low hCG, elevated prolactin and lack of optimum utilization of hCG by its receptors in the corpus luteum, resulted in low progesterone leading eventually to a missed abortion. This case underscores the need for a preconception regulation of thyroid function, early detection of pregnancy and progesterone supplementation in such patients. Further studies are warranted to elucidate a precise interrelationship of prolactin, thyroid function and gestational thyrotoxicosis in the management of infertility.

The autoimmune disease related to TSH receptor[9] has been extended to the autoantibodies against gonadal antigens in infertility[10]. Irvine in 1968[10] reported the presence of ovarian antibodies in patients with autoimmune disease and POF. Since then, multiple reports appeared in the literature in the early 1980 citing the presence of POF in patients with both endocrine and nonendocrine autoimmune disorders[11,12]. Ovarian antibodies have been found in patients with POF with the incidence ranging from 18-60%[10]. These antibodies are specific for various sites within the ovary including the interstitium, granulosa cells, thecal cells, corpus luteum and the oocyte. The antigenic sites on the ovarian cell membranes include both FSH and LH receptors. Caldwell *et al.*[13] have reported the presence of a LH-hCG receptor antibody in a patient with POF while Charreau *et al.*[14] identified antibodies specific for the FSH receptor. Contradictory reports exist regarding the effect of these antibodies function, with some demonstrating an agonist response[15], others an antagonist[16,17] response and, still others, no effect[18]. Recently, we have demonstrated lutropin receptor antibody in POF patient's serum using more specific assays[19].

In this study, monoclonal antibodies to the LH-receptor used as positive control showed a dose response in progressive inhibition of ^{125}I-hCG binding to the receptor (Fig. 32.2). An immunoprecipitation assay was used to demonstrate that up to 200 mIU LH/ml in the patient's serum did not interfere in the evaluation of the incidence of lutropin receptor antibodies in patients with POF (Fig. 32.3). Eighteen women with POF and 10 normal cycling age-matched controls were evaluated for the presence of circulating lutropin receptor antibodies. The mean age for the controls was 30.9 ± 4. They were all normal cycling with proven fertility. The mean age of the POF patients was 32.6 ± 4. Criteria for POF included age < 40 years at the onset of ovarian failure, persistent elevation in

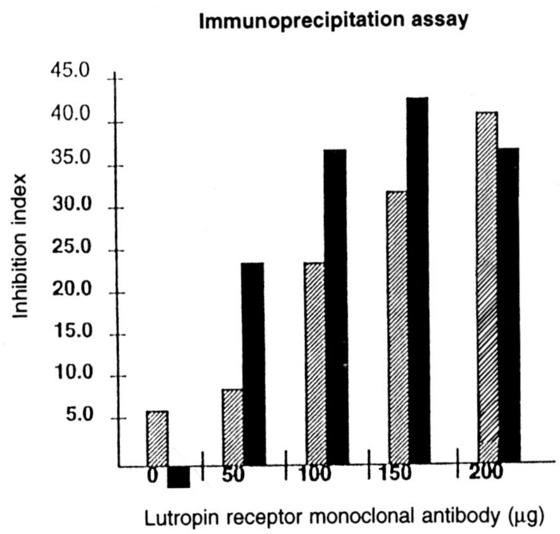

Fig. 32.2. Progressive inhibition of ^{125}I-hCG binding to the receptor in the presence of increasing amounts of antibody.

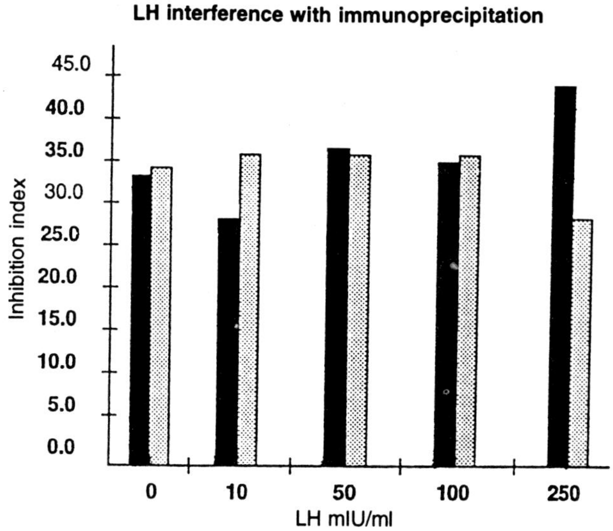

Fig. 32.3. Lack of interference by exogenous LH up to 200 mIU in the immunoprecipitation assay.

LH and/or FSH levels (LH and FSH > 50 mIU/ml), E_2 levels < 60 pg/ml and a normal karyotype. Neither patients nor controls received any exogenous steroids or immunosuppressants for one month prior to or during the study. Thirteen out of the 18 POF patients were nulligravidas, 1 had been a recurrent aborter, 1 had 3 previous elective abortions and 3 had successful pregnancies prior to developing POF. Menstrual histories revealed that majority had either irregular or regular cycles prior to the onset of menopause, only 5 had primary amenorrhoea.

Four of the patients with POF had autoantibodies present, two of which presented with clinical manifestations. One patient was diagnosed with Grave's disease, the other with Hashimoto's thyroiditis. Five patients other than the ones with autoimmune diseases had a family history of autoimmune disease. Therefore, a total of 9 of 18 patients, 50% (P = 0.001), had either a significant autoimmune history or family history.

Blood was collected by venipuncture and serum was separated by centrifugation at 3,000 rpm at room temperature. FSH and LH levels were determined by an ELISA kit (Boeringer and Mannheim, Co.). The LH receptor antibodies were determined by (a) inhibition of ^{125}I-hCG binding to bovine corpora lutea plasma membrane; (b) immunoprecipitation; and (c) immunoblotting.

Binding inhibition assay[20] : As shown in Table 32.2, six of 18 POF patients tested positive to lutropin receptor antibodies with a mean inhibition index of 32.4 (1 – percent receptor bound ^{125}I-hCG over maximum

Table 32.2. Patients with premature ovarian failure tested for serum autoantibodies against lutropin-receptor

Subjects	*Inhibition index*		*Immunoprecipitation index**	
Control	5.9 ± 4.7	(10)	12.6 ± 5.8	(10)
Positive	32.4 ±	(6)	35.5 ±	(6)
Negative	3.6 ±	(30)	0	

* Average, SEM and number

bound × 100). Of these, only 2 had autoimmune factors. One had a positive ANA with history of recurrent abortions while the other had a mother with diabetes. All 5 had a menstrual history with 3 of 5 having irregular menses. There was no correlation with gravity or autoimmune factors.

Immunoprecipitation assay : The principle of immunoprecipitation is described previously[19]. As shown in Fig. 32.3, serum LH levels below 200 mIU/ml did not show significant interference in the ^{125}I-hCG binding to the LH-receptor, suggesting that gonadotropins do not need to be removed prior to performing this assay. Fig. 32.2 demonstrates a progressive inhibition of ^{125}I-hCG binding in the presence of 50, 100, 150, 200 µg of the LH receptor monoclonal antibody as positive control. As shown in Table 32.2 immunoprecipitation confirmed the presence of the LH receptor antibodies in the same 6 samples as in the inhibition assay with an immunoprecipitation index of 35.5 (1 – percent receptor immunoprecipitated over percent total receptor bound × 100). None of the control samples showed any LH-receptor antibodies in their serum samples.

An immunoblot of a serum sample from a patient with a high titre of LH-receptor antibody, identifying a LH-receptor oligomer of, approximately, 140 Kd in presence of sodium dodecyl sulphate (SDS) alone and reduced moieties of, approximately, 77 Kd and 60 Kd of the LH-receptor in the presence of SDS and dithiotreitol (DTT).

Caldwell *et al.*[13] have suggested that gonadotropin receptors may be a site of action for immunoglobulins in POF patients. Moncayo[22] further investigated the presence of lutropin receptor antibodies in infertility patients, demonstrating the major isotype to be IgG2. Even without a full understanding of autoimmune based POF various modalities have been noted to intermittently reverse this state. Pregnancies have been reported in several patients, where corticosteroid therapy for autoimmune adrenal failure[21,22] and for severe asthmatic attack[2] has been administered. Furthermore, similar to thyroid disorders where anti-idiotype antibodies have been developed, this may be a treatment option in the future for these patients. Our data and the data of others[14,23,24] suggest that gonadotropin receptor antibodies may affect gonadotropin interaction with the receptor site and may, thus, interfere ultimately with ovarian function. Obviously, detection of autoantibodies against gonadotropin receptor may provide more focussed management of POF patients.

Endocrine, metabolic and autoimmune factors may also be the cause of unexplained male infertility. For the last three centuries, the classic approach to the investigation of male fertility and infertility has been the light microscope[25,26]. However, the light microscope is limited by low magnification, and the use of the light microscope enables only surface exploration. It gives little evaluation of the subcellular elements or the sperm cell organelles, which is most important in the evaluation of overall fertility status of the male[26]. Recently, defects in the ultrastructure of sperm has been directly related to the sperm function using scanning electron microscopy (SEM) and transmission electron microscopy (TEM) of the sperm which provides three- dimensional view of the sperm.

The quantitative ultramorphology approach determines three-dimensional views of the sperm organelles via electron optics using the transmission electron microscopy (TEM) and the scanning electron microscopy (SEM). TEM and the appropriate staining techniques make it possible to view cross-sections of the sperm cell, giving a two-dimensional view of ultrafine anatomical details. However, because of the lack of the third dimension, the overall view of the sperm structure is missing. This limitation is overcome by SEM.

Semen analysis (SA) is performed. The accessory gland function is assessed by measuring semen volume, pH, seminal Zn^{2+}, Ca^{2+}, citric acid and fructose levels. The semen analysis fertility index was calculated for each participant as follows :

Semen analysis index = [total count ($\times 10^6$ sperm cells/ejaculate) $\times$ 0.002] + [motility (%) $\times$ 0.016] + [normal forms (%) $\times$ 0.045] – [volume (ml) $\times$ 0.350] – 1.03[3].

For TEM, sperm cells are separated from seminal plasma by centrifugation at 1650 g_{max} for 15 min. and fixed in 2% formaldehyde, 2% glutaraldehyde in 0.1 M phosphate buffer solution pH 7.2 for 2 hr. at room temperature. The cells are post-fixed in osmium tetroxide. Thin sections are cut using an LKB ultratome (Bromma, Sweden), and are examined using a Joel 100 C TEM (Joel Ltd., Tokyo, Japan) at a magnification of $\times$ 15,000 and at a magnification of $\times$ 35,000. For SEM, sperm cells are separated from their plasma and fixed as for the TEM preparation. They are examined with a Joel JSM 35 SEM at a magnification of $\times$ 12,000. The ultramorphological status of each of the following sperm subcellular organelles namely, acrosome, post-acrosomal lamina, nucleus, neck, axonema, mitochondrial and fibrous sheaths, is assessed in parallel by TEM and SEM. The incidence of each ultramorphological state is assessed quantitatively for 100 cells per sample (Fig. 32.4).

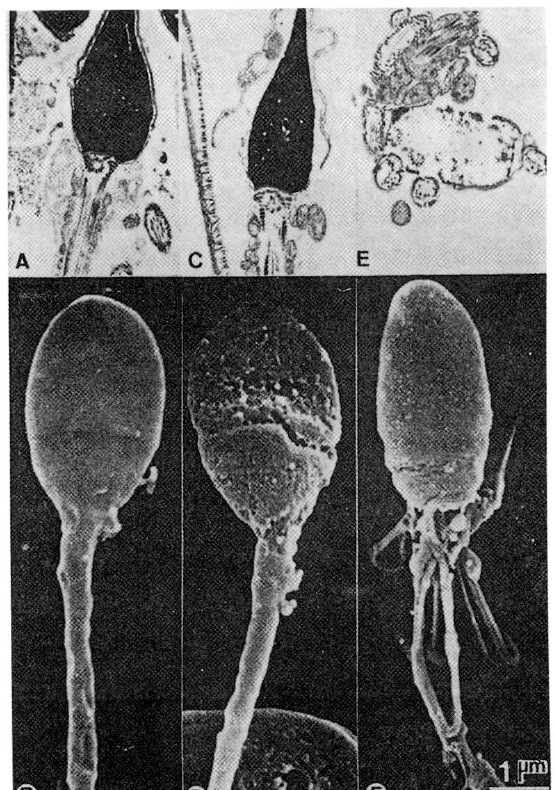

Fig. 32.4. Electronmicrographs of the sperm cell organellar ultramorphological states included in the quantitative ultramorphology (QUM) index : Intact nucleus : (A) TEM; (B) SEM, acrosomal malformation; (C) TEM, (D) SEM, outer dense fibre malformation; (E) TEM; (F) SEM, Magnification $\times$ 12,000.

The infertile group had significantly more malformations of the head and tail regions as compared with the fertile group. In all, the intact state of six subcellular organelles (except mitochondria), as well as 12 pathological ultramorphological states were found to differ significantly ($P \leq 0.01$) between the fertile and the infertile males. Using the quantitative ultramorphological (QUM) index, 88% of the fertile and 76% of the infertile males included in the study groups were classified correctly. A combination of the SA and QUM was performed to evaluate the sperm quality (SQ). Ninety percent of the fertile and 84% of the examined infertile cases were classified correctly.

These studies support the claim of Zamboni[27] that the ultrastructural pathology of sperm subcellular elements is an important component of the overall fertility evaluation. The major candidates for quantitative ultramorphology analysis are, apparently, the males whose fertility status cannot be predicted by routine semen analysis. Dr. Bartoov, of Bar-Ilan University, has developed a computer profile which provides the prediction of the male fertility potential[3].

With further understanding of the above factors it will be possible to design more focussed and improved therapeutic strategy, for each infertile couple.

Acknowledgement

Collaboration of Dr. Ricardo Asch in studies on Lutropin receptor antibodies in patients with POF is greatly acknowledged.

REFERENCES

1. Saxena BB. Measurement and clinical significance of preimplantation blastocyst gonadotropins. Journals of Reproduction and Fertility 1989, Suppl. 37 : 115-119.
2. Luborsky JL, Visintin I, Boyers S, Asari T, Caldwell BV, DeCherney A. Ovarian antibodies detected by immobilized antigen immunoassay in patients with premature ovarian failure. Journal of Clinical Endocrinology and Metabolism 1990; 70 : 69-75.
3. Bartoov B, Eltes F, Pansky M, Langzam J, Reichart M, Soffer Y. Improved diagnosis of male fertility potential via a combination of quantitative ultramorphology and routine semen analysis. Human Reproduction 1994; 9 (11) : 2069-2075.
4. Morris PL, Saxena BB. Dose- and age-dependent effects of prolactin (PRL) on luteinizing hormone- and PRL-binding sites in rat leydig cell homogenates. The Endocrine Society 1980; 107 (5) : 1639-1645.
5. Saxena BB. Human Prolactin. In Fuchs F, Klopper A (Editors). Endocrinology of Pregnancy, New York : Harper and Row, 1977 : 222-245.
6. Jovanovic L, Dawood MY, Landesman R, Saxena BB. Hormonal profile as a prognostic index of early threatened abortion. American Journal of Obstetrics and Gynecology 1978; 130 : 274-278.
7. Lazarus JH. Pregnancy, hCG, thyrotoxycosis and hyperemesis gravidarum. Clinical Endocrinology 1993; 38 : 343.
8. Kimura M, Amino N, Tamaki H, Ito E, Mitsuda N, Miyai K, *et al.* Gestational thyrotoxicosis and hyperemesis gravidarum. Possible role of hCG with higher stimulating activity. Clinical Endocrinology 1993; 38 : 345-350.
9. Smith BR, McLachlan SM, Furmaniak J. Autoantibodies to the thyrotropin receptor. The Endocrine Society 1988; 9 (1) : 106-121.
10. Irvine WJ, Chan MMW, Scarth L, *et al.* Immunologic aspects of premature ovarian failure associated with idiopathic Addison's disease. Lancet 1968; 883.
11. Alper MM, Garner PR, Seibel MM. Premature ovarian failure : current concepts. Journal of Reproductive Medicine 1986; 31 : 699-708.
12. Kreiner D, Droesch K, Navot D, Scott R, Rosenwaks Z. Spontaneous and pharmacologically induced remissions in patients with premature ovarian failure. Obstetrics and Gynecology 1988; 72 : 926-928.
13. Caldwell BV, Laborsky JL, Kase N, Behrman HR. A functional LH agonist and LH receptor antagonist in serum from a patient with premature ovarian failure syndrome. The Endocrine Society 1978; 250 : 199.
14. Charreau EH, Chiauzzi V, Cigorraga S, Escobar ME, Rivrola M. Immunoglobulin anti-FSH receptor in the resistant ovary syndrome. Recent developments in fertility research, Part A. Developments in Reproductive Endocrinology 1982; 111.
15. Dattatreyamurty B, Zhang S, Reichert LE. Polyclonal antibodies against follitropin (FSH) receptor interfere with hormone binding, but mimic the effects of FSH. Endocrinology 1990; 126 : 1318-1326.
16. Van Weissenbrich MM, Hock A, Van Vlietbleeker I, Schoemaker J, Drexhage H. Evidence for existence of immunoglobulins that block ovarian granulosa cell growth in vitro. A putative role in resistant ovary syndrome? Journal of Clinical Endocrinology. Metabolism 1991; 73 : 360-367.
17. Chiauzzi V, Cigorraga S, Escobar ME, Rivarola MA, Charreau EH. Inhibition of follicle-stimulating hormone receptor binding by circulating immunoglobulins. Journal of Clinical Endocrinology and Metabolism 1982; 54 : 1221-1228.
18. Austin GE, Coulam CB, Ryan RJ. A search for antibodies to luteinizing hormone receptors in premature ovarian failure. Mayo Clin Proc 1979; 54 : 394-400.
19. Singh M, Saxena BB, Kaali O, Asch RH. Anti LH-receptor antibodies in idiopathic ovarian resistance. The 38th Annual Meeting of the Pacific Coast Fertility Society; 1990; Los Angeles (CA).

20. Saxena BB, Dattatreyamurty B, Ota H, Rathnam P, Isolation of disulfide linked non-identical subunits of the LH-hCG receptor from bovine corpora lutea. Biochemistry 1986; 25 : 7943-7950.

21. Finer N, Fogelman I, Bottazzo G. Pregnancy in a women with premature ovarian failure. Postgraduate Medical Journal 1985; 47 : 985-995.

22. Cowchock FS, McCabe JL, Montgomery BB. Pregnancy after corticosteroid administration in premature ovarian failure (polyglandular endocrinopathy syndrome). American Journal of Obstetrics and Gynecology 1988; 158 : 118-119.

23. Moncayo H, Moncayo R, Benz R, Wolf A, Lauritzen C. Ovarian failure and autoimmunity. Journal of Clinical Investigation 1989; 84 : 1857-1865.

24. Dias JA, Gates SA, Reichert Jr. LE. Evidence for the presence of follicle-stimulating hormone receptor antibody serum. Fertility and Sterility 1982; 38 : 330-338.

25. McLeod J. Human seminal cytology as a sensitive indicator of the germinal epithelium. International Journal of Fertility 1964; 9 : 281-287.

26. World Health Organization (1992) Laboratory Manual for the Examination of Human Semen — Cervical mucus interaction. 3rd edn. Cambridge University Press, Cambridge, UK, pp. 43-45.

27. Zamboni L. The ultrastructural pathology of the spermatozoan as a course of infertility : the role of electron microscopy in the evaluation of sperm quality. Fertility and Sterility 1987; 48 : 711-734.

CHAPTER

33

Hysterosalpingography and Hysteroscopy in Infertility

Gautam Allahbadia and Champa Nariani

Introduction

Hysterosalpingography (HSG) provides a useful, albeit indirect, image of the uterine cavity and remains one of the first steps in its evaluation and that of the tuboperitoneal factor in the infertile woman. Modern hysteroscopy has two major applications in infertility, the diagnosis and management of intrauterine defects. As a diagnostic tool, hysteroscopy can be performed alone or in conjunction with other methods, such as hysterosalpingography, vaginal ultrasound, laparoscopy, and dilatation and curettage.

The direct view of the uterine cavity afforded by hysteroscopy (Figs. 33.1 and 33.2) offers a significant advantage over other diagnostic methods, as these other modalities offer only a "blind" or indirect view of the cavity. Abnormal hysteroscopic findings usually found include intrauterine adhesions (Figs. 33.8 to 33.11), endometritis (Figs. 33.12 and 33.13) and endocervicitis. The above intrauterine abnormalities were detected in 34-62% of infertile women in some studies[1-3]. Taylor[4] advocated the use of hysteroscopy alone in infertility, whereas Sciarra and Valle[5] suggested a combination of hysterosalpingography and hysteroscopy.

The accuracy of hysterosalpingography and hysteroscopy in detecting uterine pathology has been compared by various authors. It is generally agreed that hysteroscopy is more accurate because of the false positive and false negative rates associated with HSG, although the magnitude of this discrepancy is controversial.

The advantages of HSG include the ease of the study, its safety and its lesser expense in comparison with hysteroscopy. Several disadvantages are inherent in the technique, however, including exposure to ionizing radiation, exposure to iodinated contrast material, and often a great deal of discomfort for the patient. In addition, looking at the shadows or the filling defects of the uterine cavity (Figs. 33.14 to 33.17) can lead to misleading results, as shown by a 24% rate of false positive and false negative findings as stated by Siegler[6].

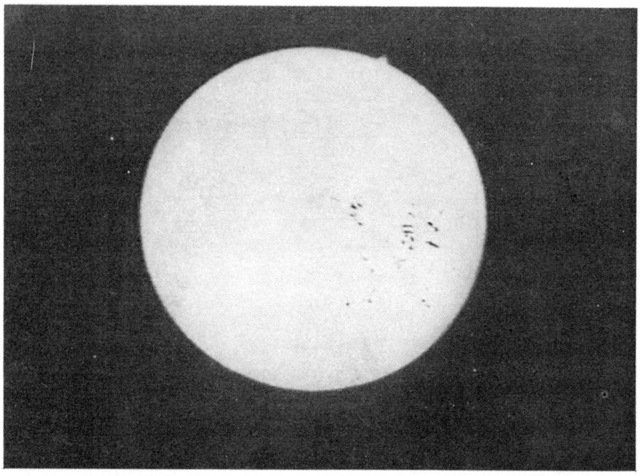

Fig. 33.1. Hysteroscopic picture. Normal tubal ostium. Early proliferative phase.

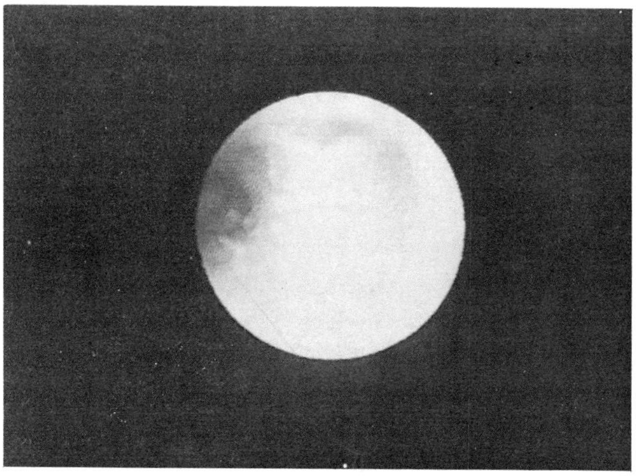

Fig. 33.2. Hysteroscopic picture. Normal right tubal ostium. Secretory phase.

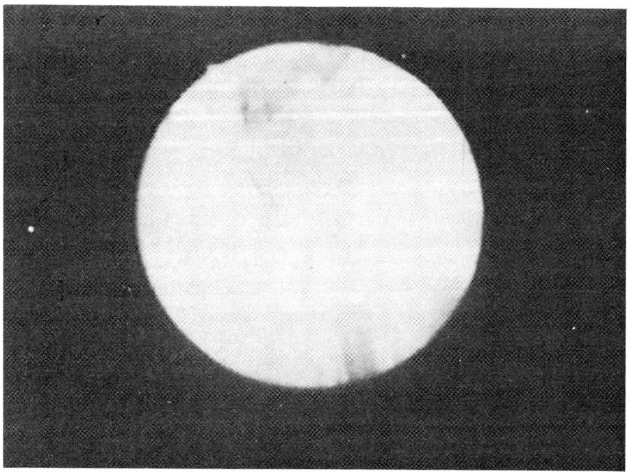

Fig. 33.3. Hysteroscopic picture. Intrauterine synechiae.

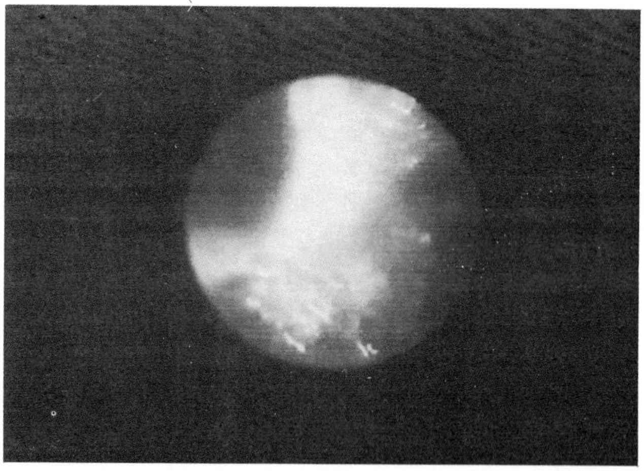

Fig. 33.4. Hysteroscopic picture. Septate uterus with both cavities and septum seen clearly.

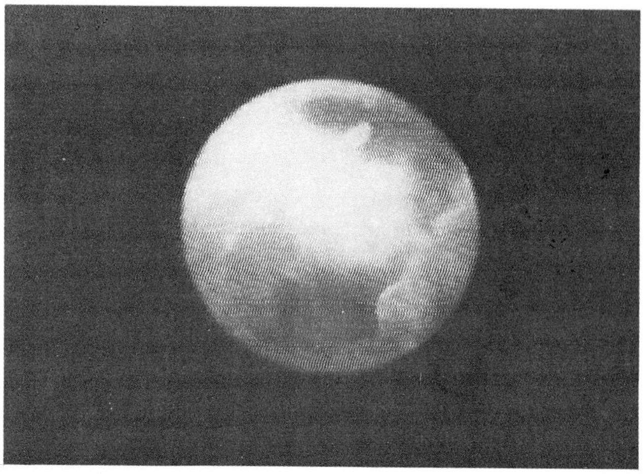

Fig. 33.5. Hysteroscopic picture. Complete bicornuate uterus. View from the level of internal os.

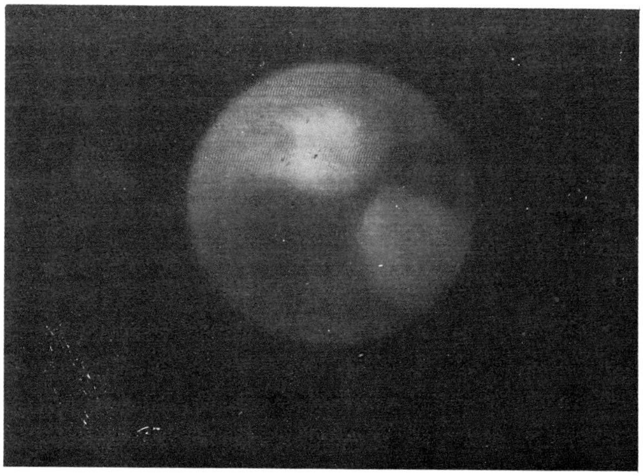

Fig. 33.6. Hysteroscopic picture. Two endometrial polyps seen clearly.

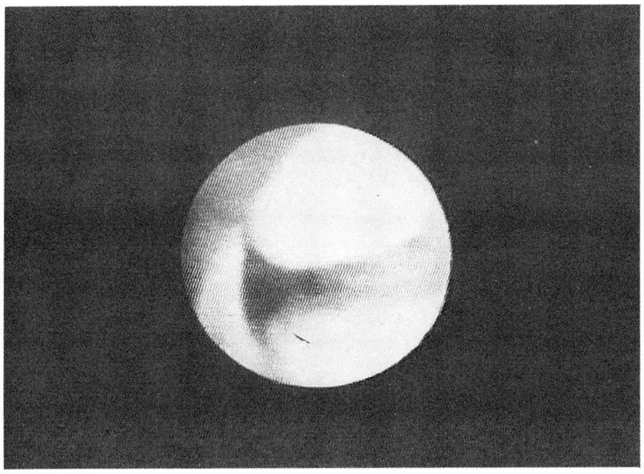

Fig. 33.7. Hysteroscopic picture. A large solitary endometrial polyp near the right ostium.

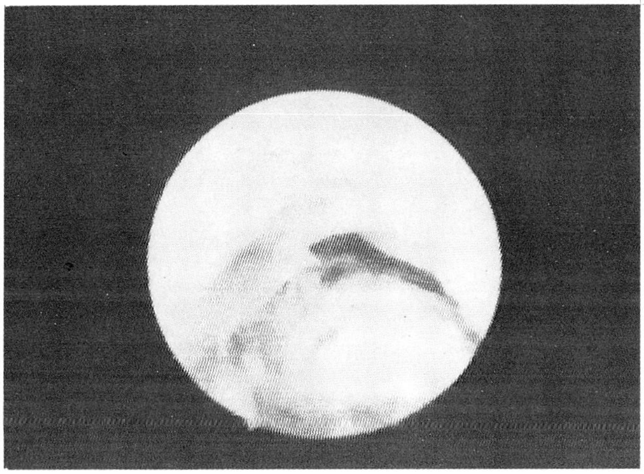

Fig. 33.8. Hysteroscopic picture. Solitary submucous fibroid on the posterior wall.

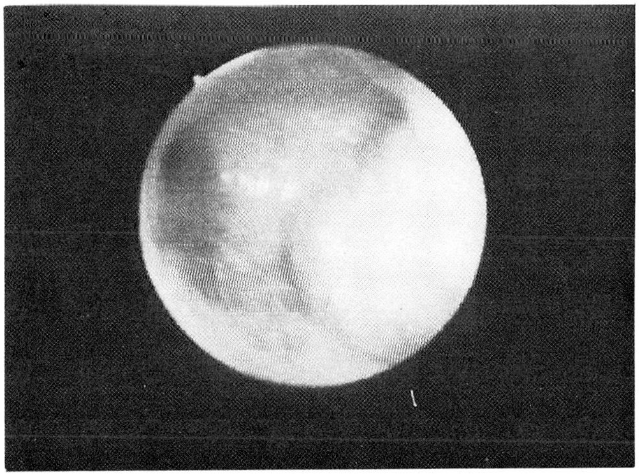

Fig. 33.9. Hysteroscopic picture. Pedunculated single submucous fibroid. Picture shows the base of the pedicle originating at the level of fundus near the right ostium.

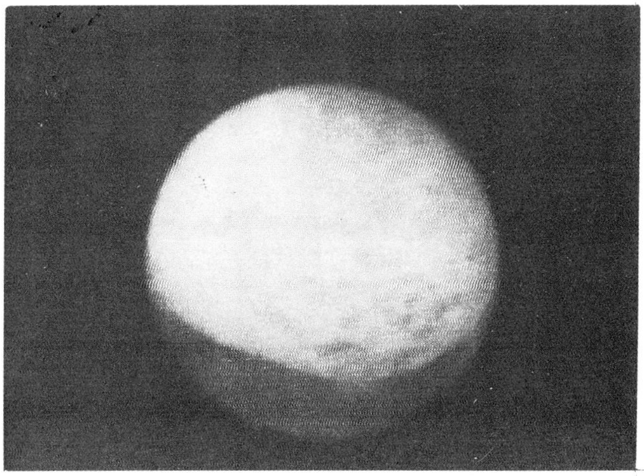

Fig. 33.10. Hysteroscopic picture. Solitary anterior wall submucous fibroid. Neovascularity seen over surface.

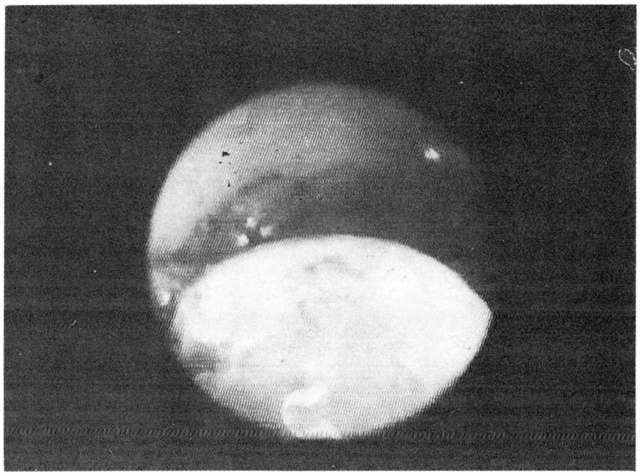

Fig. 33.11. Hysteroscopic picture. Single posterior wall submucous fibroid seen.

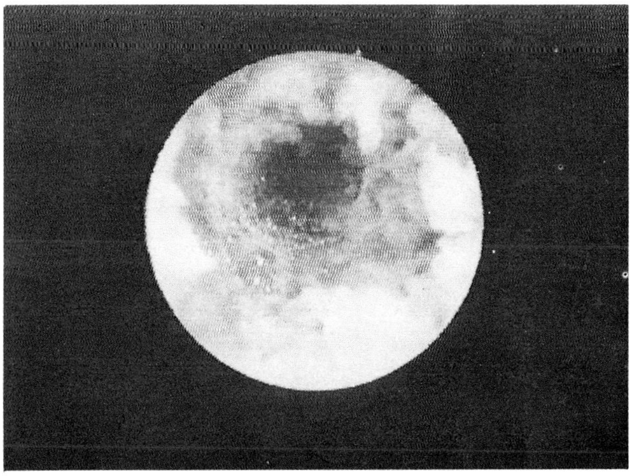

Fig. 33.12. Hysteroscopic picture. Area of endometritis seen clearly around the left ostium. Histopathologically proven TB.

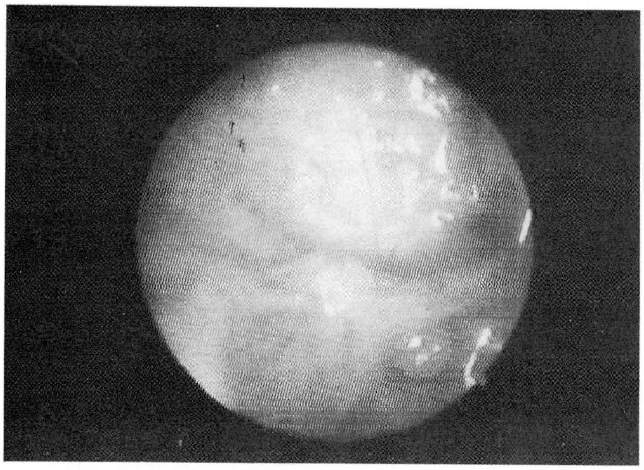

Fig. 33.13. Hysteroscopic picture. Close-up of a small caseous deposit on the posterior wall of uterus near the right ostium. Histopathologically proven TB.

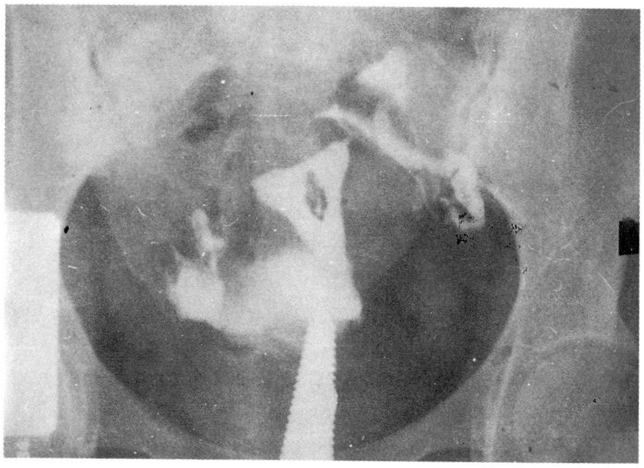

Fig. 33.14. HSG. Partial Ashermann's syndrome with bilateral free spill.

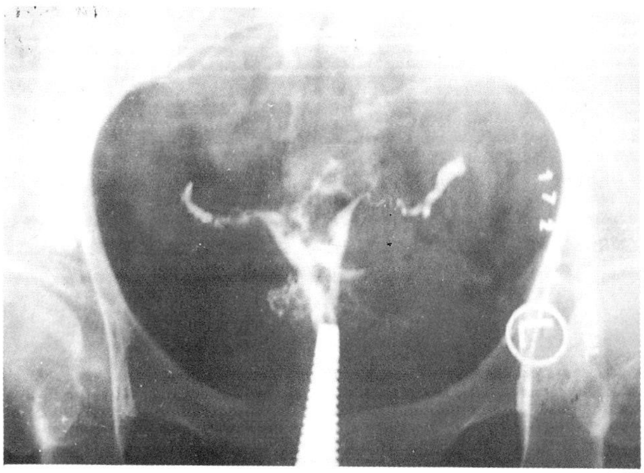

Fig. 33.15. HSG. TB endometritis with bilaterally affected fallopian tubes.

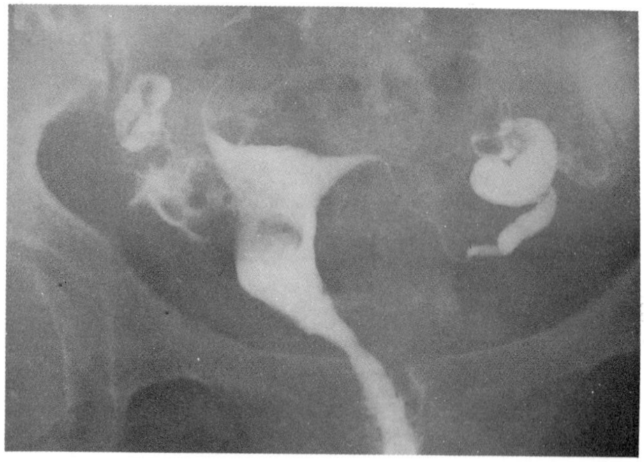

Fig. 33.16. HSG. Filling defect with loss of contour of the right uterine wall. Hysteroscopically proved submucous fibroid.

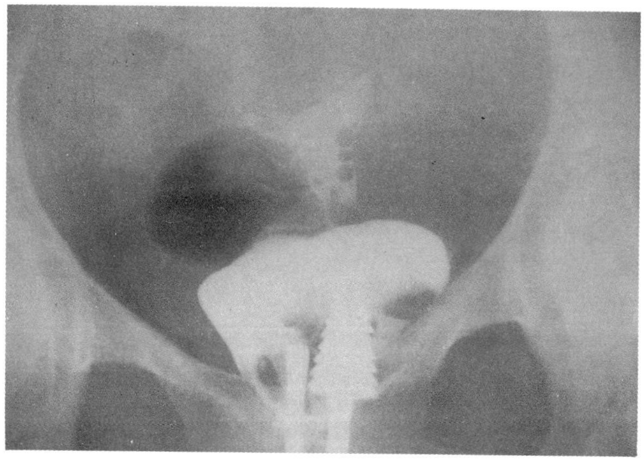

Fig. 33.17. HSG. Air bubbles as artifacts with inadvertent leakage of dye into the vagina.

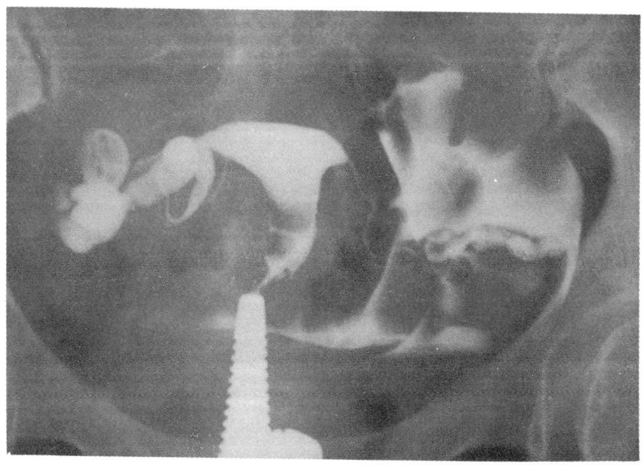

Fig. 33.18. HSG. Normal uterine cavity with bilateral free peritoneal spill.

The utility of hysteroscopy in infertility evaluation has been the subject of much discussion and has been well summarized by Taylor & Hamou[7]. Whereas Valle[8] and Kessler & Lancet[9] have demonstrated the increased accuracy of hysteroscopy over HSG, Snowden[10] found the hysterosalpingogram to be more reliable.

A more unifying approach was supported by Fayez *et al.*[11], who found HSG to be as accurate as hysteroscopy in the diagnosis of normal (Figs. 33.18 and 33.19) or abnormal cavities (Figs. 33.20 and 33.21), whereas the nature of the intrauterine filling defects was revealed accurately only by hysteroscopy (Figs. 33.22 and 33.23). The same authors, in a study of 400 cases, stated that hysteroscopy seems to be of more value than HSG in the diagnosis of some specific pathological conditions, *e.g.*, intrauterine adhesions (Fig. 33.24), submucous myomas (Fig. 33.25) and endometrial polyps (Fig. 33.26). Otherwise, HSG was found to be as accurate as hysteroscopy in the diagnosis of a normal uterine cavity and Mullerian defects.

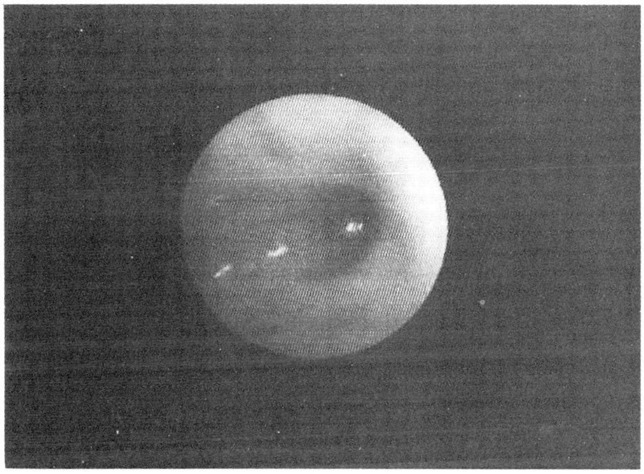

Fig. 33.19. Hysteroscopic view. Normal uterine cavity with normal left ostium seen.

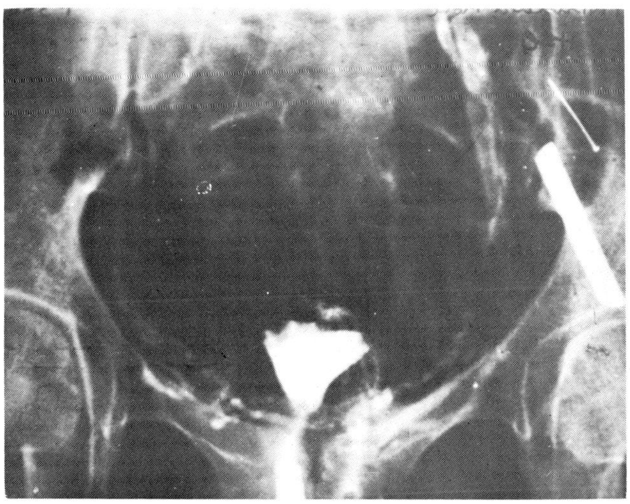

Fig. 33.20. HSG. Irregular cavity with cornual filling defects with bilateral block. Intravasation of dye seen. Genital TB.

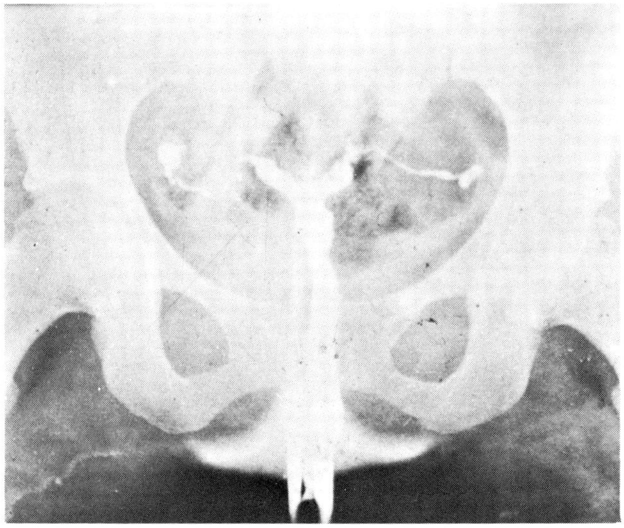

Fig. 33.21. HSG. Irregular uterine margins with fundal filling defect with bilateral terminal block. Genital TB.

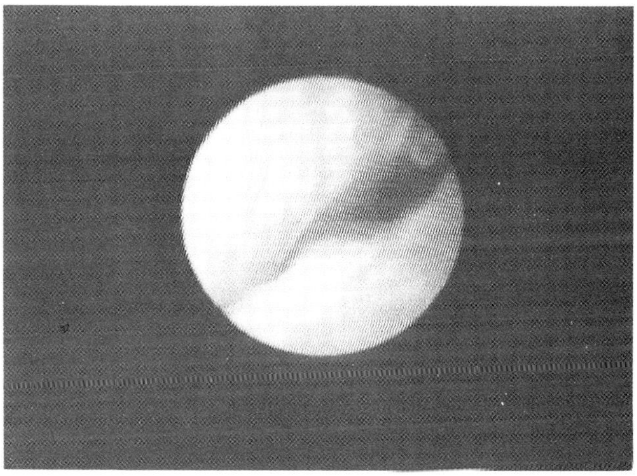

Fig. 33.22. Hysteroscopic view. Margins of a solitary submucous fibroid seen clearly.

Discussion

We agree with the published data of other authors in that hysterosalpingography is an important screening procedure even today for the study of the uterine cavity and whenever it is combined with hysteroscopy the two techniques are complementary in their application to female infertility (Figs. 33.27 to 33.34). Although transvaginal sonography in our opinion remains the primary imaging modality for gynaecological diseases,

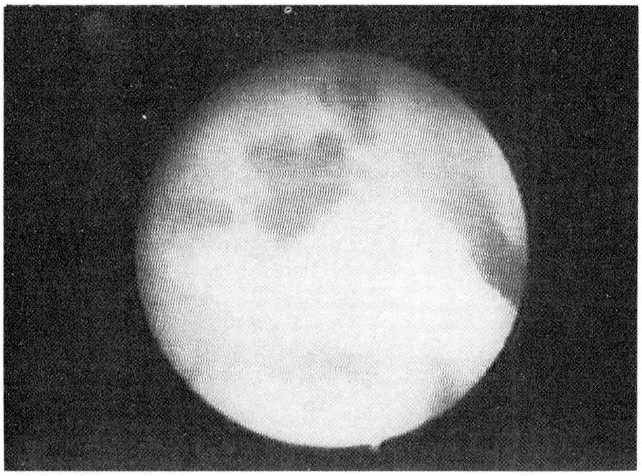

Fig. 33.23. Hysteroscopic view. Single endometrial polyp seen with few small blood clots in the foreground.

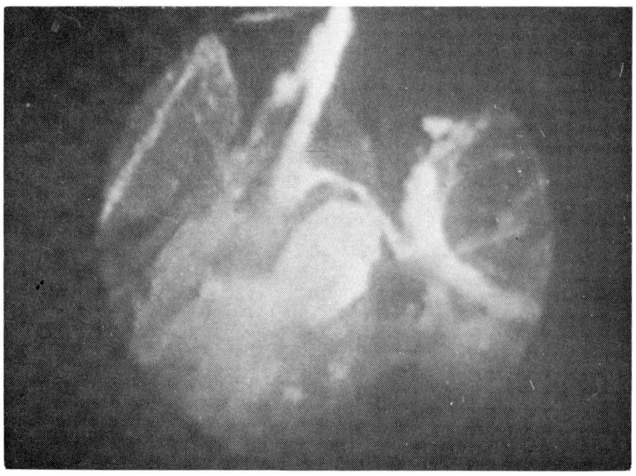

Fig. 33.24. Hysteroscopic view. Intrauterine adhesions.

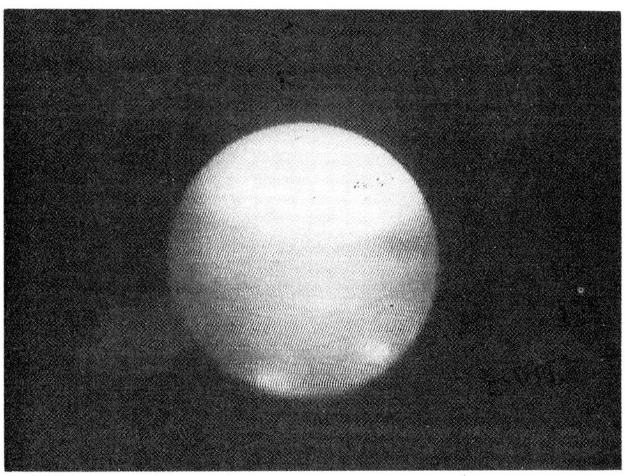

Fig. 33.25. Hysteroscopic view. Surface of a single submucous fibroid seen.

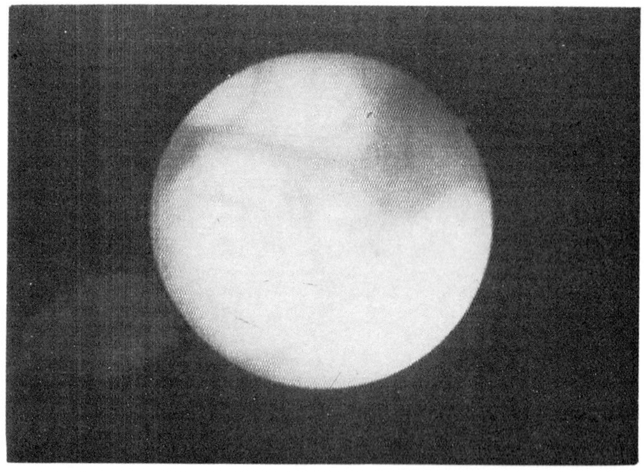

Fig. 33.26. Hysteroscopic view. Endometrial polyps with blood vessels running across their surfaces seen.

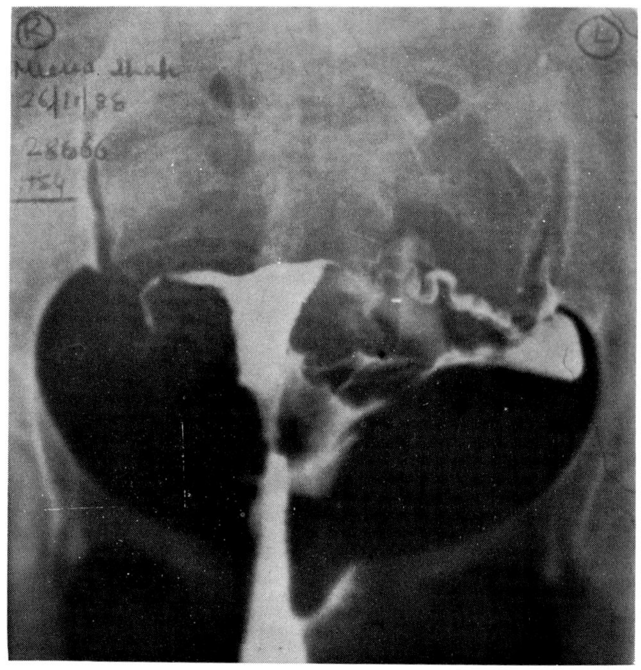

Fig. 33.27. HSG. Normal uterine cavity with left sided free spill with right sided midsegment block. Proved pelvic TB.

HSG is the study most helpful in suggesting the diagnosis of genital TB in patients being examined for infertility[12] (Figs. 33.35 to 33.40). The primary focus of genital TB is the fallopian tube. Spread from the fallopian tube to the uterus can occur in up to 50% of patients with tubal infection[13]. Plain films of the pelvis may show calcification of the tubes or ovaries. Although it has been stated that genital calcification is rare and must be differentiated from calcified presacral nodes, calcified uterine myomas, pelvic phleboliths and the opaque teeth found in ovarian dermoids[14], it is not

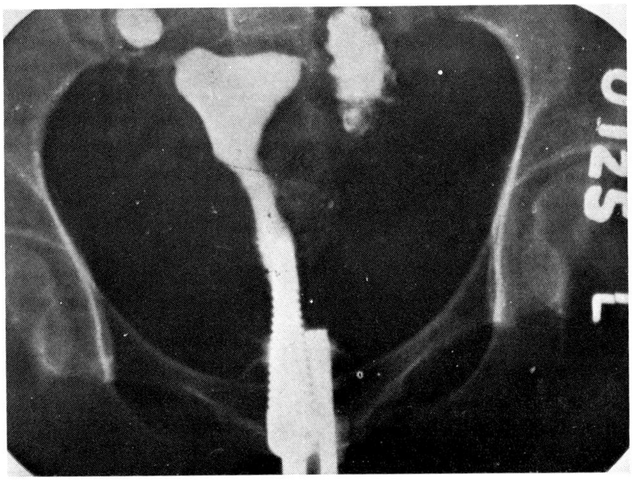

Fig. 33.28. HSG. Normal uterine cavity with bilateral hydrosalpinges. Proved pelvic TB.

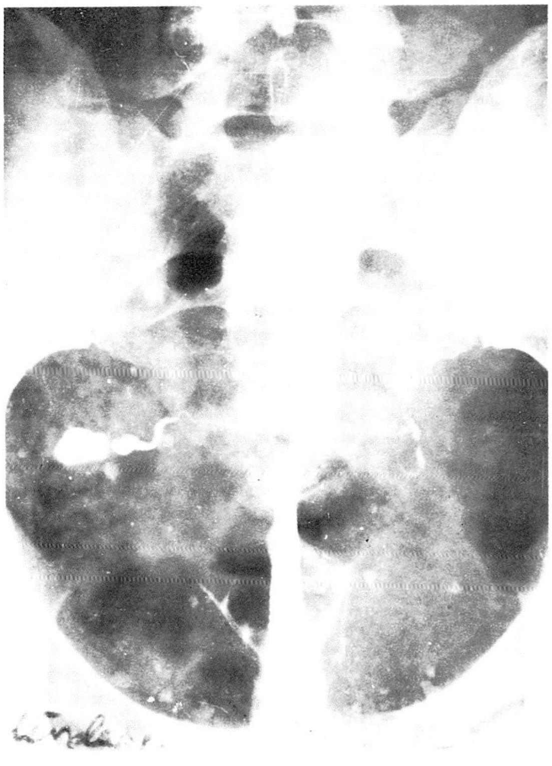

Fig. 33.29. HSG. Small uterine cavity with bilateral blocked and fixed fallopian tubes with right sided terminal hydrosalpinx. Pelvic calcification also noted. Proved pelvic TB.

so difficult to identify and differentiate such calcification, especially when it is tubal in location. Tubal calcification can take the form of linear streaks which lie in the course of the fallopian tube or appear as faint or dense tiny nodules. The former appearance is virtually diagnostic of tuberculous affection.

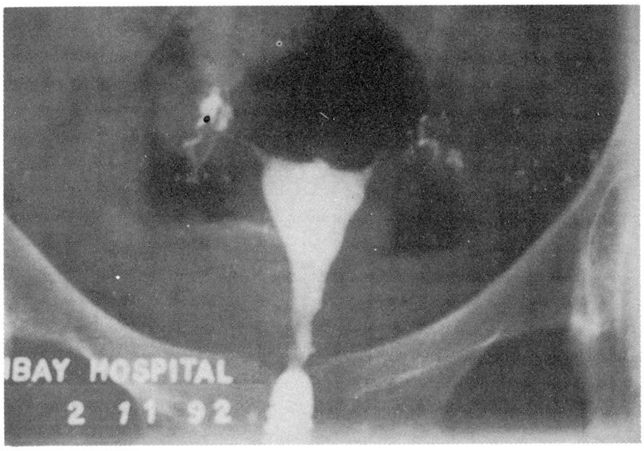

Fig. 33.30. HSG. Normal sized uterine cavity with left sided terminal block with right sided terminal dilatation and partial spill. Both tubes appear fixed and immobile with pelvic adhesions. Proved pelvic TB.

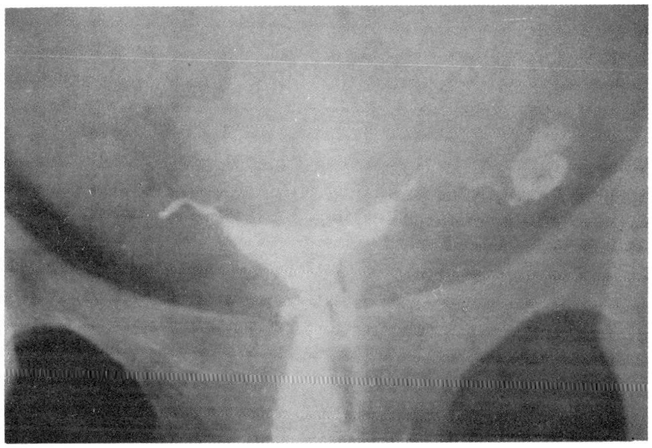

Fig. 33.31. HSG. Right sided midsegment block with left sided terminal block. Proved pelvic TB.

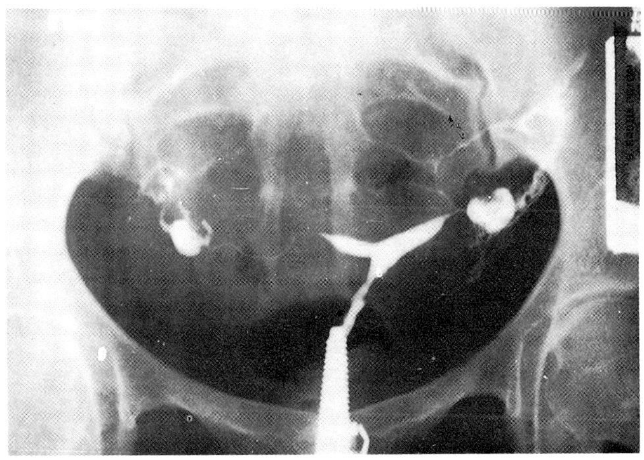

Fig. 33.32. HSG. Bilateral terminal hydrosalpinges with pelvic venous intravasation of dye seen. Proved pelvic TB.

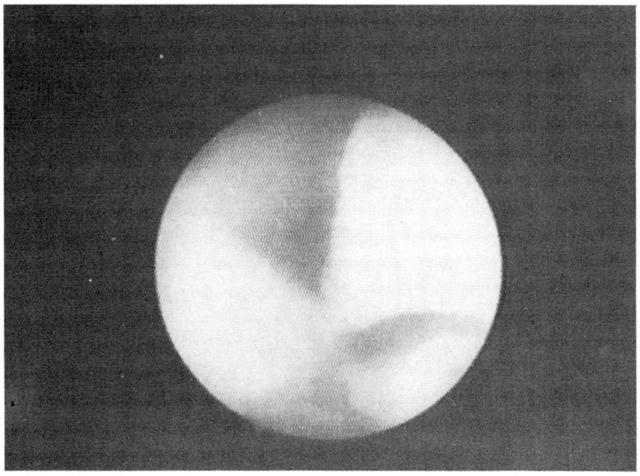

Fig. 33.33. Hysteroscopic view. Hyperplastic endometrium covering the left tubal ostium.

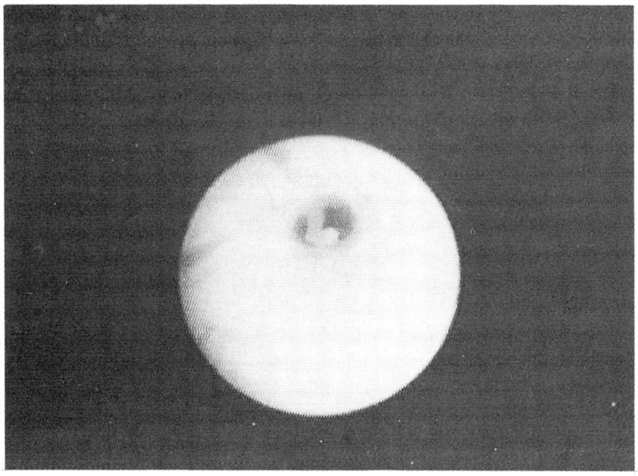

Fig. 33.34. Hysteroscopic view. Endosalpingeal polyps seen in the left tubal ostium. Cavity appears normal.

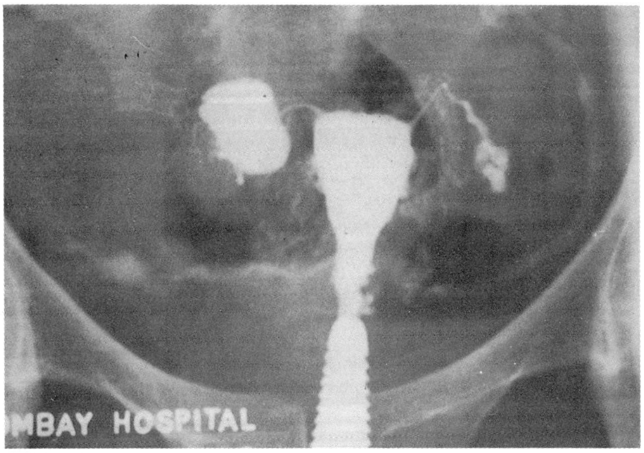

Fig. 33.35. HSG. Irregular uterine margins with right sided large terminal hydrosalpinx with left sided terminal block with pelvic intravasation. Proved pelvic TB.

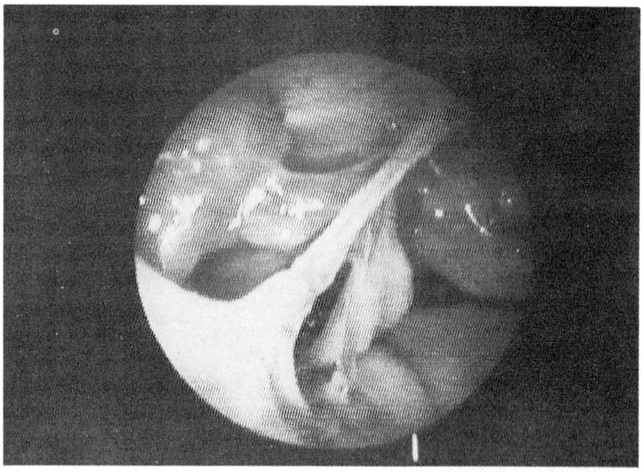

Fig. 33.36. Laparoscopic view of the same case as in Fig. 33.35. Pelvic tuberculous adhesions seen crossing the proximal portion of the right tube.

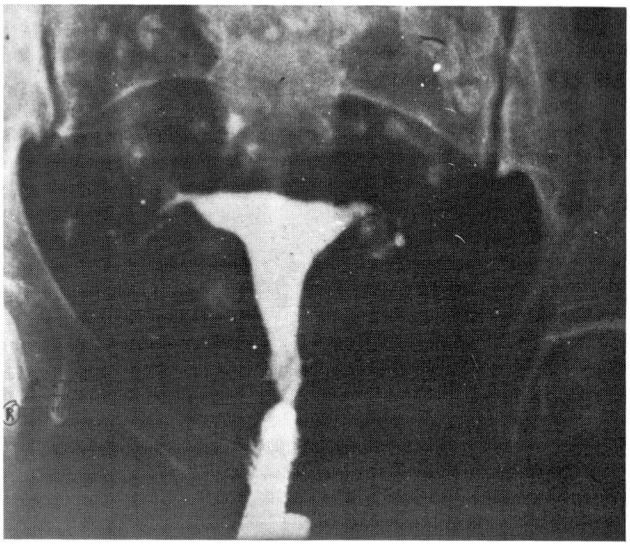

Fig. 33.37. HSG. Bilateral beaded and blocked tubes. Proved pelvic TB.

Tuberculous tubal abnormalities are almost always bilateral but not symmetrical[14]. Fallopian tube narrowing, occlusion and fistula formation have all been observed. Caseous ulceration of the mucosa produces ragged contours and diverticular out-pouchings of both the isthmus and the ampulla[12]. Although hydrosalpinx is very uncommonly noted in the western literature[14], it is a very common finding in our country (Figs. 33.39 and 33.40). Diverticular cavities may surround the ampulla and give it a characteristic tufted appearance. As TB heals, the entire tube becomes encased in a heavy connective tissue scar and the lumen develops a beaded, rigid, pipestem

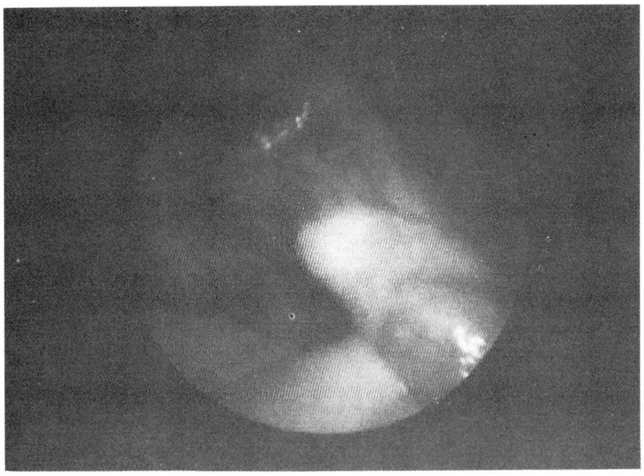

Fig. 33.38. Laparoscopic view. Close-up of the caseous deposit on the surface of the left tube in the same case as in Fig. 33.37.

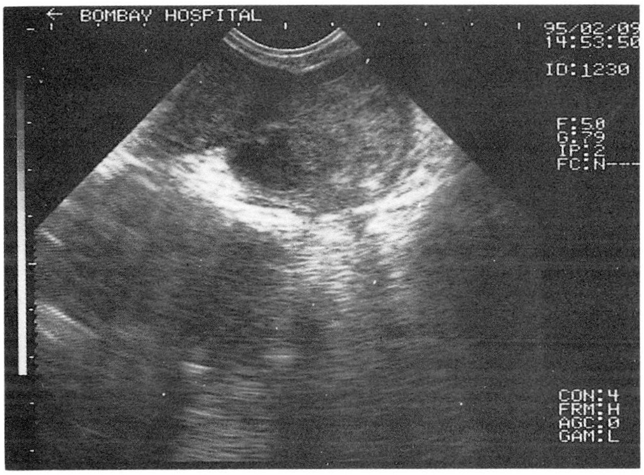

Fig. 33.39. Transvaginal sonogram. Tubo-ovarian mass on the left side. Proved pelvic TB.

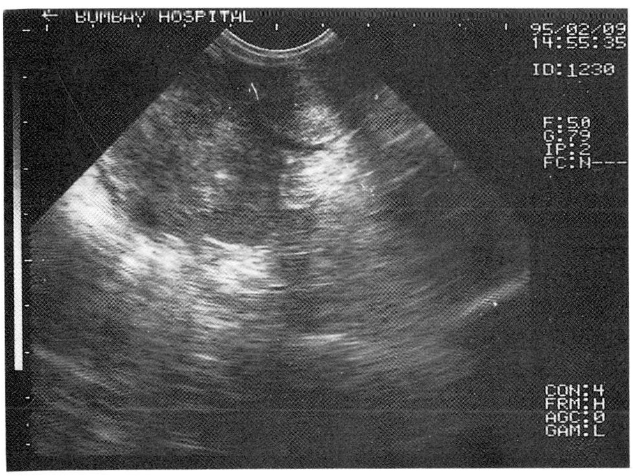

Fig. 33.40. Transvaginal sonogram. Tubo-ovarian mass on the right side. Same patient as in Fig. 33.39. Proved pelvic TB.

appearance. Isthmic obstruction is very frequent and is characterised by an irregular-patulous lumen. Tubal TB spreads to the endometrium in approximately one half of the cases. This has been reported to have a non-specific appearance on HSG, commonly characterised by synechiae, distorted uterine contours and lymphatic intravasation[12,14]. Synechiae or intrauterine adhesions are characteristically irregular, angulated and stellate with well demarcated borders. They present as filling defects due to adhesion or apposition of the walls of the uterus with failure of distension of the lumen. Adhesions vary markedly in their density and size, ranging from filmy adhesions to complete obliteration of the cavity.

Conclusion

The diagnosis of intrauterine conditions that may cause infertility should be made by a complementary evaluation of both HSG and hysteroscopy. A point to be remembered is that there is a negligible risk of infection associated with hysteroscopy[7]. This is in contrast to the significant infection rate of up to 2.9% associated with HSG[15]. Hence, all aseptic precautions should be taken when performing an HSG as it may well jeopardise the fertility status of an unsuspecting patient. HSG does not help to clarify abnormalities of tubal ostium function or shape[16,17] or confirm that ostial patency occurs only after excessive intrauterine pressure[16]. We recommend an initial screening with HSG; with hysteroscopy advised to patients with long-standing infertility. Hysteroscopy is a must for all patients undergoing workup for ART.

REFERENCES

1. Lindemann HJ, Mohr J. CO_2 hysteroscopy, diagnosis & treatment. Am J Obstet Gynecol 1976; 124 : 120-133.
2. Gallinat A. Hysteroscopy as a diagnostic and therapeutic procedure in sterility. *In* Siegler AM and Lindemann HJ (eds.), Hysteroscopy; Principles & Practice, Lippincott, Philadelphia, Pa, 1984, pp. 180-185.
3. Siegler AM. Hysterography & hysteroscopy in the infertile patient. J Reprod Med 1977; 18 : 143-146.
4. Taylor PG. Correlations in infertility : symptomatology, HSG & hysteroscopy. J Reprod Med 1983; 8 : 339-345.
5. Sciarra JJ, Valle RF. Hysteroscopy : A clinical experience of 320 patients. Am J Obstet Gynaecol 1977; 127 : 340-348.
6. Siegler AM, HSG. Fertil Steril 1983; 40 : 139-145.

7. Taylor PG, Hamou JE. Hysteroscopy. J Reprod Med 1983; 28 : 359-64.

8. Valle RF. Hysteroscopy in the evaluation of female infertility. Am J Obstet Gynecol 1980; 137 : 425-431.

9. Kessler I, Lancet M. Hysterography & hysteroscopy : A comparison. Fertil Steril 1986; 46 : 709-10.

10. Snowden EU, Jarett JC, Dawood MY. Comparison of diagnostic accuracy of laparoscopy, hysteroscopy & HSG in the evaluation of female infertility. Fertil Steril 1984; 41 : 709-714.

11. Fayez JA, Mutie G, Schneider PG. The diagnostic value of HSG and hysteroscopy in infertility investigation. Am J Obstet Gynecol 1987; 156 : 558-560.

12. Elkin M. Urogenital tuberculosis. *In* Pollack HM (ed.) Clinical Urography, WB Saunders, Philadelphia, 1990; pp. 985-86.

13. Greenberg JP. Tuberculous salpingitis : A clinical study of 200 cases. John Hopkins Hosp Rep 1921; 21 : 97-100.

14. Yoder IC. Hysterosalpingography and pelvic ultrasound — Imaging in infertility & gynecology. Boston : Little, Brown & Company, 1988; pp. 66-72.

15. Stumpf PG, March CM. Febrile morbidity following HSG. Fertil Steril 1978; 30 : 733-7.

16. Finikotis G. Abnormal cornual ostia & infertility. Aust NZ J Obstet Gynaecol 1989; 29 : 425-9.

17. Venturini N, Tantini C, Bargelli G. Hysteroscopy for evaluation of tubal ostium pathology. Acta Eur Fertil 1987; 18 : 61-5.

CHAPTER

34

Critical Evaluation of IVF-ET

Sadhana Desai

The data[1] show that more than 30,000 IVF babies are born since Edwards and Steptoe made world history with the birth of Louise Brown in 1978. The world collaborative report on the results of assisted reproduction released in the 8th World Congress of IVF-ET and Assisted Reproduction held in Kyoto, Japan, September, 1993 shows that in 1991, the pregnancy rate was 18.1% per ovarian puncture and the delivery rate was 13.5%. 760 centres from 46 countries participated in the study. A total of 138,238 ovum pickups were performed and 19,319 IVF deliveries took place in one year (1991)[2]. Our own results are elaborated in Table 34.1.

Table 34.1. IVF-ET results (1989-1992) Fertility Clinic, Bombay

No. of ovum pickups (OPU)	1033
No. of embryo transfers (ET)	901
No. of oocytes obtained	12,598
No. of embryos transferred	2,268
No. of clinical pregnancies	252
Preg. rate/OPU	24.39%
Preg. rate/ET	27.97%

The main indication for IVF-ET remains blocked fallopian tubes or altered tubal function. With passage of time the indications for doing IVF-ET are changing and the treatment of IVF-ET is getting simplified (Tables 34.2 and 34.3).

The use of GnRH analogues in induction of controlled ovarian stimulation has made monitoring of the cycle much more convenient and the ultrasound-guided oocyte recovery technique has made IVF-ET into an ambulatory procedure. Results of IVF-ET are improving every year (Table 34.4). The results get further improved by frozen embryos[3].

In considering the success of IVF-ET one must consider the age of the woman (Table 34.5), number of embryos transferred (Table 34.6) and the cumulative delivery rate after at least four treatment cycles (Table

Table 34.2. Indications of IVF-ET (1989-1991) — Fertility Clinic, Bombay

	No. of OPU	*No. of pregnancies*	*% of pregnancies*
Tubal	400 (60.6%)	89	22.5
T.B.	67	12	
Endometriosis	90	20	22.2
Unexplained	87	24	27.5
Male	43	6	13.9
Failed induction	21	11	52.3
Failed AID	19	3	15.7
	660	153	

Table 34.3. Oocyte donation (Types of ovarian failure and pregnancy) Fertility Clinic, Bombay

Type of failure	*No. of patients*	*Pregnancies*
Primary ovarian failure	7	6
Secondary ovarian failure	22	8
with amenorrhoea	6	0
with irregular periods	6	2
menopausal	10	6

Table 34.4. Fertility Clinic results

	Other protocols	*Use of GnRH analogues*	
	1987-1988	*1989*	*1990*
Cycles	120	150	233
No. of oocytes	6.3	11.4	12.9
No. of embryos	4	6.5	7
Cleaving embryos	3.2	5.6	6.6
Pregnancies	10%	21.3%	23.6%

Table 34.5. Age and pregnancy wastage (IVF-ET) Fertility Clinic, Bombay (1989-91)

Age	*OPU*	*Pregnancy*	*Preg/OPU*	*Abortions*
20-29	186	55	(29.5%)	9 (16.3%)
30-35	364	81	(22.5%)	25 (30.8%)
36-42	156	24	(15.3%)	10 (41.6%)

34.7). The delivery rate declines after 35 years of age. The cumulative delivery rate is 40% after four treatment cycles[4].

Table 34.6. Embryo transfer (1989-91) Fertility Clinic, Bombay

	No.	*Pregnancies*	*Percentage*
1-3	166	26	15.6
4-6	390	114	29.2
> 6	23	6	26.0
	579	146	25.2

Table 34.7. IVF pregnancies (1989-91)

	No. of patients	*No. of pregnancies*
One attempt	523	134
Repeat attempt	55	12
Replacement of frozen embryos	100	7
Total	578	153 (26.4%/patient)

Absolute indications of IVF-ET

At present the absolute indications for doing IVF-ET are in women with absent fallopian tubes or irreparably blocked fallopian tubes, women with frozen pelvis, women with ovarian failure or absent uterus, men with severe oligoasthenoteratozoospermia and congenital absence of vas deferens[5]. Genital tuberculosis is also an indication for IVF-ET in developing countries (Table 34.8).

Table 34.8. Results of IVF-ET in genital T.B.

No. of patients	54
No. of attempts	74
No. of clinical pregnancies	14*
No. of bioclinical pregnancies	1

27.7%/patient and 20.2%/OPU

* 1 ectopic, 1 abortion, 12 deliveries

Egg and embryo donation have given new hope to women well past their reproductive period. Micromanipulation techniques such as SUZI (Sub zonal insemination) or ICSI (intra cytoplasmic sperm injection) finally offer a treatment to all kinds of male infertility including severe degrees of oligoasthenoteratozoospermia where the sperm count is 0.5 millions/ml and are not acceptable for conventional IVF treatment. With ICSI, artificial insemination with donor sperm can only be restricted to the most resistant cases of complete azoospermia.

In couples where azoospermia is present due to the congenital absence of vas deferens, sperms can be aspirated from the caput of epididymis or testes and used for either conventional IVF-ET procedures or by micromanipulation[6]. A pregnancy rate of 14% per pickup and 28% per transfer in 2916 cases of congenital absence of vas deferens (CAVD) was reported by Asch in the 8th World Congress of IVF-ET in Japan, 1993[2].

Relative indications for IVF-ET

Relative indications for IVF-ET are women with long-standing infertility where conventional medical and surgical treatments have failed to achieve pregnancy. In considering the relative indications for IVF-ET one must consider the age of the woman, the type of treatment and duration of treatment taken in the past, local experience and success rate of IVF-ET (not international experience), risks and potential hazards of IVF versus that of conventional surgical or medical treatment offered, the wish of the couple and the cost of treatment offered.

Altered tubal function

It is found that women with history of previous tuboplasty, women having distal tubal diseases (other than those requiring adhesiolysis or fimbrioplasty), have poor pregnancy rate following microsurgery. In these cases IVF should be considered complementary and not competitive to surgical treatment.

Unexplained infertility

The chances of women conceiving spontaneously after five years of unexplained infertility are only one percent per cycle[6]. If a patient fails to conceive after 3-4 cycles of controlled ovarian stimulation and intrauterine inseminations (COH + IUI), she should be considered for IVF-ET/GIFT treatment. In women with unexplained infertility, IVF-ET is not only therapeutic but also a diagnostic tool as it gives an insight into the quality of oocytes and sperms.

Endometriosis

Women with early endometriosis having a normal anatomy of reproductive organs are to be treated like women with unexplained infertility. Women with severe endometriosis who fail to conceive after surgical or medical therapy, women having a frozen pelvis or elderly women with endometriosis should be considered for IVF-ET. Inclusion of GnRH analogues (long protocol) in ovarian stimulation improves the pregnancy rate in these group of women.

Failed AID or failed induction of ovulation

Women with anovulatory cycles and women requiring donor inseminations have better chances of success with IVF-ET than women with associated endometriosis or altered tubal function[7].

Contraindications for IVF-ET

Emotionally and psychologically unstable couples, elderly women with history of hypertension, diabetes or risk of thromboembolism should be discouraged to undergo IVF-ET. Severe intrauterine adhesions are also a contraindication for IVF-ET.

Conclusion

Credible advances in therapeutic treatments of infertility have occurred. One has to use discretion in selecting the treatment modality keeping in mind the best interest of the patient.

REFERENCES

1. Nazar A, Shaw R. A critical appraisal of assisted reproduction techniques. Hum Reprod 1993; 8 : 168-173.
2. 1991 results from the Society for Assisted Reproductive Technology generated from The American Fertility Society Registry, Society for Assisted Reproductive Technology, The American Fertility Society, Birmingham, Alabama. Fertil Steril 1993; 59 : 956-62.
3. Hammitt DG, Syrop CH. Comparison of concurrent pregnancy rates for in vitro fertilization — embryo transfer, pronuclear stage embryo transfer and gamete intra-fallopian transfer. Hum Reprod 1990; 5 : 947-54.
4. Trounson O, Alan J, Wood C. IVF and related technology, the present and the future. Med J Australia 1993; 158 : 2-6.
5. Hull MGR, Fahy U. Expectations of assisted conception for infertility. BMJ 1992; 304 : 1465-9.
6. Craft I. Factors affecting the outcome of assisted conception. Br Med Bulletin 1990; 40 : 769-82.
7. March M, Charles U. Update : The teratogenic effects of ovulatory agents. Endo Fertil Forum 1988; 11 : 1-6.

CHAPTER

35

Medically Assisted Procreation : Current Scenario and Needs for the Future

M.R. Bharucha

Introduction

There have been dramatic developments in the investigation and treatment of infertility in the last 20 years or so. These developments have been in such diverse areas as surgery, culture media, endoscopic instrumentation, male factor infertility, surrogacy, microassisted fertilization, reproductive endocrinology, etc. Techniques are being continuously refined and higher success rates are being achieved every day. Thousands of children have taken birth through these techniques. With most techniques, there have been no genetic deformities. Children born through these techniques have been known to lead a normal life. One of the reasons for the rapid proliferation of this modern technology has been the public interest, which doubtlessly has been inspired by improving success rates.

Medically assisted procreation or conception has many ramifications. It has opened new vistas in the field of reproductive endocrinology, genetics, pre-natal diagnosis, fertility control, genetic manipulation of human gametes, etc., and time is not far off when the human ovary and testes will be genetically manipulated to produce results as per need of the hour.

The etiology of infertility is of paramount importance, besides age of the female, for designing the therapeutic model for each couple. Regardless of the diagnosis, infertility is a problem of the couple and not of the individual partner. Approximately about 8-10% of couples experience some form of infertility during their reproductive lives.

Psychological aspects

The process of investigations and treatment of infertility have profound impact on the life of the infertile couple. It can provoke complex psychosocial problems in either or both partners. There is considerable concern among experts in the field about the type of feelings experienced by these couples. Menning has said that there is developmental regression of reactions like disbelief, denial, anger, isolation, guilt, grief and resolution.

Infertility may be confronted by the couples with a feeling of impotence and frustration. The female is often looked down as being responsible for the problem. For many, it affects the most productive years of life. Inability to procreate and the process of diagnosis and treatment together bring a lot of stress on both the partners and this may further complicate the issue. Stress is often seen in the way of response to various investigative procedures and treatment. Appropriate counselling by a trained professional in this field may provide the necessary safety valve to overcome their barriers.

Social, ethical and legal issues

Certain fundamental issues need to be addressed while considering medically assisted conception (MAC) for a couple. These are : respect for the human dignity, security of the genetic material, quality of services offered, and so on. Such medical procedures as embryo cryopreservation, embryo reduction, donor insemination, donor egg or donor embryo programmes, surrogacy, senile parenthood have attracted indulgence from the orthodox including the clergy. There is an urgent need to integrate services offered to the infertile couple in the National Health Care Policy. Various possibilities of human gametes and oocytes being manipulated during and after the lifetime of the progenitor in areas of banking, selecting, freezing, splitting and transferring, raise the issue of security of the human material down to the very DNA of the human cell.

Quality of service

Top priority must be given to the quality of services offered to the infertile. Accessibility, medical and economic criteria for its application, standardization of procedures and equipment, adequate training of the staff, etc., deserve attention.

A certain degree of disciplined approach is needed for improvement in quality of services. Needless to say that if the consumer does not get what he pays for, the science of infertility, and especially MAC services may get a serious jolt. The approach may be on the following lines :

- Self regulation in the development of new techniques.
- Auditing and accreditation of services offered to ensure quality and record-keeping.
- Promotion of a scheme to allow data exchange both within the country and at international level.

Medically assisted procreation or conception involves a number of techniques and procedures, commonly practised amongst which are ovulation induction, artificial insemination with or without husband or donor semen [AIH (D)], gamete intrafallopian transfer (GIFT), and similar techniques, in vitro fertilization/ embryo transfer (IVF/ET), donor oocyte and donor embryo programmes, and the more recently developed microassisted fertilization techniques. These will be discussed individually.

Ovulation induction

The technique of inducing ovulation in anovulatory subjects has achieved remarkable progress. Most of the anovulatory disorders such as ovulatory dysfunction (Group II, WHO) including the most common one polycystic ovarian disease (PCOD), hypogonadotropic hypogonadism, hyperprolactinaemia (HPRL), etc., are reversible. Modern ovulation inducing agents like clomiphene citrate (CC), human menopausal gonadotropin (hMG), pure follicle stimulating hormone (pFSH), the recently introduced in the European market, highly purified FSH, bromocriptine have been able to induce unifolliculogenesis or multiple folliculogenesis, as required, and achieve pregnancies. There is virtually no substitute for bromocriptine. It has been able to reduce prolactin (PRL) and induce ovulation in 95% of cases. In the remaining 5% it may have to be supported by other drugs like thyroxin (T_4), hMG, FSH, or even CC to induce ovulation. Bromocriptine is a safe drug and it can be used safely even during pregnancy, if it is found to be necessary.

CC (Siphene, Serum Institute) despite its drawbacks is undoubtedly the first choice in most cases of ovulatory dysfunction. Though it is able to induce folliculogenesis and ovulation in about 70% of the cases, pregnancy rates with CC therapy are significantly low. This discrepancy between ovulation rates and pregnancy rates is on account of the following :

(a) In many cases because of multiple folliculogenesis there is inappropriate rise of the gonadotropin levels during stimulation, viz., LH and FSH, leading to either lack of fertilization or subclinical abortion.

(b) Typical antiestrogenic action at the endometrial level leading to failure of implantation.

(c) The adverse impact on cervical mucus rendering

sperm transport difficult, leading to failure of fertilization.

(d) In women with elevated basal LH with or without PCO, it is unable to reduce the LH.

hMG (Pergonal, Serono) has been able to induce ovulation in women with hypogonadotropic hypogonadism in most of the cases. hMG is also being used by some, with or without intra-uterine insemination (IUI), in such cases as unexplained infertility and assisted technique procedures. The major disadvantage with hMG is that when it is used in higher dosage it may produce premature luteinization, and it has also been shown to produce dissynchronization of follicular growth with endometrial maturity, consequent to which the endometrium gets advanced and it becomes rather late for the fertilized zygote to implant. It is also one of the important reasons for higher early pregnancy wastage with hMG.

Pure FSH (Metrodin, Serono) is the drug of choice for women with PCO. This includes women refractory to CC therapy, and those in whom CC has not been used. The major advantages of pure FSH are the following :

(a) Produces unifolliculogenesis.

(b) Promotes synchronization between follicular development and endometrial maturity.

(c) Keeps the basal LH low or reduces LH during periovulatory phase.

Monocomponent therapy, *i.e.*, only the FSH therapy, is gradually gaining importance, not only in ovulation induction cases, but also in inducing multiple folliculogenesis in assisted techniques with or without hMG.

Dexamethasone (DXM) therapy helps in inducing ovulation in a certain subclass of women with nonclassical or classical adrenal hyperplasia, either associated with PCOD or unassociated. The dosage in most cases is 0.5 mg at bed time for 1-6 months.

Primary hypothyroidism leading to anovulation is amenable to thyroxin therapy. T_4 in the dose of 0.25 mg twice or thrice daily for 1-2 months may suffice.

Artificial insemination by husband/donor semen

AIH (D) is a popular technique used for inducing pregnancy in women with cervical factor, immunological infertility, unexplained infertility, and male factor alone (mild to moderate). Attempts have been made to induce pregnancy with the help of this technique in unstimulated cycles. However, greater number of pregnancies has been achieved with stimulated cycles with significant statistical differences. The stimulation in such cases is carried out by hMG, or FSH, or a combination of hMG and FSH, followed by hCG (Profasi, Serono). CC has also been used for stimulation for AIH (D), however, pregnancy rates have not been very encouraging. About 25% or pregnancies induced by AIH (D) are known to result in early abortion. Hence, luteal support in the form of hCG on D-3 and D-6 in the form of 2000 IU is preferred.

Gamete intrafallopian transfer (GIFT) and similar techniques

The GIFT technique first reported by Asch *et al.* in 1984 achieved popularity as it is claimed to be more physiological than IVF, as the fertilization and embryo development occur in vivo. This technique does not need an embryology laboratory. Intact tubal function as assessed by HSG and/or laparoscopy is an important pre-requisite for the success of this technique.

This is a process by which both female and male gametes (after preparation in vitro) are introduced into the fallopian tube laparoscopically through the fimbrial end, either in both tubes or in a single tube. The cycles are hyperstimulated to produce good quality oocytes. These procedures are employed in such cases as unexplained infertility, women with male factor alone, and in women with endometriosis. Insofar as endometriosis is concerned, GIFT is performed irrespective of the stage, but taking care that such subtle tubal factors as tubal convolutions, phimosis or agglutination, diverticulae, sacculations, and subtle peritubal adhesions are not present[1]. It has been observed in many studies that in women with such subtle factors, irrespective of the stage of endometriosis, pregnancies do not occur. Hence, these women ultimately go in for IVF-ET.

GIFT is also being used in oocyte donation programmes, for women with premature ovarian failure. The pregnancy rate/treatment cycle reported in good centres has been around 25%, spontaneous abortion rate about 24%, ectopic pregnancy rate about 4-6% and the multiple pregnancy rate is about the same as what it is with IVF when up to 4 oocytes are transferred[2,3].

Zygote intrafallopian transfer (ZIFT) first reported by Paul Devroey in 1986 in a patient with sperm antibodies, is another procedure similar to GIFT, performed in conditions as Unexplained Infertility, male factor alone and in infertility due to immunological causes. Results with ZIFT are better than with GIFT or IVF/ET in cases of unexplained infertility, ZIFT — 48%, IVF/ET — 22%, GIFT — 30%[4].

Pronuclear stage transfer (PROST), tubal embryo transfer (TET), and fallopian replacement of eggs delayed intrauterine insemination (FREDI) are other techniques with limited applications. Published reports are inadequate to draw any conclusions regarding their efficacy in terms of pregnancy rates.

In vitro fertilization-embryo transfer (IVF-ET)

This is a rapidly proliferating and developing technology with promise to achieve better pregnancy rates than those with natural spontaneous cycles today. The technology of IVF-ET is mainly indicated in the following categories of patients :

Female : Tubal factors
Endometriosis
Cervical factors [failed AIH (D)]
Immunological causes
Premature ovarian failure (POF)

Male : Severe oligoasthenozoospermia/ oligoasthenoteratozoospermia
Azoospermia (extension of standard IVF)

Multifactorial infertility
Unexplained infertility.

The selection of patients for IVF-ET is conventionally based on the following criteria :

1. Women above 40 to be explained clearly that their chances of carry home baby are poor (except under oocyte or embryo donation programme). Women with normal basal FSH have been known to be better responders than those with higher FSH levels.
2. Women must have normal uterine cavity. If any abnormality likely to interfere with implantation process is seen by hysteroscopy, it should be corrected, preferably in the same procedure, and their endometrial response to E_2 and P evaluated in a dummy cycle by endometrial biopsy and/or P levels and found to be normal (normal secretory endometrium and mid-luteal P $\geq$ 10 ng/ml).
3. Ovulation must occur spontaneously or be readily inducible.
4. The woman must be in good physical and mental health to sustain pregnancy till term.
5. Both the partners have been explained the reasons for IVF-ET and given the full background of various procedures involved and their written consent in the specially designed form obtained.

The entire manoeuvre of IVF-ET is composed of the following procedures :

1. Pre-treatment screening for diagnostic and prognostic purposes.
2. Controlled ovarian hyperstimulation (COH) for recovery of targetted number of oocytes.
3. Oocyte recovery, timed appropriately under ultrasound guidance.
4. In vitro identification of oocytes, sperm preparation and fertilization of oocytes.
5. Development of well-cleaved embryos and embryo cryopreservation.
6. Embryo transfer procedure (blind or under ultrasound guidance).
7. Post-transfer monitoring and luteal support.

Each of the above procedures is dealt with briefly.

Pre-treatment screening

The pre-treatment screening involves consideration of history of the type and duration of infertility, age, occupation of the couple, etc.

Indication for which the couple is under consideration for the IVF manoeuvre would help determine the strategy for COH and serve as a prognostic marker too. Ovarian status needs to be assessed by assaying basal FSH and LH along with basal ultrasound of the ovaries and the endometrium. Endometrial status may also be assessed in suitable cases by assaying mid-luteal P and mid-luteal or late-luteal biopsy.

Basic seminal parameters for assessment of the male factor form the necessary pre-screening procedure in the very early stage before aggressive line of investigations is planned and executed on the female. If impairment of the basic semen parameters in the male is observed, the male is subjected to further investigations for diagnosis and possible treatment. It is important to consider correction of these impaired parameters in the male, if possible, and give a chance to the couple for at least six months after normal parameters are established, to conceive in the natural way if preliminary clinical examination, history of the female and ovulation status are all normal. Hence, all efforts must be made to correct the male partner and only after this stage and the couple not managing to conceive for six months after that, the female is taken up for further and aggressive line of investigation.

Controlled ovarian hyperstimulation

This vital procedure based on a number of criteria like the indication, age, basal FSH, LH levels, presence or absence of the associated female or the male factor, etc., goes a long way in achieving success or failure in terms of pregnancy. Several protocols, most of which involving the use of LHRH analogue, have been in use. The correct strategy in stimulation, individualized for each patient, aimed at recovering the required number of mature oocytes and timing the administration of hCG such that the maturity of the follicles intended to be aspirated synchronizes with the right type of endometrial maturity, has far reaching implications in terms of establishing effective implantation of the appropriately cleaved good quality embryos and achieving clinical and a viable pregnancy. The selection of the actual embryos and the number of embryos is another important consideration contributing to the success or failure of the manoeuvre.

Oocyte recovery (OR)

Oocyte recovery, usually timed 36-38 hrs after administration of hCG is now almost universally carried out under ultrasound guidance, without anaesthesia and as an outpatient procedure. The laparoscopic procedure is hardly being practised. We have now progressed to real-time images on vaginal scanning capable of detecting minute cumulus-oocyte complexes in mature follicles. Even the ovarian and uterine blood flow can be measured by colour Doppler imaging. Ultrasound guided OR, started in 1981 by Lenz and colleagues gives the same recovery rate as the laparoscopic procedure with fewer complications and easier access to ovaries. The transvaginal route practised by most IVF units today has a number of advantages. It is easy to learn and use. The transducer is in close proximity to the ovary. Patient compliance without anaesthesia is assured. Before the advent of transvaginal technique, other techniques such a transabdominal-transvesical ultrasound-directed oocyte recovery (TUDOR), transabdominal-transvaginal ultrasound-directed oocyte recovery and transabdominal-perurethral ultrasound-directed oocyte recovery were also practised. With these techniques, patient discomfort, complications such as haematuria, inaccuracy in needling of the follicles with transabdominal probe, etc., have been frequent and these considerations have now given way to the current technique of transvaginal ultrasound oocyte recovery.

Fertilization of oocytes with prepared sperm

Mature oocytes, with pregnancy potential, recovered, are fertilized by prepared sperm and allowed to grow in vitro. Though the methods used for sperm preparation, insemination, culture of oocytes and embryos are straightforward, many variables intrinsic to the laboratory set-up are crucial to the overall success. Regular checking and maintenance of equipment, vigilance on media quality, culture conditions like maintenance of temperature, pH and osmolarity are all important. Normal fertilization of mature oocytes, observed for 12-20 hours post-insemination, is indicated by the appearance of two pronuclei. Abnormally fertilized oocytes, indicated by one, three or more pronuclei, and the resulting embryos are not transferred[5], delayed fertilization, after 20 hours, is associated with abnormal chromosomal arrangement in about 87% of embryos[6].

Embryo development and cryopreservation

Embryos dividing evenly, regularly and rapidly are the ones associated with pregnancy. Based on morphological characterization, embryos are graded as Gr. 1, Gr. 2, Gr. 3, Gr. 4 as under :

Gr. 1	Even blastomeres with no fragmentation.
Gr. 2	Uneven blastomeres with 10% cytoplasmic fragmentation.
Gr. 3	Uneven blastomeres with 10-50% cytoplasmic fragmentation.
Gr. 4	Uneven blastomeres with > 50% cytoplasmic fragmentation.

When more than 3 or 4 embryos are available for transfer, they are selected for transfer and the rest are either discarded or cryopreserved, or both, or donated as fresh embryos if a recipient is waiting on the programme. Embryo selection for transfer is done on the basis of embryo scoring in some centres and those embryos whose cumulative embryo score falls between 32-35 are known to give highest pregnancy rates.

Embryo cryopreservation technology is fairly advanced. It is a routine adjuvant to IVF in many centres. One to three day old embryos with one to eight cell cleavage are frozen in a controlled biological chamber with sub-zero temperature. Cryoprotectants like propandiol, glycerol, dimethyl sulfoxide, are used in the freezing process. Such embryos, after thawing are then transferred either to the same patient at a future date or any other recipient. Thawed embryos, before transfer at a later date, are assessed for their viability in terms of number of intact blastomeres and cytoplasmic fragmentation. Generally, frozen-thawed embryos with half the number of intact blastomeres, are capable of establishing pregnancy. The subsequent embryo transfer cycle may be a natural cycle or stimulated one or the one in which hormone replacement therapy (HRT) is given[7].

Embryo transfer

Embryo transfer (ER) procedure has hardly changed over time. It is carried out at 48-50 hrs after OR which is about 44-48 hrs after insemination of the mature oocytes. Most centres transfer 3 embryos to women up to 35 and 4 to those above 35, each at 2-4-cell cleavage for optimizing pregnancy. The stiff catheter, that is loaded with embryos and the medium (usually patient's own serum), attached to the tuberculin syringe, is introduced through the cervix so that its tip is at the fundus of the uterus. The procedure is performed as easily as possible. Leeton *et al.*[8] have classified transfers as easy, difficult and very difficult. Highest pregnancy rates have been reported in the easy transfer group. The ET procedure is usually a blind one, ultrasound-guided ET has not yielded higher pregnancy rate[9].

Post-transfer monitoring and luteal support

Oocytes, fertilized in vivo, are known to implant 5-7 days after ovulation. The embryos, developed, in vitro, are placed in the uterine cavity 48-50 hrs after OR. Hence, the embryos in IVF procedure are transferred relatively early. There is also asynchrony between the endometrium and the maturation stage reached by the embryos when placed in the cavity. Ovarian stimulation regimens lead to altered luteal function resulting in imbalance between E_2 and P levels. There is evidence that the luteal hormonal mileu in IVF cycles is different from the one in natural conception cycle[10]. Attempts are made to correct this imbalance by providing effective luteal support by either hCG or P, or both. It is suggested that the crux of the issue lies in establishing the right ratio of P : E_2 after the transfer. The dosage of hCG, dosage of P, the type of P used and the route of administration, all have the impact on the levels of P and E_2 and consequently the P : E_2 ratio.

Oocyte donation

In the last 5-8 years, centres around the world have set up programmes of oocyte donation. Pioneering work has been done by Alan Trounson and colleagues from Australia in 1983.

Appropriate counselling, ethical and legal issues involved, age of the recipient, thorough screening of the donor, future of the offsprings, etc., all need to be considered in their proper perspectives.

There are different indications for which the oocyte donation programme can be undertaken such as POF, gonadal dysgenesis including Turner's syndrome, ovarian failure secondary to chemotherapy or radiology, surgical oophorectomy, repeated failures with standard IVF procedure, carriers of genetic diseases, carriers of chromosomal abnormalities and poor responders to COH in standard IVF.

Commendable success has been achieved out of transferring embryos developed from donated oocytes, fertilized by spouse's semen or donated semen, and donated embryos, fresh or cryopreserved. Agonadal recipients have better pregnancy rates than donors. Pregnancy rates of 15%[11] and above per treatment cycle have been reported with oocyte donation and 24% with donated embryos[12].

Various steroid replacement schedules administered to both agonadal and cycling recipients along with the oocyte or the embryo quality of a young donor of proven fertility potential form the backbone of higher successes reported.

Microassisted fertilization

The world's first pregnancy with microassisted or microsurgical fertilization (MF) was reported in 1988 by S.C. Ng and colleagues from Singapore. Subsequently, the first live birth by this process was reported by Simon Fishel from Nottingham, U.K., in 1990. Ever since then, several techniques have been developed for the treatment of severe male factor who failed to conceive after standard IVF. The world survey of 1990[13] reported that the MF centres in Europe, United States, Australia and Singapore (as of August 1993) practise such techniques as sub-zonal insemination (SUZI), partial zona dissection (PZD) and intracytoplasmic sperm injection (ICSI) commonly. The other techniques lesser used are laser zona dissection (LZD), micro-injection fallopian transfer (MIFT), and microdrop insemination (MI).

The survey of 1993[13] revealed that the main selection criterion of patients by most centres practising this technology is the total motile sperm count (TMC). The dividing line between the 'male factor' and 'severe male factor' is still undecided, but based on recent data, one may suggest that the cut-off line between these two could be 300,000-500,000 TMC in the pre-treatment sample. Below this level, patients may be referred to micro-assisted procedure. If the recent successes with ICSI reported from world's two of the leading centres, at Nottingham by Simon Fishel and his colleagues in failed SUZI cases, and van Steirteghem and his colleagues at Belgium, are any indicator for things to come in the foreseeable future, it can be said that microassisted fertilization has come to stay and a new chapter in andrology has been opened.

Current research directions

The current gonadotropins used during controlled ovarian hyperstimulation (COH) are known to yield unpredictable responses with significant intercycle variations, possibly because of the presence of impurities like other non-specific proteins. Probably, recombinant FSH and LH could provide the answers. These highly purified substances may provide better oocyte recovery rates in poor responders and a better control in high responders.

Preimplantation genetic diagnosis is beginning to be a reality in the clinical setting. Embryos can now be evaluated before transfer for specific gene defects within the time frame. Gene therapy now appears to be a promising prospect. It can be logically deduced that the human genome will be sequenced and catalogued which in turn may make gene therapy limitless. Once the normal gene is cloned, the same gene could be used to treat all patients with a specific disorder. Further advances in genetics are likely to give us further insight into understanding oocyte loss by way of atresia of follicles, not only in natural cycles but also in conditions like Turner's syndrome and premature menopause.

The etiology of PCOD needs to be better understood. It is likely to turn out to be a genetic disorder. The possibility of ooplasmic transfusion from mature oocytes to aged or atretic oocytes may be extended to restore their functional capabilities.

IVF is an effective strategy for women with impaired tubal function. Work is on for artificial tubes. The rabbit model has shown promising outcome on short-term basis. Once placed inside the human body, it may provide a good chance for pregnancy.

Surgical treatment of ectopic pregnancy should be the thing of the past. Methotrexate, which may not provide all the answers, could be the harbinger of things to come.

As we understand the physiology of pregnancy and placental working better, it may be possible for a woman without uterus to bear pregnancy insider the abdomen.

Needs for the future

As a matter of priority, the implantation problem needs to be addressed. Implantation and endometrial reactivity are real problems today. The molecular events that lead to failures in implantation must be aggressively tackled and translated into meaningful outcome. There is urgent need to understand more precisely the window of implantation and the place of immunomodulation and pregnancy related proteins and the role of endometrium in successful implantation. We also must know the precise role of tubal mucosa in the early support of the embryo. There is also urgent need to reassess the role of endometrial thickness at the time of oocyte recovery as a marker for successful implantation as today's clinical opinion appears somewhat divided.

It is observed that today, 50% of the oocytes resulting from ovulation induction have abnormal chromosomal pattern[14]. We need to understand this phenomenon better for improving this important biological requirement.

Cryopreservation technology has made some strides insofar as the embryo freezing is concerned. Oocytes are frozen but the spindle and the zona pellucida develop defects. Chromosomal defects have been observed. This is another area where improvements are desirable.

Investigation of the species-specific sperm surface receptors for zona including epitope localization is of vital importance in understanding fertilization process better.

Most reports today indicate structural or numerical chromosomal aberrations on normal sperm, but hardly any similar studies have been reported on abnormal sperm.

Embryo development, in vitro, needs to be perfected. There are studies, small in number, which demonstrate that addition of platelet activating factor (PAF) to the growth media favours maturation of viable embryos. This is a potential finding as this finding is analogous to the observation of transient thrombocytopenia in spontaneous early pregnancy.

Advances in genetic technology have made possible precise diagnosis of genetic disease. It is possible now to remove just one blastomere during early biopsy and analyse for specific genetic defect. But today we have been able to detect these defects in only two of the more than 200 known recessive X-chromosome linked diseases.

Clinical reports on the role of pure FSH in improvement of sperm morphology are beginning to come in. Further large, randomized, controlled studies are needed to confirm this potential development.

REFERENCES

1. Fakih H, Marshall J. Subtle tubal abnormalities adversely affect gamete intrafallopian transfer outcome in women with endometriosis. Fertil Steril (1994); 62 : 4, 799-801.
2. Medical Research International, Society of Assisted Reproductive Technology & the American Fertility Society. In vitro fertilization/embryo transfer in the United States : 1987 results from the National IVF-ET Registry. Fertil Steril (1989); 51 : 13-19.
3. National Perinatal Statistics Unit, Fertility Society of Australia. IVF and GIFT pregnancies, Australia and New Zealand 1987, Sydney, University of Sydney, 1988.
4. Devroey P, *et al.* Zygote intrafallopian transfer as a successful treatment for unexplained infertility. Fertil Steril (1989); 52 : 246-249.
5. Plachot M, *et al.* Impairment of human embryo development after abnormal in vitro fertilization. Annals of the New York Academy of Sciences (1985); 442 : 336-341.
6. Plachot M, *et al.* Chromosome analysis of human oocytes and embryos. Does delayed fertilization increase chromosome imbalances? Hum Reprod (1988); 3 : 125-127.
7. Testart J, *et al.* High pregnancy rate after early human embryo freezing. Fertil Steril (1988); 46 : 268-272.
8. Leeton J, *et al.* The technique for human embryo transfer. Fertil Steril (1982); 38 : 156-161.
9. Strickler RC. Ultrasound guidance for human embryo transfer. Fertil Steril (1985); 43 : 54-61.
10. Hutchinson-Williams KA, *et al.* Human chorionic gonadotropin, estradiol, and progesterone profiles in conception and non-conception cycles in an in vitro fertilization programme. Fertil Steril (1989); 52 : 441-445.
11. Serhal PF and Craft IL. Ovum donation — a simplified approach. Fertil Steril (1987); 48 : 265-269.
12. Devroey P, *et al.* Establishment of 22 pregnancies after oocyte and embryo donation. Br J Obstet Gynaecol (1989); 96 : 900-906.
13. Tadir Y. Microsurgical fertilization : World survey, 1993. J Assisted Reprod & Genetics, (1994); 11 : 1, 5-13.
14. Wransby H, *et al.* Chromosome analysis of human oocytes recovered from preovulatory follicles in stimulated cycles. New England J of Med (1987); 316 : 121-124.

CHAPTER

36

Prognostic Markers for Successful Implantation in Assisted Techniques

Kamini Rao

Introduction

Any modern technology is assessed in terms of the results it produces at a workable cost. In vitro fertilization/embryo transfer (IVF/ET) is one such technology practiced all over the world for the last seventeen years or so, ever since the birth of the first baby, Louise Brown at the hands of Patrick Steptoe. This technology has experienced a rather bumpy ride, even from a few of its practitioners with a common criticism that it has failed to produce the expected results, not to speak of the costs involved. These critics, both from within the practitioners and outside, overlook the tremendous contributions, IVF/ET has made to other relevant and equally important areas such as understanding of the human menstrual cycle, the process of and physiological functions involved in, sperm transport, oocyte quality, the fertilisation process, the process of embryological development, the implantation process, understanding of pregnancy loss, etc., besides giving children to so many barren couples, who otherwise would have continued to remain with their miseries. No doubt, the actual results produced so far, in terms of carry-home baby rate are unsatisfactory.

In the complex technology as IVF/ET, we deal with a number of variables right from screening stage to the stage of establishing viable pregnancy and a successful term delivery, thereafter. These variables, singly or in combination with others, contribute, to a large measure, to the success of this manoeuvre. Correct understanding of these variables, in turn, could serve as milestones on the road to success. These variables or milestones could then be translated quantitatively and/or qualitatively and defined with greater precision. The observation of these variables, alternately described as markers, may help to predict success or failure of the procedure in terms of the desired results and may further contribute to achievement of higher success rates.

This chapter is an effort in that direction. I have reviewed my own data generated over the last few years of my experience in this technology in India besides reviewing the world experience in respect of these markers.

These milestones or the markers which indicate the prognosis, to be called, hereafter, as prognostic markers, can be broadly divided into two categories — clinical and laboratory. The clinical markers are dealt with during such procedures as the initial screening of the patients (both female and male), indication for which the patients are being taken up for IVF/ET, controlled ovarian hyperstimulation (COH), ultrasound (U/S) studies during COH, follicular aspiration, follicular flushing, embryo transfer and nature and quantum of luteal support provided. The laboratory markers constitute gonadotropin and steroidal levels, and assessment of basic seminal parameters during the screening procedure, gonadotropin and steroidal levels during COH, examination of oocyte quality, sperm preparation, the insemination procedure, the embryonic development, in vitro, and post-transfer monitoring.

In the interest of lucidity of presentation and easy comprehension, these prognostic markers are dealt with under each procedure during the IVF programme.

Initial screening before recruitment

History

Such aspects of history as age of the woman, duration of infertility, type of infertility like primary or secondary (previous pregnancy either through the same or another partner), genetic disease, previous failures in IVF/ET treatment, presence of tubal pathology with or without previous tubal surgery, associated male factor, etc., are all known to have prognostic implications on the outcome of IVF/ET treatment, to a variable degree. Age, type of infertility, duration of infertility are all known to have inverse relationship with the outcome of IVF. A Dutch study[1] over a period of two years consisting of over 3000 treatment cycles from five different centres demonstrated an on-going pregnancy rate per started treatment as 13.6% in women of < 30 years age and 3.9% in those with > 40 years. Similarly these rates were 13.7% in women of ≤ 3 years of infertility and 8.4% in those of ≥ 6 years of infertility. In women with secondary infertility the ongoing pregnancy rate per started treatment was 12.6% as against 9.4% in women with primary infertility. The overall clinical pregnancy rate/transfer in the study was 20%. These data are in conformity with data reported from other centres and from our centre in respect of these parameters.

Indication

The indication for which the patient is being take up for IVF/ET has an important bearing on success or failure. Women with PCO, endometriosis, associated male factor, male factor alone, are known to respond poorly in terms of pregnancy rates (PRs) whereas women with tubal factor, unexplained infertility (≥ 80% fertilization rates), recipient women with donated oocytes are known to yield optimal pregnancy rates (PRs). The Dutch study[1] cited above, demonstrated highest pregnancy rate per started cycle as 13.4% in women with unexplained infertility, 11.4% in women with tubal factor, 5.2% in male factor alone, in endometriosis it was reported as 8.2%. The French national IVF registry in their analysis of data from 1986-1990 indicated similar trend[2]. In this data analysis, women with tubal factor alone showed the cumulative pregnancy rate/transfer as 22.7%, tubal and male factors (spouse's semen) as 21.9%, women with male factor as 23.7%, and women with endometriosis only as 24.8%. Here the male factor patients have surprisingly shown respectable pregnancy rates. The same 5 year French data revealed, in these patients, the increasing cumulative clinical pregnancy rate, with 3 years age span, with number of cycle attempts, the highest being with ≥ 9 cycles. The glaring impact of the male factor on the outcome of IVF/ET is also evident from the report on assisted reproductive technology (ART) from the U.S.A. and Canada[3]. Out of the total number of 13,564 retrievals performed during 1991 in the U.S.A. and Canada in women < 40 years with no male factor, the number of pregnancies achieved was 3016 giving the delivery rate/retrieval as 18.0%, whereas in women of the same age group with associated male factor, the corresponding figures were 270 and 8.0% respectively. In our centre, during 1993, the corresponding figures were :

Number of retrievals — 323

Pregnancies achieved (no male factor) — 58

Delivery rate/retrieval (no male factor) — 15.40%

Pregnancies achieved (associated male factor) — 20

Delivery rate/retrieval — 7.10%

The question whether bilateral salpingectomy compromises ovarian function has remained unsettled. The analysis of our data indicates that in women having undergone bilateral salpingectomy,

the ovarian response to stimulation in an IVF programme does not appear to get compromised. In this regard, a small but elegant study by Paul Devroey and his team[4] adequately demonstrates that the pregnancy rates, implantation rates, number of days of stimulation, number of hCG ampoules used, pre-ovulatory estradiol concentrations, and the number of oocytes retrieved were identical both in the study group and in the control group.

About 25% of women with polycystic ovarian disease (PCOD/PCO) are known to go for alternate procedures like IVF/ET. The outcome of these patients with IVF treatment is highly erratic, they are known for either under-response or over-response. Fertilization rates and implantation rates are rather disappointing in spite of normal sperm parameters probably because of poor oocyte quality. Consequently, the clinical pregnancy rates are not so encouraging. The use of LHRH analogues (LHRHa) during COH with the objective of keeping high basal LH low has certainly improved the success rates in this class of patients.

Ovarian status

Though most women recruited in standard IVF programme are ovulatory or perhaps in some cases oligoovulatory, it is prudent to confirm their ovulation status. Further, their ovarian status is assessed by carrying out basal FSH on D3. If the level is < 15 mIU/ml, she is likely to be a poor responder during COH. Pregnancy rates are also better in the former than in the latter. In a large study[5] from Norfolk, the ongoing pregnancy rates were 17% in the former and 3.6% in the latter. These groups also differ significantly in their response to the stimulation. In the same Norfolk study[5], the mean number of follicles aspirated in the former was 7.4 (+/- SE) as against 4.1 (+/- SE) in the latter. The mean number of pre-ovulatory oocytes retrieved were 3.7 (+/- SE) in the former as against 1.6 (+/- SE) in the latter. In our centre, the corresponding numbers during 1992 and 1993 were 3.4 (+/- SE) and 1.2 (+/- SE).

Endometrial status

Assessment of endometrial status routinely during screening, especially in women with secondary infertility and repeated GIFT/IVF failures has been rewarding. Even in women with long-standing primary infertility with suggestive pelvic factor this must be carried out in view of the high incidence of tuberculous infection. This assessment can be made by hysterosalpingography (HSG) and/or hysteroscopy.

The small, unrandomized, but systematic, controlled studies by Frydman and Eibschitz[6] and Glass and Gollus[7] have adequately demonstrated the utility of this procedure as a routine. In the former study, in the unsuspected group, 21.8% of patients were found to harbour unsuspected lesion. When their lesion was treated hysteroscopically, prior to IVF the pregnancy rate of 10.8% per transfer was achieved. In the latter study, in retrospection, there was visual evidence compatible with diagnosis of endometritis in 22 patients and in 8 of them, chlamydia infection was confirmed by serology-titre of > 1/32. All 22 patients received doxycycline 200 mg daily for 21 days prior to next IVF. In this group, there were three spontaneous pregnancies prior to IVF and seven in the remaining 19 patients (28%).

Mid-luteal endometrial biopsy and/or progesterone (P) may yield useful information regarding possible existence of luteal phase defects. In our centre, we routinely perform mid-luteal progesterone as part of the screening process and if the level is ≥ 10 ng/ml, the patient is regarded as having no luteal problem. If less, appropriate screening is carried out and the fault corrected.

Basic seminal parameters

Assessment of semen parameters before and after wash, provides useful guideline to the likely course of the IVF treatment cycle. From our experience, it can be said that post-wash parameters give definite indication of the likely fertilization rate, the possible number of pre-ovulatory oocytes that one should target at and the number of embryos one would require for transfer depending upon the availability and the need for freezing of the embryos. This exercise enables the clinician to chalk out appropriate strategy for COH to achieve the targetted number of oocytes and good quality embryos, which ultimately reflect on the outcome of the IVF manoeuvre.

Controlled ovarian hyperstimulation (COH)

Selection of the stimulation protocol

In my well considered and candid opinion, this is the most vital part of the IVF programme, once the patient is selected and informed consent obtained. There are two important objectives, viz., obtain the required number of good quality oocytes to produce optimal rate of fertilization and consequently the required number of good quality embryos, for transfer and generate the most ideal endometrial status at the time of oocyte recovery (OR) for effective implantation. Achievement of both these objectives, to run concurrently, demands a high degree of precision in adopting the right strategy for stimulation, monitoring of the patient and judgement for timing of hCG injection prior to OR. Needless to say, therefore, that the stimulation protocol so selected, individualized for each patient, is likely to reflect the success or failure of the procedure in each patient.

In my experience, five important considerations such as the age, the basal endocrine profile (FSH, LH), indication for which the patient is being treated by IVF/ET, presence or absence of associated endometriosis and presence or absence of associated male factor determine the final option out of several stimulation protocols at the disposal of the clinician. Cyst, if present, may be aspirated, as per guidelines given later and stimulation for IVF/ET and associated endometriosis and male factor has been dealt with. The importance of basal LH is dealt with below.

Basal LH on D3 gives yet another useful marker which helps in deciding the right strategy for COH. This is regardless of whether the patient has ultrasonically proven PCO or not. Women with D3 LH ≥ 8 mIU/ml need a different strategy during COH employing LHRHa in short or long protocol. The need in these patients is to keep the LH low at < 8 mIU during COH. LH is thus controlled during periovulatory phase through the use of suitable dosage. It has been adequately demonstrated that in women with high LH levels (≥ 8 mIU/ml) during periovulatory phase, the oocyte recovery rates, fertilization rates, and implantation rates are low.

Basal ultrasound scan helps in detecting the presence of cysts. It is our experience that if the cyst is ≥ 25 mm and if estradiol (E_2) is ≥ 25 pg/ml, it interferes with the ovarian response to stimulation. Hence aspiration of such a cyst prior to stimulation is known to entail a better ovarian response to the stimulation protocol in our centre.

The secret of reaching four important benchmarks, viz., the targetted number of oocytes for recovery, targetted fertilization rate, targetted number of good quality embryos and effective implantation, lies in touching four vital milestones during COH and these are synchronization of follicular growth with endometrial maturity, correct timing of hCG administration, selection of the right embryos for transfer, and creating the right hormonal mileu in the endometrium in terms of optimal $P : E_2$ ratio at the time of transfer. These four milestones represent the markers for prognosis. Whilst the first three are controllable to a large extent, the fourth one is difficult as we still do not know what is the right ratio. But it is certainly known that the ratio of $P : E_2$ is important and not the levels of each hormone for effective implantation. Synchronization of follicular and endometrial maturity demands very high degree of precision and understanding of endocrinological aspects from the specialist and it is possible to achieve, though difficult in many cases. For selection of the right embryos, we follow the concept of embryo scoring in our centre and this helps us in deciding which embryos to transfer and which to freeze for donor programmes. For achieving the optimal $P : E_2$ ratio at the time of transfer, a great deal will depend on the E_2 and P levels at the time of hCG administration, P administered during oocyte recovery or not, and type and degree of luteal support provided.

The adequacy of laboratory support by way of optimal culture conditions, sperm preparation techniques adopted to get maximum morphologically normal motile sperm yield, satisfactory fertilization rates, and embryo development cannot be overemphasized. These are equally important requirements for optimal PR. Reinsemination of unfertilized oocytes, in our opinion, does not help and is not being practised at our centre. It may induce polypronuclear fertilization and embryos cleaving thereby do not implant.

Associated miscellaneous markers

Clinical

Hydrosalpinx. Women with hydrosalpinx have an associated risk for ectopic pregnancy and post-aspiration infection. Repeated IVF attempts fail to result in pregnancy but salpingectomy followed by IVF/ET is known to yield pregnancy. Hence, hydrosalpinx in a woman is associated with failure of IVF programme. A recent retrospective study from Sweden[8] on 254 women with tubal lesions recruited in the IVF programme reported significantly increased pregnancy and delivery rates in women with tubal lesions but no hydrosalpinx as compared to those having one or two hydrosalpinges. These results strongly indicate the negative influence of hydrosalpinx on implantation and pregnancy rates.

Chlamydial antibodies. Chlamydia trachomatis microorganism is commonly infecting the tubes and it is asymptomatic in 75% of the women infected, producing chronic salpingitis. These women remain infertile. There are very little data on the outcome of IVF/ET in this class of women. Reports about the future of these patients after treatment with IVF/ET are controversial. The Bourn Hall Clinic has reported[9,10] that the success rates in these patients are half that of patients with other tubal lesions. Later on, another study[11] from elsewhere reported no alteration in success rates in these patients with high seropositivity to chlamydia trachomatis. This study also reported failure of doxycycline therapy in these patients to induce pregnancy. Recently another Japanese study[12] has reported that the presence of antibodies (≥ 40) to chlamydia trachomatis in women included in the programme of IVF/ET does not influence the outcome of IVF/ET. Our own experience in our centre, though limited, also indicates that the presence of these antibodies does not adversely influence the outcome of IVF/ET. We have started screening suspected population only recently.

Follicular fluid

LHRH analogues are used widely during COH. Steroid levels (E_2, P) in the follicular fluid (FF) are known to be lower in those women who are on LHRH analogues as compared to those who are on gonadotropins alone. Despite these lower levels oocyte maturation is not affected. We have no experience in this area in our centre, though we use LHRH analogues extensively.

Encounters in stimulation phase

There is much controversy regarding the levels of LH, P and E_2 during the stimulation phase. There are data, for and against high levels of E_2 and P. Majority of workers regard elevated levels of LH after D9 of stimulation as being derogatory to the outcome. In our centre, we assay LH and P daily from D9 of stimulation. Our own data analysis confirms the derogatory effects of ↑ LH and ↑ P during the periovulatory phase. Regarding E_2, we have not made any study but we are inclined to believe that high E_2 levels (say > 400 pg/ml/mean foll. vol.) on the day of hCG may adversely affect prospects of implantation. Hence we try and maintain E_2 levels on the day of hCG at around 250 pg/ml/mean foll. vol.

Prolactin (PRL) has been known to get elevated during the stimulation phase and it has been reported that this elevation of PRL has no impact on the outcome of IVF[13]. We have no experience in this regard as we do not assay PRL during stimulation phase.

Follicular flushing has been shown to be associated with reduced PRs. Indeed it has been demonstrated to reduce granulosa cell mass, thereby warranting greater luteal support. In fact, the utility of flushing itself has been questioned. A prospective randomized study[14] from Liverpool demonstrated no difference in oocyte recovery rate, fertilization rate and PRs between the two groups, one in which flushing was done and the other in which no flushing was carried out. In our centre, flushing is occasionally done, we have no analysis of data to say one way or the other.

There are reports suggesting that there should be delay in comparison to traditional criteria in administration of hCG when LHRH analogue like buserilin is used. These studies report higher clinical PRs in subjects where hCG has been delayed by 24 hours[15]. There are not many studies to backup this claim. In our centre, we administer hCG by traditional criteria.

Endometrium and the implantation window

In spite of replacing good quality embryos, 85-90% of these embryos get rejected. Obviously, the endometrium is not receptive to these so called good embryos. Though we have lots to do still in improving the quality of embryos, in the present state of technology, there is much more to do for improving the endometrial receptivity.

Identification of the most important published studies through MEDLINE involving different stimulation protocols reveals the following :

1. The relative importance of receptive endometrium has been adequately demonstrated in agonadal women receiving embryos from donated eggs.
2. Widely used stimulation protocols frequently result in endometrial imbalance, the specific reason being unknown. It is speculated that supraphysiologic E_2 and P levels may be responsible for the aberrant endometrium.
3. The data gathered are indicative of compromised capacity of the endometrium to permit implantation at the time of embryo transfer.
4. Experience gained in agonadal women, with artificial endometrial cycles with hormone replacement therapy has been rewarding.

The day of embryo transfer

In the spontaneous pregnancy, implantation is known to take place about 5-7 days after fertilization, *i.e.*, on D17 to D19. Attempts have been made to transfer embryos during this period. Retrospective data analysis has demonstrated that maximum clinical pregnancies are obtained when embryos are replaced during this period. Further evidence to this effect has been obtained from studies on recipients of egg donation programmes. Many workers prefer to replace the embryos in the recipients on D3-D5 of progesterone administration during HRT. In our centre, we try to adhere to these benchmarks and we have succeeded wherever we could.

The window of implantation

Delayed rise in hCG in some GnRHa/hMG pregnancies is a known observation and it is suggestive of a delay in implantation. hCG, which appears in maternal serum only after implantation, is the earliest reliable detectable marker for implantation. Implantation time in vivo and the time of implantation after IVF have been evaluated by many using serial hCG measurements[16,17]. A study[18] reported from Chicago, USA, estimating implantation times calculated by regression analysis of serial β-hCG measurements between D7-D16 after ET, demonstrated that GnRHa/hMG pregnancies implanted between D7-D11 whereas hMG pregnancies implanted between D7-D9, after embryo transfer. The hCG regression curve for GnRHa/hMG pregnancies revealed a delay of 1.5 days in estimated implantation time compared with hMG only group. No significant pre-transfer embryo qualities or development was in both the groups. It was concluded that the GnRHa/hMG protocol widened the implantation window, which in part, may explain the improved pregnancy rates reported with GnRHa protocols.

Laboratory

A number of factors during processes of sperm preparation, fertilization, embryo development and cryopreservation of embryos are known to influence pregnancy rates. We shall deal with important factors only.

Sperm morphology

A number of workers have noticed a correlation between fertilizing ability and sperm parameters. There is good evidence to demonstrate that morphologically normal sperm offers the best fertilizing potential, whereas increased morphologically abnormal sperm gives reduced fertilizing capacity[19,20]. Hence the method employed to recover the highest density of morphologically normal sperm is likely to determine the fertilization rate which in turn may influence the PR. We have found discontinuous Percoll technique useful for optimizing recovery.

Oocyte quality

Oocyte quality is a very important prognostic marker to determine the PR. Different qualities of oocytes are recovered in the follicular aspirates — immature, mature, post-mature. It is the mature oocyte which has the highest pregnancy potential. Immature oocytes recovered, on prolonged pre-incubation period do fertilize. These embryos whether they give pregnancies is not yet known, because whenever embryos developed out of immature oocytes have been replaced, they are transferred along with other good quality embryos developed out of mature oocytes. Hence it is difficult to say which embryo has implanted and given the pregnancy. Immaturity and chromosomal abnormalities in oocytes have been widely reported. Oocyte quality is vastly a result of stimulation protocol. Post-mature oocytes, though fertilized, do not implant. Optimal oocyte quality, by traditional criteria, as defined by Lucinda Veek, are known to develop into good quality embryos and cleavage rate.

Fertilization

Fertilization can be influenced by a number of male factors, besides oocyte quality and zona pellucida antibodies, such as morphology, presence of anti-sperm antibodies, sperm acrosin activity, etc. Standard semen analysis has never been proven to be a useful parameter for determining sperm fertility potential. Sperm fertilizing ability has received attention from clinicians and scientists alike. The development of bioassays to assess sperm function at fertilization level has enhanced our knowledge of the interaction between the sperm and the egg. A number of tests have been in use. Sperm binding capacity to zona pellucida reduced in couples with male factor has been well documented.

Acrosin, a constituent of the acrosome is involved in sperm-oocyte interaction. Sperm devoid of acrosin have no fertilizing potential, and acrosin levels have been shown to be higher in fertile men than in infertile men. Acrosin activity has been shown to be correlated with the proportion of mature oocytes fertilized and transferred as cleaving embryos. The higher the acrosin activity, the greater the likelihood of potential success in IVF.

Female antisperm antibodies have been well implicated in female infertility and females with high titers of these antibodies have proven to be failures even in IVF/ET. Incubating the oocytes of these females, in vitro, even with albumin instead of using maternal serum has proved to be insufficient. It appears that there may be greater complexity to the problem of antisperm antibodies than the simple contamination of the serum and the follicular fluid. This remains an area for further research.

Embryo development

Attempts are being made to improve the embryo quality. Platelet activating factor (PAF-acether, as is known now) or an analogue substance has been proposed as an early embryonic signal to indicate embryo viability. Mild thrombocytopaenia has been a known phenomenon during early pregnancy in the normal fertile population. PAF is secreted by the growing embryo immediately after insemination. Many studies have shown that PAF produced by early embryonic development plays a significant role in the implantation. PAF has also been measured in the embryo culture media. However, this concept has yet to find its place in the practical laboratory setting and hence it calls for further research.

Cryopreservation

The first pregnancy following frozen-thawed embryo transfer was achieved in 1983 and the first live birth following blastocyst freezing was reported in 1985. Ever since then, there has been constant improvement in this technology. Embryos can be frozen at different stages of development like bipronucleate stage, early cleavage stage. The low rates of spontaneous miscarriage reported could be due to a number of reasons, but principally, could be attributed to replacement in unstimulated cycle and the tendency of maternal age to be lower. The most common approach in ovulating women with regular cycles has been to transfer the embryos in natural cycle. Rarely has there been a need for cancelling a cycle for lack of follicular or estrogenic response in the natural cycle. Some centres follow an HRT type regimen with slight modification from what is followed in oocyte donation programme, with the view to achieving temporary hypogonadism and adequate endometrial response in women with both normal cycles and aberrant ones. One of the factors claimed to influence the embryo quality adversely, is the use of GnRHa in the generating cycle. However, remarkable similarity in pregnancy rates has been demonstrated in some centres between groups under different types of stimulation protocol in the generating cycle, with or without GnRH analogues. It has also been suggested that premature LH surge induced during stimulation protocol in the generating cycle may render the embryo sensitive to freezing and thawing giving lower pregnancy rates or survival rates.

Microsurgical (microassisted) fertilization (MF)

Different techniques such as partial zona dissection (PZD), laser zona dissection (LZD), sub-zonal sperm injection (SUZI), intra-cytoplasmic sperm injection (ICSI), microdrop insemination (MI), microinjection fallopian transfer (MIFT), etc., have been developed ever since this sophisticated technology was introduced in clinical practice in 1987 and gave the first live baby in 1990. There are arguments for and against, for the treatment of male factor infertility. A line between the male factor and the severe male factor has yet to be drawn, though discussions take place. A question is asked : Does microsurgical fertilization work at all? The first world review in 1991 by Cohen[21] demonstrated 69 clinical pregnancies following PZD (53 babies born) and 59 pregnancies following SUZI (11 babies born). A new wave of optimism has been created by ICSI, ever since the pregnancies were first reported in 1992.

Though more than 70 centres throughout the world practise MF, encouraging results are limited to a few. The most recent review[22] of results produced by centres practising MF indicates that the important factors affecting the outcome are experience, staff dedication "just for MF", good equipment, strict control of osmolarity, temperature and pH and above all, the superior results in standard IVF at ≥ 20-25% pregnancies/ET.

Conclusion

The practice of IVF/ET, both standard and applied, calls for standardized equipment, experience and above all dedication on the part of the staff. Systematic data recording and retrospective data analysis are invaluable and pave the way for further improvements. Various well-defined milestones in this rapidly developing technology have been dealt with through the world literature survey and my own experience in our centre in India, and abroad.

REFERENCES

1. Haan G, *et al.* Results of IVF from a prospective multicentre study. Human Reproduction (1991); 6 : 6, 805-810.
2. FIVNAT (French In Vitro National), French national IVF registry : analysis of 1986 to 1990 data. Fertil Steril (1993); 59 : 3, 587-595.
3. Society for Assisted Reproductive Technology, The American Fertility Society, Assisted reproductive technology in the United States and Canada : 1993 results from the Society for Assisted Reproductive Technology generated from The American Fertility Society Registry. Fertil Steril (1993); 59 : 5, 956-962.
4. Verhulst G, van der steen N, van Steirteghem AC, and Devroey P. Bilateral salpingectomy does not compromise ovarian stimulation in an in vitro fertilization/

embryo transfer programme. Human Reproduction (1994); 9 : 4, 624-628.

5. Scott R, *et al.* Follicle stimulating hormone levels on cycle day 3 are predictive of in vitro fertilization outcome. Fertil Steril (1989); 51 : 4, 651-654.
6. Frydman R, and Eibschitz I. Uterine evaluation by microhysteroscopy. Human Reproduction (1987); 2 : 481-487.
7. Glass RH, and Gollus MS. Habitual abortion. Fertil Steril (1978); 29 : 257-265.
8. Strandell A, *et al.* Hydrosalpinx reduces in vitro fertilization/embryo transfer pregnancy rates. Human Reproduction (1994); 9 : 5, 861-863.
9. Moss TR. Chlamydia trachomatis : importance in in vitro fertilization. J Soc Med (1984); 77 : 40.
10. Rowland GF, *et al.* Failure of in vitro fertilization and embryo replacement following infection with chlamydia trachomatis. J in vitro Fert Embryo Transfer (1985); 2 : 51.
11. Torode HW, *et al.* The role of chlamydial antibodies in an in vitro fertilization programme. Fertil Steril (1987); 48 : 987.
12. Tasdamir I, *et al.* Effect of chlamydial antibodies on the outcome of in vitro fertilization (IVF) treatment. J Asst Reprodn and Genetics (1994); 11 : 2, 104-106.
13. Pattinson HA, *et al.* Transient hyperprolactinemia has no effect on endocrine response and outcome in in vitro fertilization (IVF). J in vitro Fert and Embryo Transfer (1990); 7 : 2, 89-93.
14. Kingsland CR, *et al.* Is follicular flushing necessary for oocyte retrieval? A randomized trial. Human Reprodn (1991); 6 : 3, 382-383.
15. Dimitry ES, *et al.* Beneficial effects of a 24 hour delay in human chorionic gonadotropin administration during in vitro fertilization treatment cycles. Human Reprodn (1991); 6 : 7, 944-946.
16. Leeton EA, *et al.* Plasma concentrations of human chorionic gonadotropin from the time of implantation until the second week of pregnancy. Fertil Steril (1982); 37 : 773.
17. Confino E, *et al.* The predictive value of hCG beta-subunit levels in pregnancies achieved by in vitro fertilization and embryo transfer : an international collaborative study. Fertil Steril (1986); 45 : 526.
18. Tur-Kaspa I, *et al.* Ovarian stimulation protocol for in vitro fertilization with gonadotropin-releasing hormone agonist widens the implantation window. Fertil Steril (1990); 53 : 5, 859-864.
19. Pousette A, *et al.* Increase in progressive motility and improved morphology of human spermatozoa following their migration through Percoll gradients. Int J Androl (1986); 9 : 1-13.
20. Mortimer D, *et al.* Morphological selection of human spermatozoa 'in vivo' and 'in vitro'. J Reprodn Fertil (1982); 64 : 391-399.
21. Cohen J. A review of clinical microsurgical fertilization. *In :* Micromanipulation of human gametes and embryos. Cohen J, Malter HE, Talansky BE, Grifo J. (eds), 1991 : 163-190.
22. Tadir Y. Microsurgical fertilization : World survey, 1993. J of Asst Reprodn and Genetics, 1994; 11 : 1, 5-13.

CHAPTER

37

Intracytoplasmic Sperm Injection (ICSI) :

A Novel Micromanipulation Technique in Assisted Fertilisation

S. Ghosh Dastidar

Historical perspectives and review of literature

Micromanipulation of living cells is not a new concept. It was practiced to inoculate living cells nine decades ago[1]. During the last five decades, micro-surgical studies have been applied using living eggs of rat[2]; human[3]; and the mouse[4]. Most of the work to develop various techniques of micromanipulation using mouse eggs (which have a thick zona pellucida) was undertaken in the laboratory of Teh Ping Lin[5,6,7,8]. In order to perform micromanipulation, preovulatory oocytes need to be treated in a medium containing hyaluronidase enzyme (Type 8 from bovine testis, USA) to dissociate follicular cells and corona radiata cells. Chang and Bedford[9] first reported that such hyaluronidase treated eggs are still fertilisable. Most of the earlier studies with micromanipulation were not aimed at micro-fertilisation of oocytes. During 1970-1980s experiments were undertaken by Uehera and Yanagimachi[10] and Markert[11] to attempt micro-surgical injection of spermatozoa into egg cytoplasm in lower mammals. During the '80s, several varieties of micromanipulation were being attempted to assist fertilisation of human oocytes in vitro where husband's sperm quality and quantity was too inadequate for conventional in vitro fertilisation. While the initial methods like zona drilling[12], and partial zona dissection (PZD)[13], is almost abandoned, currently, subzonal insemination (SUZI)[14] and Intra Cytoplasmic Sperm Injection (ICSI)[15,16], are being practiced with reasonable rate of normal fertilisation, subsequent cleavage and pregnancy rate. While in SUZI, the damage of oocytes is relatively low, ICSI has shown higher fertilisation rate, even in patients with less than one million spermatozoa in the ejaculate or with no motile spermatozoa. Van Steirteghem *et al.* have reported higher success rate by ICSI than SUZI, in a series of 300 treatment cycles[17]. Moreover, ICSI confirms injection of single sperm in the egg cytoplasm and might benefit even those cases where SUZI has failed[18]. ICSI bypasses the final steps of fertilisation process like spermatozoon's binding to and penetration of zona pellucida and its fusion to the oolemma. Lanzendorf *et al.*[19] showed that human oocytes are capable of surviving the mechanical insertion of spermatozoa directly into the ooplasm.

Intracytoplasmic sperm injection (ICSI) : Introduction

In extreme degree male factor infertility, patients usually have a combination of multiple sperm defects and are known to have a very poor chance of conception. As already discussed even standard IVF technology is frustrating in severely oligozoospermic patients[20]. Though other assisted reproductive technologies have been attempted to treat male factor infertility, for example, Tubal Embryo Transfer; still the results are discouraging as the oocytes still need to be fertilised before transfer to the fallopian tube. Ng *et al.* first reported successful pregnancies in humans using subzonal microinjection of multiple sperm cells[14]. However, in this procedure, initial reports showed higher polyspermic fertilisation. Recent reports on improved fertilisation rate using intracytoplasmic sperm injection for severe male factor infertility[15] is encouraging. In a subsequent study of the same group, Van Steirteghem *et al.* reported significantly higher fertilisation and pregnancy rate in ICSI[17]. Thus, ICSI appears to be the most efficient method in assisted fertilisation using sophisticated micromanipulation available at present.

Indications of ICSI

1. Extreme degree male factor infertility

Most of the male factor patients have a combination of multiple sperm defects like very low count and motility and increased abnormal morphology. De Krester and co-workers have reported that such combination of multiple sperm defects in the semen significantly diminishes the chance of fertilisation in vitro to as low as 8%[20]. Thus, these group of patients have very little chance of success with standard IVF technology.

2. Previous failed fertilisation in standard IVF

Patients who have showed complete fertilisation failures in previous attempts in standard IVF technique are also candidates for the ICSI programme.

3. Failed cases of SUZI

Since SUZI has a lower fertilisation rate and it is obligatory that sperm cells have to be successful in fusion with the oolemma and penetration into the ooplasm, ICSI appears to have better prospects in such cases. Van Steirteghem *et al.*[16] have reported few successful pregnancies in cases where previous SUZI has failed.

Follicular stimulation for controlled ovarian hyperstimulation

The current practice of promoting multiple follicular growth by exogenous administration of gonadotropins is preceded by a long pituitary down regulation phase with GnRH-analogs to have total control over the ovarian cycle. Its use has been extensively reported[21,22] and has been associated with almost no cycle cancellation rate due to premature LH surge, which was a drawback of only hMG stimulation protocol practised in 1980s. However, chances of ovarian hyper-stimulation syndrome should always be borne in mind whenever a female is subjected to hMG stimulation protocol especially in cases where a feature of early polycystic changes are suspected. In short, GnRH-analog (Suprefact, Hoechst) can be taken as nasal spray or by subcutaneous injection from day 19 or 20 of previous cycle to desensitize the pituitary gonado-trophs. In our centre, we administer Suprefact sub-cutaneously as a daily dose from day 19 of previous cycle till the date of hCG injection. Multiple follicular growth is normally achieved with administration of human menopausal gonadotropin (hMG, Humegon, Organon, Holland). 150-225 IU of hMG are usually started on day 3 of cycle till adequate follicular maturation is achieved. The monitoring of morpho-logical maturation of follicles is performed by using serial transvaginal sonography using dual frequency (5/7.5 MHz) sector transducer and daily serum estradiol study from day 7 onwards. When two to three dominant follicles having transverse diameter greater than or equal to 17 mm are recorded by transvaginal sono-graphy and a serum estradiol level of around 1500 pg/ml is achieved; the stimulation is terminated and about 10,000 IU of human chorionic gonadotropin (hCG, Profasi, Serono) is administered. Oocyte recovery is planned approximately 34-36 hours following hCG administration.

Oocyte recovery

Oocyte recovery is performed using transvaginal ultrasound-guided puncture technique. In brief, a 7.5 MHz transvaginal transducer fitted with a biopsy guide (Fig. 37.1) is used. A 17 gauge single lumen aspiration needle (Casmed, UK) is used for aspiration of follicular

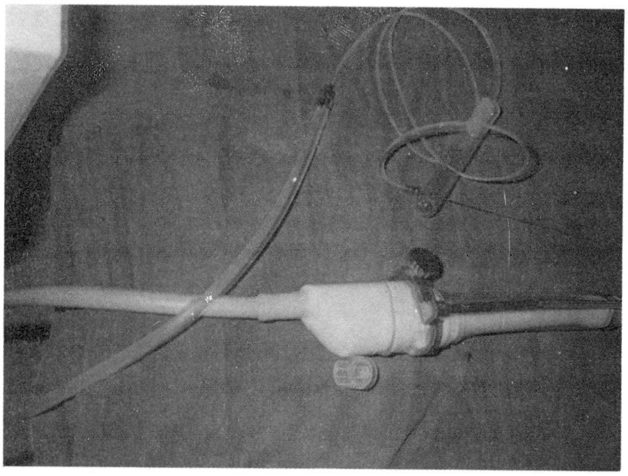

Fig. 37.1. Transvaginal transducer with guide and trap for oocyte recovery.

fluid. The negative suction pressure is kept around 120 to 160 mm of mercury produced by a foot-controlled suction pump (Crafts Suction Unit, Rockett of London, UK). Currently we aspirate 2 to 3 follicles simultaneously in a single collection tube. The oocytes are identified under low power dissecting microscope. The oocyte identification and handling are done as in standard IVF procedures. Once the oocytes are retrieved, they are graded for maturity based on the morphological study of oocyte cumulus-corona cell complexes (OCCC) as described by Veeck *et al.*[23] using an inverted phase contrast microscope at magnification × 40 or × 100. Oocytes are classified as mature (type A), hypermature (type A-1), slightly immature (type A-2) or immature (type B).

Preparation of oocytes for ICSI

The cumulus and corona radiata cells need to be dissociated for performing sperm microinjection. The cells are removed by incubation of oocytes for about 1 min in Hepes buffered Earle's medium with 80 IU hyaluronidase per ml (Type VIII, specific activity 320 IU per mg, Sigma Chemical Co., St. Louis, Mo, USA). Some centers including us, prefer to remove some of the cumulus mass by microdissection using 26 gauge needles fitted to a tuberculin syringe under dissecting microscope before hyaluronidase treatment. The removal of cumulus corona cells is normally done by aspiration of the oocyte complexes in and out of hand-drawn glass pipette with an opening of about 200 microns[16]. It needs to be mentioned that this handling should be done by a speedy but gentle manipulation to prevent any damage to the oocyte. Soon after oocytes are denuded of cumulus-corona cells, they are rinsed quickly in several changes of Hepes buffered Earle's medium and then in Menezo B-2 medium to remove the hyaluronidase enzyme and finally placed into droplets of equilibrated B-2 medium covered by light paraffin oil (International Medical, Brussels) and subjected to careful observation under inverted microscope × 200 magnification.

The oocytes are assessed by the following observations :

1. The zona pellucida is examined for its intactness.
2. The presence or absence of germinal vesicles within the oocyte.
3. The presence of first polar body in the perivitelline space. The egg cytoplasm is also examined for the presence of vacuoles or other abnormalities.

Egg incubation

The oocytes thus prepared are incubated at 37°C in an atmosphere of 5% CO_2 in air. All these oocytes are again examined at × 200 magnification using inverted microscope approximately 4-5 hours later to see whether more oocytes have extruded the first polar body. The intracytoplasmic sperm injection will be carried out only on morphologically intact oocytes which show the first polar body in the perivitelline space.

Semen handling and preparation of spermatozoa

Initial semen evaluation

All male factor patients are evaluated for their sperm count, motility, morphology and they must have completed basic treatments to improve either semen quality or have undergone intrauterine insemination for at least 3 cycles or one or two attempts of Gamete Intrafallopian Transfer (GIFT) in cases where sperm count is more than 5 million and having a progressive motility of 10 to 20%.

Pre-treatment semen evaluation for ICSI

The semen analysis is performed and the following parameters are recorded :

1. Volume of ejaculate.
2. Liquefaction time.
3. Presence of too many cellular debris.
4. Spermatozoa count and motility.
5. The sperm morphology is assessed by critical criteria described by Kruger *et al.*[24].

Sperm preparation

Isolation of good quality spermatozoa from the semen sample can be performed by several techniques.

1. Double sperm wash by centrifugation followed by swim-up.
2. Discontinuous percoll gradient separation (80%-40%).

However, no statistically significant difference in terms of fertilisation of pregnancy rate has been observed between these two different types of sperm preparation techniques.

Percoll gradient separation technique

The percoll gradients are prepared from a percoll stock solution (Percoll Pharmacia, Uppsala, Sweden). In percoll separation procedure, the sperm suspension is put on top of lowest density gradient. After centrifugation at 300 × g for 20 min. the bottom layer is aspirated with a Falcon (1 ml) individually sterile pipette (Falcon Plastics, USA) and placed into 5 ml Falcon tube. This tube is filled with medium and centrifuged for 5 min at 800 × g. The supernatant is removed and discarded with a Pasteur pipette. The pellet which is formed at the bottom of the tube is generally resuspended in 2 ml of B-2 medium. After this selection procedure the semen parameters, *i.e.*, concentration, motility and morphology are again assessed. If the concentration is more than 2 million per ml, it is diluted with addition of further B-2 medium to bring it to a concentration of 1 million per ml. This is checked by counting on a Makler chamber. However, after the percoll gradient the sperm concentration may be extremely low. In this situation a further concentration step may be performed by centrifugation at 1800 × g for 5 mins using a 1.5 ml Eppendorf tube. The supernatant is discarded and 5 to 10 microlitre of suspension is kept at the bottom of the Eppendorf tube[16]. The target is to assure that there are enough sperms available for microinjection in the sperm droplet. The sperm suspension thus prepared is kept at 37°C in an atmosphere of 5% CO_2 in air until the laboratory procedures for ICSI are ready to be performed.

Preparation of egg holding and injection micropipette for intracytoplasmic sperm injection

Egg holding and injection pipettes are made from 30 micrometre borosilicate glass capillary tubes (Drummond Scientific Co., Brumell, Pa, USA) of 78 mm length having an inner and outer diameter of 0.69 mm and 0.97 mm. The cleaning of these capillaries are performed almost on the same principle of glass pipette cleaning for standard IVF technology. First, these are sonicated for 30 mins in pure water (Milli-Q Water System — Millipore, USA) with 2% (volume by volume) tissue culture grade detergent (7 × PF — Flow Laboratories, UK) and then they are subjected to rinsing in running Milli-Q water for approximately 20-30 mins. These are dried in small glass vials with cap and then sterilised in a hot air oven at around 100°C for 6 hours. These capillary tubes are used for preparing either injection or holding pipette using micropipette puller (MXE 70174, Narishige, Japan). The holding pipette is cut and fire-polished on a micro-forge (MF-9 micro-forge, Narishige Co. Ltd., Tokyo, Japan) to obtain an outer diameter of 60 micrometre and inner diameter of 20 micrometre. To prepare the injection pipette, after the capillary tube is pulled by micropipette puller, the thin end is opened on a micro-grinder (EG-4 micro-grinder, Narishige Co. Ltd., Tokyo, Japan) to get an outer diameter of 7 micrometre and inner diameter of 5 micrometre. The bevel angle is made at around 30°. During the grinding the wet stone of the grinder is humidified by slow water drip during the process. This grinding step takes approximately 3 minutes. The micro-forge is used to make a sharp spike on the injection pipette. An individual laboratory may choose to have an angle at the edge of the holding and injection pipette. At present most of the laboratories including ours use an angle of about 45°. This will help the injection procedure in a microdrop on the petridish. Alternatively this holding and injection micropipettes can be procured commercially (Embryotech Lab., Ma, USA).

Micro-manipulation

Before the intracytoplasmic sperm injection procedure, the sperm fraction is added to approximately four to five microlitres of polyvinyl pyrrolidone (PVP) solution (w/v) in Hepes buffered Earle's medium. 10% PVP solution is made by dissolving 1 gm of PVP in 10 ml of Hepes buffered Earle's medium[15] and it is filtered through 0.8 microlitre millipore disposable filter (Millex AA, Cat No. SLAA-025PS). Aliquots of 0.5 ml are stored for use. Using the tissue petridish (Falcon Type 1006) 5 microlitres of sperm-PVP droplet is placed in the centre of the petridish and six to eight, 5 microlitre droplets of Hepes buffered Earle's medium is placed surrounding it. Approximately, 3.5 ml of lightweight paraffin oil is used to cover these droplet preparations in the petridish.

Micro-manipulation system

The intracytoplasmic sperm injection is performed on a heated stage of an inverted microscope to keep the petridish and its contents warm around 37°C. It may be emphasised that different varieties of high resolution research level microscopes are available at present. We have been using an inverted microscope from Nikon Corporation, Tokyo, Japan (Diaphot-300) (Fig. 37.2) and the magnification used is 400 ×. The microscope is equipped with a Nikon camera for still pictures and a video camera (Sony Corporation, Japan) with C.C. T.V. attachment. This is connected to a colour TV monitor (Sharpline) for documentation of the procedure as well as for teaching purposes.

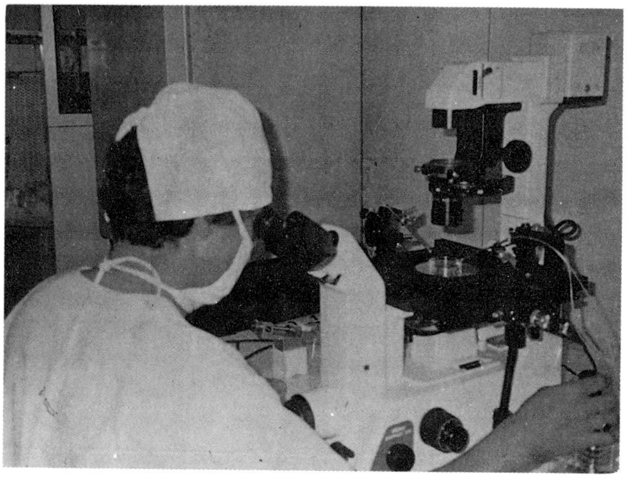

Fig. 37.2. Micromanipulator — fitted with TU Nikon inverted microscope (Diaphot 300).

The microscope is fitted with two course positioning manipulators (3-dimensional course control manipulator mm-188, Narishige, Japan) and with one, 3-dimensional hydraulic micro-manipulator (Joystick hydraulic micro-manipulator mo-202, Narishige, Japan). The micro-pipettes (holding pipette and the ICSI pipette) are fitted to a tool holder and are connected by teflon tubing (Narishige, Tokyo, Japan) to a micro-injector (IM 188, Narishige, Japan). The teflon tubing is filled with mineral oil using the syringe incorporated with the microinjector and either the negative suction or the delivery of the sperm (microinjection) is controlled via one microlitre resolution vernier micrometer using the syringe attached to the teflon tubing.

The ICSI procedure

After the installation of the micropipettes, both the holding pipette and the microinjection pipette are brought on the same line facing each other. Using the right sided injection micropipette, a single almost immotile spermatozoon is selected from the central sperm-PVP droplet[25] and is aspirated tail first into the tip of the injection pipette. By using the right-sided vertical knob (Diaphot, 300), the stage of the microscope is moved so that an oocyte in one of the droplets surrounding the centrally placed 'sperm-PVP droplet', is visualised. The next step is to fix the oocyte by slight negative pressure using the left-sided microinjector. It needs special emphasis that the oocyte is immobilised in a fashion so that the polar body is at 12 o'clock or 6 o'clock position. The microinjection pipette is mobilised towards the oocytes (Fig. 37.3 – Plate 10). It is important that the tip of the injection micropipette is parallel to the stage for proper visualisation of the sperm cell and its accurate delivery. The microinjection pipette containing a single sperm is pushed through the zona pellucida and the oolemma into the ooplasm by slow but steady pressure using the remote-controlled joystick hydraulic micromanipulator (mo-202) at 3 o'clock position and the spermatozoon is injected slowly. An indentation is seen at the place of contact and once the micropipette gets into the ooplasm, the oocyte again gets the original shape. Approximately 2-3 minutes are required for each microinjection. After the sperm is delivered with a very small amount of medium, the injection pipette is drawn out gently. The oocyte is briefly examined for its intactness and the negative suction is released to free the oocyte within the droplet. Similar technique is followed and all metaphase II oocytes are microinjected with single spermatozoon in a similar technique, as described.

At present we culture injected oocytes in B_2 medium (Inra Menzo B_2, IMV International, Minneapolis, USA). All injected oocytes are quickly washed in 2 changes of equilibrated B_2 medium covered with light weight paraffin oil. The oocytes are incubated at 37°C in 5% CO_2 air (Forma Scientific, USA).

Microscopic evaluation of injected oocytes

After the oocytes are subjected to ICSI, the subsequent steps are similar to our standard IVF technique. In our laboratory, microinjected oocytes are routinely examined at 16 hour intervals at 200 × or 400 × magnification under the inverted microscope. Special attention is given for detecting any visual damage to the oocytes and also the presence of pronuclei and polar bodies are noted. As in normal in vitro fertilisation, two distinct pronuclei are seen when fertilisation process is complete. Oocytes showing single pronucleus are examined at an interval of 4-6 hours to see whether two pronuclei are seen. Normally fertilised oocytes are examined after 24 hours of culture. Subsequently, the cleaving embryos are graded depending on the homogeneity of blastomere or presence or absence of cytoplasmic fragments. It has been reported that pre-embryos having 20-30% space occupied by cytoplasmic fragment are fit for transfer to recipients.

Embryo transfer

As in standard IVF, pre-embryos are normally transferred in the uterine cavity via cervical os. It may be transferred to the fallopian tube (tubal embryo transfer, TET or zygote intra fallopian transfer, ZIFT).

The morphologically normal pre-embryos are pooled up in a droplet of medium containing serum supplementation (either maternal or Bovine Serum Albumin, BSA, Sigma USA). Up to three embryos are loaded in a Craft Embryo Transfer Catheter (Rockett of London, UK) and transferred to the uterine cavity via cervical os, while the patient is in lithotomy position. Though uterine embryo placement is usually done at 4 to 8 cell stage, either pronucleus or 2 cell stage pre-embryos are used for tubal transfer (TET).

Luteal phase supplementation and follow-up

As in standard IVF, following embryo transfer, patients are supported with progesterone in oil as intramuscular injection during the luteal phase. Normally 25 to 50 mg of progesterone (Gestone, USA) is given daily as intramuscular injections. Patients are monitored by endocrine assay of progesterone, estradiol and hCG-beta at three days interval from D-10 following embryo transfer. Pregnancy is confirmed by hCG-beta and ultrasonographic recording of fetal cardiac activity (around sixth week from the last menstrual period). The endocrine estimations are done weekly until sixteen weeks of gestation.

Biochemical pregnancy is defined when there is a significant increase in serum hCG level (more than 10 mIU/ml between day 10 and 20 after hCG induction). Clinical pregnancies are recorded where a distinct gestational sac is observed during ultrasound examination. It is still debated whether amniocentesis should be performed for genetic counselling. The prospective follow-up of the children who are born following micro-manipulation[26] technique like ICSI and SUZI should always be maintained.

Results

The experience of different centers throughout the world indicates that the success of microinjection procedure depends on the individual worker's training, expertise and experience. Moreover, correct use of microinjection pipettes with sharp spikes are extremely useful for effective penetration through zona pellucida and also to avoid damage to oocytes.

ICSI results

Currently the fertilisation rate following ICSI varies from 30% to 60% in different centres. However, pregnancy rate per embryo transfer appears to be still lower comparable to standard IVF technology. In our experience, the fertilisation rate has been 30% while pregnancy rate has been obtained little below 10%. Van Steirteghem *et al.*[27] from Brussels have recently reported high fertilisation and implantation in ICSI. From their study it appears that higher success in terms of fertilisation and pregnancy rate is expected in ICSI in comparison to its close counterpart sub-zonal insemination (SUZI). Also dramatic improvement of results are observed when initial series are compared to their currently published series.

Discussion

The patients with severe degree male infertility are associated with lowest success rate in standard IVF methods. In addition to sperm concentration, sperm motility is extremely important and has direct correlation with human fertilisation in vitro. The methods available at present to concentrate the motile sperms available from the ejaculate are not very efficient when standard IVF method is applied. Thus,

Table 37.1. Results of ICSI from different authors

Author's name	*No. of ICSI cycles*	*% of fertilised oocytes*	*Pregnancy rate*	*Ongoing pregnancy rate*
1. Van Steirteghem *et al.*				
(a) First series	287	33.1%	20.2%	13.8%
(b) Current series	555	66.9%	38.7%	36.0%
2. Leveran D, *et al.*	117		33% per attempt	

during the last five years there has been a tremendous interest in assisted fertilisation by using micro-manipulation of gametes. This move from basic studies to clinical application is an obvious consequence of the frustrating outcome of standard IVF in severe male factor infertility. Among the two methods, *i.e.*, SUZI and ICSI practised during the last 4 to 5 years, the latter one was introduced relatively later. However, ICSI appears to be more successful even in cases where SUZI has failed[16]. Nevertheless, it needs to be addressed in detail whether such micro-manipulation which bypass many of the steps to fertilisation would have any impact on the normal growth of offspring. The process of natural selection which involves a complex and orderly process is overridden by micro-manipulation techniques and the subsequent assisted fertilisation. From the male point of view, the fertilisation appears to be highly inefficient, since millions of spermatozoa are required for normal male fertility. Keeping in mind that male ejaculates normally contain many morphologically abnormal sperms and thus several barriers which the sperm has to cross to succeed the final steps of fertilisation was thought to be an evolutionary mechanism to reduce the possibility of abnormal fertilisation. Hence, it is easily recognised that micromanipulation like ICSI circumvents the normal sequence for fertilisation and thus the possibility exists that it might increase the likelihood of fertilisation by genetically absent cells. As expected, with more centres practising and perfecting this technique like ICSI, more pregnancies will be achieved and the concern regarding possible malformation can hopefully be addressed in detail in the near future. On the other hand, in most instances, genetic aberrations will undoubtedly preclude development beyond the preimplantation stage and thus the process itself may be self-limiting to reduce the possibility of abnormal conceptions. The recent reports of a London-based clinic has raised hope in the clinical application of preimplantation genetic counselling by using the novel technology 'The Blastomere Biopsy'.

Interestingly, it again involves the novel micro-manipulation technique by which a single blastomere is taken out of early cleavage stage (*e.g.*, 8 cell stage) following ICSI and genetic study of the blastomere could effectively detect those normal pre-embryos which are fit for replacement to the recipient uterus. Since a large number of severe degree male infertility exists among the infertile patient population, it can be anticipated that in the coming years, a substantial number of babies will be born through assisted fertilisation like ICSI or SUZI. Many of the hitherto unanswered questions relating to scientific, social and ethical issues arising out of this new aggressive micromanipulation technology will hopefully be answered.

REFERENCES

1. Barbar MA. A technique for the inoculation of bacteria and other substances into living cells. J Inf Diseases; 8 : 348-360, 1911.
2. Nicholas JS, Hall BV. Experiments on developing rats. II. The development of isolated blastomeres and fused eggs. J Exp Zool; 90 : 441-458, 1942.
3. Duryee WR. Microdissection studies on human ovarian eggs. Trans NY Acad Sci II; 17 : 103-108, 1954.
4. Tarkowski AK. Experimental studies on regulation in the development of isolated blastomeres of mouse eggs. Acta Theriologica; 3 : 191-267, 1959.
5. Lin TP. Microinjection of mouse eggs. Science; 151 : 333-337, 1966.
6. Lin TP. Micropipetting cytoplasm from the mouse eggs. Nature; 216 : 162-163, 1967.
7. Lin TP. Micropipetting cytoplasm from the mouse eggs. Nature; 222 : 480-481, 1969a.
8. Lin TP. Development of a microsurgical procedure for delivery of mouse sperm into unfertilized egg. Soc study or Reprod, Sec Ann Meeting, Abstracts, No. 38, 0.19, 1969b.
9. Chang MC, Bedford JM. Fertilisation ability of rabbit ova after removal of corona radiata. Fertility Sterility, 13 : 421-425, 1962.
10. Uehara T, Yanagimachi R. Microsurgical injection of spermatozoa into hamster eggs with subsequent transformation of sperm nuclei into male pronuclei. Biol Reprod, 15 : 467-72, 1976.
11. Markert CL. Fertilization of mammalian eggs by sperm injection. J Exp Zool, 228 : 195-201, 1983.
12. Gordon JW, Grunfeld L, Garrisi GJ, Talansky BE, Richards C, Laufer N. Fertilisation of human oocytes by sperm from infertile males after zona pellucida drilling. Fertil Steril, 50 : 68-73, 1988.
13. Cohen J, Malter H, Fehilly C, Wright G, Elsner C, Kort H, *et al.* Implantation of embryos after partial opening of oocyte zona pellucida to facilitate sperm penetration. Lancet, 2 : 162, 1988.
14. Ng Sc, Bongso A, Ratnam SS, Sathananthan H, Chan CLK, Wong PC, *et al.* Pregnancy after transfer of sperm under zona. Lancet, 2 : 790, 1988.
15. Palermo G, Joris H, Devroey P, Van Steirteghem AC. Pregnancies after intracytoplasmic injection of single spermatozoon into an oocyte. Lancet, 340 : 17-18, 1992.

16. Van Steirteghem AC, Liu J, Joris H, Nagy Z, Staessen C, Camus M, Wisanto A, Liebaers, I, Devroey P. Sub-zonal insemination (SUZI) and intracytoplasmic sperm injection (ICSI). Hum Reprod, 8 : (Suppl 1), 134, 1993.
17. Van Steirteghem AC, Liu J, Joris H, Nagy Z, Janssenswillen C, Tournaye H, Derde M, Van Assche E and Devroey P. Higher success rate by intracytoplasmic sperm injection than by subzonal insemination. A report of a second series of 300 consecutive treatment cycles. Hum Repord, 8 (7) : 1055-1060, 1993.
18. Fishel S, Timson J, Lisi F, Jacobson M, Rinaldi L, Gobetz L. Micro-assisted fertilization in patients who have failed subzonal insemination. Hum Reprod, 9 (3) : 501-505, 1994.
19. Lanzendorf SE, Maloney MK, Veeck LL, Slusser J, Hodgen GD, Rosewaks Z. A preclinical evaluation of pronuclear formation by microinjection of human spermatozoa into human oocytes. Fertil Steril, 49 : 835-42, 1988.
20. De Krester DM, Yates CA, Kovacs GT. The use of in vitro fertilization in the management of male infertility. Clin Obstet Gynaecol, 12 : 767-73, 1985.
21. Porter RN, Smith W, Craft IL, Abdul Wahid NA, Jacobs HS. Induction of ovulation for in vitro fertilisation, Lancet, 2 : 284-5, 1984.
22. Neveu S, Hedon B, Bringer J, Chinchole JM, Arnol F Humeau C, *et al.* Ovarian stimulation by a combination of a gonadotropin-releasing hormone agonist and gonadotropins for in vitro fertilisation. Fertil Steril, 17 : 639-43, 1987.
23. Lucinda LV. In : Atlas of the Human Oocyte and Early Conceptus. Williams and Wilkins, Waverly Press Inc., 1986.
24. Kruger TF, Menkveld R, Stander FSH, Lambard CJ, Van der Merwe JP, Van Jiji JA, *et al.* Sperm morphologic features as a prognostic factor in in vitro fertilization. Fertil Steril, 46 : 1118-23, 1986.
25. Bongso TA, Sathananthan AH, Wong PC, Ratnam SS, Ng Sc, Anandakumar C, *et al.* Human fertilization by microinjection of immotile spermatozoa. Hum Reprod, 4 : 175-9, 1989.
26. Liebaers I, Bonduelle M, Van Assche E, Buysse A, De Smyttere S, Legein J, Devroey P, Van Steireteghem AC. Prenatal diagnosis and follow-up of children born after assisted fertilization. J Ass Reprod Gen, 10 (6 suppl) : 156, 1993.
27. Van Steirteghem AC, Nagy Z, Joris H, Liu J, Staessen C, Smitz J, Wisanto A, Devroey P. High fertilization and implantation rates after intracytoplasmic sperm injection. Hum Reprod, 8 (7) : 1061-1066, 1993.

CHAPTER

38

Medical Management of Male Infertility

Satish Tibrewala

Introduction

Advances in assisted reproductive technology (ART) have brightened the outlook for the severe male factor infertile group. However, ART remains beyond the financial reach of the majority of our population. Moreover, the success rate with micro-manipulation at present remains below 10%. On the other hand, there has been a proliferation of therapeutic modalities in the management of male infertility. The major criticism of the majority of these drugs[1,2] is that their value has not been adequately proved by proper drug trials. It is the author's opinion that if a particular drug is used in a properly selected case and the schedule adhered to, then the success rate obtained is acceptable.

Medical treatment of male infertility disorders must be based on certain guidelines[3].

Guidelines

1. Exclude all possible exogenous injurious factors such as hot baths, tight underwear, tobacco use (smoking, chewing or application on the gums), alcohol dependence, drug dependence, medications (*e.g.*, nitrofurantoin, cimetidine, chemotherapy) exposure to pesticides, fertilisers, excessive occupational heat or radiation.
2. Rule out surgical conditions such as congenital or acquired obstructive azoospermia, cryptorchidism, varicocoele.
3. Ensure that any drug prescribed to improve sperm density is given for at least 1 cycle of spermatogenesis (74 days plus an additional 10 to 14 days for epididymal spermatozoal maturation and transport).
4. Ensure that the serum FSH level is not abnormally elevated indicating severe testicular damage. The FSH level should not be higher than twice the upper limit of normal, as specified by the laboratory (*e.g.*, if the range is 2 to 8 mIU/ml then do not try therapy for males with levels over

16 mIU/ml). Reconfirm that the FSH level is high by repeating the test 4 weeks later and ensure that the male has not been on endocrine therapy for at least 4 weeks before the test.

Medical therapy

Medical therapy of male infertility may be grouped under 3 heads. Therapy that works at :

I. Pre-testicular level
II. Testicular level
III. Post-testicular level

I. Drugs acting at the pre-testicular level

These drugs are used basically to improve sperm count.

1. Anti-estrogens

A. Clomiphene citrate (CC) : CC being an anti-estrogen, binds competitively to the estrogen receptors in the hypothalamus, thereby blocking the negative feedback effect of testosterone on the hypothalamus. This increases GnRH and thus gonadotropin secretion, which is thought to improve spermatogenesis. Reports regarding its usefulness are conflicting (pregnancy rates 0 to 35%)[4,5,6] Earlier, CC was used in 100 mg and later 50 mg daily dosage. Presently, the dosage recommended is 25 mg daily for 25 days, followed by rest for 5 days; this schedule is followed for 3 months or longer. The author personally recommends no rest periods. Doses higher than 50 mg daily may depress spermatogenesis. Semen analysis is advised every 4 weeks to chart the progress. Side-effects such as loss of libido, visual disturbances, headaches, etc., necessitate its stoppage.

B. Tamoxifen : This anti-estrogen has less intrinsic estrogenic activity than CC. The dosage recommended is 20 mg daily for 3 months or longer. As with CC, its usefulness is controversial[6,7,8]. Its theoretical advantage over CC remains to be proved.

2. GnRH

It is useful in cases of hypothalamic hypogonadotropic hypogonadism (HHH) with an intact pituitary. H. Jacobs has reported pregnancies using pulsatile sub-cutaneous infusion of GnRH in a dose of 5-15 μg/pulse at intervals of 90-120 minutes for up to 18 months. Wagner has identified a group he calls 'Slow Pulsing Oligospermia' with slow pulses of GnRH, in which sperm count improves with sub-cutaneous GnRH infusion of 50 μg/pulse every 120 minutes (the dose being delivered over 1 minute). However, the cost is prohibitive and it relies highly on patient compliance.

3. Testosterone (T)

T when used in high doses (*e.g.*, Sustanon 250 mg deep i.m. fortnightly), suppresses the pituitary release of FSH and LH by its negative feedback effect, thereby suppressing spermatogenesis. In an oligozoospermic male, with normal testicular volume and normal FSH level Heller[9] has recommended continuation of the drug until azoospermia is achieved. Stoppage of T then frees the pituitary of the negative feedback of T and an enhanced endogenous release of FSH and LH which so to say whips up to the seminiferous epithelium to produce larger numbers of sperms. Other workers have failed to show this regimen working. Occasionally, a male may be rendered permanently azoospermic.

4. Bromocryptine

This drug is useful only in the occasional male who has an elevated prolactin level. This is a rare finding and may be suspected when the male complains of depressed libido or impotence. There is no evidence that treatment with bromocryptine is beneficial for men with normal or marginally elevated prolactin levels. This compound is usually administered in doses of 1.25-2.5 mg two to three times daily.

II. Drugs acting at the testicular level

1. Anti-estrogens

CC as well as tamoxifen are also thought to act directly on the testes. The dosage and schedule have been discussed earlier.

2. Human gonadotropins (hCG and hMG)

They are useful in conditions such as :

(a) Hypothalamic hypogonadotropic hypogonadism (HHH) (GnRH deficiency), *e.g.*, idiopathic HHH.
(b) Fertile eunuch syndrome (LH deficiency)
(c) Isolated FSH deficiency
(d) Acquired gonadotropin deficiency
(e) Idiopathic oligozoospermia with normal levels of FSH and LH.

hCG may be used singly or in combination with hMG as the situation demands. hCG has been used in a dosage of 2000 IU given i.m. 2 to 3 times a week for 2 months and up to a few years (as in the case of pubertal development). hMG has been used in a dose of 75 to 150 I.U. given i.m. 2 to 3 times a week (it may be dissolved in the same syringe with hCG) until the desired sperm density is achieved in the semen. Isidori from Rome reports that circulating gonadotropins (Gn) may not be biologically active and hence there is a place for exogenous Gn therapy. Lunenfeld[10] recommends a GnRH stimulation test to identify men who could benefit from Gn therapy. Further, Lunenfeld[11] has found that since malformations of the fine structure of the sperm head subcellular organelles seem to be prerequisites for the success of FSH treatment, ultramorphological examination of the sperm may serve as an indication for the probability of success with FSH. There is a universal agreement on one point that Gn therapy does not work in the presence of elevated levels of FSH and LH. Currently, a trial with recombinant human FSH is in progress to determine whether fertilisation rates can be improved in men with abnormal semen and previous poor results in IVF.

3. *Androgens*

The manufacturers of androgen preparations claim that sperm density can be improved by them, [*e.g.*, mesterolone 25 mg (Provironum) 2 t.i.d. or testosterone undecanoate[12] 40 mg (Nuvir) 1 t.i.d. for 3 months]. However, the general experience is disappointing.

III. Drugs acting at the post-testicular level

1. *Androgens*

Natural or synthetic androgens when given in small doses may improve accessory sex glandular secretions and thereby enhance sperm motility and viability (*e.g.*, testosterone 25 to 50 mg i.m. twice a week or mesterolone 1 t.i.d. for 4 to 8 weeks). However, sometimes their use may lower sperm concentration.

2. *Antibiotics*

A recent review article by Purvis[13] on infections of the reproductive tract and male infertility concludes that these inflammatory episodes are common and may be diagnosed by rectal ultrasound, chlamydia trachomatis and ureaplasma urealyticum often being the offending organism, with increasing probability of infection in the female. The author concurs with this view and recommends that both partners be treated with antibiotics simultaneously. The drugs most often used are :

A. Erythromycin 250 mg 1 q.i.d. or 400 mg 1 t.i.d. for up to 10 days (along with B complex).

B. Doxycycline 100 mg 1 b.d. for up to 10 days (along with B complex).

C. Co-trimoxazole DS 1 b.d. for 10 days followed by 1/2 b.d. for 10 to 20 days (especially useful for chronic prostato vesiculitis).

D. Norfloxacin 400 mg 1 b.d. for 10 days.

E. Ciprofloxacin 250 to 500 mg 1 q.i.d. for 7 to 10 days.

The general pointers are that prostatic smear and routine semen culture are not helpful in the management of infertile men.

The role of antibiotics is thought to be 2 fold :

(i) To combat the infecting organism, reduce macrophage activity and improve sperm motility and morphology and sometimes count.

(ii) To lower the antisperm antibody titres.

The author has found that on direct questioning, about 20% of men give a positive history of promiscuity and hence the role of antibiotics cannot be overstressed.

3. *Steroids*

Steroid use in immunological infertility is controversial. 2 regimes have been tried[14].

A. Low dose regimes : Prednisolone 5 mg t.i.d. given by Hendry to 29 patients resulted in 4 pregnancies. The improved sperm counts were attributed to reduction of epididymal inflammation and consequent relief of obstruction.

B. High dose regimes : Schulman and Schulman recommend that methylprednisolone 96 mg per day be administered to the husband for days 21 to 28 of the wife's menstrual cycle.

In view of the risk of aseptic necrosis of the hip joints and gastrointestinal haemorrhage with high dose steroid therapy, Hendry now recommends prednisolone 20 mg b.d. given to the husband on days 1 through 10 of the wife's menstrual cycle. The author has used a lower dose (Prednisolone 5 mg 1 to 2 tabs. b.d.) successfully in some couples. It is mandatory to discuss with the male the side-effects of steroid therapy.

4. *Minerals and vitamins*

Although generally branded as empirical therapy, there is a place for these in deficiency conditions as malnourishment is so prevalent in our country.

A. Iron and B_{12} in anaemia, as per requirement.

B. Zinc (50 mg b.d.) especially for those with recent illness.

C. Vitamin A and E in individuals especially with low dietary fat intake.

D. Vitamin C to those with low resistance to infection.

There has been renewed interest in antioxidant vitamins because of the finding by Aitken *et al.* in 1992 of excessive production of reactive oxygen species by spermatozoa from men with idiopathic oligozoospermia.

Conclusion

The effectiveness of medical therapy for male infertility has been clouded with uncertainty. Hargreave's[13] findings in 1983 suggest that as long as the semen contains 1 million motile sperms/ml, the percentage chance of conception for 12 months is 25% (provided that the wife has normal tubal patency and spontaneous ovulation). On the other hand, Melvin L. Taymor states that if a couple is taken as a unit then males with sperm counts between 20 to 40 million sperms/ml represent those for whom the most can be done yet who often go without treatment. In the author's opinion, careful selection of medical therapy coupled with good counselling produces acceptable results in male infertility.

REFERENCES

1. Gilbaugh JH, Lipshultz LT. Nonsurgical treatment of male infertility : An update. Urol Clin North Am; 21 (3), 1994.
2. O'Donovan PA, *et al.* Treatment of male infertility : Is it effective? Review and meta analysis of published randomized controlled trials. Hum Reprod 9 (8) : 1209-22, 1993.
3. Schirren C. Basic principles of drug therapy in andrology. Experience of 40 years' andrologic treatment. Fortschr Med; 112 (14) : 199-202, 1994.
4. Schill WB. Recent progress in pharmacological therapy of male infertility — a review, Andrologia 11 (2) : 77, 1979.
5. Sokol RZ, *et al.* A controlled comparison of the efficacy of clomiphene citrate on male infertility. Fertil Steril; 49 : 865, 1988.
6. Breznik R, Borko E. Effectiveness of antiestrogens in infertile men. Arch Androl; 31 (1) : 43-8, 1993.
7. Kotoulas IG, *et al.* Tamoxifen treatment in male infertility, 1. Effect on spermatozoa. Fertil Steril; 61 (5) : 911-4, 1994.
8. Sterzik K, *et al.* Tamoxifen treatment of oligozoospermia : A re-evaluation of its effects including additional sperm function tests. Arch Gynecol Obstet; 252 (3) : 143-7, 1993.
9. Rowley MJ, Heller CG. The testosterone rebound phenomenon in the treatment of male infertility. Fertil Steril; 23 : 498, 1972.
10. Bruno Lunenfeld, Meir Berezin. Hypogonadotropic hypogonadism with gonadotropins in current therapy of infertility, eds. Garcia, Mastroianni, Amelar, Dubin, BC Dekker, 187, 1989.
11. Bartoov B, *et al.* Sperm quality of subfertile males before and after treatment with human follicle stimulating hormone. Fertil Steril; 16 (4) : 727-34, 1994.
12. Gregoriou O, *et al.* Treatment of idiopathic infertility with testosterone undecanoate. A double blind study. Clin Exp Obstet Gynecol; 20 (1) : 9-12, 1993.
13. Purvis K Christiansen. Infections in the male reproductive tract. Impact, diagnosis and treatment in relation to male infertility. Int'l J of Andr; 16 : 1, 1993.
14. Hargreave TB. Medical treatment of the infertile male. In : Andrology, eds. John P Pryor, Larry I Lipshulz. Butterworths & Co., 261, 1987.

CHAPTER

39

Update : Sperm Function Tests

Satish Tibrewala

Introduction

It is currently well accepted that the standard parameters for semen analysis have significant limitations as indicators of fertility. Multivariate discriminant analysis using standard criteria of seminal analysis have shown that progressive sperm motility and normal sperm morphology are variables that provide significant information to categorize males as fertile, subfertile or infertile[1]. The main drawback here, however, is the inability to ascertain the functional capacity of a given semen sample to fertilize the human oocyte either in vivo or in vitro. To add to that, fertilization of the oocyte is generally looked upon as a single process, whereas, in reality a spermatozoon must be able to penetrate cervical mucus, cumulus oophorus, corona radiata and zona pellucida before it can fuse with the oolemma and enter the ooplasm for final fusion. These processes besides requiring normal sperm motility and morphology also involve complicated biochemical and morphological events.

A variety of tests have been devised to improve evaluation of the fertilizing capacity of the human sperm and hence a more accurate measurement of male fertility potential.

The ability of human sperm to fertilize human eggs would be the ideal test. Unfortunately, the routine use of human eggs has obvious practical and ethical limitations and cannot be expected to become a clinical tool. Hence, we are forced to fall back on the use of other in vitro tests to assess sperm fertilizing capacity.

The limitation of such tests are that they are indicators of the activity of a particular sperm organelle, *e.g.*, sperm plasma membrane, acrosome, nucleus, mitochondria, etc. Hence, it seems necessary to test the various sperm organelles by a variety of tests before declaring the semen sample as fertile/subfertile/infertile.

The next point to be considered is whether these tests, which are in vitro, truly represent in vivo conditions.

Another fact that raises discussion is that these tests are often performed upon the total ejaculated sperm population and compared with the human in vitro fertilisation rates. Knowing that the IVF procedure has been performed with a specific sperm population selected by procedures such as swim-up, swim-down, percoll centrifugation, etc., are we justified in comparing the test results of total sperm population against specific sperm population? On the other hand tests performed on the specific sperm populations need to be co-related with results of tests performed on total sperm populations.

Given below are some relevant sperm function tests with their methodology and discussion.

1. Sperm cervical mucus penetration test

The first barrier that the sperm encounters in the female reproductive system is the cervical mucus. Hence, it is only logical that a test be designed to study the functional capacity of the sperm to penetrate the mucus under optimal conditions (*i.e.*, a mucus score of 8 or more based on Insler's cervical score).

Method

In the capillary tube technique (Fig. 39.1), a glass slide is graduated by scoring millimetre marks along one side using a diamond pen. A sperm reservoir is made by halving the lower end of a 0.5 cm test tube and glueing one half to the graduated slide. This reservoir is filled with the semen. Ovulatory mucus is aspirated into a

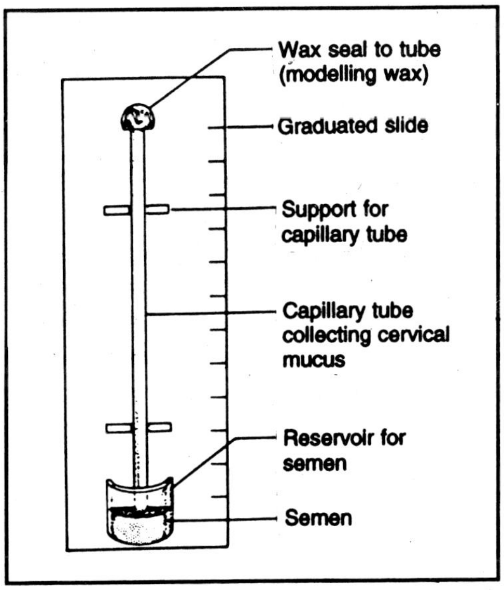

Fig. 39.1. The use of a tube containing cervical mucus into which the penetration by spermatozoa can be tested.

wide bore capillary tube. One end of the tube is sealed with non-toxic wax. The end of the tube, with the mucus protruding slightly, dips into the semen pool, as the tube is placed on the slide, on two small supports. A petridish containing a moistened filter paper (to maintain humidity) is taken, the test slide is placed horizontally in it and incubated at 37°C for 1 hour. The capillary tube is then examined to ascertain the distance travelled by the vanguard sperm, the sperm density at various distances and the percentage of sperms showing progressive motility. For details of the scoring system the reader is referred to the study by Kroeks & Kremer[1].

Discussion

If the test result is negative or poor the same should be repeated using a donor mucus with the husband's semen and also donor semen with the wife's mucus. If the husband's sperms are unable to penetrate the wife's mucus, but can penetrate the donor mucus, the sperm function is taken to be normal and the wife's mucus becomes suspect; it becoming necessary to rule out sperm antibodies in the wife's mucus. If the husband's sperm is unable to penetrate the mucus of the wife as well as the donor, the semen becomes suspect, it becoming necessary to rule out sperm antibodies in the husband's semen.

Bovine mucus is very similar to human cervical mucus in its properties, particularly its visco-elastic characteristics. Human spermatozoa can penetrate it without difficulty and their behaviour in bovine mucus has been studied by various groups. The test kit is marketed commercially as the Penetrak test (Serono Diagnostica GmbH).

Berberoglugil[2] states that a normal semen with abnormal sperm cervical mucus penetration test identifies couples with a decreased IVF ability, while a normal semen with a normal test identifies couples with a very low fertilizing failure risk. The test does not add any predictive value to sperm analysis in the case of abnormal semen analysis[2].

2. Peritoneal sperm migration test (PSM test)

This test, also known as laparoscopic sperm retrieval, is a sperm function test performed by a clinician. It is an interesting attempt to realise the in vitro benefits of the sperm cervical mucus penetration test under in vivo conditions and assesses the ability of the spermatozoa to enter and traverse the female genital tract.

Method

Infertile women at midcycle who have abstained

sexually for at least 3 days, are either instructed to have intercourse or undergo artificial insemination between 6 to 12 hours prior to the laparoscopy. Fluid that normally occupies the pouch of Douglas is aspirated, centrifuged and the sediment re-suspended in a smaller quantity of fluid (*e.g.*, distilled water). The red cells may be lysed by treating with twice the volume of 0.01% (w/v) saponin. A count is made of the number of sperms seen in the washings.

Discussion

The presence of spermatozoa in the peritoneal fluid proves that they can reach the site of fertilization. In practice, however, spermatozoa are detected in only about half the cases, due to the fact that only a small number of spermatozoa reach the fimbria of the uterine tube and their concentration gets highly diluted in the peritoneal fluid obtained at mid cycle. The timing of the test is of utmost importance, being performed at midcycle. These facts probably account for the reason why this test has not been widely adopted.

3. Hypo-osmotic swelling test (HOST)

The sperm cell is covered with a plasma membrane across which osmosis and exchange of ions takes place.

The HOS test is purported to measure the physiological integrity of the sperm plasma membrane. This test is based on the fundamental tenet that if spermatozoa are exposed to a hypoosmotic medium, there is an influx of water into the cell in an attempt to re-establish an osmotic equilibrium. This influx of water will, if the spermatozoon has an intact plasma membrane, cause the cell to swell and this, in turn, will be reflected by a progressive curling of the terminal portion of the sperm tail (Fig. 39.2). The proportion of spermatozoa exhibiting such changes in the sperm tail on exposure to hypo-osmotic media is taken to reflect the population size of sperms with physiologically normal plasma membrane.

Details of the HOS test as described by Jeyendran & Zaneveld[3] are given below :

Method

Mix equal (0.5 ml) volumes of aqueous solutions of fructose (2.7%) and sodium citrate (1.47%). Keep the mixture at 37°C for 10 mins.

Add 0.1 ml of semen sample after estimating the incidence of coiled tails during initial microscopic examination. Incubate at 37°C for 30 mins.

Take 10 µl of the incubated mixture onto a clean glass slide, place a coverglass over it and examine at least 200 spermatozoa under phase contrast microscopy using a × 40 objective.

Calculate the percentage of coiled tails (Fig. 39.3) and subtract the number of coiled tails observed in the initial microscopic examination to obtain a final figure of sperms showing a positive reaction to the HOS test.

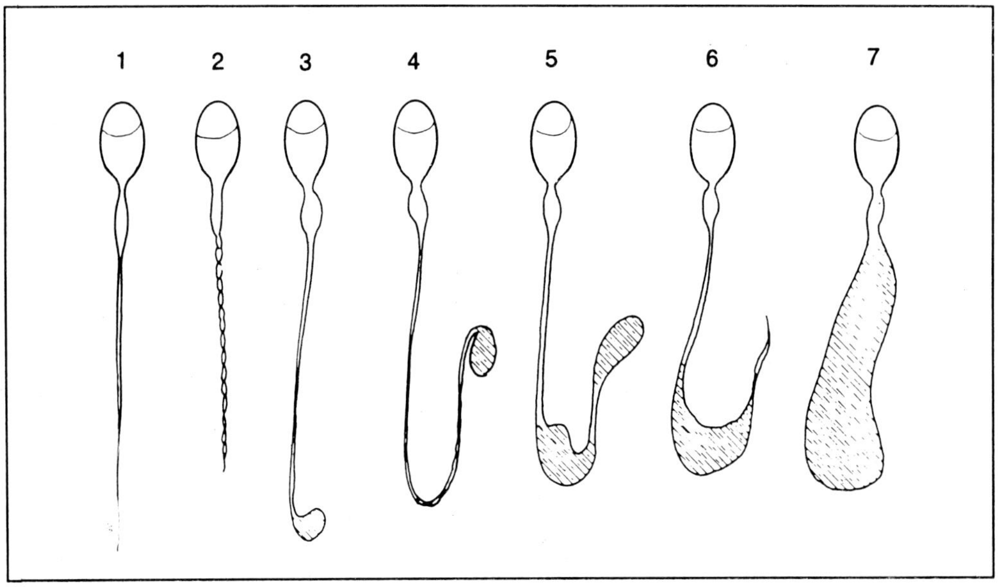

Fig. 39.2. HOS test. Diagrammatic representation of the typical morphological changes to the tail of spermatozoa under hypoosmotic conditions. **1.** No change. **2.** 'Chain-like swelling', minimal, segmented swelling of the entire tail. **3-7.** Different forms of swelling of the tail of increasing magnitude (swollen section of tail shaded).

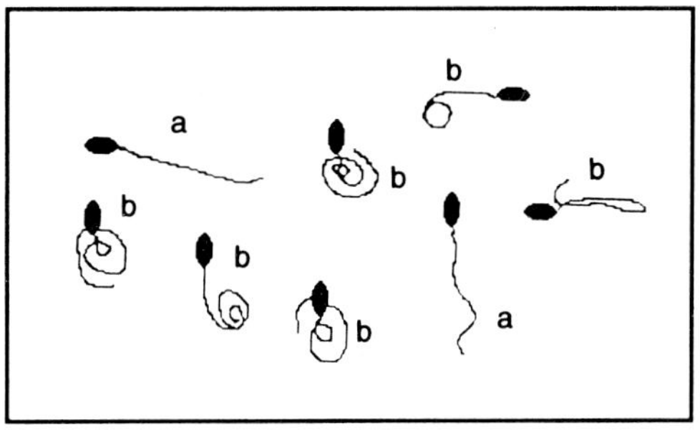

Fig. 39.3. Diagrammatic representation of spermatozoa showing a HOS –ve response (a) with uncoiled straight tails and those showing a HOS +ve response (b) with coiled tails.

Make duplicate observations of two separate preparations and take the mean of the two figures.

Discussion

Several workers[3,4] have claimed that a good co-relation exists between the incidence of spermatozoa showing a +ve HOS reaction and fertilization rates of human oocytes in IVF. Smith *et al.*[4] compared the results of zona-free hamster oocyte penetration assay with the HOS test. They found that the majority of semen samples (87.3%) showing a normal penetration rate (> 10%) also exhibited a 60% (or higher) reaction in the HOS test. They also found that the inter-assay variation of the HOS test (9.0%) was within the accepted range for this type of assay. It would be interesting to know the percentage of samples showing a 60% (or higher) reaction to the HOS test and a poor penetration rate (< 10%) on zona free hamster oocyte penetration assay.

It has been reported that a strong relationship exists between results of the sperm swelling test and fertilization of human oocytes in IVF[5,6]. No oocytes are fertilized by sperm samples in which < 60% of the sperm showed swelling. The results of the swelling test were significantly more reliable than were the results of the standard spermiogram in prediction of successful conception. Recent reports state that the sperm swelling test is of limited diagnostic value for IVF and is not significantly more useful than any of the standard semen variables[7].

According to Gopalkrishnan *et al.*[8], a semen sample showing incidence of coiled tails of :

> 60% indicates fertility
50-59% indicates subfertility
1-49% indicates infertility

4. Test for acrosome intactness

The sperm cells of all mammals cannot fertilize at ejaculation. This ability is usually developed during a period of several hours within the female reproductive tract. True acrosome reaction is described as a progressive fusion between the plasma membrane and the outer acrosomal membrane resulting in the formation of a series of vesicles[9] (Fig. 39.4). Pores between the areas of fusion allow a progressive loss of the acrosomal contents including enzymes like hyaluronidase, corona penetrating enzyme (CPE), a trypsin like enzyme (TLE) also known as acrosin and

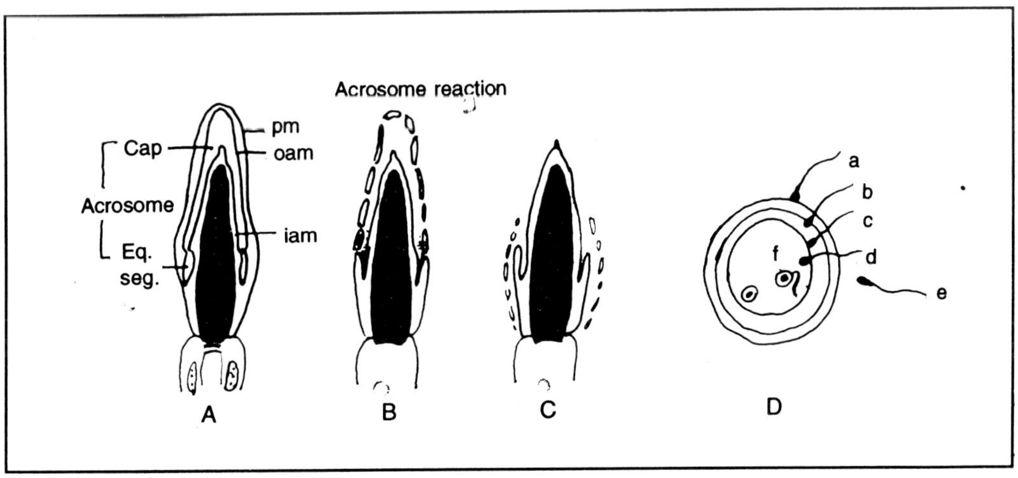

Fig. 39.4. (A) Diagram of the sperm head with condensated nucleus surrounded by plasma membrane (pm), outer acrosomal membrane (oam), acrosome and inner acrosomal membrane (iam). (B) Acrosome reaction in progress : fusion of plasma membrane and outer acrosomal membrane, formation of pores and release of proteolytic enzymes. (C) Inner acrosomal membrane exposed. (D) Diagram showing (a) zona pellucida contact, (b) zona pellucida penetration, (c) peri-vitelline space penetration, (d) vitelline membrane penetration, (e) block to polyspermy, (f) male pronucleus formation.

a neuriminidase like enzyme (NLE). These enzymes facilitate the spermatozoa to penetrate the various investments of the ovum namely the cumulus oophorus, corona radiata and zona pellucida. The NLE is apparently not involved in zonal penetration but supposedly aids in the 'zona reaction', *i.e.*, it prevents further penetration of the zona by spermatozoa and is a natural block to polyspermia[10].

In some pathological cases, the acrosome may be defective or absent and such spermatozoa lack the ability to fertilize.

Gopalkrishnan *et al.*[8] have standardised a very simple method to assess acrosome function based on the principle that the acrosomal enzymes dissolve protein (*e.g.*, gelatin). The method is described below :

Solutions

1. PBS-Glutaraldehyde solution :

   Dissolve 0.2 g of NaCl, 0.14 g of Na_2HPO_4, 0.0023 g of KH_2PO_4 in 100 ml of distilled water. Add 0.2 ml of 25% glutaraldehyde to 100 ml of PBS.

2. PBS-D-Glucose :

   Dissolve 3 g of d-glucose in 100 ml of PBS and adjust pH to 7.8 with 0.1 N HCl.

Gelatin coated slides

Spread 40 μl of warm (50°C) aqueous 5% solution of gelatin onto a clean glass slide. Keep slide horizontal for 24 hrs at 4°C. Immerse the coated slides into the 0.05% PBS-glutaraldehyde solution for 2 mins and wash twice in distilled water and store vertically at 4°C.

Method

Dilute semen twenty fold with PBS-d-glucose solution and leave it to equilibrate at 37°C for 30 mins.

Bring the gelatin coated slides to room temperature; gently smear a drop (10 to 20 μl) of the diluted semen on it and leave the slide at room temperature for 5 to 10 mins to evaporate excess moisture.

Transfer slide to a petridish containing a moistened filter paper; leave at 37°C for 2 hrs. Examine slide under phase contrast microscopy using an × 40 objective and an occulometer. Spermatozoa having intact acrosomes will show halos (Fig. 39.5).

Count at least 200 spermatozoa in different optical fields and determine the incidence of those having halos measuring 30 μm and express data as a percentage.

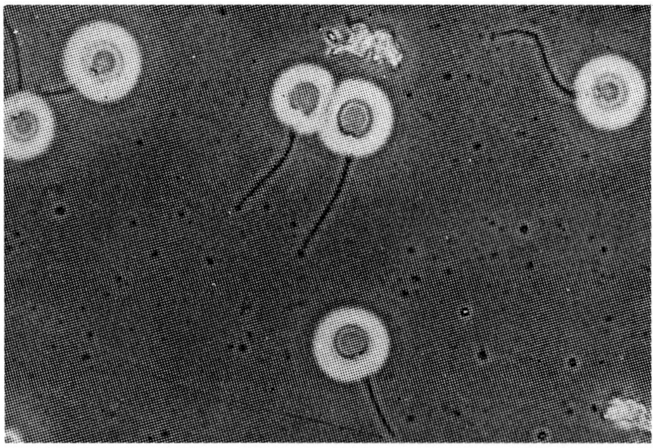

Fig. 39.5. Photomicrograph of spermatozoa showing a positive reaction (halos) to acrosome intactness test. Phase contrast microscopy × 40 objective.

Discussion

Gopalkrishnan *et al.*[8] have reported that a semen sample showing percentage of spermatozoa with halos having a diameter of 30 μm, being :

≥ 50% indicates fertility

40-49% indicates subfertility

0-39% indicates infertility

Pampiglione *et al.*[9] have reported that stimulated acrosome reaction by use of calcium ionophore A 23187 allows accurate prediction of the fertilizing ability of human spermatozoa. In their report 8 out of 16 IVF failures showed only a minimal increase (< 31.3%) in the number of acrosome reacted sperms. Hence, according to them, it can help to identify those who have a high chance of failure.

Wang *et al.*[10] have shown that assessment of acrosome reaction along with human sperm hyperactivation parameters can predict with 84% accuracy the fertility of a semen sample as judged by successful human IVF.

5. In vitro sperm nuclear chromatin decondensation test

The sperm head contains nuclear chromatin. During spermatogenesis the sperm chromatin undergoes condensation and stabilization, a process which gives characteristic properties to the sperm nucleus. Chromatin condensation is due to the presence in sperm cells of specific DNA properties and to the formation of large numbers of disulfide (S-S) bonds within the chromatin. This complicated process needs to be reversed once the sperm head enters the ooplasm. Decondensation of the sperm nuclear chromatin is a requirement for the transcription of the male genetic information to the zygote.

Sperm penetration assays, flow cytometry, acridine orange fluorescence are tests devised to study the chromatin nature of the sperm nucleus. However, these tests need expertise, expensive set-up and are time consuming. Gopalkrishnan *et al.*[11] have designed an in vitro test (described below) to evaluate the percentage of spermatozoa in a given semen sample capable of nuclear decondensation following egg penetration.

Solutions

1. 0.05 M borate buffer :
   a. 12.4 g of boric acid in 1000 ml of distilled water (0.02 M)
   b. 19.05 g of borax in 1000 ml of distilled water (0.05 M)

   Take 50 ml of 'a' add 59 ml of 'b' and make up solution to a final volume of 200 ml (pH 9).
2. EDTA-SDS mixture

   0.22% EDTA (6 ml) and 1% sodium dodecyl sulphate (SDS) in 0.05 M borate buffer.
3. Glutaraldehyde borate buffer

   2.5% glutaraldehyde in 0.05 M borate buffer.

Method

Centrifuge the semen after liquefaction at 400 g for 15 mins to separate the seminal plasma. Wash the sperm pellet twice in 0.05 M borate buffer.

To 1 vol of sample add 9 vols of the EDTA-SDS mixture. Incubate at 37°C for 60 mins. Add an equal volume of glutaraldehyde borate buffer to the incubate to arrest reaction.

Place a drop (19 to 15 µl) of this mixture onto a glass slide, place a coverslip over it and observe under phase optics using × 40 objective.

Determine the incidence of sperm heads that have decondensed and those that have not by examining at least 200 spermatozoa (Fig. 39.6) and express data as a percentage.

Discussion

According to Gopalkrishnan *et al.*[11] a normal fertile sample will show 70% spermatozoa whose nuclear chromatin has decondensed. Figures below this number suggest that the sample contains spermatozoa with a very poor nuclear chromatin decondensing ability in vitro and therefore the sample is likely to be subfertile (60-69%) or infertile (1-59%).

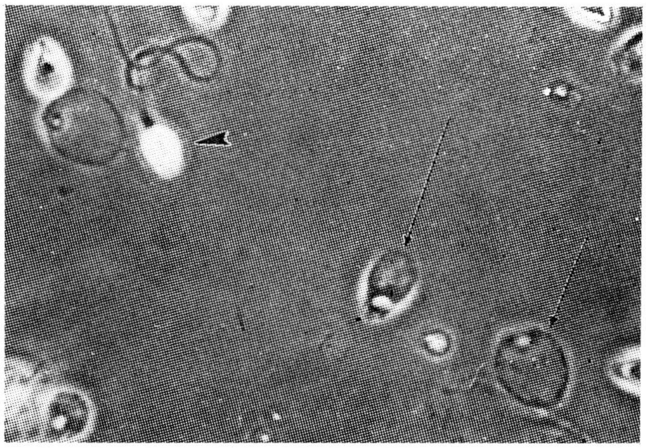

Fig. 39.6. Photomicrograph of spermatozoa subjected to in vitro nuclear decondensation test. Arrows point to those showing a positive reaction while arrow-heads indicate those that show a negative reaction. Phase contrast microscopy × 100 objective.

6. Sperm mitochondrial activity index

The midpiece of the spermatozoa contains a sheath of mitochondria which contain respiratory enzymes essential for providing energy for sperm motility. Lack of mitochondrial enzymes impair sperm motility and may thus impair fertility.

Gopalkrishnan *et al.*[12] have described a test (given below) to estimate the incidence of spermatozoa having a full complement of mitochondria.

Solutions

1. Tris HCl buffer

   7.88 g of tris HCl in 100 ml of distilled water. Adjust pH to 7.4 with 0.1 N HCl.
2. Neutral formalin

   Take 10 ml of 40% formalin in 90 ml of distilled water and add a pinch of calcium carbonate. Adjust pH to 7.0 with 0.1 N HCl.
3. Nitroblue tetrazolium (NBT)

   Dissolve 1 mg of NBT in 1 ml of tris HCl buffer.

Method

Take a drop (10-15 µl) of semen and a drop (10-15 µl) of NBT solution in a cavity slide. Cover the cavity with a coverslip and transfer the slide into a moist petridish. Incubate at 37°C for 30 mins.

Mix up the contents in the cavity using a coverslip. Prepare a wet smear of the contents on a clean slide. Air dry and fix in neutral formalin for 2 hrs.

Wash slide with distilled water and dry the slide. View under phase contrast microscopy using oil-immersion, × 100 objective.

Score spermatozoa on the basis of the amount of bluish black NBT precipitate (formazan) seen in at least 200 spermatozoa and classify them as standard, sub-standard, low, residual or nil (Figs. 39.7 and 39.8).

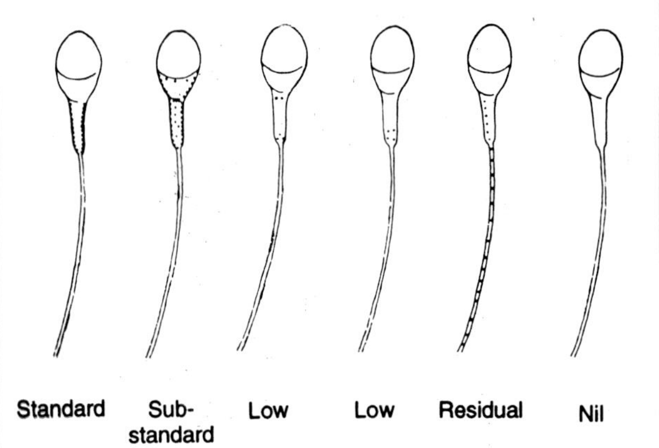

Fig. 39.7. Diagrammatic representation of the classification of extent of formazan deposit in human spermatozoa.

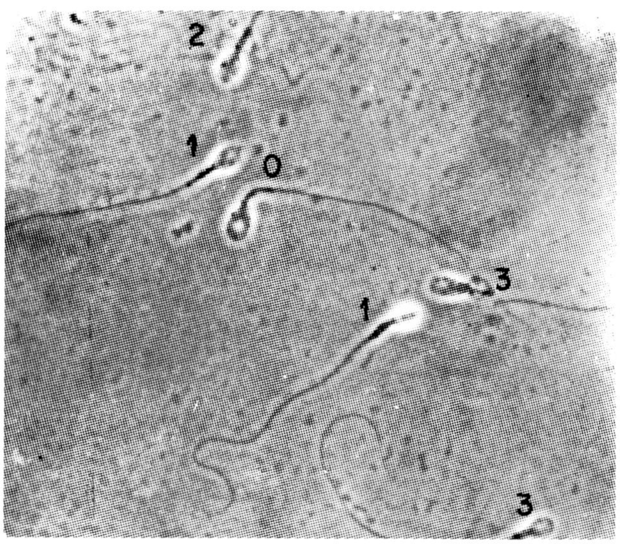

Fig. 39.8. Photomicrograph of spermatozoa subjected to mitochondrial activity test phase contrast × 100 objective. 1 = standard; 2 = sub-standard; 3 = low.

Multiply the number of sperms in each category by the figures 1, 0.7, 0.3, 0.1 and 0 which have arbitrarily been chosen respectively for standard, substandard, low, residual and nil. Total the products to determine the sperm mitochondrial activity index.

Discussion

According to Gopalkrishnan *et al.*[12], the semen sample showing sperm mitochondrial activity index (SMAI) of :

≥ 50 denotes fertility

40-49 denotes subfertility

0-39 denotes infertility

7. Hamster egg penetration assay

In the absence of easy availability of human eggs to test the biologic fertilizing potential of the human sperm, one is forced to fall back on the use of animal eggs. Hamster eggs devoid of zona pellucida can be fertilized by capacitated sperm from virtually any species. Hence, it has become one more tool to study the fertilizing ability of the sperm in the work-up of an infertile couple, under special circumstances.

Sperm mitochondrial activity index (example)

	No. of sperms	*Multiplication factor*	*Product*
Standard	70	1.0	70.0
Substandard	20	0.7	14.0
Low	5	0.3	1.5
Residual	0	0.1	0
Nil	5	0	0
Total			85.5

Method

1. Preparation of the zona-free oocytes.
   (a) The female hamster is injected intraperitoneally with 25 i.u. of pregnant mare serum gonadotropin on day 1 to induce superovulation. An intraperitoneal injection of 25 i.u. of human chorionic gonadotropin (hCG) is given on day 3 to induce follicular rupture.
   (b) At 17-22 hours the animal is killed, oviducts dissected out and the oocytes surrounded by a mass of cumulus cells attached to the ends of the oviducts, separated. The mass of cells is placed in BWW (Bigger, Whitten and Whittingham) medium containing 0.3% human serum albumin.
   (c) The cells are then placed in a BWW medium containing 0.1% hyaluronidase, which separates the cumulus cells leaving the large oocytes free in the medium.
   (d) The eggs are now washed twice in BWW, then

placed briefly in a 0.1% solution of trypsin in BWW to remove the zona pellucida, washed once again in BWW and then placed in BWW under mineral oil in a sterile plastic petridish.

2. Preparation of the human sperm

The semen is centrifuged at 600 g for 5 minutes. After 3 washes the sperms are suspended in a final sperm concentration of 10 million sperms/ml. Aliquots of 0.5 ml are made and incubated at 37°C for 18 hours. Alternatively, sperms may be prepared by the 'swim-up technique'.

3. In vitro insemination

The sperms prepared as above are added, under the mineral oil, to the medium containing the zona free eggs and the eggs and sperms are incubated together for about 2 to 3 hours. This incubation period may have to be longer if the pre-incubation period of the sperms (step 2) has been shorter.

4. Examination of the eggs

The eggs are aspirated from under the drop of mineral oil, placed on a microscope slide and a coverslip placed on it and pressed down over the eggs almost to the point of rupture. Sperm heads are seen as clear areas within the eggs with their tails attached to or associated with the heads (Fig. 39.9). Usually 40 to 50 eggs are examined per patient. Percentage penetration is the number of eggs with swollen heads divided by the number of eggs inseminated multiplied by 100.

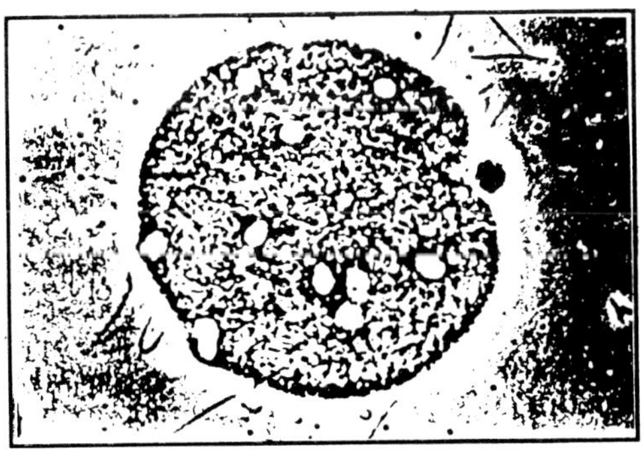

Fig. 39.9. Zona-free hamster egg with polyspermic penetration by human spermatozoa.

Discussion

It is generally accepted by most workers[4,5] in this field that a percentage penetration rate of ≥ 10 indicates fertility.

The issue of correlation between conventional semen parameters and the egg penetration results seems somewhat unclear. This may be in part due to the fact that some authors have compared the results in fertile men/semen donors while others have worked with infertile men. More recent work correlates egg penetration most significantly with motility quality and morphology[5]. On comparing human and hamster egg penetration it is found that 89% of the men who fertilized their wives' eggs also showed a positive penetration of hamster eggs (≥ 10%).

Given the difficulty of assay performance, it seems prudent to recommend sperm penetration assays only for couples with a potential male factor or unexplained infertility. A high degree of penetration of hamster eggs with no simultaneous human egg penetration could be interpreted as an egg quality problem.

Conclusion

Pregnancy is the only irrefutable proof that a sperm can fertilize. Routine semen parameters have for long been predictors of fertility in men. It is now understood that there is more to assessing the fertilizing potential of the sperm than routine analysis. Various sperm function tests have been described to test the various organelles of the sperm. This battery of tests needs to be introduced into the investigation protocol for the male partner of an infertile union.

REFERENCES

1. Kroeks MVAM, Kremer J. The role of cervical factors in infertility. In : The infertile couple (eds) Pepperell RJ, Hudson B, Wood C. Churchill Livingstone, pp 142-57, 1987.
2. Berberoglugil P. Abnormal sperm mucus penetration test predicts low IVF ability of apparently normal semen. Fertil Steril 1993; 59 : 1228-32.
3. Jeyendran RS, Zaneveld LJD. Controversies in the development and validation of new sperm assays. Fertil Steril 1993; 59 : 726-8.
4. Blanco L. Clinical tests of sperm fertilizing ability. Fertil Steril 1984; 41 : 177-92.
5. Zaneveld LJD, Jeyendran RS. Sperm function tests. In : Overstreet JW (ed) Infertility and reproductive medicine clinics of North America, Philadelphia, Saunders, pp 353-71, 1992.
6. Rogers B. Jane. The sperm penetration assay : its usefulness re-evaluated : modern trends in infertility and conception control. Arch Androl 1988; 4 : 425-44.
7. Smith R, Madariaga M, Bustos-Obregon E. Reappraisal

of the hypo-osmotic swelling test to improve assessment of seminal fertility status. Intl J Androl 1992; 15 : 5-13.

8. Gopalkrishnan K, Hinduja IN, Mehta RH, Anand Kumar TC. Laboratory manual for human semen analysis. Institute for Research in Reproduction (ICMR), 1991.

9. Pampiglione JS, Jan SL, Campbell S. The use of stimulated acrosome reaction test as a test of fertilizing ability in human spermatozoa. Fertil Steril 1993; 59 : 1280-4.

10. Wang C. Human sperm hyperactivation and acrosome reaction and their relationship to human IVF. Fertil Steril 1993; 59 : 1221-7.

11. Gopalkrishnan K, Hinduja IN, Anand Kumar TC. In vitro decondensation of nuclear chromatin of human spermatozoa : assessing fertilizing potential. Arch Androl 1991; 27 : 43-50.

12. Gopalkrishnan K, Hinduja IN, Anand Kumar TC. Assessment of mitochondrial activity of human spermatozoa : motility/viability in fertile/infertile men. Mol Androl 1991; 3 : 243-50.

CHAPTER

40

Update : Intrauterine Insemination

Vijay Mangoli

Today intrauterine insemination (IUI) is considered as the first line of treatment for male factor of infertility because it is simple, noninvasive and inexpensive as compared to more complicated and invasive procedures like varicocele surgery, tubal microsurgery, IVF or GIFT.

IUI is not a recently developed technique. The first scientifically recorded IUI was performed in London in the 1770s by John Hunter, nearly 70 years after van Leeuwenhoek first described spermatozoa in 1696. Hunter did IUI using raw, unprocessed semen samples with the help of metal catheters and faced the problem of patients having severe cramping of the uterus due to high content of prostaglandins in the seminal plasma. Since then many different groups have tried IUI with modifications in the sperm preparation and transfer techniques with varying degree of success[1,2,3,4].

Today when a couple with an infertility problem approaches a gynaecologist or an andrologist, IUI is generally considered in case of one or more of the following indications[5,6].

Female factors

(i) Anatomic defects of the vagina or cervix
(ii) Immunological infertility including antisperm antibodies in the cervical mucus
(iii) Sexual dysfunction where direct coitus is not possible

Male factors

(i) Anatomic defects of the penis
(ii) Sexual/ejaculatory dysfunctions, *e.g.*, retrograde ejaculation
(iii) High and prolonged viscosity problem
(iv) Immunological factors, *e.g.*, autoantibodies and agglutination
(v) Oligoasthenoteratozoospermia

Other factors

(i) Idiopathic infertility

(ii) Poor post-coital test

IUI can be done in a natural cycle or in a stimulated cycle[7,8,9] using different combinations of ovulatory agents. Most commonly used protocols are :

1. No drugs
2. Clomiphene citrate
3. Clomiphene citrate + hCG
4. Clomiphene citrate + hMG + hCG
5. GnRHa + FSH + hCG

The monitoring of the cycle is done by :

(i) Ultrasonography for follicular development

(ii) Blood tests for hormonal regulation of E_2, P & LH

Methodology

Today the main aim of the conventional methods used for sperm preparation is to recover maximum motile sperms and separate them from dead sperms, debris and seminal plasma[10,11].

Most of the laboratories use either swim up techniques or discontinuous percoll gradient method.

Swim up is the most simple method based on the natural tendency of live sperms to migrate from denser pellet to the above layered liquid medium for their free movement[12]. In brief, the liquefied sample is mixed with sperm wash medium and centrifuged at 300 g for 5 minutes. The supernatant is removed and the pellet is layered with about 0.5 ml medium. The tube is kept in CO_2 incubator at 37°C for 30 minutes. The supernatant is removed, checked and used for IUI.

Percoll gradient is based on separation of different cells according to their differential densities. Percoll consists of colloidal silica particles of 15-30 nm diameter. It forms self-generated gradients which trap cells of different sedimentation coefficient. Live sperms settle at the bottom and leucocytes, pus cells, debris, dead sperms and seminal plasma remain in between the gradient layers[13].

Other less commonly used methods include :

(i) Albumin gradient separation which involves layering of washed sperms over HSA or BSA in a vertical column allowing progressively motile sperms to swim into two or more discontinuous albumin gradients. The albumin medium acts as a filter and after a period of 30 minutes, progressively motile sperms are obtained. However, this method reduces the total sperm count[14].

(ii) Glass wool separation. Here a Pasteur pipette is filled with glass wool. On the top of the column liquefied semen sample is placed. After about 30 minutes, motile sperms with improved fertilizing potential are obtained. Cervical mucus penetration is also increased. However, retention of glass fibres in the sample, inability to remove seminal plasma completely and ultrastructural damage to the membrane restricts its use routinely[15].

(iii) Glass bead column separation. Chemically treated small glass beads are used in a column and dilated semen sample is poured on top of it. As dead sperms stick to the glass beads, only live sperms move downwards. This method also yields much less motile sperms in the final recovery and hence is not used routinely[16,17].

General precautions

(i) Collection of sample. Split ejaculation method is preferred over single ejaculation. This is very useful particularly when :

(a) Patient has severe oligospermia. The whole semen sample is formed by successive addition of components from different glands at different times. First 2-3 spurts contain maximum sperm concentration which can be collected in the first split.

(b) Patients having highly viscous sample. If sperms and prostatic secretions are separated from the then following seminal plasma which contains proteins and enzymes responsible for clotting, then trapping of motile sperms in the coagulum can be avoided.

(c) Patients having autoantibodies. Many times sperms themselves act as antigens with their antibodies like proteins present in the seminal plasma. Collection of sample by split ejaculation can avoid their contact, thus preventing agglutination. This can be further reduced by collecting the sample in a container having sperm wash medium.

(ii) Type of container. If a plastic container is used, it has to be of polypropylene. Other plastics may turn out to be toxic to sperms. If the glass bottles are used, then borosilicate glass is preferred, which is to be tissue cultured, washed and heat sterilized. Contact of rubber with the sample is to be totally avoided.

(iii) Type of medium used. Many types of media can be used, *e.g.*, Tyrod's solution, Earl's balanced salt solution, HF10, HF12, Whittingham's BWW. Care has to be taken of proper protein supplement and proper concentration of calcium, sodium and potassium which are essential for natural progress of events leading to hyper-activation of the sperms, induction of acrosome reaction and fertilization[18].

(iv) Alkaline pH range between 7.1 and 7.4 of the medium should be maintained. Osmolarity between 220 and 380 mOsm/lit. is acceptable for IUI procedures.

(v) Addition of antibiotics to sperm wash medium. Penicillin, Gentamicin or Streptomycin can be used in a limited range of concentration. Higher concentration may have adverse effect on glycoproteins of the sperm head membrane thus impairing selective permeability and fertilizing ability of the sperm[19].

(vi) Day of treatment. IUI is generally done when leading follicles reach size of 18-20 mm and the day when they rupture. The sperms have the ability to survive in vivo up to 72 hours in the fertilizable conditions.

(vii) Type of catheter use. Catheter should be non-toxic, with smooth inner and outer surface and should be able to reach near the fundus without disturbing the endometrium.

(viii) Site of insemination. It is better to measure the utero-cervical length (UCL) before insemination. This is to avoid touching the fundus which may result in contraction of muscles and thus repulsion of the inseminated fluid.

(ix) Volume. 0.3 to 0.8 ml of prepared sample can be inseminated. Recently published papers prefer more volume to be inseminated. Patient is kept under head low position for 15-20 min.

New approaches and developments

Although the 20th century can be considered as a milestone in the treatment of infertility by giving birth of the test tube baby in 1978, looking retrospectively at the progress made in the field of male factor associated infertility, it can be realized that very little success is achieved in actually improving fertilizing ability of the spermatozoa.

Now it is proved beyond doubt that a successful fertilization and cleavage can be achieved in vitro even by using dead sperms by injecting DNA from the nucleus of the sperm head into the cytoplasm of the oocyte by micromanipulation techniques like SUZI (sub zonal insemination) and DISCO (direct insemination of spermatozoa into cytoplasm of the oocyte).

To date, attention was given mainly to improve the motility of the spermatozoa. Although motility is an important factor which allows sperms to reach the vicinity of the oocyte, there are many subsequent steps which lead to fertilization, *e.g.*, digestion of cumulus and corona by enzymes released during acrosome reaction, attachment of sperm head to zona pellucida, fusion of the two membranes and decantation of the DNA from the sperm head nucleus into the ooplasm. Recent research is therefore concentrated to improve all these factors for better fertilization rate in vivo as well as in vitro.

Some of the new ideas with encouraging results are :

1. Use of Methylxanthine derivatives like pentoxy-fylline and caffeine. These derivatives are known to inhibit phosphodiesterase activity. When phosphodiesterase activity is suppressed, more cAMP is available which acts as a second messenger in extracting energy from ATP. This energy is supplied to the tail portion of the sperm to enhance the motility. Methylxanthine derivatives are also known to boost up the acrosome reaction by altering the influx of calcium ions; the indigenous threshold concentration of which induces the reaction[20].
2. Exposure of the sperm with the sperm wash medium containing follicular fluid increases the fertilizing potential.
3. For severe oligospermic patients, cryoaccumulation of the sperm is done by preserving the husband's samples with abstinence of 4-5 days and then pooling them together at the time of IUI treatment.
4. Exposure of sperms to the combination of ATP with progesterone has been found to increase penetration in vitro[21].
5. Use of Forskolin, an adenylate cyclase activator, induces acrosome reaction without increasing cAMP content in the sperm in hamsters[22].
6. Prostaglandins trigger acrosome reaction by increasing influx of extracellular calcium. Follicular fluid, progesterone and prostaglandins cause increase in flow of cytosolic free calcium concentration in the human sperm. PGE1 and PGE2 induce calcium influx through the dihydropyridine insensitive calcium channel which may play an important role in triggering the acrosome reaction[23].
7. In mice, co-culturing granulosa cells or oviductal cells with sperms is found to accelerate the fertilization rate due to an increase in sperm motility and facilitation of acrosome reaction[24].

Assisted reproductive techniques like IUI combined with modifications in sperm preparation techniques aid the fertilizing ability thereby improving pregnancy rates. Before I close I would like to present our own results (Tables 40.1 to 40.4).

Fertility Clinic results

Table 40.1. Patients (n = 170)

	No. of cycles	
COH + IUI	154	345 cycles
CC + IUI	191	
IUI	47	
	392	

No. of pregnancies = 30

Table 40.2. Male Factor — Semen and stimulation protocol

No. of patients = 90
No. of cycles = 239
No. of pregnancies = 13 (14.4%)

Count (millions/ml)	*IUI*	*CC + IUI*	*COH + IUI*	*Pregnancy/ cycle*
< 1	8	14	2	0/24
1-3	7	49 (1 pregnancy)	17	1/73 (1.4%)
> 3 - < 10	18	67 (4 pregnancies) (4.9%)	57 (8 pregnancies) (14.0%)	12/142 (8.6%)

Table 40.3. Age of patients

	No. of patients	*No. of pregnancies*
< 30	82	21 (25.6%)
30-35	63	7 (11.1%)
36-40	25	2 (8.0%)

Table 40.4. Male factor — method of semen preparation

Count < 10×10^6

	No. of cycles	*No. of pregnancies*
Swim up	171	6 (3.5%)
Pentoxyfylline	68	7 (11.8%)

REFERENCES

1. Hanson FM, Rock J. Artificial insemination with husband's sperms. Fertil Steril 1951; 2 : 162-4.
2. Barwin BN. Intrauterine insemination using husband's semen. J Reprod Fertil 1974; 36 : 101-3.
3. Cohen MR. Intrauterine insemination. Int J Fertil 1962; 7 : 235-9.
4. White RM, Glass RH. Intrauterine insemination with husband's semen. Obstet Gynecol 1976; 47 : 119-23.
5. Scammell GE, Stedronska J, Dempsey A. Successful pregnancies using human seroalbumin following retrograde ejaculation : a case report. Fertil Steril 1982; 37 : 277-9.
6. Nachtigall R, Faure N, Glass RH. Artificial insemination of husband's sperms. Fertil Steril 1979; 32 : 141-5.
7. Muasher SJ, Garcia JE, Rosenwaks Z. The combination of follicle stimulating hormone and human menopausal gonadotropin for the induction of multiple follicular maturation for IVF. Fertil Steril 1985; 42 : 62-9.
8. Serhal PF, Katz M, Little V, Woronowski H. Unexplained infertility : the value of Pergonal superovulation combined with intrauterine insemination. Fertil Steril 1988; 49 : 602-7.
9. Shelden R, Kemmann E, Bohrer M, Pasquale S. Multiple gestation is associated with the use of high sperm number in the intrauterine insemination specimen in women undergoing gonadotropin stimulation. Fertil Steril 1988; 49 : 607-11.
10. Baerthlein WC, Muechler EK, Chaney K. Simplified sperm washing techniques intrauterine insemination. Obstet Gynecol 1988; 71 : 277-82.
11. Arny M, Quagliarello J. Semen quality before and after processing by a swim-up method : relationship to outcome of intrauterine insemination. Fertil Steril 1987; 48 : 643-7.
12. Windt ML, Menkveld R, Kruger TF, Van der Merwe JP. The effect of sperm washing and swim-up on antibodies bound to sperm membrane : Use of immunobed/ sperm cervical mucus contact tests. Arch Androl 1989; 22 : 55-9.
13. Acosta AA. Human spermatozoa in assisted reproduction. Arch Androl 1990; 23 : 264-7.
14. Dmowski WP, Gaynor L, Lawrence M, Rao R. Artificial insemination homologous with oligospermic semen separated on albumin columns. Fertil Steril 1979; 31 : 58-63.
15. Van der Ven HH, Jeyendran RS, Tunnerhoff A, Hoebbel K. Glass wool column filtration of human semen : relation swim-up procedure and IVF outcome. Hum Reprod 1988; 3 : 85-9.
16. Rhemrev J, Jeyendran RS, Zaneveld LJD. Selection of

viable spermatozoa by glass wool filtration or percoll density gradient centrifugation. J Androl 1988; 9 : 23-7.

17. Edward RG. Human conception in vitro. Proceedings of the 1st Bourn Hall Meeting, London, 1985.
18. Purdy Jean M. Human conception in vitro. Proceedings of the 1st Bourn Hall Meeting, London, 1985.
19. Alexander NJ, Steven B, Ackerman M. Evaluation and preparation of spermatozoa for intrauterine insemination. Arch Androl 1990; 25 : 262-6.
20. Yovich JL. The role of methylxanthine derivatives for sperm enhancement. (Proceedings of 8th World Congress on IVF and alternate assisted reproduction, Japan) J Asst Reprod Gen 1993; 10 : 58-9.
21. Tomiyama T, Ohashi K, Tsutsui T. Acrosome reaction of human sperm induced by ATP and progesterone. (Proceedings of 8th World Congress on IVF and alternate assisted reproduction, Japan) J Asst Reprod Gen 1993; 10 : 118-9.
22. Oshio S, Ishda K, Tomomasa H, Yazaki T. Forskolin stimulates human sperm penetration into zona free hamster oocytes in vitro. (Proceedings of 8th World Congress on IVF and alternate assisted reproduction, Japan) J Asst Reprod Gen 1993; 10 : 117-8.
23. Shimizu Y, Kubota T, Sakamoto S. Prostaglandins induce calcium influx in human sperm. (Proceedings of 8th World Congress on IVF and alternate assisted reproduction, Japan) J Asst Reprod Gen 1993; 10 : 119-20.
24. Bongso A, Fong CY, Rathnam SS. Human sperm and embryo behaviour in human oviduct and endometrial coculture systems. (Proceedings of 8th World Congress on IVF and alternate assisted reproduction, Japan) J Asst Reprod Gen 1993; 10 : 54-5.

CHAPTER

41

Management of Male Infertility : A Surgeon's View

S. Thatte

Approximately 15% of the the couples attempting their first pregnancy meet with failure. It is believed that approximately 30% is solely secondary to male factors, while in another 20% both partners have detectable abnormalities. Therefore in approximately 50% of infertile couples male factor is partially responsible for infertility.

Treatment of male infertility offers more hope to childless couples today than ever before. Techniques of assisted reproduction for achieving pregnancy in cases of male factor have been successful in many cases when all other treatments have failed. The surgical therapies have shown higher chances of success with the introduction of the operating microscope.

The surgical procedures that may be needed to be performed upon the subfertile male fall into two headings — diagnostic and therapeutic. The diagnostic procedures done are testicular biopsy and vasography. The therapeutic surgical procedures are undertaken for hydrococele, varicocele, undescended testis, vasovasostomy, vasoepididymostomy, transurethral incision of the ejaculatory duct (TURED), microsurgical epididymal sperm aspiration (MESA) and placement of artificial spermatococele for subsequent aspiration.

Testicular biopsy

With the advent of sophisticated laboratory techniques, including cytogenetics and radio-immunoassay, it is not necessary to perform testicular biopsy in most subfertile males. There are, however, specific indications for this procedure — azoospermia or severe oligozoospermia in presence of normal size testis and normal gonadotropin levels. If one testis is quite small and the other is normal in size, the few sperms that are found may be coming from the small testis, as there may be a complete obstruction on the contralateral side. In this instance, a bilateral testicular biopsy should be performed. In most cases when the testes are of equal size and consistency, only one testis needs to be biopsied. The biopsy can be performed by an open method or percutaneous needle biopsy. Biopsy material should be placed in Bouin's solution and not in formalin. For the electron microscopic study, glutaraldehyde solution is to be used.

Vasography

This is of particular importance if the patient has had prior inguinal surgery or if the seminal volume is relatively small (< 1 ml) and clinically the vas is palpable or thickened which is suggestive of ejaculatory duct obstruction. Patency of the vas needs to be confirmed prior to vaso-epididymal-anastomosis and this should be undertaken at time of definitive surgery rather than pre-operatively to avoid latrogenic block at the site of vasography.

Hydrococele

This condition is very commonly seen in a surgical practice and can contribute to the infertility in the male and in certain patients surgical correction would help in improving the sperm parameters. The hydrococele depresses the spermatogenesis by the disturbed heat exchange mechanism because of the fluid filled within tunica vaginalis. If the fluid quantity is large (tense hydrococele) it can cause pressure atrophy and also lead to separation of the epididymis from the testes.

Infertility may be caused due to surgery undertaken for hydrococele as during surgery there would be inadvertent trauma to epididymis or vas deferens, surgery may lead to fibrosis or post-operative infection may cause the damage.

When undertaking surgery for hydrococele in young males it is advisable to avoid surgery for small hydrococele, avoid prophylactic surgery on the contralateral side and always carry out a testicular biopsy along with hydrococele surgery in cases of azoospermia or severe oligozoospermia. To avoid injury to the epididymis or vas during hydrococele surgery one should stay away from these structures.

Varicocele

Varicocele is still considered the most common correctable cause of infertility. It is estimated that 8-16% of unselected population would have a varicocele. It is also seen that approximately 40% of men who visit infertility clinics have varicocele. Presence of varicocele does not automatically indicate infertility as in 50% of these patients the semen analysis would be normal.

Varicocele in the face of abnormal semen analysis would be significant but the exact mechanism which leads to the abnormal count is still not well understood. The various theories put forward are, there is increase in the testicular temperature due to increased arterial blood flow, hypoxia of the germinal epithelium and reflux of the toxic substances due to incompetent valves in the gonadal veins.

The diagnosis of a varicocele can be made by clinical examination with the patient standing and the Valsalva manoeuvre. One can also detect a smaller varicocele with the help of Doppler stethoscope and use of colour Doppler.

Varicocele ligation is one of the most commonly performed surgeries in the treatment of male infertility[1].

Even when a varicocele is detected in a man with abnormal semen count, controversy exists as to whether correction of the varicocele will improve the semen count to an extent that pregnancy will be possible, some authors claim that varicocele ligation is no more effective than medical therapy in improving male infertility[2,3]. Various studies have demonstrated improvement in the semen analysis in 35-85% of patients after varicocele surgery and the pregnancy rate achieved is around 40%. Results of the surgery depend on combination of several factors.

A variety of techniques have been described to ligate or obliterate the dilated veins. Since the report of Tulloch[4] in 1952, treatment of varicocele has primarily been by surgical ligation. The open surgery can be carried out through either inguinal, retroperitoneal (high ligation) or subinguinal or scrotal incision. With all the surgical techniques it is important to preserve the testicular artery and lymphatics in order to be sure that testicular function is not further compromised. Microsurgical varicocelectomy and intra-operative application of vasodilator like papavaerine or lignocaine will allow for direct visualisation of the testicular artery in every case and more precise ligation of the accompanying veins.

Urological surgeons have attempted to employ their newly acquired laparoscopic skill to varicocelectomy. Recently presented data has shown that unilateral laparoscopic varicocelectomy was two times costlier than surgical procedure. As experience increases operative time will decrease. This will also reduce the cost.

It is also shown that there is no benefit relating to recovery parameters such as analgesic requirement or rest required before returning to work. There is a possibility of damage to the testicular artery during the laparoscopic procedure. Therefore laparoscopic varicocelectomy appears not to offer any advantages and has a theoretical disadvantage when compared to the open surgical procedure.

Percutaneous sclerotherapy was first reported by Limas *et al.*[5] in 1978. Since then, various techniques such as sclerotherapy, coils and detachable balloons have been used by the femoral or jugular venous approach to occlude the spermatic vein. Each technique has its own advantages or disadvantages. Sclerosing therapy can occlude small collateral vessels but extent of the sclerosing agent cannot be controlled; recanalisation is a possibility and there is pain during the procedure. Balloon occlusion can be accurately placed beyond the collateral veins but these are expensive, coils are inexpensive but placement is relatively difficult. Overall complication rate is around 11% and only reported major complications are two embolisations of balloons to the lung without detectable sequelae. Minor complications are extravasation, contrast reaction, testicular thrombophlebitis, venous spasm. Overall occlusion rate is 73% but varies from 50-100% on left side varicocele. The overall recurrence rate is 50%. Percutaneous embolisations are necessary as treatment for surgical failures, primarily because of their advantage in locating and treating collaterals that were missed or developed after surgical ligation.

Obstruction azoospermia

Obstruction of the male reproductive tract may represent another correctable cause of infertility. Obstructive azoospermia could be due to epididymal obstruction or ejaculatory duct obstruction.

The most common causes are vasectomy. Infection specially smallpox, congenital block including congenital vasal agenesis and rarely latrogenic obstruction due to surgery for hydrococele, or inguinal herniorrhaphy.

Vasovasostomy

In 1915, Quinby reported the first vasovasostomy performed on a man requesting restoration of his fertility after vasectomy. Since that time, many procedures have been performed with varying degree of success. The only factor which predicts the success for vasectomy reversal has been the time interval since vasectomy. The longer the interval since the vasectomy, the less likely sperms would return to the ejaculate and less likely the fertility would ensue.

The macrosurgical technique consisted of anastomosing the vas over a nylon splint. In experienced hands, even this relatively crude technique could achieve patency rates of 70-90% and pregnancy rates of 30-55%[6]. However the newer microsurgical techniques give better results with regard to patency and pregnancy as compared to nonmicroscopic techniques. With microsurgical procedures the patency rates are 85-97% and pregnancy rates are 50-75%[7].

In the two layer method, mucosa is anastomosed to mucosa using 10.0 nylon, and the muscle is anastomosed over with 8.0 nylon to achieve a leak-proof anastomosis. In the single layer technique, the vas is anastomosed using 6 full thickness stitches that include muscle and mucosa and the anastomosis is then made leak-proof by placing additional stitches through seromuscular layer. Recent studies have shown that both carefully performed anastomosis have resulted in similar success rates. The important principle in vasovasostomy is accurate approximation of the mucosal edge, lack of tension, anastomosis to be carried out on straight vas, and to check that the proximal cut end of vas shows presence of sperms, if sperms are absent from the fluid then vasoepididymal-anastomosis should be carried out.

Vaso-epididymal-anastomosis

Azoospermia secondary to epididymal obstruction may result from congenital or acquired lesions. Each epididymis measures approximately 1 × 1 × 5 cm in size and if unfolded, the entire tubular length would be about 4 metres with a diameter of about 0.2-0.3 mm. The causes of epididymal obstruction can be either inflammatory (smallpox, TB) congenital, post-vasectomy or traumatic.

Whatever the cause, diagnosis of epididymal obstruction should not be difficult when presented with an azoospermic patient with active spermatogenesis, a normal semen volume and no prior surgery in the scrotal or inguinal area.

In vaso-epididymal-anastomosis the vas is rejoined to the epididymis proximal to the site of obstruction.

As the diameter of the tubule is only 0.2-0.3 mm, in the conventional method (macroscopic VEA) the surgeon is unable to anastomose the epididymal ductule to the vas directly hence after incision in the epididymis, slit open vas is sutured to the fascia surrounding the epididymal ductule and create a sperm fistula and the sperms coming out of ductule will find their way into the vas. The patency and pregnancy rates are low.

The new microsurgical techniques which use the magnification of an operative microscope are prepared to achieve a direct anastomosis between the epididymal ductule and the vas mucosa. Two techniques are popular :

1. End to end technique of Silber[8]. The epididymis is transected and the cut end of the vas is sutured to the cut end of the ductule.
2. End to side technique[9]. A loop of epididymal ductule is dissected free and a side hole is made in it and the cut end of the vas is sutured to this opening.

The end to side anastomosis to a single loop of the epididymal tubule seems, currently, the most popular method of VEA. The lumen of the vas is carefully sutured to the opened, unroofed epididymal tubule using five 10.0 nylon sutures. The muscularis and adventia of the vas deferens are then sutured to the tunica of the epididymis with interrupted 9.0 nylon sutures.

Several studies have now shown that the microsurgical technique of direct anastomosis has better results than the conventional method[10,11]. Microsurgical VEA achieves patency rates of 50-85% and pregnancy rates between 37-51%.

Ejaculatory duct obstruction

Azoospermia or oligozoospermia can be caused by complete or partial obstruction of the ejaculatory ducts or obstruction to the terminal portion of vas where it is joined by seminal vesicles. The obstruction may be congenital, inflammatory or iatrogenic.

These patients usually present with small semen volume (less than 1 ml), the semen is often acidic in nature with pH around 6 and with some or no fructose present. Physical examination shows normal size testis with full epididymis and palpable vas.

Diagnosis is confirmed by transrectal ultrasound or vasography. Marked dilatation of the seminal vesicle and ejaculatory ducts can be seen. There may be presence of Mullerian duct cyst — a congenital condition causing obstruction[9]. The obstruction exists at the end of ejaculatory ducts but there may be associated obstruction within the epididymis similar to the "blow out" that occurs in some cases after vasectomy due to high pressure. The more distal obstruction should be taken care of first before VEA is performed in these cases.

The technique for unroofing the obstruction is to undertake vasography and cystoscopy in a lithotomy position on a X-ray table. The vas is canulated and fluid aspirated for identification of sperms and a mixture of contrast material and small amount of indigo carmine is then injected into vas. With the resectoscope loop the bulge seen proximal to veru is opened up. One has to be careful in not damaging the bladder neck and the external sphincter. As the ejaculatory duct is opened up the blue colour of indigo carmine is immediately seen. Minimal cauterisation is to be carried out in order to prevent subsequent scarring of the area. Patients are on indwelling catheter for 24 hours and advised to abstain from intercourse for 2-3 weeks and do semen analysis after 6 weeks.

If the transurethral endoscope resection is not feasible then sperm could be aspirated from the vas and IUI of IVF could be carried out.

Artificial spermatocele

Bilateral congenital absence of vasa deferentia is seen in about 1% of men with azoospermia. Clinical diagnosis is confirmatory and surgical exploration or testicular biopsy in these cases of azoospermia is not required.

Semen analysis shows azoospermia, low semen volume and absent fructose, a doubtful palpable vas is an absent vas.

Creating an artificial spermatocele to aspirate sperms repeatedly have not been successful. Various techniques and materials have been used with only a minimum success. In 1968 Schoysman described the technique of using a segment of saphenous vein sutured to an open epididymis from which sperm could be aspirated. He reported four pregnancies but the vein graft showed early obliteration within days to week after implantation. Wagenknecht used silicon prosthesis but with minimum success. In 1986 Belker compiled the results of 91 patients who underwent 130 spermatocele implantation, only seven pregnancies resulted, three of which ended in miscarriage. Recently Moni and Lalitha[12] described four patients in whom the epididymal tubule was left open, draining into tunica vaginalis as a sort of natural spermatocele, which was subsequently aspirated for sperms, one pregnancy resulted. This method needs to be further evaluated in order to see whether it is able to be used for multiple aspiration of sperms.

Microsurgical sperm aspiration (MESA)

In 1985 it was reported by Temple-Smith[13] and associates that sperm aspirated from the epididymis could be used for in vitro fertilization (IVF) with successful pregnancy. Recently published combined results of 217 cases having undergone epididymal aspiration with IVF have shown 23 pregnancies (11%).

All wives underwent IVF — some with micromanipulation.

Technique of MESA is similar to that of vasoepididymostomy without the anastomosis. Under operating microscope, the epididymis is visualised and tunica overlying the epididymal tubule is incised, exposing and isolating single loop of epididymis, loop is incised and fluid is examined for sperms, the fluid is aspirated with a micropipette and specimen handed over to the reproductive biologist. The loop of tubule is closed with 10.0 nylon suture. The tunica overlying the loop is closed with running 9.0 nylon to minimize scarring and to make it more easily accessible if another procedure needs to be performed in the future.

Undescended testis

To maintain spermatogenic functions an undescended testis should be brought down by age of 2 years. It has been shown that an unilateral atrophied testis may have a negative immunological effect on the normal testis thus causing infertility.

Improvement in the semen quality after removal of unilateral atrophied testis is seen but response is unpredictable. If unilateral undescended testis is small and atrophied and even if it can be brought into the scrotum it is advisable to remove it.

In summary there are number of surgical procedures which will help infertile male to achieve fatherhood but one should subject these men for surgical procedures only with appropriate indications. Microsurgical techniques will help in achieving higher success rates. Microsurgical aspiration of sperms from epididymis or even testis with micromanipulation will be the only hope in number of infertile couples to achieve pregnancy.

REFERENCES

1. Dubuin L, Amelar RD. Varicocelectomy : 986 cases in a year study. Urology 10, 446, 1977.
2. Nilsson S, Edvinsson A, Nilsson B. Improvement of semen and pregnancy rate after ligation and division of the internal spermatic vein : Fact or fiction? Br J Urol 51, 591, 1979.
3. Vermeulen A, Van de Weighe M. Improved fertility after varicocele correction : Fact or fiction?. Fertil Steril 42 : 249, 1984.
4. Tulloch WS. Varicocele in subinfertility : Results of treatment. Br Med J. 2 : 356, 1955.
5. Lima SS, Castro MP, Costa OF. A new method for the treatment of varicocele. Andrologia 10 : 103, 1978.
6. Phadke GM, Phadke AG. Experiences in the reanastomosis of the vas deferens. J Urol 97, 888, 1967.
7. Silber SJ. Microscopic vasectomy reversal. Fertil Steril 28, 1191, 1977.
8. Silber SJ. Microscopic vasoepididymostomy, specific microanastomosis to the epididymal tubule. Fertil Steril 30, 565, 1978.
9. Fogdestam I, Fall M, Nilsson S. Microsurgical epididymovasostomy in the treatment of occlusive azoospermia. Fertil Steril 466, 925, 1986.
10. Hendry WF. The long-term results of surgery for obstructive azoospermia. Br J Urol 53, 664, 1981.
11. Niederberger C, Ross LS. Microsurgical epididymovasostomy : Predictors of success. J Urol 149, 1364, 1993.
12. Moni VN and Lalitha PA. Moni's window operation : A new surgical technique to create a sperm reservoir in congenital vasal agenesis. J Urol 148 : 843, 1992.
13. Temple-Smith PD, Southwick GJ, Yates CA *et al.* Human pregnancy by in vitro fertilization (IVF) using sperm aspirated from the epididymis. J In Vitro Fert Embryo Transf 2 : 119, 1985.

CHAPTER 42

Critical Appraisal of Tubal Surgery in Infertility

Kusum Zaveri

Introduction

Tubal occlusion is the principal cause of 25-30% of female infertility. The success of tubal surgery is dependent upon both the nature and extent of tubal damage as well as the expertise of the surgeon. Before the initiation of surgical repair, a thorough evaluation of the fallopian tube is therefore requisite to accurately make a post-surgical prognosis. With the advent of in vitro fertilization (IVF) and embryo transfer (ET), the infertility surgeon has an alternative recommendation should the probability of surgical reproductive restoration be less than the pregnancy rate attainable in IVF-ET.

Tubal blocks are divided into three categories based on their site of occurrence: cornual or proximal block, mid block, and terminal block.

Proximal block

Approximately 20% of tubal surgery is performed for occlusion of the proximal portion of the fallopian tube[1].

Diagnosis

The diagnosis of proximal tubal occlusion has remained controversial. Hystero-salpingography (HSG) over-diagnoses proximal tubal occlusion in as many as 42% of the patients. Laparoscopy and HSG do not give accuracy of diagnosis of proximal tubal occlusion as they cannot differentiate a spasm from an occlusion.

Pathology

The concept of intraluminal tubal plugs as a cause of proximal occlusion has risen only recently. In a convincing study, Sulak *et al.*[2] demonstrated that crystallized tubal secretions can cause obstruction of the proximal part of the oviduct. Recent reports suggest that in most cases this abnormality is caused by amorphous intraluminal debris, light adhesions or muscular spasms[2]. It is more correct to record this finding less specifically as 'Proximal Tubal Injection Failure' without hypothesizing as to the cause.

In light of this consideration, selective osteal salpingography is an effective tool to differentiate functional from organic obstructions of the fallopian tube.

Treatment

The traditional approach to the correction of a cornual occlusion has been cornual implantation. In the mid 1970s, Gomel recommended a microsurgical tubo-cornual anastomosis for proximal tubal block with improved results over cornual implantation. In the 1980s, selective salpingography or transcervical tubal cannulation gained popularity because of high recanalisation success rates.

Several investigators have pioneered techniques to relieve proximal tubal obstruction caused by luminal debris using tubal catheterisation, thus avoiding surgery (Table 42.1).

Table 42.1.

	Patency rate	*Pregnancy rate*	*Recanalisation procedure*
Confino *et al.*[3]	92%	34%	Transcervical balloon plasty
Novy *et al.*[4]	84%		Fluoroscopy
	92%		Hysteroscopy
Dietrich *et al.*[5]			Tactile sensation
Lisse & Sydow[6]	84.2%	31%	Ultrasonography

Confino *et al.*[3] reported the cannulation and opening of the fallopian tube by a balloon catheter in a multi-centric study where 92% patency rate and a 34% intrauterine pregnancy rate was attained in 77 patients.

Novy *et al.*[4] demonstrated that fluoroscopic and hysteroscopic catheterisation resulted in 84% and 92% patency rates respectively. The positioning of the catheter by a tactile technique has been reported by Dietrich *et al.*[5], who reported that characteristic discomfort was experienced by patients when the tubes were successfully catheterised. Lisse and Sydow[6] reported that fallopian tube catheterisation and recanalisation under ultrasonic observation was successful in 91% of the fallopian tubes with pregnancy resulting in 31% of the patients. They used direct visualisation by laparoscopy to confirm the success of their technique.

Until recently, investigators have had to rely primarily on the more indirect methods of HSG and hydrochromotubation under laparoscopic observation for assessing tubal patency, stricture formation, dilatation or obstruction. More recently, fluoroscopic tubal catheterisation, hysteroscopically directed tubal cannulation, and transcervical balloon tuboplasty have been used. Recently, falloposcopy which provides direct visual evidence of the site, nature and extent of tubal epithelial defects, is considered to be very important for improving the results. Kerin *et al.*[7] report falloposcopy on 74 patients which was in concurrence with HSG and laparoscopy in 74% of the cases. Falloposcopy is a safe technique for both diagnostic and therapeutic purposes. A falloposcopic classification and scoring system has been developed to characterise and qualitate the site, type and severity of endotubal disease, and to co-relate such a scoring system with endotuboplasty results and pregnancy outcomes[7].

Colour Doppler

Stern *et al.*[8], in 49 patients used colour Doppler ultrasound, HSG and laparoscopy for proximal tubal block diagnosis. The frequency of agreement between colour ultrasound and chromopertubation was 82%, and with HSG 57%.

Digital Road Mapping Technique (DRM)

The road map technique is also used to improve the safety factor and efficacy of fluoroscopic transcervical tuboplasty. Out of 10 patients, catheterisation was achieved in all with 3 pregnancies within 3 months[9].

Re-occlusion

Thurmond and Rosch[10] reported re-occlusion after recanalisation in 50% of cases after a year. The recanalisation procedure ought to be repeated to rule out recurrent obstruction after a year.

Conclusion

In conclusion, several new techniques are currently available for evaluation of proximal block. Transcervical selective salpingography is less invasive than surgery, requires no general anaesthesia, and is useful for diagnosis and treatment. Hence, after HSG and laparoscopic diagnosis, selective salpingography is a popularly used technique for proximal tubal occlusion diagnosis.

Tubal surgery for proximal block has changed from cornual implantation to microsurgical tubocornual anastomosis yielding results from 23% to 56%. From laparotomy it has changed to selective osteal salpingography giving 92% patency and 34% intrauterine pregnancy (IUP) rates. In very selective cases where falloposcopy shows extensive tubal damage, IVF will be the only treatment available to the patient.

Mid block

Reversal of sterilization forms the major group in this category, whereas tubotubal anastomosis for the correction of tubal occlusion secondary to the pathologic event is rare.

Diagnosis

1. Laparoscopy
2. HSG
3. Falloposcopy

Preoperative laparoscopic evaluation will give the information about types of sterilization, tubal length, peritubal and paraovarian adhesions, presence of fimbria and associated pathology. This helps in the selection of the patient and facilitates the prognosis.

Performance of a microsurgical anastomosis for mid-block specially in reversal of sterilization has given satisfactory results. Cost containment pressure as well as a desire to reduce patient morbidity are the main reasons for the exploration of new techniques. Initial attempts at developing techniques for outpatient reversal of tubal sterilization by a purely laparoscopic approach have not yet met with success. Sedban and co-authors[11] reported on 5 cases performed with fibrin glue with no subsequent pregnancies. Reich[12] reported on 20 cases with laparoscopic suturing techniques. There were 2 subsequent term pregnancies and 3 ectopic pregnancies. Conversely Berger[13] reported a 73% intrauterine pregnancy rate in 26 women who had been followed for at least 1 year after outpatient sterilization reversal by laparotomy. Outpatient microsurgical reversal of tubal sterilization by a combined approach of laparoscopy and mini-laparotomy has good theoretical potential for safety. Silva and co-authors[14] have shown in a prospective study of 17 cases of microsurgical reversal of tubal sterilization by a combined approach of laparoscopy and mini-laparotomy, 71% success rate with a significant reduction in cost and time as compared with standard techniques. Hence, for mid-blocks, laparotomy reversal has not changed technically over the years.

Distal block

Distal tubal occlusion with varying degrees of dilatation and mucosal damage can be a result of acute pelvic infection, intra-abdominal or appendicular infection, pelvic surgery or endometriosis.

In 1970, Young *et al.*[15] suggested that the pregnancy rate in patients with distal occlusion when normal rugae were observed at the time of HSG was 60% as opposed to a 7.3% success rate when rugae were absent.

Classification

Rock *et al.*[16] classified distal tubal block into mild, moderate and severe disease, taking account of :

1. Quality of tubal mucosa at HSG
2. Degree of distal tubal dilatation
3. Extent of associated adhesions

Similarly, Bruhat *et al.*'s classification[17] was based on a scoring system using :

1. Appearance of mucosal folds at HSG
2. Degree of distal occlusion
3. Appearance of tubal wall evaluated at laparoscopy

Adhesions were classified using the scoring system (filmy, vascular and dense)[17].

Both the above classifications help to establish a system for prognosis for successful outcome in patients undergoing distal neo-salpingotomy.

Salpingoscopy

Endoscopic evaluation of the endosalpinx has been shown to provide information that directly correlates to the reproductive outcome after surgery, independent of the information obtainable by HSG or laparoscopy. Salpingoscopic observations differed from the findings noted on routine external examination of the fimbriae in 23.5% of the patients[18]. Salpingoscopy therefore provides a diagnostic modality of obvious importance to reproductive surgeons and may prove to be an indispensable tool in the evaluation and in the subsequent treatment of distal tubal disease.

Treatment

The outcome of surgery for distal tubal obstruction using conventional techniques by a number of authors ranged from 20% to 35% with 10-50% of these pregnancies being tubal ectopics. The concept of microsurgical techniques was introduced in the 1960s in an attempt to improve surgical results. Many studies using microsurgical techniques have been published showing crude pregnancy rates in the range of 30 to 40%, again with 10-30% of these being tubal ectopics[19,20,21]. Significant advances in the laparoscopic treatment of tuboperitoneal infertility have been made in the last 10 years. The first reports of laparoscopic distal tuboplasty appeared promising. The Pregnancy

Rates (PR) were 44% and 26% in the studies of Gomel[22] and Mettler *et al.*[23] respectively. Bruhat *et al.*[24] found no difference in PRs between microsurgery and laparoscopy, and reported 33.3% PRs with laparoscopic distal tuboplasty. Dubuisson and Joliniere[25] also reported 27.7% PR following the laparoscopic approach (Table 42.2).

Table 42.2. Laparoscopic pregnancy rate in terminal salpingostomy

	No. of cases	*No. of pregnancies (%)*
Mettler *et al.*[23]	38	10 (26%)
Gomel[22]	9	4 (44%)
Fayez[26]	19	2 (10%) (Ectopic)
Bruhat *et al.*[24]	87	29 (33.3%)
Dubuisson *et al.*[25]	65	22 (27.7%)

When compared with classical procedures performed by laparotomy, laparoscopic surgery has several widely accepted advantages including minimal physical stress, shorter hospitalization time and reduced costs. Furthermore, when using laparoscopy, diagnosis and treatment are always achieved during the same operative procedure. Laparoscopic procedures limit the risk of postoperative adhesions. Nevertheless, operative laparoscopy requires a laparoscopist well trained in endoscopic procedures and tubal surgery. For mild distal tubal lesions laparoscopy may be an alternative to microsurgery, and in severe disease, IVF-ET may be the right choice.

CO_2 Laser

The use of the CO_2 laser represents another generation of surgical breakthroughs in the treatment of distal tubal occlusion.

Fayez[26] as well as Mage and Bruhat[27] have reported that the term pregnancy rate was 16.6% with the use of electrosurgery, whereas that with the use of the CO_2 laser was 23.7%. This difference was not significant and hence the CO_2 laser has no magical advantage over electrocautery[27].

Using the salpingoscope, patients with very mild mucosal damage can be selected for laparoscopic or microsurgical neosalpingostomy. Improved selection of patients and the prognosis of salpingostomy can be significantly improved by preoperative salpingoscopy.

Tubal transplant

Tubal transplantation cases are reported but still remain case reports, and are not part of routine surgery.

In animal experiments, a synthetic tube is transplanted as conduit and is found to be working. The same experience remains to be transferred to the human being.

Ectopic pregnancy

Although the management of ectopic pregnancies does not fall strictly under the purview of tubal surgery, it is relevant to examine the effects of treatment of such ectopic pregnancies, since they directly affect the fallopian tube, as well as future reproduction. Ectopic gestation accounts for 1% of all reported pregnancies[28,29]. To reduce post-operative morbidity and to preserve child-bearing ability, improvements in the treatment of ectopic gestation have been sought. Recent improvements in diagnostic modalities, operative laparoscopy and microsurgical instrumentation have enabled the widespread use of conservative techniques.

Management

Oral administration or injection of methotrexate (MTX) into the gestational sac under ultrasonographic guidance, laparoscopic linear salpingostomy, with or without suturing, or laparoscopic salpingectomy are carried out as compared to laparotomy.

Medical management

Non-surgical treatment for ectopic pregnancies including transvaginal intra-tubal administration of MTX does not require anaesthesia, major surgery or prolonged hospitalisation, and majority of patients do not require future intervention.

MTX can be given orally, parenterally, or locally in an individualised dose schedule. Menard *et al.*[30] reported a 50 mg single dose in 17 patients with complete resolution in 13 cases. Oral and local MTX has a few disadvantages such as prolonged follow-up time, close clinical monitoring with β-hCG and USG, and hence is not cost-effective. Again, the long-term fertility after local MTX remains subject to further study.

Local MTX has the advantage over systemic MTX of no side effects like dermatitis, alopecia, pleuritis, vomiting, diarrhea and hepatic or bone marrow toxicity (24% of cases in oral therapy)[31].

Surgical management

Several studies have shown that laparoscopy appears to be safe and effective when compared with laparotomy for the treatment of ectopic pregnancies.

Vermesh *et al.*[32] in a prospective randomised trial comparing laparoscopy with laparotomy for treatment of unruptured ectopic pregnancies by linear salpingostomy reported significant decrease in estimated blood loss and length of hospital stay with no difference in patency of the tube and the intrauterine pregnancy rate.

Tulandi & Melvin[33] showed a higher incidence of intrauterine pregnancies after conservative treatment than after salpingectomy, and intrauterine pregnancies occur earlier after salpingostomy without suturing than with suturing (Table 42.3)[33].

Table 42.3. Laparoscopic management of ectopic pregnancy[33]

	No. of cases	*IUP within 12 months*	*IUP within 24 months*
Salpingostomy w/o suturing	15	45%	45%
Salpingostomy with suturing	19	21%	47%
Salpingectomy	24	21%	26%

Dubuisson *et al.*[34] reported laparoscopic salpingectomy in 241 cases. Only 2 patients developed complications. The pregnancy rate was 46.9% when the contralateral tube was normal, and 25.6% when the contralateral tube was abnormal. The procedure is simple, readily performed and post-operative complications are rare. Tuomivaara & Kaupilla[35] also reported an IUP rate of 64% in the laparoscopic salpingectomy group.

Conservative treatment for the second ectopic has little value. It may predispose to a high risk of recurrence (Table 42.4).

Table 42.4. Reproductive potential after two consecutive ectopic pregnancies (EP)

	No. of cases	*% of IUPs*	*% of EPs*
Vermesh *et al.*[32]	10	20%	66.7%
Pouly *et al.*[36]	27	11.1%	57%
DeCherney *et al.*[37]	13	30.8%	20%

Conclusions

There have been significant changes in the diagnostic and therapeutic approach to proximal and distal tubal blocks. From laparotomy, we have progressed to minimally invasive and non-invasive treatment. On the other hand, treatment of mid-block has not changed much except for the transition from being an inpatient to an out-patient procedure.

REFERENCES

1. Musich JR, Behrman SJ. Surgical management of tubal obstruction of the uterotubal junction. Fertil Steril 1983; 40 : 423-41.
2. Sulak PJ, Lettesie GS, Coddington CC. History of proximal tubal occlusion. Fertil Steril 1987; 48 : 437-9.
3. Coufino E, Tukarspa I, DeCherney AH. Transcervical balloon tuboplasty — A multi-centre study. JAMA 1990; 264 : 2079-82.
4. Novy MJ, Thurmond AS, Patton P, Uchida BT. Diagnosis of cornual obstruction by transcervical fallopian tube cannulation. Fertil Steril 1988; 50 : 434-5.
5. Dietrich K, Banner O, Warner A. Transvaginal intratubal embryo transfer : A new treatment of male infertility. Hum Reprod 1991; 6 : 672-5.
6. Lisse K, Sydow P. Fallopian tube catheterization and recanalization under ultrasonic observation : a simplified technique to evaluate tubal patency and open proximally obstructed tubes. Fertil Steril 1991; 56 : 198-201.
7. Kerin JF, Pearlstone AC, Williams DB. Falloposcopic classification and treatment of fallopian tube lumen disease. Fertil Steril 1992; 57 : 731-41.
8. Stern J, Peters AJ, Coulam CB. Colour Doppler ultrasonography assessment of tubal patency — a comparison study with traditional techniques. Fertil Steril 1982; 58 : 897-900.
9. Eckstein N, Orron DE, Vagman I. Digital road mapping image — a novel fluoroscopic real time guide for selective transcervical cathcterization in the treatment of proximal tubal obstruction. Fertil Steril 1992; 58 : 850-3.
10. Thurmond AS, and Rosch J. Non-surgical fallopian tube recanalization for treatment of infertility. Radiology 1990; 174 : 371-5.
11. Sedbon E, Delajolinieres JB, Boudouris O, Madelenat P. Tubal desterilization through exclusive laparoscopy. Hum Reprod 1989; 4 : 158-62.
12. Reich H. Laparoscopic reversal of sterilization. (Abstr.) Presented at the Second World Congress of Gynaecologic Endoscopy, Clairemont-Ferrard, France, June 5-8, 1989.
13. Berger GS. Outpatient sterilization reversal. Presented at the 44th Annual Meeting of the American Fertility Society, Atlanta, Georgia, Oct. 10-13, 1988. Published by the American Fertility Society in the Program Supplement pp 106, 1988.
14. Silva PD, Schaper AM, Meisch JK, Schauberger CW. Outpatient microsurgical reversal of tubal sterilization

by a combined approach of laparoscopy and mini laparotomy. Fertil Steril 1991; 55 : 696-9.

15. Young PE, Egan JE, Barlow JJ, Mulligan WJ. Reconstructive surgery for infertility at the Boston Hospital for women. Am J Obstet Gynecol 1970; 108 : 1093-5.
16. Rock JA, Katayama KP, Martin EJ. Factors influencing the success of salpingostomy techniques for distal fimbrial obstruction. Obstet Gynecol 1978; 52 : 591-3.
17. Bruhat MA, Mage G, Manhas H, Sonalhat C, Ropert JF, Pouly JL. Laparoscopic procedures to promote fertility : ovariolysis and salpingolysis. Results of 93 selected cases. Acta Eur Fertil 1991; 56 : 616-21.
18. Shapiro BS, Diamond MP, DeCherney AH. Salpingoscopy : An adjunctive technique for evaluation of the fallopian tube. 1988; 49 : 1076-9.
19. Lubor K, Beeson CC, Kennedy JF, Villaneurea B, Young PE. Results of microsurgical treatment of infertility and early tubal secondary look laparoscopy in the post-pelvic inflammatory disease patients : implications for in vitro fertilization. Am J Obstet Gynecol 1986; 154 : 1264-9.
20. Kitchin III JD, Nunley Jr WC, Bateman BG. Surgical management of distal tubal occlusion. Am J Obstet Gynecol 1986; 155 : 524-6.
21. Jacobs LA, Thie J, Patton PE, Williams TJ. Primary microsurgery for post-inflammatory tubal infertility. Fertil Steril 1988; 50 : 855-7.
22. Gomel V. Salpingostomy by laparoscopy. J. Reprod Med 1977; 18 : 265-9.
23. Mettler L, Giesel H, Semm K. Treatment of female infertility due to tubal obstruction by operative laparoscopy. Fertil Steril 1979; 32 : 384-6.
24. Bruhat MA, Dubuisson JB, Pouly JL, Bouguet de Joliniere J, Mage G, Madelenat P, Aubriot FX, Cauis M, Manhes H. La Coeliochirurgie, In Encycl Med Chir, Techniques Chirurgicales, Urologie Gynaecologie, Vol 6, Paris, France, pp 38, 1989.
25. Dubuisson JB, Aubriot FX, Barbot J. Traitement microchirurgicaldes lesions tubo-peritoneales. Resultats des platies distales : a propos de 135 cases. J Gynaecol Obstet Biol Reprod 1985; 14 : 641-5.
26. Fayez JA. An assessment of the role of operative laparoscopy in tuboplasty. Fertil Steril 1983; 39 : 476-9.
27. Mage G, Bruhat MA. Pregnancy following salpingostomy : comparison between CO_2 laser and electrosurgery procedures. Fertil Steril 1983; 40 : 472-4.
28. Westrom L, Bengtsson LPH, Mardh PA. Incidence, trends and risks of ectopic pregnancy in a population of women. Br Med J 1981; 282 : 15-8.
29. Centres for Disease Control, Ectopic Pregnancies, United States, 1987, MMWR. 1990; 39 : 24-7.
30. Menard A, Hanny JP, 'Crequat J. Treatment of unruptured tubal pregnancy by local injection of methotrexate under transvaginal sonographic control. Fertil Steril 1990; 54 : 47-50.
31. Sauer MV, Gorill MJ, Rodi IA, Yeko TR. Non-surgical management of unruptured ectopic pregnancy : an extended trial. Fertil Steril 1987; 48 : 752-5.
32. Vermesh M, Silva PD, Rosen GP, Stein AL, Fossum GT, Sauer MV. Management of unruptured ectopic gestation by linear salpingostomy : a prospective randomized clinical trial of laparoscopy versus laparotomy. Obstet Gynecol 1989; 73 : 400-4.
33. Tulandi T, Melvin J. Treatment of tubal ectopic pregnancy by salpingotomy with or without tubal suturing and salpingectomy. Fertil Steril 1991; 55 : 53-5.
34. Dubuisson JB, Bruel D, Aubriot FU. Reproductive outcome after laparoscopic salpingectomy for tubal pregnancy. Fertil Steril 1990; 53 : 1004-7.
35. Tuomivaara L, Kauppila A. Radical or conservative surgery for ectopic pregnancy? A follow-up study of fertility of 323 patients. Fertil Steril 1988; 50 : 580-8.
36. Pouly JL, Malines H, Mage G, Cauis M, Bruhat MA. Conservative laparoscopic treatment of 321 ectopic pregnancies. Fertil Steril 1986; 46 : 1093-7.
37. DeCherney AH, Silidker JS, Mezer HC, Tarlatzis BC. Reproductive outcome following two ectopic pregnancies. Fertil Steril 1985; 43 : 82-5.

CHAPTER

43

Modern Trends in Tubal Catheterisation Procedures

John Anderson

Developments in cannulation of the fallopian tubes from the vagina and the invention of endoscopes just 0.5 mm in diameter have made it possible to reach, to look and to operate where the great majority of human lives have begun : the fallopian tube's lumen. (The ovulated oocyte is normally collected in its sticky cumulus oophorus by the tube's fimbrial end, and travels down the ampulla in about 30 minutes; fertilisation normally takes place at the junction of the ampulla with the isthmus, where the developing embryo will remain for several days, before the isthmus is quickly transited for the embryo to reach the endometrial cavity of the uterus and to implant.)

Much was learned in the 1970s of the physiological mechanisms in the fallopian tube that control these movements of the oocyte and the embryo[1]. But because of its narrow medial lumen and its anatomical remoteness, positioned on each side between the ovary and the uterus, information on the tube's internal functioning could only be obtained indirectly, and then usually through inference from mammals other than humans. The late 1980s and early 1990s, however, have seen thoroughly simultaneous development of (a) ultrasound-guided tubal catheterisation for gamete and embryo transfer[2,3] (Figs. 43.1, 43.2 and 43.3), (b) radiographically-controlled tubal dilatation for diagnosis and treatment of obstruction[4-6], and (c) fallopian tube endoscopy (falloposcopy)[7]. In each case the tube has been approached from its uterine end, using procedures conducted through the vagina and the uterine cavity.

In principle, catheters, flexible wires and endoscopes can be positioned in the fallopian tube from the vagina by any of several real-time methods of imaging or sensing : (1) radiography (particularly fluoroscopy); (2) hysteroscopy, either with a fluid medium for distension or with carbon dioxide (Figs. 43.4 and 43.5); (3) transvaginal ultrasound; and (4) so-called *tactile sensation*, in which a characteristic feeling of lateralized discomfort is experienced by the patient and a smoothly overcomeable resistance is felt by the

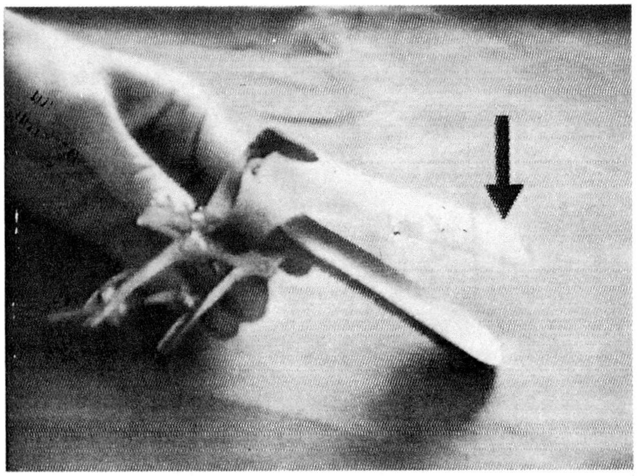

Fig. 43.1. A special bivalve speculum designed with a notch anteriorly for USG-guided or tactile tubal catheterisation.

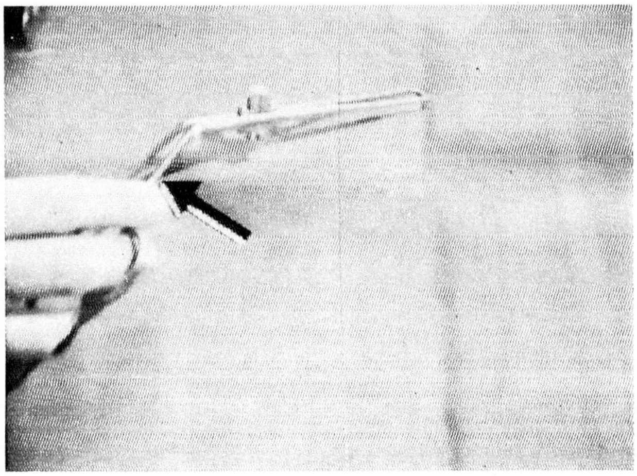

Fig. 43.2. A special tenaculum that is complementary to the speculum shown in Fig. 43.1.

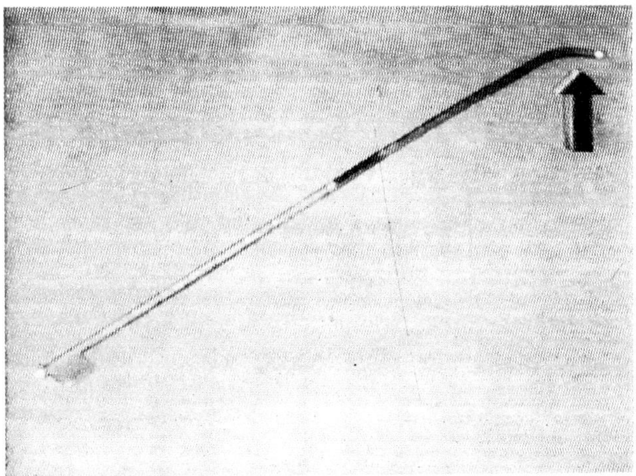

Fig. 43.3. A memory guide which is sonoreflective and through which the fallopian tube catheter passes.

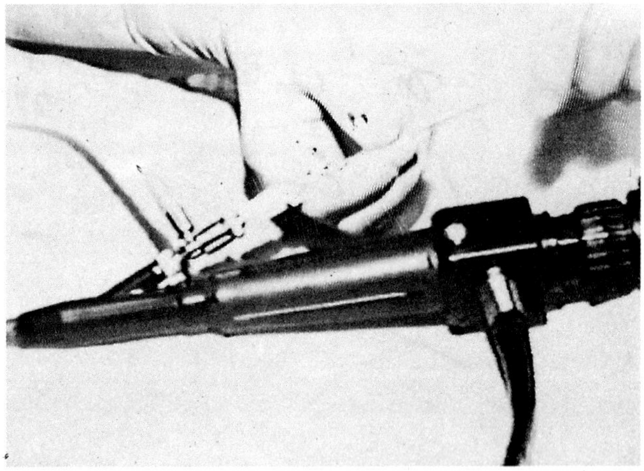

Fig. 43.4. A flexible hysteroscope with a fallopian tube catheter being loaded down its operative channel.

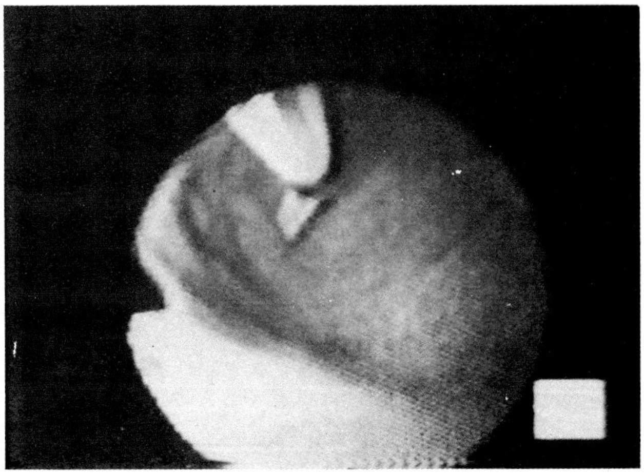

Fig. 43.5. An hysteroscopic view of the catheter passing through the uterine tubal ostium.

operator, and which is then relied on exclusively for proper placement. Of these, only ultrasound provides an objective means of confirming intratubal placement with no transport of introduced fluid down the fallopian tube's lumen.

If the fallopian tubes are normal, it is appealing to use them when conception is to be assisted clinically. The advantages are probably several. First, an early intratubal location for gametes or embryos provides a better, or at least a more reliable, environment for embryonic development than might be expected with fertilisation and embryo culture in vitro. Second, the timing of embryo entry into the uterus will be determined more by endocrine events affecting the genital tract than by the operator's judgement. And third, the direction of entry of embryos into the uterus will be from the tubes, not, as is usually the case with in vitro fertilisation (IVF), from the cervix. Several studies have shown that gamete intrafallopian transfer (GIFT), as well as early embryo transfer to the tubes, as conventionally practised through the fimbrial end of the tube at laparoscopy, produce higher rates of pregnancy than do embryo transfers through the cervix to the uterus[8,9].

Despite the advantages of tubal transfers of gametes or embryos at laparoscopy, clinical IVF since 1984 has rested more and more on transvaginal, ultrasound-guided follicle aspiration for obtaining oocytes, often with local anaesthesia alone, rendering IVF and uterine embryo transfer an ambulatory, outpatient procedure in most clinics. Having to revert to laparoscopy and general anaesthesia for gamete or embryo transfer to the tubes therefore perpetuates a disadvantage.

The catheter system we described in 1987[2] allowed gamete and embryo transfer procedures to be undertaken in an ambulatory care setting. We and others subsequently reported pregnancies following transvaginal intratubular insemination, GIFT and embryo transfer[3,10]. Pregnancy rates with transvaginal gamete or embryo transfer procedures, however, have been slow to become established[11], and are about two-thirds of those to be expected : we have not yet demonstrated that results can equal or exceed comparable tubal cannulations through the tube's wider, fimbrial end at laparoscopy. It does seem, though, that transvaginal-GIFT is a reasonable alternative to other ambulatory, non-anaesthesia-requiring forms of assisted conception, such as ovarian stimulation and washed-semen intrauterine insemination[12] and follicle aspiration with direct intraperitoneal sperm and oocyte transfer[13]. For the limited number of eggs transferred at TV-GIFT, the pregnancy rate is at least comparable and the hazard of occasional high-multiple pregnancy can be avoided.

It has been known for generations that the pressure required to *open* the uterine end of the tube to perfusing fluid is often greater than that needed subsequently to sustain the flow of fluid down its length. Rubin in the 1920s made kymographic tracings of tubal inflation pressures and wrote that "tubes were found to be patent after an initial high pressure (150-190 millimetres mercury) was required to force the gas through them".[14] His conclusions are as apt today as they were then.

Total obliteration of its (the intramural part's) lumen is very infrequent and when present is part of more extensive tubal disease. 'Isthmospasm' as an entity has not been definitely demonstrated but tubal contractions can be seen with the aid of intra-uterine lipiodol injection and the fluoroscope. The uterotubal junction (intramural portion) appears to be the site of predilection of spasm or hypertonicity in a relatively small proportion of the cases examined.

Ever since, fallopian tube surgeons have known that a variable but significant proportion of patients who come to resection of the intramural and adjacent isthmic part of the fallopian tube for apparent obstruction do not have organic abnormality demonstrated histologically in the removed bits of tube[15], the percentage reported as normal ranging from 2%[16] to 60%[17]. Pregnancies have long been reported among patients with untreated and apparently bilateral proximal tubal occlusion.

This experience lays a sceptical foundation for therapeutic fallopian cannulation based solely on salpingographic or laparoscopic diagnosis of medial tubal obstruction. No doubt there are cases of mild organic tubal occlusion able to be overcome by either balloon dilatation[5,18] or passage of a coaxial wire[19,20]. The tube has a trumpet shape, with cilial and muscular action in the wide ampulla highly convergent medially onto the narrow isthmus, where flow of secretions and transport of early embryos will probably happen uneventfully irrespective of the condition of its mucosa, provided proper patency is present. The first report of such dilatation of the proximal tube from the vagina to overcome obstruction without resorting to operation dates from the mid-nineteenth century[21].

It is easy to exaggerate the number of women who on the one hand would not have conceived given more time, while on the other have their truly organic pathology permanently overcome by retrograde tubal dilatation. In one study of 157 women with apparent bilateral proximal tubal obstruction on at least two conventional hysterosalpingograms, investigated by selective salpingography by retrograde catheterisation carried out by other than the original proponents of these methods[22], fully 61 (39%) had tubes that in fact were normally patent. Catheter dilatation successfully *recanalized* the proximal tube in 79 (82%) of the remaining 96. Pregnancy was achieved in just 11 of the 157 patients : 5 among those in whom selective salpingograms showed patent tubes : 6 among those whose obstructions were overcome by catheter dilatation. These results are modest but probably realistic. It can be sensibly argued, though, that these women at least were spared laparotomy and tubal resection.

The retrograde falloposcope is typically a 0.5 mm-diameter flexible endoscope. Its successful use was first described by Professor John Kerin, now at Flinders University in Adelaide[7]. Placement of the falloposcope can be by way of coaxial catheterisation of the tube[7] or with a linear averting balloon catheter positioned at the uterotubal junction[23].

Obtaining images by falloposcopy demands sophisticated attention to detail. In the ampullary-isthmic junction and in the isthmus, images are usually made while the falloposcope is being withdrawn. A point of complete obstruction is thus peculiarly difficult to see, and a diagnosis of complete obstruction in the absence of other confirmatory evidence can be wrong. What constitutes a clinically important abnormal appearance of the endosalpingeal mucosa on falloposcopy is still under evaluation. Nonobstructive adhesions and polyps have been documented in cases with reportedly normal salpingograms[24], but how important such lesions are to the later chance of intrauterine pregnancy is not clear, and is obscured further by the likely therapeutic effect of having passed the falloposcope.

The condition of the ampullary endosalpinx is better seen by endoscopy from the fimbrial end, a procedure that was called salpingoscopy when introduced in 1987 by Brosens *et al.*[25] Provided that the tube receiving attention is mobile, flexible or rigid, endoscopes with a 3 mm-diameter are passed readily at laparoscopy. The cross-sectional view such salpingoscopy provides is more than an order of magnitude better than obtainable from retrograde falloposcopy.

In summary, the advent of safe retrograde cannulation of the fallopian tubes from the vagina means that the anatomy and the physiology of where the huge majority of human conceptions take place will be ever less mysterious — open to direct inspection and diagnostic sampling. Further development will enable endoscopic surgeons, working from within, to operate on the fallopian tube's mucosa when it is abnormal, and to place gametes or embryos there when it is normal and conception needs assisting. Knowledge of isthmic tubal secretions during the menstrual cycle will lead endoscopic physiologists and biochemists better to understand the tube's normal function and, in turn, to better duplicate its internal environment in the laboratory when conception needs to take place in vitro.

This manuscript is based closely on two previously published works[26,27].

REFERENCES

1. Jansen RPS. Endocrine response in the fallopian tube. Endocr Rev 1984; 5 : 525-51.
2. Jansen RPS, Anderson JC. Catheterisation of the fallopian tubes from the vagina. Lancet 1987; ii : 309-10.
3. Jansen RPS, Anderson JC, Sutherland PD. Non-operative embryo transfer to the fallopian tube. N Engl J Med 1988; 319 : 288-91.
4. Platia MP, Krudy AG. Transvaginal fluoroscopic recanalization of a proximally occluded oviduct. Fertil Steril 1985; 44 : 704-6.
5. Confino E, Friberg J, Gleicher N. Transcervical balloon tuboplasty. Fertil Steril 1986; 46 : 963-6.
6. Thurmond AS, Novy M, Uchida BT, Rosch J. Fallopian tube obstruction : selective salpingography and recanalization. Radiology 1987; 163 : 511-4.
7. Kerin J, Anderson R, Daykhovsky L. Falloposcopy : A microendoscopic technique for visual exploration of the human fallopian tube from the uterotubal ostium to the fimbria using a transvaginal approach. Fertil Steril 1990; 54 : 390-400.
8. Yovich JL, Yovich JM, Edirisinghe WR. The relative chance of pregnancy following tubal or uterine transfer procedures. Fertil Steril 1988; 49 : 858-64.
9. Jansen RSP, Anderson JC, Birrel WRS. Outpatient gamete intrafallopian transfer : 710 cases. Med J Aust 1990; 153 : 182-8.
10. Jansen RPS, Anderson JC. Transvaginal versus laparoscopic GIFT : a case-controlled retrospective comparison. Fertil Steril 1993 (In Press).
11. Bustillo M, Schulman JD. Transcervical ultrasound-guided intrafallopian placement of gametes, zygotes and embryos. J In Vitro Fert Embryo Transfer 1989; 6 : 321-4.
12. Silverberg KM, Burns WN, Johnson JV, Schenken RS, Olive DL. A prospective, randomized trial comparing two different intrauterine insemination regimens in controlled ovarian hyperstimulation cycles. Fertil Steril 1992; 57 : 357-61.
13. Stack PS. Ovarian hyperstimulation syndrome. Am J Med 1991; 90 : 766-7.
14. Rubin IC. Observations on the intramural and isthmic portions of the fallopian tubes with special reference to so-called 'isthmospasm'. Surg Gynecol Obstet 1928; 4 : 87-94.
15. Jansen RPS. Tubal resection and anastomosis in isthmic salpingitis. Aust NZ J Obstet Gynecol 1986; 26 : 300-4.
16. Fortier KJ, Haney AF. The pathologic spectrum of uterotubal junction obstruction. Obstet Gynecol 1985; 65 : 93-8.
17. Sulk PJ, Letterie GS, Coddington CC, Hayslip CC, Woodward JE, Kelin TA. Histology of proximal tubal occlusion. Fertil Steril 1987; 48 : 437-40.
18. Confino E, Friberg J, Gleicher N. Preliminary experience with transcervical balloon tuboplasty. Am J Obstet Gynecol 1988; 159 : 370-5.
19. Novy M, Thurmond AS, Patton P, Uchida BT, Rosch J. Diagnosis of corneal obstruction by transcervical

fallopian tube cannulation. Fertil Steril 1988; 50 : 434-40.

20. Thurmond AS, Rosch J, Patton PE, Burry KA, Novy M. Fluoroscopic transcervical fallopian tube catheterization for diagnosis and treatment of female infertility caused by tubal obstruction. Radiographics 1988; 8 : 621-40.
21. Tyler Smith W. New method of treating sterility by the removal of obstructions of the fallopian tubes. Lancet 1849; i : 529-31.
22. Lang EK, Dunaway HE Jr., Roniger WE. Selective osteal salpingography and transvaginal catheter dilatation in the diagnosis and treatment of fallopian tube obstruction. Am J Radiol 1990; 154 : 735-40.
23. Scudamore IW, Dunphy BC, Cooke ID. Outpatient falloposcopy : Intraluminal imaging of the fallopian tube by trans-uterine fibre-optic endoscopy as an outpatient procedure. Br J Obstet Gynecol 1992; 99 : 829-35.
24. Kerin JF, Pearlstone AC, Williams DB, Grundfest WS, San Roman GA, Surrey ES. Falloposcopic classification and treatment of fallopian tube lumen disease. Fertil Steril 1992, 57 : 731-41.
25. Brosens I, Boeck W, Delattin PH, Puttemans P. Salpingoscopy : a new preoperative diagnostic tool in tubal infertility. Br J Obstet Gynecol 1987; 94 : 768-73.
26. Jansen RPS. Medicine and surgery inside the fallopian tube. Med J Aust 1993; 158 : 799-800.
27. Jansen RPS. Diagnostic and therapeutic cannulation of the fallopian tubes. Bom Hosp J 1993; 35 : 71-8.

CHAPTER

44

Laparoscopic Management of Myomas

Shashi Goyal and P.B. Pai Dhungat

When experience has been gained in endoscopic adhesiolysis, a surgeon can then proceed with advanced laparoscopic surgeries. Laparoscopic myomectomy is one of the advanced laparoscopic surgical procedures.

Patient selection and preparation. Subserous, pedunculated single myomas are best tackled laparoscopically[1]. For deep intramural multiple myomas, consent for laparotomy must always be taken. Preoperative administration of GnRh analogues will reduce uterine blood flow and hence bleeding during the procedure[2].

Instruments. Special instruments include claw forceps; tissue punch morcellator, electric morcellator if available, myoma screw and unipolar spatula. Regular instruments for operative video laparoscopy and coagulative units are also required.

Subserous pedunculated fibroids can be easily removed laparoscopically. If it is pedunculated, hold the myoma with grasping forceps and coagulate the pedicle with bipolar cautery (Figs. 44.1 – Plate 10, and 44.2 – Plate 11). If it is a thick stalk, it can be coagulated and then cut with scissors in 2-3 sessions. Remove excised fibroid through a 10 mm sheath (Fig. 44.3 – Plate 11) but if it is larger, one can morcellate it by using a tissue punch morcellator or electric morcellator. Alternatively colpotomy can be done and a fibroid removed vaginally. Suction irrigation is done to remove blood and to prevent adhesions.

Intramural fibroids are the ones which require technically expert and advanced laparoscopic surgery[3]. Select the site of incision. If preferred inject vasopressin in the area of incision and bed of the fibroid. Serosa is coagulated for the incision and then incised by unipolar electrocautery point (or laser point if available) till the fibroid is seen. Fibroid is caught in grasping forceps or myoma screw and fixed. With the help of spatula, blunt probe, scissors and aquadissection fibroid is dissected. Countertraction is applied with grasping forceps during dissection from the bed. Base of the fibroid is coagulated with bipolar forceps and it is excised. Never pull the base as it can avulse the endometrium. Fibroid is parked anteriorly over the uterus and the myoma bed is checked for bleeding. Coagulation is done by bipolar forceps. Irrigation suction will help to establish haemostasis. If additional myomas are found, they should be removed through same incision by retracting the serosa over uterus[4,5].

When a big myoma is removed and depth is more than half of the uterine wall, it requires suturing[6]. One has to use suture material like 1.0 vicryl or 1.0 P.D.S. on a regular needle. It is introduced through the second puncture. Uterine myometrium and edges are approximated by mattress sutures and knotting is done by intracorporeal techniques. Excised fibroid is removed either by colpotomy or electric morcellator[7,8]. Haemostasis can also be achieved by point coagulator at 100-120°C temperature.

Laparotomy is required if long and deep incision has been done or if endometrium is exposed.

Post-operative care

Laparoscopic myomectomy patients should be hospitalized for 24-48 hours and post-operatively haemoglobin, fever and abdominal distension should be watched to ensure the safety and well-being of the patient. Unsuspected bowel injury and bowel adhesion to large uterine defect is a cause of worry to the endoscopist.

Use of Hyskon, Ringer lactate and early second look laparoscopy are advocated for prevention and lysis of adhesions[9].

We need to do comparative study of laparoscopic versus abdominal myomectomy. Open myomectomy is the procedure of choice for multiple, large and deep myomas.

REFERENCES

1. Murphy AA. Operative laparoscopy. Fertil Steril 1987; 47 : 1-18.
2. Semm K, Mettler L. Technical progress in pelvic surgery via operative laparoscopy. Am J Obstet Gynecol. 1980; 138 : 121-127.
3. Gordon AG, Lewis BV (eds.) Gyn. endoscopy. JB Lippincott, Philadelphia. 1988 : 8.9-8.10.
4. Bradley S. Laparoscopic myomectomy. Springer-Verlag. p. 125-136.
5. Alan G, Gordon B, Victor Lewis. Gynaecological endoscopy.
6. Kutz BR, Deniell JL, Abstract of 21st AAGL Meeting Chicago Santa Fe CA 1992 : 91.
7. Semm K. Pelviscopic enucleation of myomas. Operative manual for End Abd Surgery 1987, 184-188.
8. Semm K. Enucleation of myoma in pelviscopic op guiderz. Edited and published by K Semm, Kiel, 1992.
9. Operative laparoscopy and hysteroscopy. Dr. SD Khandwalla.

CHAPTER

45

Laparoscopic Management of Endometriomas

Rakesh Sinha

Introduction

The first case of an ovarian endometrioma published by W.W. Russel in 1899 gave a detailed description of the ovary 'enveloped in adhesions to the posterior face of the broad ligament' and 'the presence of areas which were an exact prototype of the uterine glands and interglandular connective tissue'. However, it took more than two decades before the relationship between the haemorrhagic cyst of the ovary and the ectopic endometrium was established. In 1920 Cullen suggested that active endometrium was involved in the pathogenesis of the 'ovarian haematoma'. It has been the merit of Sampson (1927) to introduce the idea that the small blood-spots on the surface are the first commonly visible sign of ovarian endometriomas. Several authors have subsequently held the view that ectopic endometrium eats its way into the ovary like insects eating into an apple or that chocolate cysts are situated in ovarian follicles or lying wholly in the medulla of the ovary. In 1957 the role of the adhesions in endometrioma formation was clarified by Hughesdon. His work was based on serial sections of ovarian endometriomas and confirmed that 'even in the most advanced lesions the ectopic endometrium never in fact leaves the surface : it remains on, and is never in the ovary'. In 90% of the cases the inner cystic wall could be identified as ovarian cortex. Owing to stretching, the inner cortex is not always uniform and recognizable as is the case in large endometriomas. In many cases the ovary does not invaginate centrally but remains on one side as a more or less definite mass and the cavity is surrounded on the other side by a relatively flat wall.

Gross appearance

The term 'chocolate cyst' was coined to describe the endometrial cysts of the ovary, but is purely descriptive and may be misleading if one only notices the chocolate content of a cyst. Aspiration of a cyst is therefore not a reliable diagnostic tool as a similar content can be found in haemorrhagic functional cysts and even in some neoplastic tumours.

The gross features of the endometrial cyst are very familiar to the gynaecological surgeon. Several of these characteristics are explained by its particular structure. First, the adhesions are an essential feature. The inversed ovarian cavity is sealed by adhesions to form a cystic structure. In many cases the ovary is adherent to an adjacent structure which can extend from the lateral pelvic wall to the back of the uterus. This explains the difficulty of mobilizing the cyst without opening or rupturing it and spilling its content. In some cases the ovary can be free but adhesions and scarification are present and are usually located on the lateral side of the ovary. Second, the cysts of modest size have a thick wall as the wall is the ovary itself. Enlargement of the cyst tends not to produce a general expansion as with other benign, truly intraovarian cysts. As the flattening of the wall usually occurs on the medial side, the remaining ovarian structure is usually found on the lateral side.

Laparoscopic management

Ovarian cystoscopy was described by Brosens and Puttemans (1989) as a tool to investigate the ovarian cysts which are not suspected of malignancy at the time of laparoscopy and to avoid unnecessary ovarian surgery. The haemorrhagic functional cyst can be simply aspirated. The technique is based on inspection and exploration of the cystic wall using a second endoscopical system. After aspiration and flushing, the cyst is entered by the cystoscope, which has a 5 mm diameter. A saline drip connected with the operating channel of the cystoscope is used to expand the wall of the cyst which would otherwise collapse when a large incision is made. A biopsy forceps can then be introduced through the operating channel of the cystoscope and biopsies are obtained from selected areas. Using this technique the benign characteristics can be confirmed and functional cysts such as an haemorrhagic follicular cyst or a cystic corpus luteum can be discerned from endometrial cyst.

Inspection of the endometrial cyst shows a great variation in the degree of vascularization and the presence of endometrial implants. In some cysts large parts of the wall consist of a uniformly dark, non-vascularized tissue which represents pigmented fibroreactive tissue. In some, probably young, endometriomas the pearl-like surface of the ovarian cortex can still be identified. Endometrial tissue can be identified by its vascularization and sometimes mucosal appearance. Again, young or very active endometriomas consist of free, mucosa-like implants covering ovarian cortex from which they can be easily separated, while in older endometriomas much of the wall is fibroreactive tissue with interspersed vascularized implants. Irregular congested vessels are frequently noted close to the ovarian hilus.

The rationale for endo-ovarian laparoscopic surgery is that the lesion causing the endometrioma is located superficially and can be identified using the described technique of ovarian cystoscopy. This technique is minimally invasive and allows localization of the implants. This is proven by the high rate of positive biopsies, while in up to one-third of resected endometriomas only tissue compatible with endometrioma, *i.e.*, fibroreactive tissue with pigmentation, is found.

Laser treatment for endometriomas

Advanced operative laparoscopy techniques for laser adhesiolysis and vaporization of endometriotic implants have been developed, and laser surgeons are now able to remove endometriosis from the reproductive structure with precision. There are at least three advantages of laser laparoscopy over conventional operative laparoscopy : precise destruction of diseased tissue, minimal bleeding and minimal damage to the adjacent normal tissue. Tissue reaction and post-operative adhesion formation have been shown to be no greater than with conventional methods.

Laser surgery

The endoscopic use of the laser is not new in medicine, and several types of operative procedures have been carried out with the CO_2 laser laparoscope for the treatment of reproductive pathology. The most frequent indication is endometriosis, which can be vaporized by means of CO_2 laser laparoscopy with highly satisfactory postoperative pregnancy rates[1]. Laser surgeons have removed endometriosis with great precision from the reproductive structure. But vaporization of the endometriotic peritoneal lesion or of the endometriotic cyst wall provokes residual carbon charring. Expensive high-power operating lasers are required for the vaporization of tissue without residual carbon charring. The SwiftLase allows a char-free ablation, even when using a 30 W operating laser.

Peritoneal endometriotic implants

In general, a power setting of 40-50 W is used. The debulking of endometriotic implants is best performed using a continuous firing mode. If a lesion is overlying a vital structure such as the ureter, urinary bladder, colon, or larger blood vessels, a retroperitoneal injection of fluid (aquadissection and aquaprotection) provides safer vaporization of the lesions. This duration allows a 100-200 μm depth of vaporization, thus substantially limiting the depth of penetration. Vaporizing an endometriotic implant provokes the bubbling of old blood, followed by a curdy white material representing vaporization of the stromal layer. After the endometriotic lesion has been vaporized, retroperitoneal fat is encountered, and the appearance of bubbling confirms the complete vaporization of the lesion. Absorption of the CO_2 laser by water (contained in fatty tissue) for a few seconds after the complete destruction of the implant prevents deeper penetration of the laser beam.

Ovarian endometriosis < 3 cm (Figs. 45.1 to 45.4 – Plate 11, and 45.5 – Plate 12)

Ovarian endometriosis is treated during first-look laparoscopy if a penetration of no more than 3 cm into the ovary is observed and if the cyst diameter is no longer than 3 cm.

Small (< 1 cm in diameter) endometriotic implants of the ovary are vaporized until follicles containing fluid are encountered or no further pigmented tissue is seen. Large (< 3 cm in diameter) endometriomas are destroyed as follows. A 3-4 mm portion of the top of the cyst is excised, the chocolate-colored material is aspirated, and the cyst is washed out with irrigation fluid. After washing, the interior wall of the cyst is examined carefully to confirm the absence of any intracystic lesion suspected to be malignant (ovarian cystoscopy). With a power setting of 40 W and continuous mode application, the interior wall of the cyst is then vaporized to destroy the mucosal lining of the cyst. The vaporization continued until no further pigment can be seen. After copious irrigation, the ovaries are left open.

Ovarian endometriosis > 3 cm (Figs. 45.6 to 45.10)

During diagnostic laparoscopy, the endometrial cyst is washed out with irrigation fluid (saline solution), and a biopsy is taken. Then, gonadotropin releasing hormone (GnRh) agonist therapy is given for 12 weeks to decrease the cyst size. A decrease of 50% in cyst diameter is observed after drainage followed by a 12-week course of a GnRh agonist. Drainage alone (if not associated with GnRh agonist) is ineffective; indeed, 12 weeks after drainage, the ovarian cyst

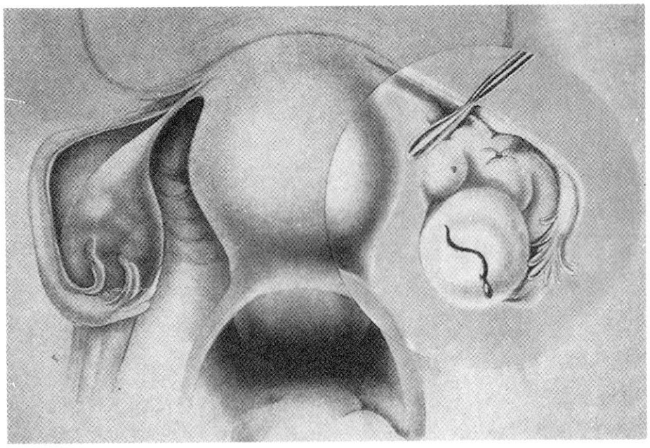

Fig. 45.6. Ovarian endometrioma > 3 cm. Linear incision on dependent part.

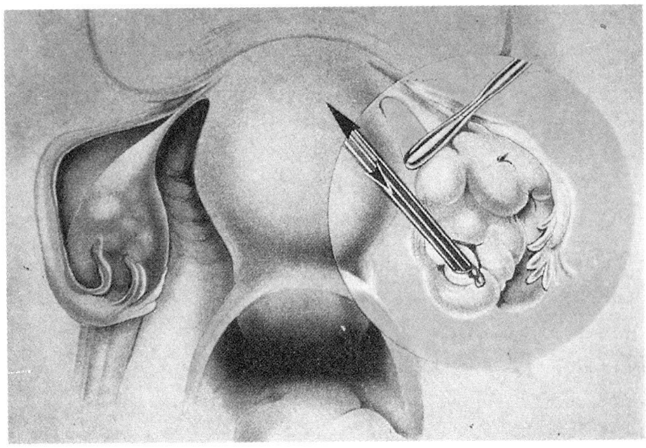

Fig. 45.7. The ovarian cyst is washed out with saline solution.

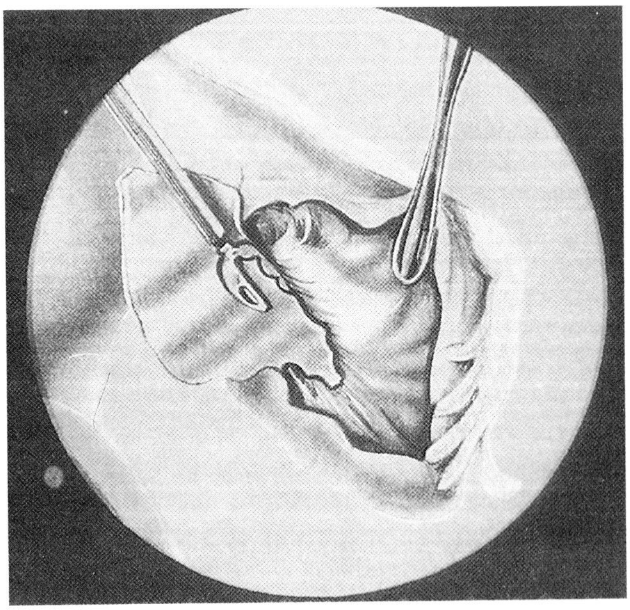

Fig. 45.8. The mucosal lining of the cyst wall is vaporised or cauterised. The cyst wall removed is sent for biopsy.

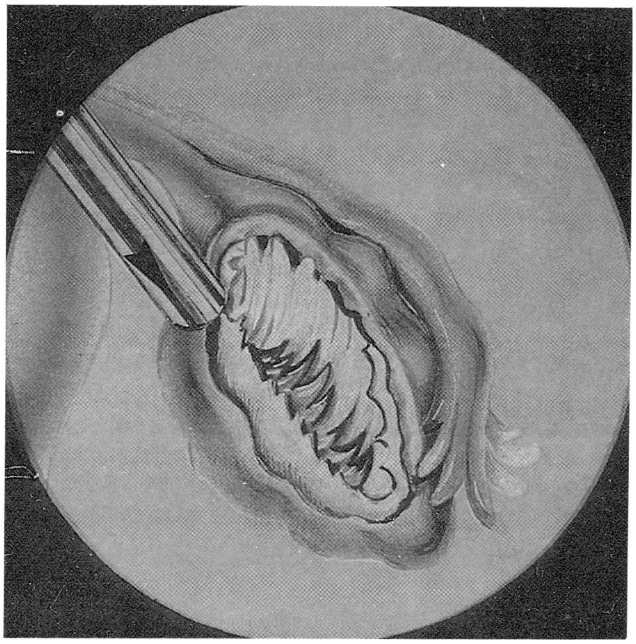

Fig. 45.9. Residual endometrial cyst wall is vaporised or coagulated. Swiftlase permits a char-free ablation, layer by layer. It reduces the carbonization and the thermal damage to the normal ovarian cortex.

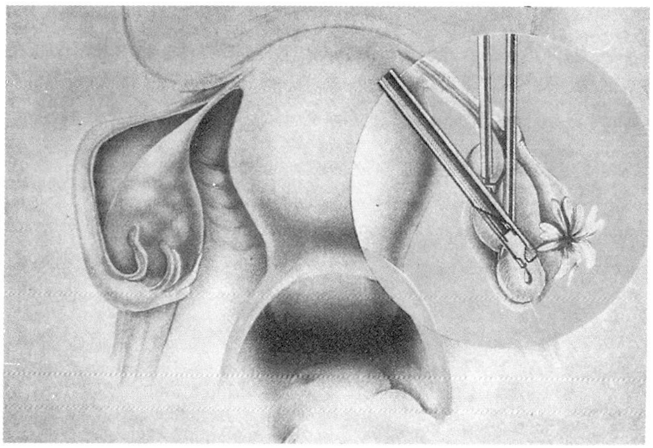

Fig. 45.10. Ovarian edges can be left alone, sutured or closed with titarium clips — as shown here.

diameter is found to be unchanged when compared to the diameter observed before drainage.

Thereafter, a second-look laparoscopy is carried out. If the diameter of the residual endometrial cyst is < 3 cm after GnRH agonist therapy, the interior wall of the cyst is vaporized as previously described. If the diameter of the residual cyst was < 3 cm after GnRH agonist therapy another technique is proposed. A portion of the ovarian cyst is first removed by making a circular cut over the protruded ovarian cyst portion, using the CO_2 laser or electro-surgery. Partial cystectomy is then carried out. Ovarian cystoscopy is performed for evaluation of the interior cyst wall, and a biopsy is taken. The residual endometrial cyst wall is then vaporized with the CO_2 laser. The ovary is left open. To close the ovary, Tissucol (fibrin sealant) (Immuno AG, Vienna, Austria) is injected trans-abdominally into the intraovarian vaporized area, and the edges of the ovarian cyst are approximated with atraumatic forceps for 2-3 minutes. (After clotting occurs, further mechanical stress should be avoided for 3-5 minutes.) At the end of the procedure, copious irrigation of the pelvic cavity is carried out to prevent deposits of carbon and glue. Thereafter, 100-200 ml of 32% Dextran 70 is instilled into the peritoneal cavity in all patients. Recently, the closure of the ovarian edges has been performed using special new titanium clips. The clips permit an excellent approximation of ovarian edges. Very often, two or three clips are sufficient to close the ovary.

Pregnancy rates

The cumulative pregnancy rates were analyzed in a consecutive series of 407 patients with ovarian endometriosis [American Fertility Society (AFS) — moderate, n = 305; severe, n = 102].

A pregnancy rate of more than 55% was achieved in moderate endometriosis and 44% in severe endometriosis. The majority of pregnancies occurred during the first 10 months after surgery[2].

Ovarian cystectomy (Figs. 45.11 to 45.17)

Ovarian cystectomy, a frequently performed procedure, can be accomplished laparoscopically in most cases. The procedure begins with adhesiolysis. Once the cyst is mobilized, the cortex is grasped with a forceps introduced through a second trocar. The cortex is incised using laser or scissors. The cyst wall is then exposed. The incision is enlarged with scissors, and aquadissection can be used to separate the cyst wall from the ovarian stroma. If the cyst is opened and spillage occurs, peritoneal irrigation must be performed in order to remove the chocolate-coloured fluid. Sometimes, ovarioscopy and careful evaluation of the internal cyst wall allow the surgeon to exclude the presence of malignant lesions. The ovary usually does not require suturing.

Conclusion

CO_2 laser laparoscopy offers several advantages over cautery. With the CO_2 laser, the laparoscopist is able to

DISSECTION OF ENDOMETRIOMA

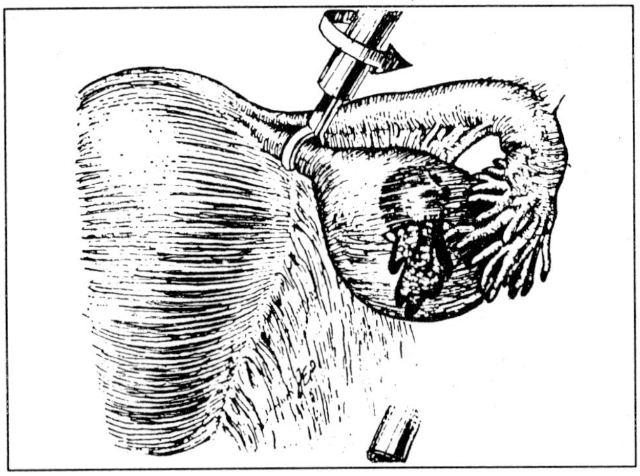

Fig. 45.11. Elevate and rotate ovary to expose the thinnest portion of capsule. Rupture usually occurs at this point releasing 'chocolate'.

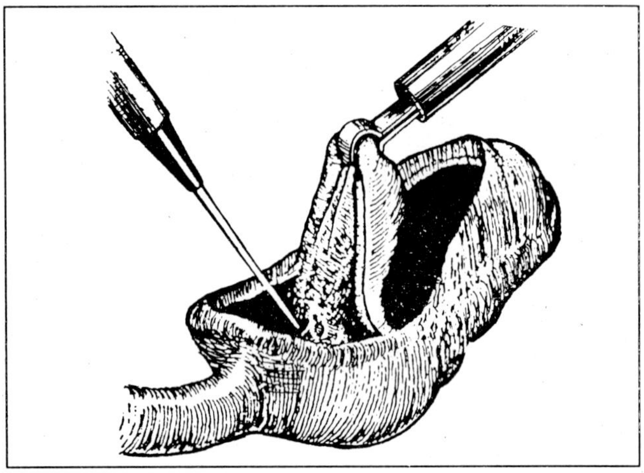

Fig. 45.14. Incise edge of ovary-capsule to identify cleavage plane. Additional retraction may be needed.

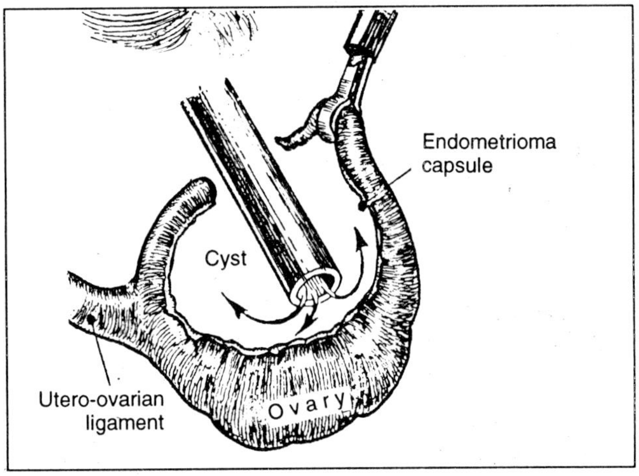

Fig. 45.12. Grasp upper edge, irrigate cyst until clear. Opening usually tears — cyst begins collapsing.

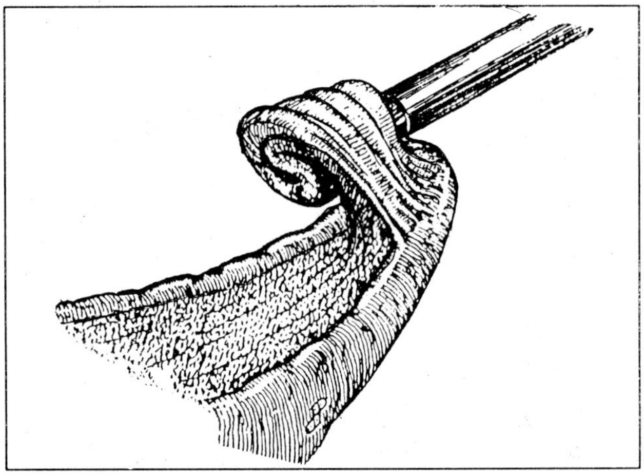

Fig. 45.15. "Spaghetti-roll" to control large capsule. Bleeding usually minimal.

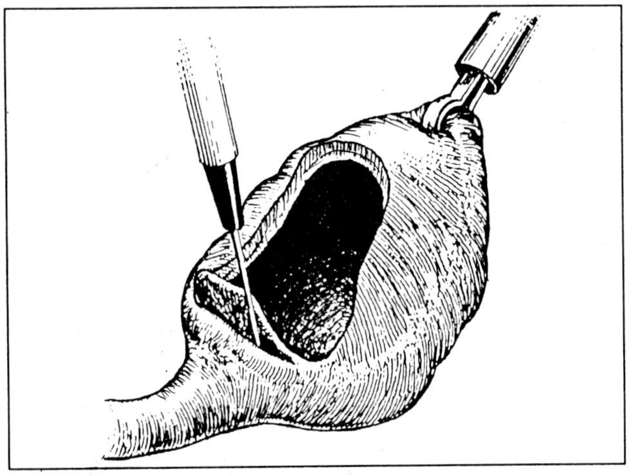

Fig. 45.13. Electroknife, laser or scissors on capsule edge closest to the utero-ovarian ligament, to work away from the utero-ovarian blood supply.

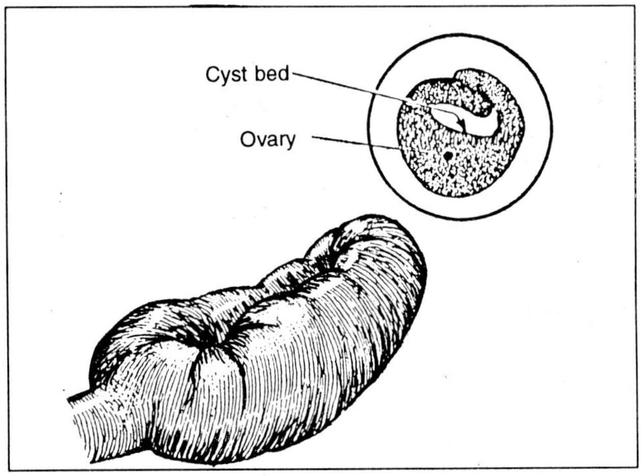

Fig. 45.16. After hemostasis, ovarian edges usually close. Sutures for approximation are rarely necessary.

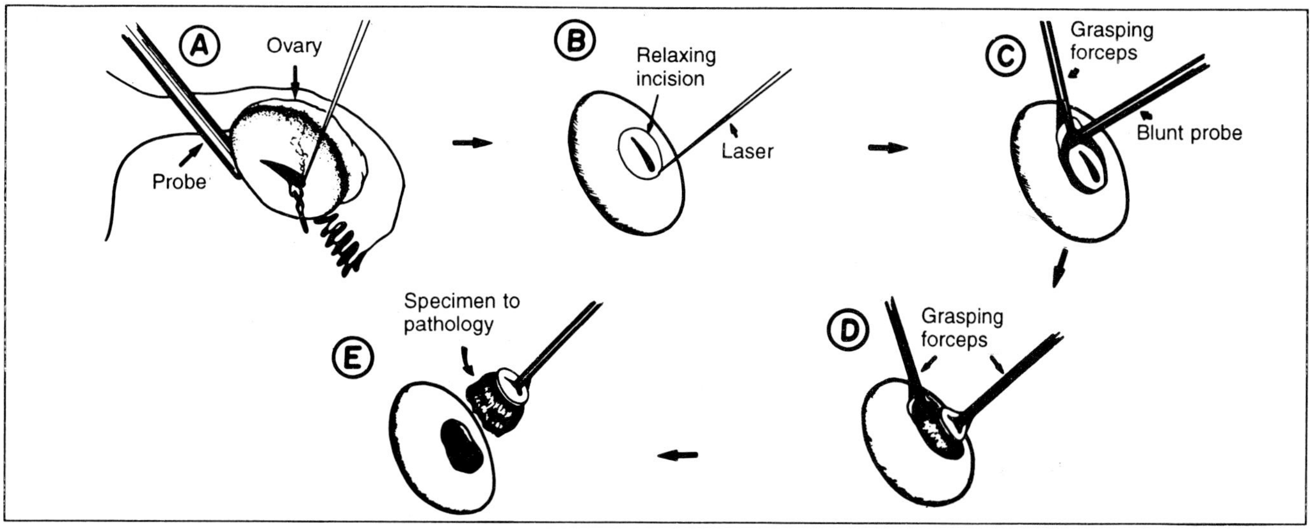

Fig. 45.17. Resection of an endometrioma : **A.** An incision is made on the most dependent portion of the ovary. **B.** A relaxing incision is made circumferentially — after drainage and irrigation of cyst wall lining. **C.** A plane of dissection is established with either a blunt probe or forceps. **D.** Dissection is carried out bluntly or sharply. **E.** The entire cyst wall is sent for histopathology.

control the process of vaporization by seeing the three-dimensional boundaries of the lesion.

In a previous study[3] significantly different pregnancy rates according to the stage of endometriosis were found. Severe endometriosis had the poorest prognosis in terms of pregnancy rates. For this reason, a preoperative hormonal (gonadotropin releasing hormone agonist) therapy was given to patients with very large ovarian endometriomas (> 3 cm). The release of a GnRh agonist by a biodegradable implant is effective in reducing endometriotic size to a greater extent than other drugs, and permits a decrease in pelvic inflammation.

In cases of vaporization of a very large cysts (> 3 cm), the risk of post-operative adhesions was found to be high in our study if the ovary was left open. Dense and fibrous periovarian adhesions between the vaporized area and other pelvic structures were diagnosed in eight out of nine patients who underwent a laparoscopy in the 3 months after vaporization, although periovarian adhesions were not frequently observed after vaporization of small endometriotic implants.

To decrease the risk of post-operative adhesions between the ovary and other pelvic structures, a fibrin glue was used. It was injected transabdominally through a catheter. A third-look laparoscopy proved the absence of periovarian adhesions.

Recently, the SwiftLase[4] has been used, the SwiftLase is a miniature optomechanical scanner compatible with any CO_2 laser. It enables a very rapid, homogeneous, single-layer char-free ablation even at low power levels. It increases the visual control of tissue destruction and permits a layer-by-layer ablation, reducing the carbonization and the presence of carbonized particles in the tissue.

REFERENCES

1. Nezhat C, Crowgey SR and Garrison CP (1986). Surgical treatment of endometriosis via laser laparoscopy. Fertil Steril, 45, 778-83.
2. Donnez J, Nissole M, Anaf V, Smets M, Bassil S and Roux FC. Endoscopic management of peritoneal and ovarian endometriosis. An Atlas of Laser Operative Laparoscopy and Hysteroscopy. The Parthenon Publishing Group, 1994.
3. Donnez J, Nisolle M and Casanas-Roux F (1990). Endometriosis-associated infertility : evaluation of preoperative use of danazol, gestinone and buserilin. Int F Fertil, 42, 128.
4. Donnez J, Zair E, Reich H, Nisolle M and Slatkine M (1994). SwiftLase : a new technology for endometriosis management. Fertil Steril, submitted for publication.

CHAPTER

46

Laparoscopic Management of Extrauterine Pregnancy

Shashi Goyal and P.B. Pai Dhungat

Introduction

Incidence of ectopic pregnancy has increased four-fold since 1970. It has been due to tubal surgery, increased incidence of pelvic inflammatory diseases and assisted reproductive techniques. Thanks to transvaginal sonography and β-hCG hormonal assay which has made it possible to diagnose ectopic pregnancy at an early stage when it is possible to perform conservative surgery and to retain fertility of such patients. Laparoscopy was considered to be a reliable diagnostic method yesteryear, has now become a therapeutic modality (Figs. 46.1 to 46.4 – Plate 12). Depending upon the general condition, site and status of ectopic pregnancy, different therapeutic modalities can be performed through laparoscopic surgery.

Diagnosis

Early diagnosis is the mainstay of conservative treatment of ectopic pregnancy. Diagnosis of ectopic pregnancy before the tubal destruction and significant haemorrhage will help the endoscopist to salvage the tube. To diagnose ectopic pregnancy early, clinician must subject the high risk patient to newer modalities of investigations. High risk patients for ectopic pregnancy are the ones who have history of previous tubal surgery, previous pelvic inflammatory disease, previous ectopic pregnancy and pregnancy after assisted reproductive techniques. All these patients should be advised serial serum β-hCG measurements and transvaginal sonography with colour Doppler to exclude or to confirm the diagnosis. If the initial β-hCG is below 1000 mIU/ml repeat estimation is done after 48 hours. For intrauterine pregnancy, β-hCG increase should be 66%. Any variation on lower side or plateau of β-hCG level denotes either spontaneous abortion or ectopic pregnancy. On transvaginal sonography absence of intrauterine gestational sac and presence of complex adnexal mass is highly suggestive of ectopic pregnancy, serum β-hCG levels will clinch the diagnosis in the said circumstances.

With this strategy, diagnosis of ectopic pregnancy

can be done at such a stage where tubal damage is not extensive and fertility potential can be salvaged. A ruptured extrauterine pregnancy with severe abdominal pain, bleeding and collapse is classical clinical triad of ectopic pregnancy. A leaking tubal abortion will present with irregular bleeding P/V, lower abdominal pain and signs of peritoneal irritation.

Prerequisites for laparoscopic surgery

1. Skilled and experienced laparoscopist.
2. Stable patient.
3. Tube must be mobile and tubal pregnancy accessible.
4. Size of ectopic pregnancy must be less than 3 cm.
5. General anaesthesia with full muscle relaxation.
6. Pneumoperitoneum maintenance during the whole procedure is important which can be done by Laparoflator.
7. Video laparoscopy helps in active participation of assistants.

Instruments

Appropriate laparoscopic instruments such as '0' degree telescope with video and monitor, Hydromet for suction and irrigation, traumatic and non-traumatic forceps, unipolar and bipolar electrocautery (laser energy if available), three additional 5 mm trocar and cannula and laparoscopic scissors are needed. D & C instruments and instruments for removing resected tissue should be handy.

Surgical technique

Under general anaesthesia and proper dorsal lithotomy position, laparoscope is introduced and blood is washed out of the pelvis and fallopian tube is held, using atraumatic forceps and site, size and status of ectopic pregnancy is visually judged. If the tube is intact and patient is desirous to conserve fertility status, it can be treated with four methods.

1. Methotrexate injections;
2. Linear salpingostomy;
3. Salpingotomy;
4. Fimbrial aspiration.

1. Methotrexate injections

Special needle is used for injection. Tube is held up with non-traumatic forceps and needle is inserted into the gestational sac, aspiration of blood is done and then 50 mg of methotrexate is injected into the sac. Needle is withdrawn through the protective sheath.

2. Linear salpingostomy

Unruptured isthmic and ampullary ectopic pregnancies of small size can be tackled by this method.

Tube is gently held proximal to the implantation site with nontraumatic forceps. Depending on availability, unipolar needle electrode or laser energy is used for incising the tube.

Blended current is used for electrocautery. First coagulate the antimesentric border of ectopic site and then the coagulated tube is incised with scissors. Non-traumatic forceps can compress the tube and pregnancy is extruded. With the help of forceps, dissection of sac can be done. Gentle suction can also help in removing the sac. Additional coagulation may be required to achieve haemostasis. Lavage with warm ringer lactate will confirm haemostasis and remove clots. It has been observed that leaving the tube open will restore tubal function rapidly. When it heals by secondary intention, longitudinal folds of tube are maintained. In the study done by Tulandi in 1991, his result showed that the intrauterine pregnancy rate at 12 and 24 months was 45% and 45% without suturing, while with suturing I.U.P. at 12 and 24 months were 21% and 44%. Second look laparoscopy has found no difference in degree of adhesions with and without suturing. If one wants, 4/0 P.D.S. suture with intracorporeal technique can be used.

Limitations of conservative methods

1. Possibility of persistent trophoblastic tissue which may require additional surgical or medical line of treatment.
2. Recurrent ectopic pregnancy rate is minimally increased.
3. Repeated serum β-hCG assays are required at weekly intervals.

Tubal aspiration

It was used for the management of terminal ampullary ectopic pregnancy. Results are not encouraging as patient worsened in many cases and required laparotomy. If fertility is required, salpingotomy extending up to fimbria is best. If fertility is not required, one can perform segmental resection or salpingectomy.

Segmental resection

When patient of ruptured isthmic or proximal ampullary pregnancy desires conservative surgery, segmental excision of tube followed by reanastomosis at a later date is the only alternative. Ectopic pregnancy is held up with grasping forceps, tube is coagulated distal and proximal to the ectopic pregnancy and coagulated area is transected with scissors. Ectopic pregnancy is held up proximal to the transection line and a series of burns and cuts are placed progressively along the mesosalpinx from distal to proximal end of tube. Excised segment of tube is held with grasping forceps and advanced towards the tip of telescope which is gradually withdrawn from laparoscopic cannula. Under vision, excised portion of tube with gestational sac is kept into the lower part of the principal cannula. First telescope is removed and by railroad technique excised portion can be removed through principal cannula. If need arises it can be minced into smaller pieces by a morcellator. One can also remove it by using Kocher's forceps directly through one of the puncture sites. Rarely posterior colpotony is required to remove it. Irrigation and suction is done to remove any remaining tissue.

3. Salpingectomy

It is indicated when tube is markedly destroyed either by rupture or by chronic ectopic pregnancy and fertility is not desired. To begin with fimbriated end is coagulated and then successive coagulation and cutting of mesosalpinx is done till the isthmus. Tubal isthmus proximal to ectopic is coagulated effectively before dividing. Endoloop also can be used from fimbrial side. Three loops are placed proximal to ectopic pregnancy site and tube is transected.

Excised tube can be retrieved by the earlier two methods.

Interstitial or cornual ectopic pregnancy

In recent advances, if interstitial pregnancy has been detected early, sonographic guided injection of methotrexate or KCl will be method of choice. One can also try medical therapy of oral methotrexate in the dosage of 0.3 mg/kg for four days, maximum dose is 25 mg/day.

Alternatively if surgeon is experienced and patient is settled, one can try laparoscopic surgery. Tube is coagulated and cut distal to the site of ectopic pregnancy and then coagulation and dissection of mesosalpinx is extended towards uterus. Myometrial dissection is done by laser or cautery depending on availability. Resected part is removed through the primary 10 mm cannula, or tissue may be removed piecemeal. After removal of tissue, thorough irrigation and aspiration is done to remove any trophoblastic tissue.

Cervical pregnancy

Since I.V.F. and E.T. are becoming more and more prevalent, incidences of cervical pregnancies are also increasing. It is best treated by medical therapy or local injection of methotrexate. As a last resort it can be treated by hysterectomy.

Ovarian ectopic pregnancy

Incidences of ovarian ectopic pregnancy are less. Experienced and patient laparoscopic surgeon can treat ovarian ectopic by dissecting ectopic pregnancy with laser or unipolar needle cautery. Subsequently haemostasis is achieved and ovarian closure is not done.

In case it is not possible to differentiate ectopic pregnancy from normal ovary, laparoscopic oophorectomy can be performed as below.

1. Identify the course of ureter and infundibulo-pelvic ligament after irrigation and suction.
2. Coagulate utero-ovarian ligament with bipolar forceps and at the same time apply medial traction on the ovary with tooth or claw forceps.
3. Coagulate vessels entering ovarian hilum from infundibulo-pelvic ligament.
4. Cauterised area should be about 5 mm in width.
5. Incise utero-ovarian ligament and proceed by coagulating and cutting mesoovarium with continued traction over ovary.

Instead of coagulation three loop ligatures can be put over, taking care of not including or kinking ureter in the ligature.

Because of pregnancy, vascularity is increased in ovarian vessels hence it is important that the procedure is done by experienced and trained laparoscopic surgeon.

Complications of laparoscopic surgery

1. Haemorrhage due to increased vascularity during pregnancy. It can be taken care of by prior injection of vasopressin locally. If required coagulation by cautery, laser coagulation or ligature, and laparotomy as last resort can tackle haemorrhage.
2. Damage to adjacent structures like ureter, omentum and bowel, specially if adhesions are present.
3. Any conservative procedure for ectopic has danger of persistent trophoblastic tissue and hence all these patients need to be followed up by weekly serums β-hCG levels till it nullifies. If required methotrexate or actinomycin therapy

can be given. Sometimes it may be necessary to do radical surgery by laparoscopy or by laparotomy, if need arises.

In conclusion, benefits of laparoscopic surgery for ectopic pregnancy are mainly two :

1. Conservation and enhancement of fertility status of patient.
2. Reduction in hospital stay and resuming normal activity.

In early diagnosed cases of ectopic pregnancy laparoscopic conservative and radical surgery remains the method of choice.

REFERENCES

1. Reich H, Reich F. Laparoscopic of 109 consecutive ectopic pregnancies. Journal Reprod Med 1988; 33 : 885-889.
2. Tulandi T. Fertility Sterility 1991; 51 : 53-58.
3. Paurstein CJ. Anatomy & Pathology of Tubal Preg. Obstet Gynaecol 1986; 67 : 301-308.
4. Meck H, Semm K. Results of operative pelviscopy in 202 cases of ectopic pregnancy. International Journal Fertility 1989; 34 : 93-100.
5. Stovall TG. Single dose methotrexate. Obstet Gynaecol 1991; 77 : 754-757.
6. Shapiro HI. Excision of an ectopic pregnancy. American Journal Ob Gyn 1973; 117 : 290-293.
7. Pouly MA. Fertility Sterility Journal 1988; 46 : 1093-97.
8. Nager CW. 46 Annual Meeting 1990, Washington DC Abtc. — 0-099.
9. Ana Alvarel Murphy. Operative laparoscopy & hysteroscopy. 9 : 79-90.

CHAPTER

47

Hysteroscopic Surgery in Infertility

Prakash Trivedi

Introduction

Of all the miracles which the human body shows us, none is more marvellous and admirable than the uterus. In 1869 the impossible barrier of the cervix was crossed by Panteleoni[1] who did the first hysteroscopy and diagnosed intrauterine pathology.

Due to lack of proper distension systems and instruments hysteroscopy did not really get any recognition. It is only with the advent of video camera, continuous flow resectoscope and operative hysteroscopy equipment, hysteroscopy has now enjoyed a resurgence and has gained a growing number of enthusiasts.

In this age of advanced endoscopy it is surprising that gynaecology is the only speciality still blindly inserting the instruments into the body cavity. It is very difficult to separate a gynaecologist from the curette. However the days of blind curettage are over. Operative hysteroscopy allows us to diagnose and treat small or large intrauterine lesions responsible for infertility or abnormal uterine bleeding or recurrent abortion. The primary principle of hysteroscopic surgery is "why open the door when the job can be done through the keyhole?".

Indications

Though hysteroscopy has been advised for all infertile patients, however, the yield in terms of intrauterine pathology is variable from 15-42%. In an infertile patient hysteroscopy is particularly indicated if :

1. There is an abnormal HSG suggestive of uterine cavitary problem.
2. Suspected intrauterine adhesions or old kochs or endometritis.
3. Suspected intrauterine fibroid or intrauterine septum.
4. For extended sperm migration test or trans-cervical GIFT.

5. For tubal cannulation, salpingoscopy and transcervical balloon tuboplasty.

Instrumentation

The progress of hysteroscopic surgery was definitely delayed due to non-availability of proper instruments.

The instruments needed for operative hysteroscopy are :

A. Semirigid or flexible instruments like grasping forceps, biopsy forceps, scissors usually of 7 French calibre, hence with limited strength these instruments are commonly used for adhesiolysis, septal incision, etc.
B. Rigid or optical instruments : These are stronger group of instruments which go around the telescope like a sheath, however they remain at a optically fixed distance from telescope and also block 25-30% of the vision.
C. A bilamellar or continuous flow operating sheath usually of 21 or 24 French size allowing adequate distension of uterine cavity and also clearing the debris or blood stained fluid.
D. Resectoscope (Fig. 47.1 – Plate 12) with Collin's knife cutting loop and point electrode specially useful to incise intrauterine septum or resect cavitary fibroids.
E. Hopkins II telescope with 30° forward oblique vision.
F. Fluid distension systems like C-infusor pump, Quinones pump, hysteromat or endomat are preferred since CO_2 gas media have poor vision due to smoke or inability to clear blood from surgical site.
G. Diode or Nd-YAG laser though used less frequently in infertile patient for adhesiolysis, etc., since it can damage normal endometrium also.
H. Video camera is essential as operative field is magnified, operator is in comfortable position and for involvement of entire nursing staff and such recording serves as an excellent media for documentation and teaching.

Hysteroscopic surgery for intrauterine adhesion

Intrauterine adhesions have been found in 15-32% of infertile patients specially more frequently in secondary infertility. Patients of intrauterine adhesion may present with infertility, amenorrhoea, hypomenorrhoea, dysmenorrhoea or repeated abortions. Intrauterine adhesions can be diagnosed by HSG (Fig. 47.2) or hysteroscopy (Fig. 47.3). Intrauterine adhesions are classified by Sugimoto[2] according to their tissue characteristics (Table 47.1) or by Wamsteker[3] depending on their severity and visibility of ostia (Table 47.2).

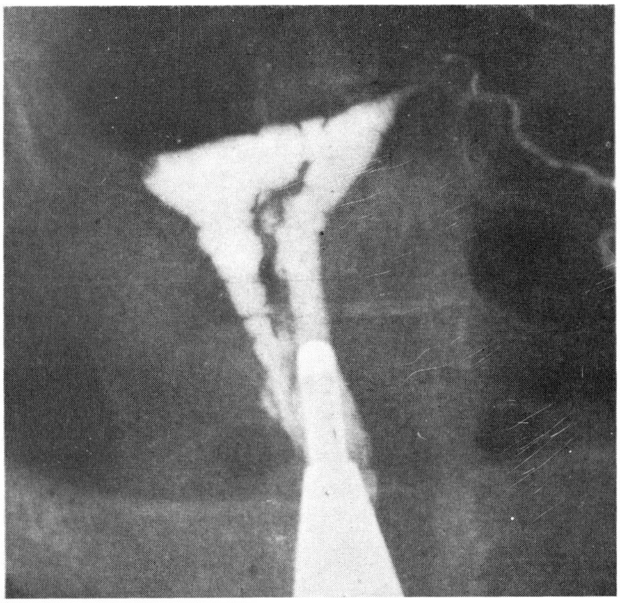

Fig. 47.2. Intrauterine adhesion on HSG.

Table 47.1. Sugimoto's classification of intrauterine adhesions by tissue characteristic

Endometrial	Easily lysed without bleeding.
Myofibrous	Thin cover of endometrium requires more force to break, fragments reddish.
Connective	Ischaemic, tough pale.

Table 47.2. Wamsteker's classification of intrauterine adhesion

Grade I	Thin filmy adhesiolysis by hysteroscope possible, uterotubal ostia normal.
Grade II	Single firm adhesiolysis by hysteroscopic sheath not possible, uterotubal ostia normal.
Grade III	Multiple adhesions with unilateral obstruction of uterotubal ostium.
Grade IV	Agglutinations of wall with bilateral obliteration of uterotubal ostium.

In 1948, Asherman[4] described a specific type of amenorrhoea an traumatica after a curettage done in postabortal or postpartum period. Sugimoto[2] evaluated 258 patients of intrauterine adhesion and found 14% were after puerperal curettage, 35% after incomplete

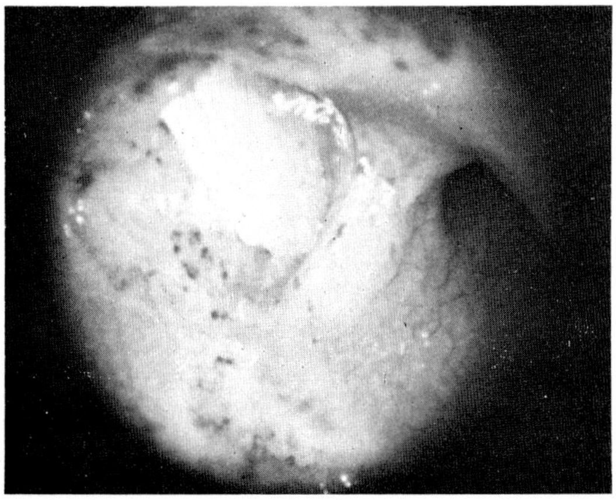

Fig. 47.3. Intrauterine adhesion on hysteroscopy.

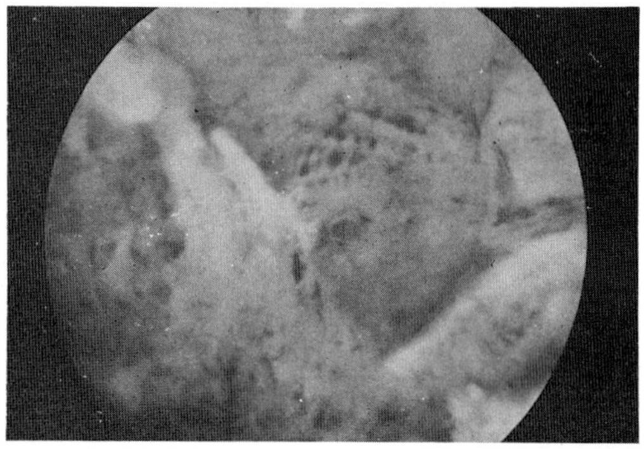

Fig. 47.4. Hysteroscopic adhesiolysis (final view with ostral opening).

abortion, 24% after induced abortion, 6% after molar pregnancy, 2% after myomectomy and 2% after caesarean section.

Hysteroscopic treatment of intrauterine adhesions can be done by the tip of the outer sleeve of hysteroscope in mild cases or by blunt dissection with grasping forceps or by cutting with scissors and in case of dense adhesions by Collin's knife or point electrode with current set at 30-40 watts only to reduce tissue necrosis and damage. Coagulating current should be avoided since it leads to charring and adhesions.

Diode or Nd-YAG contact lasers can be used for lysis of adhesions, however wattage should be very low to avoid tissue damage.

A grade III or grade IV intrauterine adhesion can be more challenging even to an experienced hysteroscopist, since there is loss of anatomy and there are high chances of uterine perforation. Laparoscopic control is necessary and safe. A novice hysteroscopist should not deal with more than mild to moderate intrauterine adhesion.

There is no better modality of treatment than hysteroscopic surgery for intrauterine adhesions specially for infertile patient.

After lysis of adhesions IUCD insertion is preferred by few hysteroscopist, however we do not find it to be extremely useful as an IUCD occupies only a small area. We prefer to give high doses or conjugated estrogen (Premarin) 1.25 mg twice a day for 3 cycles with progesterone added from 22nd - 26th day of therapy.

Results (Fig. 47.4) in terms of menstrual improvement depends on severity of adhesions and varies from 73-92%. Rafael Valle & Sciarra[5] reported a term pregnancy rate of 62.5% in mild intrauterine adhesions, 33.3% in moderate and 17% in severe intrauterine adhesions. The adhesions recurred in 25% of moderate and 53% of severe adhesions. 2 perforations were reported out of 61 patients treated.

Sugimoto[2] reported an overall pregnancy rate of 42% in 258 patients treated hysteroscopically with more than one third ending with spontaneous abortion.

Hysteroscopic treatment of cavitary fibroid in an infertile patient

Recently there is a growing concept that a cavitary fibroid (Figs. 47.5 and 47.6) does as much harm to the fertility of a women as comparable to an IUCD. This is further supported by the fact that out of so many caesarean sections done by obstetrician almost no one has come across a fibroid in the cavity. Hence it is logical to assume that a fibroid in uterine cavity can lead to infertility. If there is no other cause for infertility then such myomas should be resected by hysteroscope (Fig. 47.7). However at least more than 50% of the fibroid should be projecting in the cavity to perform a safe hysteroscopic myoma resection.

The author prefers to use pure cutting current set at low wattage to reduce damage to normal endometrial lining. The base is demarcated and vessels are coagulated. Fibroid should not be more than 6 cm in size. GnRH agonists injection can be given 3-4 weeks prior to surgery, this reduces the size on an average by 38% and also reduces the vascularity (Donnez *et al.*[6]). It is necessary to remember that GnRH agonists makes

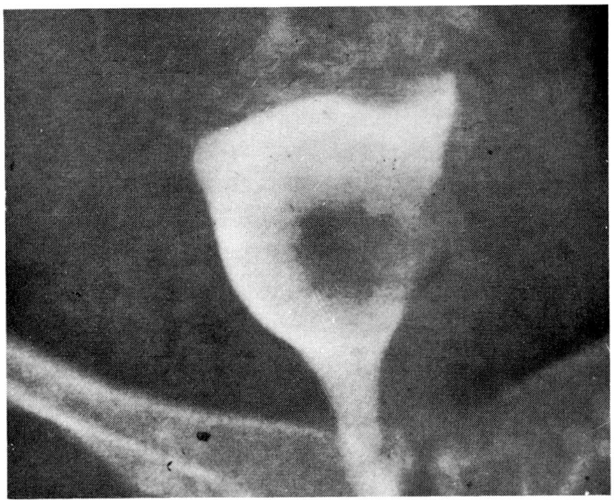

Fig. 47.5. Intracavitary fibroid (HSG view).

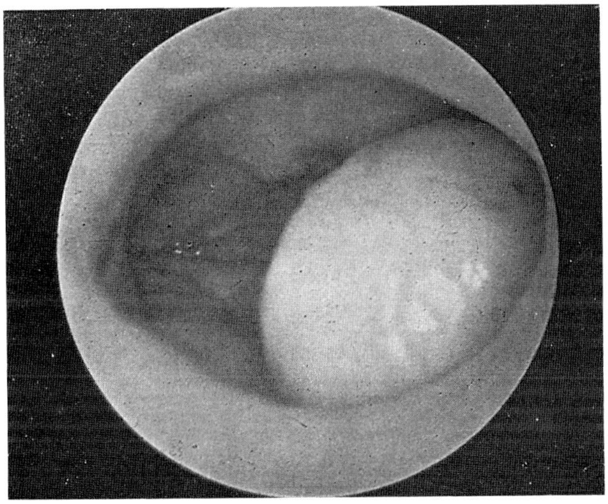

Fig. 47.6. Intracavitary fibroid (hysteroscopic view).

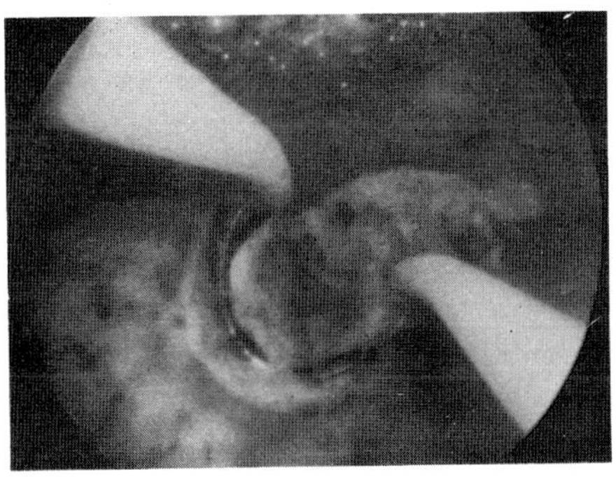

Fig. 47.7. Hysteroscopic myoma resection.

the patient hypoestrogenic and can predispose intrauterine adhesion later.

Donnez 1990[7] achieved 66% pregnancy rate in 24 cases of cavitary fibroid desirous for conception.

Fluid overload, bleeding and uterine perforation should be watched for in case of large fibroids.

Hysteroscopic intrauterine septal incision in infertile patient

There has been few studies justifying the hysteroscopic incision of septum (Figs. 47.8 and 47.9) in infertile patients, where no other obvious cause is detected. However apart from patients who are on IVF programme such surgical approach may be debatable. However in cases of secondary infertility with no other obvious cause, incision of an intrauterine septum is justified. It has been noticed that after delivery or abortion uterus which is more muscular involutes better than a fibrous septum, thus making the septum occupy more space in the uterus and contributing to reduction in fertility.

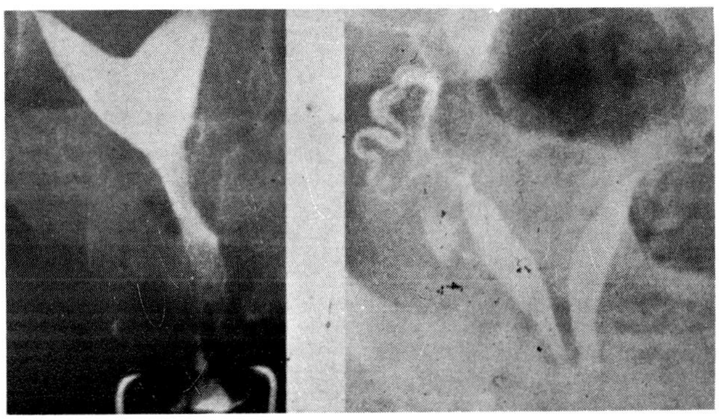

Fig. 47.8. Intrauterine septum (HSG view).

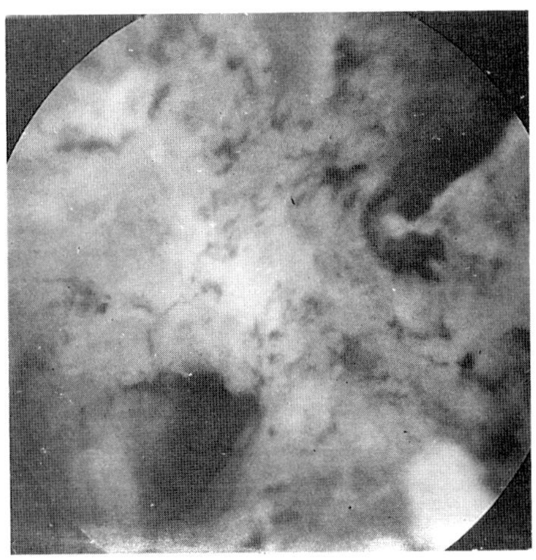

Fig. 47.9. Intrauterine septum (hysteroscopic view).

The author[8] prefers to incise an intrauterine septum with a Collin's knife or a point electrode set at 30-40 watts of pure cutting current. Septum is incised till both the tubal ostia are seen equidistant from the upper end of incision which is 0.5-1.0 cm away from ostia. Laparoscopic control is useful for wide septum and to rule out possibility of a bicornuate uterus.

Out of 63 hysteroscopic septal incision done by the author, 12 cases had infertility of which 5 cases were referred from IVF centres and remaining had secondary infertility with no other obvious cause.

The author and all leading hysteroscopist of the world find no justification for doing an open surgery for intrauterine adhesions, myoma and septum. The obvious advantages of hysteroscopic surgeries are shown in Table 47.3.

Table 47.3. Advantages of hysteroscopic surgery

1. Avoid exploration and its aftermath.
2. Avoid opening uterus which could be a risk for future conception.
3. Reduces possibility of caesarean section in future pregnancy.
4. Reduces hospital stay.
5. Less morbidity.
6. Rapid recovery.

Hysteroscopic surgery for proximal tubal occlusion

In recent years there is a great deal of interest for treatment of proximal tubal occlusion either under fluoroscopic, sonographic or hysteroscopic guidance. The transvaginal tubal cannulations (Fig. 47.10) have been primarily developed for :

1. Overcoming proximal tubal occlusion from reversible blocks due to intraluminal debris or plugs or adhesions.
2. Diagnosing intraluminal disease.
3. Deposition of sperms, embryos, oocytes.

The major advantage of such approach is avoiding the need of incisional surgery, reducing the use of anaesthetic agents and greater convenience to the patient.

Various authors, *viz.*, Lisa *et al.*[9], Sweeney *et al.*[10] have studied the intramural oviduct in post-hysterectomy specimens and have found cannulation techniques to be of a little value and probably traumatic. However, Corfman[11], Kerin[12] and others pointed out that such conclusions were due to artifactual changes due to myometrial contraction in special which is not the same as experienced by in vivo cannulation, provided the cannula is flexible smooth-walled, coaxial or a linear eversion balloon type system.

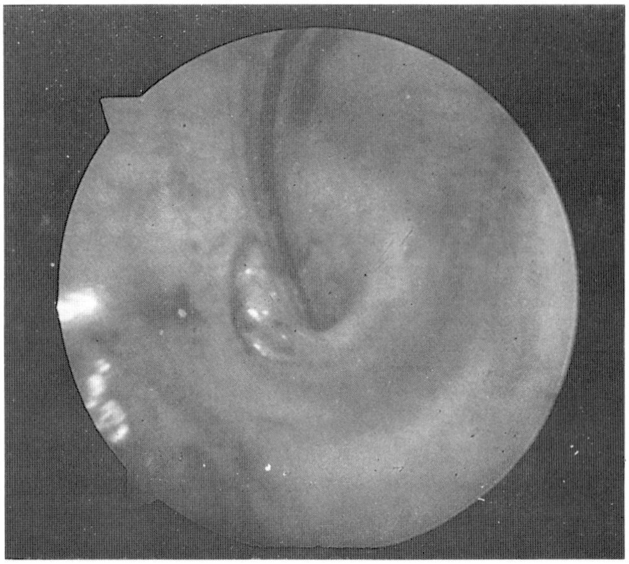

Fig. 47.10. Transcervical hysteroscopic tubal cannulation.

A clear knowledge of oviduct anatomy and physiology is mandatory and these details would probably go beyond the scope and purpose of this chapter. A small flexible hysteroscope with an outer diameter of 3.5-5 mm and an operating channel of 2-5.5 mm is suitable. However, if there is failure to advance the guide-wires possibility of tubal blocks secondary to debris, adhesions, stenosis, sharp bend or fibrotic occlusion should be considered. A falloposcope with irrigating channel is useful for proper vision, however one should keep falloposcope within the cannula and avoid pushing against resistant white areas to avoid perforation or tubal damage.

Reversible non-obstructive and obstructive lesions are treated by aquaflushing and endotuboplasty with balloon catheters. However, if the block is severe, therapeutic effect is reduced. In a multicentric study of 77 balloon tuboplasty under falloposcopic and laparoscopic monitoring, 3% had a small perforation without clinical consequences. The currently available linear eversion catheter systems for tubal cannulation approved by FDA bypasses the need of hysteroscopic visualisation and even fluoroscopic-sonographic. Tactile approach is acceptable.

The debate over genuineness of a pathological or functional proximal tubal block still prevails and such techniques could still be considered experimental.

In conclusion the author feels that today no

gynaecologist can be called thoroughly trained without being exposed to this modality of surgical treatment. Guiding principles of hysteroscopic surgery are accuracy, familiarity and persistent training to achieve maximum benefit with minimal discomfort to the patient.

REFERENCES

1. Pantoleoni D (1869). On endoscopic examination of the cavity of the womb. Med Press. Circ. 8, 26.
2. Sugimoto O, Ushiroyama T and Fukuda Y (1984). Diagnostic and therapeutic hysteroscopy for traumatic intrauterine adhesions. *In* Siegler AM and Lindemann HJ (eds.) Hysteroscopy, Principles and Practice, pp. 186-192. J.B. Lippincott, Philadelphia.
3. Wamsteker K (1984). Hysteroscopy in Asherman's syndrome. *In* Siegler AM and Lindemann HJ (eds.) Hysteroscopy, Principles and Practice, pp. 198-203, J.B. Lipincott, Philadelphia.
4. Asherman JG (1948). Amenorrhoea traumatica (atretica). J Obstet Gynecol Br Empire 55, 23-30.
5. Valle RF, Sciarra JJ (1988). Intrauterine adhesions, hysteroscopic diagnosis, classification treatment and reproductive outcome. Am J Obstet Gynecol. 158 : 1459-70.
6. Donnez J, Schrurs B, Gillerot S, Sadow J, and Clerckx F (1988). Treatment of uterine fibroids with implants of gonadotropin releasing hormone agonist; assessment by hysterography. Fertil Steril, 51, 947.
7. Donnez J, Gillerot S, Bourgonjon D, Clerckx F and Nisolle M (1990). Neodymium : YAG laser hysteroscopy in large submucuous fibroids. Fertil Steril, 54, 999.
8. Trivedi PH, Langdana F and Chhatre S. J Obstet and Gynec. India, 44, 625-630, 1994.
9. Lisa JR, Gioia JD, Rubin IC. Observation of the interstitial portion of the fallopian tube. Surg Gynecol. 1954; 99 : 159-60.
10. Sweeney WJ, The interstitial portion of the uterine tube : Its gross anatomy, course, and length. Obstet Gynecol. 1963, 19 : 3-8.
11. Corfman RS. Falloposcopy : Frontiers realized a fantastic voyage revisited. Fertil Steril 1990; 54 : 574-6.
12. Kerin J, Daykhovsky L, Segalowitz J *et al.* Falloposcopy : A microendoscopic technique for visual exploration of the human fallopian tube from the uterotubal ostium to fimbria using a transvaginal approach. Fertil Steril 1990, 54 : 390-400.

CHAPTER

48

Lasers in Gynaecology

Asha Singhal

LASER is an acronym of Light Amplification by Stimulated Emission of Radiation.

In 1985, Daikuzona and Joffe gave this definition : A laser device produces and amplifies visible and near visible light to create intense and coherent electromagnetic energy beam which is passed through air and reflected off mirrors to bring it to a precise point.

In USA in 1960, the first laser was produced using a ruby rod. Later on other materials like gases, dyes, rare elements (*e.g.*, Neodymium) were used. The different materials produce different types of beams with different effects on biological systems. Therefore no single laser is suitable for all purposes.

The laser beam is a highly directional beam of a special kind of light which can be focussed to a very small spot. The laser beam has varied applications in diagnosis and treatment because of special properties listed below :

1. Coherent light : It has single frequency so behaves as one single wave.
2. Precision : It is a parallel beam. This precision is up to a few micrometres. The beam can be accurately focussed on a very small spot (*e.g.*, to open blocked canal of Schlemm in glaucoma, use in microsurgery).
3. Directional.
4. Monochromatic beam.
5. Dose can be controlled. Finer beam and shorter time leads to less tissue damage of sore areas. Intense and longer lasting beam leads to more tissue damage.
6. Absolutely no touch technique so asepsis is perfect.
7. Biological effects of laser and their local advantages. When it falls on tissues the electromagnetic energy is converted into intense heat which causes either cell destruction or explosive evaporation. The advantages of this explosive evaporation are that

   (a) there is complete haemostasis;

(b) minimum tissue debris and discharge;
(c) healing is rapid;
(d) there is no tissue ischaemia (Lucrano (1989);
(e) the adhesions are minimum;
(f) the post-operative pain is less because after laser the nerve endings are blunt, whereas after knife cut they become broom-like.

During this procedure some plume (smoke) is produced and this is sucked away by simultaneously used suction (laser plumes).

Applications of Laser in Obstetrics & Gynaecology (Diagnostic, Therapeutic)

Diagnostic applications of laser

1. Diagnosis of diseases and defects at morula stage. Laser slicing of one cell from morula for studies.
2. Diagnosis of early malignancy
   — by noting laser florescence
   — by taking biopsies and excision biopsies, *e.g.*, biopsy from surface cancers of vulva, vagina and cervix (*e.g.*, cone biopsy).

   The laser conisation seals the vascular spaces so less bleeding and less tissue embolisation.
   — No post-operative discharge.
   — Better specimen for histopathology — the tissue margins are adequate because thin spot beam makes narrow precise incision. The incision is speedy and there is minimal thermal damage.

Therapeutic applications of laser

1. Medical.
2. Surgical.
3. Photocoagulation.
4. Photoradiation therapy.

1. Medical uses

1. Phototherapy of skin lesions.
2. Photoradiation therapy (PRT) for recurrence of gynaecological cancers and breast cancer :
   — external cancers — cancer of cervix, vulva, vagina
   — PRT — via endoscope for cancer of internal organs.

2. Surgical uses (ultramicrosurgery/microsurgery/surgery)

A. Ultramicrosurgery at cellular level : for gene slicing, chromosome slicing.

In IVF
— to make a microhole in zona so that sperm can go in
— for slicing away the defective gene or chromosome
— for introducing a gene.

B. Microsurgery of organs (special advantage — shorter surgery to conception interval).

(a) Tubes

adhesiolysis : excellent results, provided there is no damage to muscle and mucosa. A relook scopy shows tubes patent and without adhesions;

tubal anastomosis : for removing the blocked segment;

neosalpingostomy : aim only at serosa 5 mm from margin of tube.

Results : Daniel U.K. 1984 — He is also a microsurgeon. His results with laser and microsurgery are same. In over 190 cases — intrauterine pregnancies 28% and tubal pregnancies 15%.

(b) Ovaries

P.C.O.D. : drill 25-30 holes in ovary by Nd-YAG or argon laser to drain out androgenic fluid (one can use cautery for same results).

Results : In 6 months — 75% spontaneous ovulation, 50% got pregnant, ovaries become sensitive to clomid. (Duration of effect 9-15 months.)

C. Surgery

(a) Uterus

cone biopsy, conisation (laser has no role in primary treatment of carcinoma cervix)

laser cutting of septum via hysteroscopy

hysteroscopic ablation of endometrium for cases of menorrhagia

hysteroscopic removal of surface lesions like polyps, fibroids.

Drawbacks of endometrial ablation
— Troublesome post-laser bleeding, recurrence due to regeneration of some endometrium, even after endometrial ablation, the associated hyperestrenism and adenomyosis is still there.
— Myomectomy, laparoscopic hysterectomy
— Laser neurectomy for severe dysmenorrhoea.

Problems in laser neurectomy are :

— Difficulty in identification of utero-sacral ligament if it is flat and thin;
— Difficulty in identification of big veins lateral to utero-sacrals;
— Difficulty in identification of ureter;
— Bleeding
— Large amount of smoke disturbs the view.

(b) Uterosacral ligaments

Endometriosis of uterosacral ligaments — the lesions can be 11 mm deep. Use a probe to feel for nodularity.

Treatment

Lase it deep enough to remove all nodularity, otherwise pain will return.

Luna results with CO_2 laser for dysmenorrhoeas due to endometriosis — 86% cases improve.

Primary dysmenorrhoea — Laser neurectomy treatment — excise the utero-sacral ligaments at uterine attachment. This means division of Lee Frankenhauser plexus which is in and along utero-sacrals. The principle is same as Doyle's procedure done surgically.

Post-operative : The first menstruation may be painful due to oedema in healing phase. Therefore careful counselling is important.

(c) Tubes

Unruptured uncomplicated ectopic :

The tube is opened by bloodless incision, sac separated and sucked out. The cut is left as such or sutured (Kurt Semm). Put the drain for 4 hours.

(Results — repeat ectopic rate is 5.8%).

N.B. : In case the pregnancy falls out in peritoneal cavity and if it is difficult to suck it out still there is no need to do laparotomy. Keep her under observation. Do weekly β-hCG. If it is not falling then give her methotrexate, actinomycin.

Removal of fimbrial cyst.

(d) Ovaries

Laser use enables saving of ovarian tissue

Wedge resection; Oophorectomy;

Laser excision of benign ovarian tumours;

Endometriosis.

(e) Surface lesions surgery

(i) Cervix, vagina, vulva — Condyloma and other genital lesions can be treated by CO_2 laser. Vaporisation, brushing or excision is done. (Result — 90% cure. Also the laser eliminates the virus from neighbouring skin too.)

(ii) S.I.L. (Squamous Intra-epithelial Lesions) (CIN, VIN, VAIN)

Biopsy, excision biopsy, total excision of lesion, conisation is done by laser. After laser vaporisation, the healing occurs in 3 weeks.

(iii) Invasive Gynaec Cancer — laser biopsy

Laser surgery in endometriosis

The types of lesions seen in endometriosis are :

(a) Burnt out lesion — hemosiderin deposits;
(b) Angry patch — haemorrhage and telengiectasis;
(c) Non-pigmented patch (scarring — very painful area)

Laser management of these lesions

For a, b, c type lesions, the laser therapy is good as the endometriotic deposits do not penetrate through the fat. Lasing destroys the patches and coagulates the blood vessels. If the blood vessels are left behind, then the chances of recurrence increase. The results are good as the histopathological examination of residual pigmented areas shows only carbon granules surrounded by foreign body giant cells.

For adhesiolysis : The laser management is almost bloodless.

For type d lesion (endometrioma)

Big size : Open by small elliptical incision and drain chocolate cysts and invert the cyst; vaporise the inner lining superficially. Now revert and suture.

Small size : It is better to do photocoagulation by Nd-YAG or KTP laser, as the CO_2 laser does not work in fluid. Besides, the endometriosis causes moderate to dense adhesions.

Results : Guildford Laser Laparoscopy Project October 1992 for Endometriosis.

70% better/relapse 17% in only 2 patients at the same site. Rest at some new site.

Pregnancy rate 80% (take home baby — 2/3 cases).

3. Photo-coagulation therapy

Indications

Endometriosis of vascular tumors (as haemangioma cervix).

4. Photo-dynamic therapy (P.D.T.)/Photoradiation therapy (P.R.T.)

Indications

(i) Solid malignant tumors of vulva, vagina and their superficial recurrence;

(ii) Recurrence of breast tumour after mastectomy.

Principle : To use photosensitive dye (HpD or DHE)

Dye — Haemarto-porphyrin derivative (HpD) or its tumour active component (DHE)

Dose — 2 mg/kg body weight in 250 cc of fluid i.v. infusion;

After i.v. injection, the dye is cleared from serum and normal tissues in 2 -3 days, but is selectively retained in (a) dysplastic or tumour cells (because these cells are rich in DNA (b) around vascular stroma.

After 3-6 days a peak differential exists between normal cells and tumour cells. The cells with dye concentrated are called sensitised cells, and are reactive to red light.

Now (*i.e.*, after 3-6 days), the porphyrin in tissues is photochemically activated by means of exposure to visible light, (derived generally from a dye laser system emitting a bright red light at 630 to 640 nm. The light activated porphyrin transfers the energy to endogenous oxygen of tissue to make nascent (or singlet) oxygen. The singlet oxygen destroys the cells by causing photo oxidation and bursting. When this oxygen is quenched or enhanced, the tumour cell destruction is quenched or enhanced.

Results

After light exposure : Within a few hours the tumour becomes devoid of blood. First there is red cell coagulation within the blood vessels. Next within a few hours, there is complete vascular collapse and rupture. Thus up to 5-15 mm of tumour cells are destroyed.

N.B. — The normal tissue is less photosensitive, so only mild reaction occurs but still after injection, for safety, the patient after treatment must be kept away from sunlight or any bright light for 30 days as there may be small amount of dye in some normal cells like liver.

Endoscopic use of laser

Laser hysteroscopy

Laser used are Argon, Nd-YAG, Krypton, KTP.

Distending medium : It is better to use 1.5% glycine solution as it does not caramelize. The caramalization is troublesome as it damages laser fibers which have to be repaired or replaced. This delays the procedure and also increases the cost.

Use only bare fibres. The CO_2 conducting fibres may cause bubbling of medium leading to poor visibility and gas embolism.

Pre-operative treatment with GnRH analogue for 8 weeks dries up the endometrium and uterus hence operative bleeding is less.

Laser laparoscopy

With CO_2 a coincident Helium Neon (HeNe) laser is used. This provides a visible red spot, on to which the laser beam can be directed.

Constant irrigation with Ringer Lactate (add 5,000 units of Heparin per litre). This keeps the tissues moist and prevents fibrin deposition.

Pitresin (Vasopresin) : 1 : 30 diluted, amount 1-2 cc only. This is injected in mesosalpinx to reduce bleeding. (Caution : It may cause serious complications.)

Power setting

(a) For septum cutting — Power density (P.D.) 1,000 W/cm^2 or less, at intermittent time exposure of 1-2 seconds.

(b) Lysis of adhesions — Power setting 5-15 W/cm^2.

(c) Ovarian excision — Power setting 20-30 W/cm^2.

(d) Vaporization of implants — Power setting 2-5 W/cm^2. Time exposure 0.1 seconds intermittent or continuous. Spot size 0.2-0.4 mm.

Insert more instrument in abdominal cavity to enable constant traction and countertraction while making the incision. This protects surrounding tissues from heat damage and allows rapid dissection.

Accessories : Use moistened wood spatulas for manipulations and use back stop to absorb stray laser energy.

After the procedure : Leave in pelvis 100-200 cc of 32% Dextran to minimize adhesion formation.

Future of laser

With continued advances the laser has more and more to offer in diagnostic and therapeutic fields.

1. Advances in laser devices : More compact and computerized devices with better delivery systems, available in different wavelength.
2. With more advances the organ conservation would be feasible as it selectively destroys dysplastic and malignant cells.

It would be useful in disseminated malignancy also.

Use with other accessory instruments with endoscope and with phototherapy.

REFERENCES

1. Michael S. Baggish. Basic and Advanced Laser Surgery in Gynecology. (ACC) Appleton Century Crofts, Norwalk/Connecticut 1985.
2. Jacques Donnez. Laser Operative Laparoscopy and Hysteroscopy. University of Louvain, Brussels, Belgium 1989.
3. Fertility and Sterility. Vol. 6, No. 4, p. 81, April 1994.
4. Am J O and Gyn. 161 (1) 1989; 60-68. CO_2 laser in CIN.
5. Carson. Am J O and Gyn 1989 160 (3) 718. Laser in endometriosis.
6. Davis. Br J Obs and Gyn 1989 96 (8) 928-32. Endometrial ablation.
7. Goldrath NH, *et al.* Laser photovaporization of endometrium for the treatment of menorrhagia. Am J Obst and Gyn 1981; 140 : 14.
8. Negro AG. Comparison of microsurgical suture and CO_2 laser welded anastomosis of rabbit uterine cornua. Laser Surg Med 1987; 6 : 533.
9. Newton. Br J Obst and Gyn. 1989. Jan. 96 (1) 102-4. Uterine adhesions.
10. Shapiro AG, *et al.* Conventional reanastomosis versus laser welding of rat uterine horns. Am J Obs and Gyn. 1987; 156 : 1006-9.
11. Nezhal. Fert. Sterility, 1989; 52 : 237-40. Video laseroscopy.
12. Shirk. Am J Obst and Gyn. 1989; 160 (6) : 1344-51. Laser in endometriosis.

U

V

W

Professor and Head,